Diseases of the Bronchioles

DISEASES OF THE BRONCHIOLES

Editor

Gary R. Epler, M.D.

Associate Clinical Professor
Boston University School of Medicine
Chairman, Department of Medicine
New England Baptist Hospital
Boston, Massachusetts

Raven Press New York

Raven Press, Ltd., 1185 Avenue of the Americas, New York, New York 10036

Made in the United States of America

Library of Congress Cataloging-in-Publication Data

Diseases of the bronchioles / edited by Gary R. Epler.
p. cm.
Includes index.
ISBN 0-7817-0123-6
1. Bronchioles—Diseases. I. Epler, Gary R.
[DNLM: 1. Bronchial Diseases—pathology. WF 500 D611 1994]
RC776.B75 1994
616.2'3—dc20
DNLM/DLC
for Library of Congress 93-36029
CIP

The material contained in this volume was submitted as previously unpublished material, except in the instances in which credit has been given to the source from which some of the illustrative material was derived.

Great care has been taken to maintain the accuracy of the information contained in the volume. However, neither Raven Press nor the editor can be held responsible for errors or for any consequences arising from the use of the information contained herein.

9 8 7 6 5 4 3 2 1

To my wife, Joan
and children, Gregory and Brett

Contents

Section 4. Bronchiolar Diseases Among Children

Contributing Authors

Connor M. Burke, M.D.
Consultant Respiratory Physician
James Connolly Memorial Hospital
Blanchardstown
Dublin #15, Ireland

Charles K. Chan, M.D.
Associate Professor of Medicine
Director, Pulmonary Fellowship Program
University of Toronto
Consultant in Respiratory Medicine and Critical Care Medicine
Wellesley and Princess Margaret Hospitals
Suite 242, Jones Bldg.
160 Wellesley Street East
Toronto M4Y1J3, Ontario, Canada

Andrew M. Churg, M.D.
Department of Pathology
University of British Columbia
2211 Westbrook Mall
Vancouver V6T 2B5, British Columbia, Canada

Thomas V. Colby, M.D.
Department of Surgical Pathology
Mayo Clinic
200 First Street
Rochester, Minnesota 55905

Jean-Francois Cordier, M.D.
Professor of Pneumology
Hôpital Louis Pradel
Claude Bernard University
BP Lyon Montchat
69394 Lyon Cedex 03, France

Paul A. Corris, M.B., B.S., F.R.C.P.
Consultant Respiratory Physician
Associate Medical Director
Department of Cardiopulmonary Transplantation
Regional Cardiopulmonary Centre
Freeman Hospital
High Heaton
Newcastle Upon Tyne, NE7 7DN, England

Manuel G. Cosio, M.D.
Professor of Medicine and Director, Respiratory Division
Royal Victoria Hospital and McGill University,
687 Pine Avenue W
Montreal H3A 1A1, Quebec, Canada

Ulrich Costabel, M.D.
Ruhrlandklinik
Tüschener Weg 40
D-4300 Essen 16, Germany

David B. Coultas, M.D.
Associate Professor of Medicine
Pulmonary and Critical Care Division
New Mexico Tumor Registry, Cancer Center
University of New Mexico School of Medicine
900 Camino de Salud, NE
Albuquerque, New Mexico 87131

William W. Douglas, M.D.
Department of Internal Medicine
Division of Thoracic Diseases
Mayo Clinic
200 First Street
Rochester, Minnesota 55905

Gary R. Epler, M.D.
Associate Clinical Professor
Boston University School of Medicine
Chairman, Department of Medicine
New England Baptist Hospital
125 Parker Hill Avenue
Boston, Massachusetts 02120

Richard A. Finkelstein, M.D.
Fellow of the Canadian Lung Association
McGill University
Montreal, Quebec, Canada

Linda M. Funk, M.D.
Department of Medicine
Pulmonary and Critical Care Division
University of New Mexico School of Medicine
900 Camino de Salud, NE
Albuquerque, New Mexico 87131

Duncan M. Geddes, M.D.
Royal Brompton National
Heart and Lung Hospital
Sydney Street
London, SW3 6HP, England

D. M. G. Halpin, M.D.
Royal Brompton National Heart and Lung Hospital
Sydney Street
London, SW3 6HP, England

Karen A. Hardy, M.D.
Pediatric Pulmonary Medicine
California Pacific Medical Center
P.O. Box 7999
San Francisco, California 94120

Thomas E. Hartman, M.D.
Department of Radiology
University of British Columbia
and
Vancouver General Hospital
855 W. 12th Ave.
Vancouver, British Columbia V5Z 1M9
Canada

Ank A. W. Ten Have-Opbroek, M.D., Ph.D.
Department of Surgery
School of Medicine
University of California
Davis, California 95616
and
Department of Pulmonology
School of Medicine
University of Leiden
P.O. Box 9602
2300 R.C. Leiden
The Netherlands

James C. Hogg, M.D.
University of British Columbia Research Laboratory
Pulmonary Division
St. Paul's Hospital
1081 Burrard Street
Vancouver V6Z 1Y6, British Columbia, Canada

Helen M. Hollingsworth, M.D.
Director, Allergy Clinic
Division of Pulmonary and Critical Care Medicine
University of Massachusetts Medical Center
55 Lake Avenue
Worcester, Massachusetts 01655

Masatoshi Iwata, M.D.
Chief, Department of Respiratory Medicine
Haibara General Hospital
2887-1 Hosoe, Haibara-cho, Haibara-gun
Shizuoka 421-04, Japan

Takateru Izumi, M.D.
Clinical Director
Department of Medicine and Environmental Respiratory Disease
Chest Disease Research Institute
Kyoto University
Shogoin-Kawaramachi 53
Sakyo-ku, Kyoto 606-01, Japan

T. Bernard Kinane, M.D.
Pediatric Pulmonary Unit, Children's Service
Massachusetts General Hospital
Fruit Street
Boston, Massachusetts 02114

R. Loire, M.D.
Department of Pathology
Hôpital Louis Pradel
Claude Bernard University
69394 Lyon, France

Joseph P. Lynch, III, M.D.
Associate Professor, Internal Medicine
Division of Pulmonary and Critical Care Medicine
University of Michigan Medical Center
3916 Taubman Center
Ann Arbor, Michigan 48109-0360

Fernando J. Martinez, M.D.
Associate Professor, Internal Medicine
University of Michigan Medical Center
3916 Taubman Center
Ann Arbor, Michigan 48109-0360

Janet R. Maurer, M.D.
Department of Medicine
Division of Respirology
The Toronto Hospital
University of Toronto
10-220 Eaton Wing TGH
200 Elizabeth Street
Toronto M5G 2C4, Ontario Canada

Theresa C. McLoud, M.D.
Chief, Thoracic Radiology
Department of Radiology
Massachusetts General Hospital
Fruit Street
Boston, Massachusetts 02114

Nestor L. Müller, M.D.
Department of Radiology
Vancouver General Hospital
855 W. 12th Avenue
Vancouver V5Z1M9, Canada

Jeffrey L. Myers, M.D.
Department of Laboratory Medicine and Pathology
Mayo Clinic
200 First Street
Rochester, Minnesota 55905

S. Peyrol, M.D.
Cellular Pathology Laboratory
CNRS URA 602
Institut Pasteur
69007 Lyon, France

Charles G. Plopper, Ph.D.
Department of Anatomy and Cell Biology
School of Veterinary Medicine
University of California
1321 Harring Hall
Davis, California 95616

Atsuhiko Sato, M.D.
Associate Professor
Second Division
Department of Internal Medicine
Hamamatsu University School of Medicine
3600 Handa-cho, Hamamatsu-shi
Shizuoka 431-31, Japan

Daniel C. Shannon, M.D.
Chief, Pediatric/Pulmonary Unit
Massachusetts General Hospital
Fruit Street
Boston, Massachusetts 02114

Stephen J. Swensen, M.D.
Department of Diagnostic Radiology
Mayo Clinic
Rochester, Minnesota 55905

Eero Taskinen, M.D.
Associate Director of Pathology and Cytology
Transplantation Laboratory
University of Helsinki
Haartmaninkatu 3
00290 Helsinki, Finland

Pentti Tukiainen, M.D.
Associate Director
Department of Pulmonary Medicine
Helsinki University Central Hospital
Haartmaninkatu 4
00290 Helsinki, Finland

Mary Ellen Beck Wohl, M.D.
Professor of Pediatrics
Harvard Medical School
Chief, Division of Respiratory Diseases
Pulmonary Division
Children's Hospital
300 Longwood Avenue
Boston, Massachusetts 02115

Samuel A. Yousem, M.D.
Department of Pathology, NW 625
Montefiore University Hospital
University of Pittsburgh
School of Medicine
3459 Fifth Avenue
Pittsburgh, Pennsylvania 15213-3241

Preface

There have been intermittent reports about bronchiolitis obliterans since the early 1900s. In the middle 1980s, there was an explosion of articles about the bronchiolar syndromes. This proliferation was caused by the discovery of new syndromes and the life-threatening nature of obliterative bronchiolitis as a complication of organ transplantation. As these new developments occur, it is imperative to maintain a systematic perspective of these disorders. This book has been written as a reference text designed to give a comprehensive review of the clinical and pathological findings of each bronchiolar disorder. In addition, it should provide a basis for developing clinical and cellular biological research.

The reader will be able to learn the clinical, physiological, radiographic, and pathological findings of each of the bronchiolar disorders. Patient management and prognosis are also discussed. The book is intended for the practicing clinician in general medicine and pulmonary medicine, as well as for pathologists and others in related medical and surgical specialties. It is also designed to be used for the education of physicians and surgeons as part of their study of pulmonary medicine.

The first section includes a review of the historic perspective and general aspects of the bronchiolar disorders. An anatomical classification and histological description of the normal bronchioles, essential for the understanding of the bronchiolar diseases, is given. The unique findings of the chest radiograph and high-resolution chest CT scan are described. The histological and clinical classifications and the base for these classification systems are described.

The second section is a review of bronchiolar lesions that result in airway abnormalities and airway obstruction, including an important chapter regarding small airway disease in smokers and a possible breakthrough in the understanding of one of the specific types of emphysema. The finding of life-threatening obliterative bronchiolitis as a complication of bone marrow transplantation is also discussed.

The third section is a review of the bronchiolar interstitial disorders including chapters on respiratory bronchiolitis-interstitial lung disease and idiopathic bronchiolitis obliterans organizing pneumonia (BOOP).

The last section reviews bronchiolar disorders in children.

Gary R. Epler

Acknowledgments

Fulfilling the goal of making this the most useful reference text for the bronchiolar disorders has been made possible by the excellence and thoroughness of the contributing authors. It has been a pleasure working with every one of them, and I thank them for their outstanding contributions. I thank Sandra Smith for her technical assistance, thorough review of the manuscripts, and organizational assistance. The assistance of Klaus W. Korten in the translation of the early German manuscripts was essential for the development of the historical discussion. Paul Woodard of the New England Baptist Hospital Health Sciences Library was extremely helpful in his thorough search of the literature and in obtaining the ancient references for review. I also thank Shari Regen of the Health Sciences Library for her assistance in literature search and translation of the French literature. I thank Edward A. Gaensler and Gordon L. Snider for their encouragement and assistance in developing my interest in the bronchiolar disorders. I would like to acknowledge all of my patients who courageously dealt with their bronchiolar disorders, and to Mary Emerson and her family who provided a lasting inspiration in the long siege against polymyositis-related BOOP. Finally, I thank Lisa Berger, Senior Medical Editor, and her colleagues at Raven Press for their energetic assistance.

SECTION 1

The Bronchioles

Diseases of the Bronchioles, edited by
Gary R. Epler. Raven Press, Ltd.,
New York © 1994.

1

Historic Perspective of the Bronchiolar Disorders

Gary R. Epler

Associate Clinical Professor, Boston University School of Medicine. Chairman, Department of Medicine, New England Baptist Hospital, 125 Parker Hill Avenue, Boston, MA.

The historic events with regard to the bronchiolar disorders began during the early part of the nineteenth century, when Dr. Reynaud described obliteration of small airways in a dissertation in 1835. Dr. Wilhelm Lange first documented bronchiolitis obliterans in 1901 with the description of an idiopathic respiratory illness in two patients. During the next few years, the same lesion was described after toxic fume exposures and infections. There were scattered reports for the next half century, until the 1980s, when a burst of reports resulted in the description of new syndromes, causes, and associated disorders. This chapter is a review of the historic beginning of study of bronchiolar disorders and concludes with the present perspective and issues.

In 1835, Dr. Reynaud (1) described the anatomical obliteration of airways in a 50-page dissertation. The report was written to fill in the gaps of the anatomy of the lung up to that time. Several types of obliteration of the airways were noted, one of which occurred in the vicinity of tumors. Some of the obliteration was diffuse in all airways, whereas other obliterative lesions were localized. The report noted that the bronchioles, like the smaller blood vessels, are obliterated or destroyed by the same cause as the underlying disorder. These descriptions were obtained from dissection of the airways as far into the lung as possible, with accompanying drawings. Microscopic findings were not described. The dissertation concluded with the note that the importance of the subject probably did not deserve such a lengthy discourse; however, in view of the uniqueness of these observations, that the reader would pardon the digressions of the author and consider these efforts in a beneficial manner.

In 1901, Dr. Wilhelm Lange (2) first used the term *bronchiolitis obliterans* in a report that described an idiopathic respiratory illness that resulted in the deaths of two patients. The first was a 22-year-old woman with a week-long flu-like illness who died from respiratory failure in several days. Autopsy revealed lungs studded with small miliary nodules, distributed diffusely in both lungs. These foci were close to each other—about 1 to 2 mm separated them. They were rounded, linear, forked-like, or in the shape of a clover leaf, with a size of 1 to 5 mm. They were not seen directly under the pleural surface. These lesions represented small airways—the end branches of the bronchial tree. They started where the bronchi lost their cartilage in the walls. Microscopically, the lumina of the bronchioles were irregularly narrowed because of a structure that reached into the airway. Depending on the width of the base, this structure looked like a mushroom or a cone, and was made up of spindle cells and young granulation tissue. In the plugs with a broader base, structures resembling real capillaries could be seen. In addition to the young connective tissue cells, leukocytes, eosinophils, and plasma cells were found in the plug. Epithelial cells mixed with leukocytes and red blood cells could be seen in the remaining part of the lumen. The lumina of some bronchioles were completely obliterated—only the granulation tissue plug was seen. Foci of 10 to 15 alveoli, adjacent to the obliterated bronchioles or free in the lung, were filled with a cellular exudate in the center, similar to the bronchiolar plugs that obliterated the airway. The septa were widened with a leukocyte infiltration. When the bronchiole was cut lengthwise, the connective tissue could be followed from the bronchiole into the alveoli. Growth of the young connective tissue plugs originating from the alveolar walls into the alveoli could not be documented. The second patient was a 32-year-old wallpaper hanger with 6 months of pulmonary distress followed by a 4-week progressive course with sudden respiratory failure and death in 3 days. Autopsy of this patient revealed lungs studded with small miliary nodules that microscopically showed scarring of small airways with foci extending into alveoli.

The next year, Fraenkel (3) described bronchiolitis obliterans in a patient who died from inhalation of nitric acid fumes. He also described three stages of the illness. First, the patient developed "stormy initial symptoms" of cough, dyspnea, and rust-colored sputum for 9 days. Second, during a 1-week interval symptoms diminished but fever gradually developed. Third, 1 week before death, the original symptoms increased, followed by death from respiratory failure. The physical findings had a similar pattern: crackles initially, then minimal findings, then crackles during the final stage. In 1903, this obliterative lesion was also reported (4) from the autopsy findings of a 24-year-old etcher.

In 1904, postinfectious bronchiolitis obliterans were reported in patients after measles (5,6) and pertussis (6). Thus, within a brief time, three categories of bronchiolitis obliterans had been described: idiopathic, postinhalation of toxic fumes and postinfection.

An additional report (7) was written in 1906 about three patients with fume-related bronchiolitis obliterans as a result of nitric acid, sulfuric acid, and ammonia fume inhalation. Two survived. The third died 26 days after exposure, and this patient also had the three-stage progression of the illness as described by Fraenkel (3).

In 1908, there was a report (8) of a 3-year-old child who developed respiratory distress with dyspnea and cyanosis after aspiration of a prune pit. There was stabilization initially, but the child died on day 56. Autopsy showed the prune pit in the trachea. The major and moderate sized bronchi were filled with purulent masses. Most airways of about 1 mm in diameter were completely filled with plugs of exudate. These exudative plugs consisted of leukocytes, occasional epithelial cells, and no fibrin; however, the small airways up to the respiratory bronchioles showed a totally different picture. The airway wall was often disrupted. Strange plugs reached into the lumina of the airway and filled them almost completely. The plugs had a different appearance than the exudates of the bronchi and consisted of newly built connective tissue, which grew into the lumen from the bronchiolar wall. This young connective tissue consisted of long spindle cells, usually at the periphery of the plugs, and parallel fibrils; elastic fibers were missing completely. Cells rich in cytoplasm were predominant, while spindle cells and collagen were less common, resulting in the appearance of granulation tissue. Fibrin was not found in these plugs.

Four additional patients with bronchiolitis obliterans were described in a lecture published by Fraenkel (9) in 1909; the disease in two was related to nitric acid fume exposure and in two was idiopathic. Thus, within the first decade of the twentieth

TABLE 1. *Bronchiolitis obliterans: the first decade of the twentieth century*

Year	Cause	Patients	Lesion	Reference
1901	Idiopathic	2	Bronchiolitis obliterans	(2)
1902	Nitric acid	1	Bronchiolitis fibrosa obliterans	(3)
1903	Etching	1	Pneumonia desquamative obliterans	(4)
1904	Measles	2	Bronchiolitis obliterans	(5,6)
1904	Pertussis	1	Bronchiolitis obliterans	(6)
1906	Nitric acid	1	Bronchiolitis fibrosa obliterans	(7)
1906	Sulfuric acid	1	Bronchiolitis fibrosa obliterans	(7)
1906	Ammonia	1	Bronchiolitis fibrosa obliterans	(7)
1908	Prune pit	1	Bronchitis obliterans	(8)
1909	Idiopathic	2	Bronchiolitis obliterans fibrosa	(9)
1909	Nitric acid	2	Bronchiolitis obliterans fibrosa	(9)

century, there were reports of at least 15 patients with bronchiolar obliterative lesions of unknown cause or related to toxic fume exposures, infections, or aspiration (Table 1).

Several additional reports appeared during the next two decades (Table 2). In 1917, bronchiolitis obliterans was described (10) in a 39-year-old man who was accidentally involved in a chemical explosion and exposed to various chemicals as part of the preparation of trinitrotoluene. The three-phase illness occurred as described by Fraenkel in 1902: a fit of coughing at the time of exposure, dyspnea 3 days later, with progressive and severe dyspnea and cyanosis leading to death 3 weeks later. The next year, bronchiolitis obliterans was described in a patient who had previously developed influenza (11).

In a 1929 report (12), bronchiolitis obliterans was defined as a disease characterized by connective-tissue proliferation in the bronchioles in response to local injury. The authors described five patients who died from bronchiolitis obliterans. The char-

TABLE 2. *Bronchiolitis obliterans: two centuries of events*

Year	Event and description	References
1835	Anatomic description of a small airway obliteration	(1)
1901	Idiopathic bronchiolitis obliterans	(2)
1902	Toxic fume bronchiolitis obliterans, three-stage illness	(3)
1904	Postinfection bronchiolitis obliterans	(5,6)
1956	Silo filler's bronchiolitis obliterans	(16)
1973	Cigarette smoking respiratory bronchiolitis	(27)
1977	Connective tissue related bronchiolitis obliterans	(29)
1977	Drug-related bronchiolitis obliterans	(29)
1982	Bone marrow obliterative bronchiolitis	(33)
1983	Diffuse panbronchiolitis	(36)
1983	Mineral dust respiratory bronchiolitis	(37)
1984	Heart–lung transplant obliterative bronchiolitis	(39)
1985	Idiopathic bronchiolitis obliterans organizing pneumonia (BOOP)	(40)
1985	Connective tissue related BOOP	(40)
1987	Respiratory bronchiolitis–interstitial lung disease	(44)
1989	Lung transplant obliterative bronchiolitis	(50)
1989	HIV infection related BOOP	(58)
1989	Drug-related BOOP	(59,60)
1990	Stevens-Johnson related obliterative bronchiolitis	(63)
1990	Viral-induced BOOP	(69)
1990	Radiation therapy induced BOOP	(70)
1990	Myelodysplastic syndrome related BOOP	(71)
1990	International Congress on BOOP	(88)

acteristic pathologic lesion consisted of an injured bronchiole whose lumen was partially or completely obliterated by organizing granulation tissue, and whose wall was surrounded by an irregular growth of newly formed fibrous tissue. The first patient was an 18-year-old who had a "cold" two weeks before admission, developed dyspnea and cyanosis, and died 1 week after hospitalization. The second patient had a mild episode of scarlet fever, then varicella infection within a few days, and 5 weeks later a diagnosis of pertussis was made. The patient died 11 weeks after admission. The third patient was a 46-year-old who had asthma for 2 ½ years and had experienced an episode of influenza 9 years before. The fourth patient was a 73-year-old man who had no associated infections or exposures, and the fifth was a 42-year-old patient who had had influenza 3 years before. In 1938, bronchiolitis obliterans was found at autopsy in a 22-year-old medical student after a 3-week illness; the diagnosis had been considered but had no effect on the clinical outcome (13).

In 1941, LaDue (14) reported bronchiolitis obliterans in a 20-year-old patient who died 9 days after hospitalization. The chest radiograph showed bilateral, small nodular opacities, and the lung at autopsy showed obliteration of the bronchiolar lumen by fibrin and partial organization of the exudate. There was no apparent cause of the illness. The disease was noted to be exceedingly rare, having been found in only 1 of 42,038 autopsies performed by members of the pathology department at the University of Minnesota Medical School since 1899. This report also contained an important summary of the literature at that time and mentioned the lesion resulting from exposure to chlorine and phosgene in laboratory animal studies in 1920. Poison gas exposure was implicated as a cause of bronchiolitis obliterans in a 1936 report. Three categories of bronchiolitis obliterans were recognized: after inhalation of irritant fumes, as a complication of infection, and of unknown etiology.

In 1955, there was another updated review (15) of the literature and a report of a 38-year-old man who died with extensive bronchiolitis obliterans after exposure to nitrogen dioxide. Histologically, the characteristic lesion involved with bronchioles, and the lumen was virtually obliterated by organizing exudate, which often projected in a polypoid fashion. The next year a breakthrough report (16) was published establishing nitrogen dioxide as a cause of bronchiolitis obliterans in "silo-filler's disease." That report also established that corticosteroid therapy could save lives: two of the four patients treated with antibiotics died, whereas two treated with corticosteroid therapy survived. Therapy was given in the form of intramuscular prednisone at 30 mg three times daily; prompt and striking improvement was seen During the next 3 years, McLean (17–19) described the pathology of bronchiolitis in the adult by examining 20,000 cut sections.

In 1963, acute bronchiolitis was described (20) in nine patients as a result of the 1962 London fog; all patients recovered as the fog cleared. The next year, infectious obstructing bronchiolitis was reported (21) as a febrile illness in seven adult patients aged 29 to 64 years. In 1966, the histological findings (22) at autopsy of a 56-year-old man showed bronchiolitis obliterans with concentric rings of fibrosis typical of constrictive bronchiolitis. The interstitium was spared and the cause was idiopathic. The next year, acute bronchiolitis as a result of an upper respiratory tract infection was described (23) as a cause of chronic airflow obstruction in two adults. That same year, during a symposium in Boston, Liebow and Carrington (24) described bronchiolitis obliterans and diffuse alveolar damage as bronchiolitis interstitial pneumonia (BIP) in a discussion of the interstitial pneumonias published in 1969. In this disorder, the changes in the bronchioles appeared to be the same as those of the alveoli.

In 1971, chronic obstructive disease of small airways was described (25) in seven patients with chronic airflow obstruction, all with reticular pattern on their chest roentgenograms, and chronic hypercapnia in four. In 1973, Gosink and colleagues (26) described the radiographic and pathologic findings in 52 patients with bronchiolitis obliterans. The disorder developed after pneumonia or chronic pulmonary infection, after toxic inhalation, or was of unknown etiology. The radiographic patterns were classified as nodular densities, alveolar opacities, and, rarely, hyperinflation. Two types of bronchiolitis obliterans were described pathologically. Most commonly, the respiratory bronchioles were filled with masses of organized exudate. Less frequently, peribronchial and mural infiltration by mononuclear cells and granulation tissue resulted in constrictive bronchiolitis.

In 1974, respiratory bronchiolitis due to cigarette smoking was described from a study (27) of the autopsies that resulted from the sudden deaths of 39 cigarette smokers.

Three years later, there was a report (28) of a 48-year-old woman who developed rhinorrhea, sore throat, and nonproductive cough, followed 2 weeks later by dyspnea. She was admitted to the hospital 6 weeks later for a biopsy. The chest film showed patchy infiltrates at the bases; the lung biopsy showed polypoid masses of granulation tissue filling many of the small bronchioles; and the photomicrograph showed an organizing pneumonia component. The patient returned to normal health after a course of corticosteroid therapy.

In 1977, connective tissue disease–related bronchiolitis obliterans was established when Geddes and colleagues (29) reported an association of bronchiolitis obliterans with rheumatoid arthritis. Drug-related bronchiolitis obliterans was also recognized in patients with rheumatoid arthritis who had received penicillamine in the same report and in a report two years later (30).

A burst of reports and new findings occurred in the decade of the 1980s and into the 1990s (Fig. 1).

In 1981, obliterative bronchiolitis in adults was established (31) in 10 patients on the basis of clinical criteria that included a forced expired volume in one second (FEV1) of 60% predicted or less, and several exclusion criteria, such as asthma, chronic bronchitis, and emphysema. The same year, two additional patients with rheumatoid arthritis were reported (32) to have developed obliterative bronchiolitis while receiving penicillamine.

In 1982, bronchiolitis obliterans was reported (33) in a 22-year-old patient who received an allogeneic bone marrow transplant for aplastic anemia. The patient developed graft-versus-host disease in 3 months, followed by cough and dyspnea 9 to 12 months after transplantation. Crackles were heard on examination, and the chest film showed hyperinflated lungs without infiltrative opacities. Five months later, the patient died of severe respiratory failure. At autopsy, the lungs showed widespread necrotizing obliterative bronchiolitis. The same year, a report (34) of the radiographic findings of 13 patients with cryptogenic obliterative bronchiolitis indicated diminished middle and lower zone vasculature with evidence of mild overinflation. There was also a report (35) of bronchiolitis obliterans in a 66-year-old man who had ulcerative colitis and had been taking sulfasalazine for 6 months. The lung biopsy also showed chronic interstitial pneumonia; the patient responded to corticosteroid therapy.

In 1983, diffuse panbronchiolitis was described by Japanese investigators (36). Chronic sinusitis, a unique finding, developed in 75% of patients. Pseudomonas infection was a late and bad prognostic sign, with only 30% survival at 10 years.

In 1983, small airway lesions were reported (37) in the lungs of seven workers exposed to nonasbestos mineral dust. The lesions were seen in the walls of membranous and respiratory bronchioles and alveolar ducts, those in the last two being significantly different when compared to a matched population of persons with no dust exposure, suggesting predominantly a respiratory bronchiolitis. Also in 1983, there

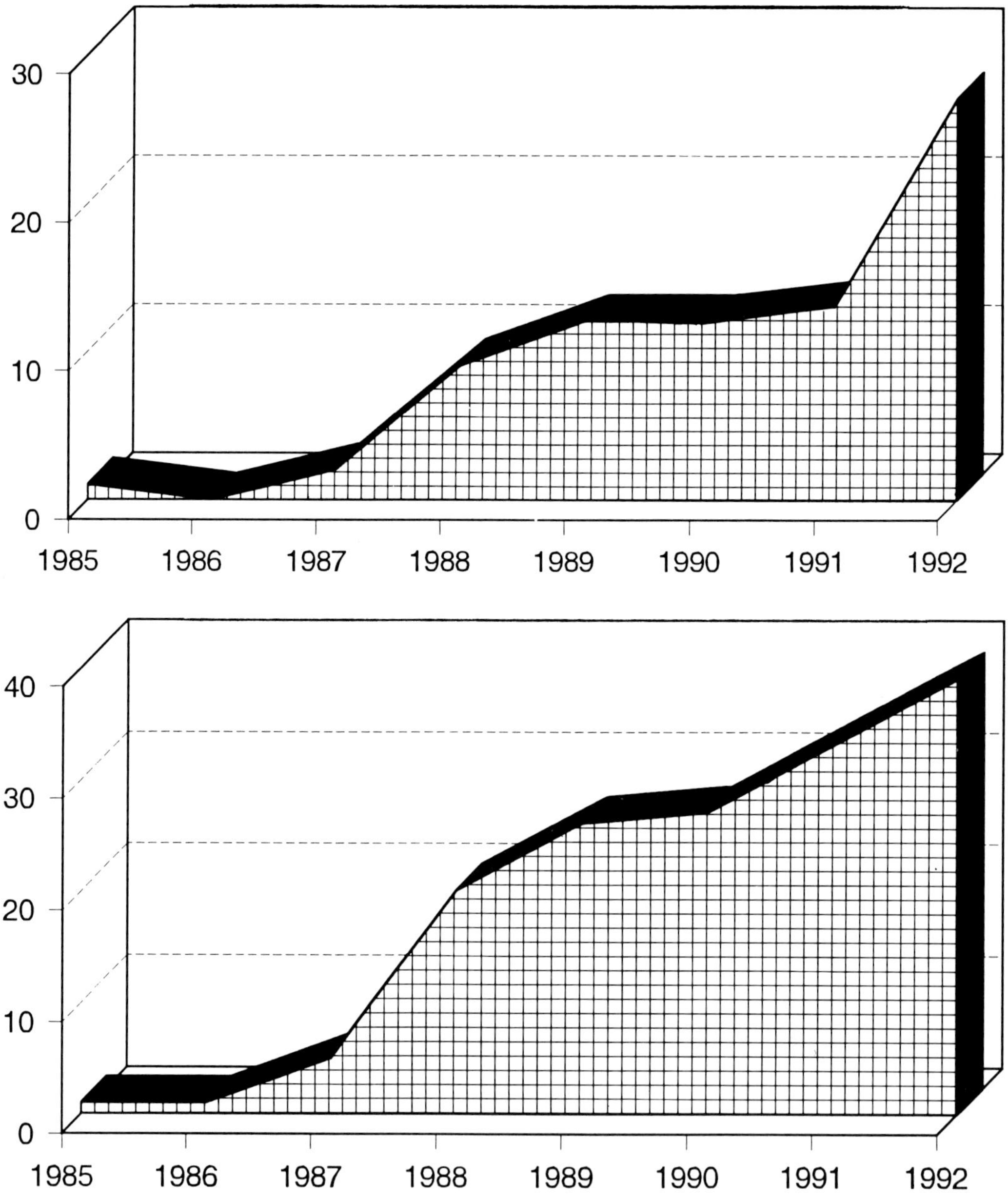

FIG. 1. (Top) The number of articles in which bronchiolitis appeared as "bronchiolitis obliterans," "obliterative bronchiolitis, or "bronchiolitis obliterans organizing pneumonia" in the title of articles in English and non-English, adult and pediatric literature obtained from a Medline search 1985 to 1992. (Bottom) The number of articles in which the term "bronchiolitis obliterans organizing pneumonia (BOOP)" appeared in the title. From the same literature search.

was a report (38) of a 65-year-old woman with rheumatoid arthritis who was treated with gold injections and died of respiratory failure 11 months later. Autopsy findings indicated widespread bronchiolitis, mild bronchopneumonia, and end-stage thyroiditis.

In 1984, 5 of 19 long-term heart–lung transplant survivors developed irreversible airflow obstruction; 3 had biopsy-proven obliterative bronchiolitis. The patients developed cough and dyspnea, sometimes associated with fever. These symptoms began from 3 to 28 months after transplantation. Typical signs of chronic graft-versus host disease were not present. The chest roentgenogram showed patchy infiltrates or bilateral nodular opacities, and the physiological studies showed severe, irreversible reductions in the FEV1. Prognosis was poor at the time: death or disabling pulmonary symptoms often occurred in patients with established obliterative bronchiolitis.

In 1985, bronchiolitis obliterans organizing pneumonia (BOOP) was described (40) in 50 patients with an idiopathic illness responsive to corticosteroid therapy. It was defined as granulation tissue plugs within lumina of small airways, sometimes with complete obstruction of small airways, and granulation tissue extending into alveolar ducts and alveoli. The architecture of the lung was maintained. The bronchiolitis obliterans component of BOOP is the proliferative bronchiolitis obliterans lesion. Idiopathic BOOP is distinctly different from the airway lesion of constrictive bronchiolitis because it is an interstitial process with crackles on examination, patchy infiltrates radiographically, and abnormal diffusing capacity, and is responsive to steroid therapy. It was also noted in this report that this BOOP lesion occurs in lupus erythematosus; 1 year later, it was noted (41) with polymyalgia rheumatica.

Also in 1986, there was a report (42) of a 37-year-old man who developed *Mycoplasma*-related bronchiolitis obliterans that resolved after treatment of infectious pneumonia. There was also a report (43) of a 44-year-old woman with rheumatoid arthritis who developed bronchiolitis during the fifth month of oral gold treatment (43).

In 1987, respiratory bronchiolitis-interstitial lung disease was described (44) in six patients as a distinctive syndrome occurring in smokers. It was the second bronchiolar disorder found to occur in smokers. Histologically, the lesion is characterized by pigmented macrophages within respiratory bronchioles and neighboring alveolar ducts. The alveolar septa show a chronic inflammatory cellular infiltrate. The illness is reversible if the patient stops smoking, although some patients may require corticosteroid therapy. Free-base cocaine was found to be the cause of BOOP in a 32-year-old man in 1987 (45). The same year, there was a clinical comparison (46) of 16 patients with BOOP, 9 patients with small airway disease, and 18 patients with usual interstitial pneumonia. The characteristic radiographic finding in BOOP was patchy airspace consolidation, a finding that was not present in the other two disorders. The radiographic differential diagnosis between BOOP and usual interstitial pneumonia was also discussed in a similar report (47) regarding these patients. The next year, BOOP responsive to corticosteroid therapy was reported (48) in a 20-year-old woman with ulcerative colitis. In 1988, the ultrastructural findings of BOOP were described (49) in nine patients, who showed the presence of extensive epithelial damage involving peribronchiolar alveolar septa with necrosis and sloughing of alveolar lining cells.

In 1989, obliterative bronchiolitis was reported (50) as a complication of lung transplantation in one of three patients. This patient was a 54-year-old man who had had a single lung transplant for pulmonary fibrosis with a successful postoperative course and was able to walk 5 miles per day with improvement up to 3 months after transplantation. Then he developed progressive dyspnea and decrease in the vital capacity and diffusing capacity. Lung biopsy at 4 months showed obliterative bronchiolitis; 2

months later, he had a second lung transplant but died in 3 weeks. Autopsy showed severe rejection of the newly transplanted lung and severe obliterative bronchiolitis of the previously transplanted lung.

Also in 1989, bronchoalveolar lavage studies (51) in 16 patients with airflow obstruction due to bronchiolitis indicated that patients who responded to corticosteroid therapy initially had a high percentage of neutrophils in the lavage fluid, with a mean of 46% neutrophils compared to patients who did not respond, who had a mean of 6% neutrophils. Lung permeability studies (52) in 10 patients with obliterative bronchiolitis showed increase in clearance and patchy peripheral deposition of technetium. There was also a report (53) of a 16-year-old patient who was given activated charcoal for a drug overdose and had a seizure 10 minutes later. She was in coma, survived mechanical ventilation, and was discharged in 2 weeks. One week later, she developed dyspnea, late inspiratory crackles, and an FEV1 of only 0.64. She died 10 weeks after this admission and 14 weeks after the overdose. Autopsy showed extensive charcoal deposition along the airways with bronchiolitis obliterans and fibrous obliteration and stenosis of most small airways. A 1989 report (54) indicated the success of a double-lung transplant for management of bronchiolitis obliterans.

Several reports concerning BOOP were published in 1989. A report (55) of five patients with idiopathic BOOP indicated that the chest roentgenograms may show peripheral infiltrates similar to chronic eosinophilic pneumonia. In England, there was a report (56) of two patients with an acute, apparently infectious illness and BOOP; both responded to corticosteroid therapy. In France, focal BOOP as a single alveolar opacity was reported in 16 patients with idiopathic BOOP. It was also noted that patients with interstitial opacities at the lung bases had a poor response to corticosteroid therapy. Furthermore, the bronchoalveolar lavage fluid in patients who responded to corticosteroid therapy showed a high percentage of lymphocytes, with a mean of 38%, compared to 6% in those who did not respond as well. Bronchiolitis obliterans organizing pneumonia was described (58) in a 40-year-old man with HIV infection. This patient responded completely to corticosteroid therapy. Drug-related BOOP was reported in patients receiving bleomycin (59), acebutolol (60), and amiodarone (60). A review (61) of bronchiolar disorders noted the differences in idiopathic BOOP and idiopathic pulmonary fibrosis or usual interstitial pneumonia. Clinically, fever and upper respiratory tract infection were more common in BOOP, while dyspnea was less common. Pulmonary function indicated that airflow obstruction was seen in 20% of both disorders. The radiograph showed air-space opacities in BOOP but not in usual interstitial pneumonia, while honeycombing was frequently seen in usual interstitial pneumonia but not in BOOP. Histologically, the lesions in BOOP were patchy, predominantly involved air spaces, were of a uniform and recent temporal appearance, were a fibroblastic type of fibrosis with little collagen deposition, and contained foamy macrophages; whereas the lesion associated with usual interstitial pneumonia was diffuse and random, predominately interstitial, varying in temporal appearance, had a mature, collagen type of fibrosis, and honeycombing.

In 1990, a review (62) of the methyl isocyanate explosion tragedy in Bhopal implicated the pyrolysis product hydrogen cyanide as the cause of the irreversible airflow disorder characterized as fibrosing bronchiolitis obliterans. Stevens-Johnson syndrome was associated (63) with bronchiolitis obliterans in a 41-year-old woman who died from an irreversible airflow disorder. Autopsy indicated a loss of the bronchial epithelium, which was replaced by fibrous granulation tissue, and bronchiolar obliteration without associated findings of BOOP.

Idiopathic BOOP was reported from Singapore (64). The chest CT findings were reported in 15 patients with obliterative bronchiolitis (65) and in 14 patients with BOOP (66). Connective tissue related BOOP was reported among 14 patients with polymyositis and dermatomyositis (67) and in a 52-year-old man with Sjogren's syndrome (68). Bronchiolitis obliterans organizing pneumonia was described (69) in a 31-year-old man who had received an allogeneic bone marrow transplant 4 months after developing cytomegalovirus pneumonia. Radiation therapy induced BOOP was described (70) in a 61-year-old man who had small cell carcinoma and received 5,600 rad to the left hilum and mediastinum. The patient died despite large dosages of methyprednisolone. Myelodysplastic syndrome related BOOP was reported (71) in a 58-year-old man who developed hypoxemia, crackles, radiographic patchy infiltrates, and fever with resolution in a few days with prednisone at 1.5 mg/kg.

In a 1990 study (72) of idiopathic BOOP, French investigators suggested three distinct cell-matrix patterns of the intra-alveolar bud evolution: fibrinoid inflammatory cell clusters, desmin-containing fibroblasts, and fibrotic buds in which myofibroblasts organized a loose connective matrix composed of fibronectin and type III collagen.

During the next 2 years, three additional patients from Spain with idiopathic BOOP were described (73); all responded to corticosteroid therapy. Two forms of bronchiolitis obliterans were reported (74) to occur in heart–lung transplant recipients. Three of seven developed the airflow obstructive lesion characterized by acellular concentric fibrosing process limited to the terminal bronchioles, most like secondary to chronic lung allograft rejection. Four of the seven patients had BOOP that was related to infection: cytomegalovirus in three and adenovirus in one. There was also a review article (75) regarding BOOP that suggested that the patchy alveolar opacities, migrating and relapsing, are the most responsive to corticosteroid therapy. An additional review article described (76) the differences between bronchiolitis obliterans and BOOP. Bronchiolitis obliterans organizing pneumonia was also described in a 73-year-old woman with rheumatoid arthritis (77) and associated with common variable immunodeficiency syndrome (78). An abstract (79) regarding a rapidly progressive form of BOOP in six patients was published in 1991. The patients had underlying disorders or exposures, such as rheumatoid arthritis, dermatomyositis, or nitrofurantoin use. These patients were treated with high-dose corticosteroid therapy and additional therapy with cyclophosphamide or azathioprine, but they developed rapid respiratory failure. Most died within 1 month after onset of the illness.

In 1992, the findings (80) of the two types of bronchiolar lesions were confirmed in lung-transplant recipients, with obliterative bronchiolitis occurring in 9 of 50 single-lung transplants and in 5 of 40 double-lung transplants; whereas BOOP occurred in 3 of the single-lung recipients and in 2 of the double-lung recipients. Lupus-related BOOP was also confirmed in a 54-year-old man who responded to corticosteroid therapy and a 28-year-old woman who died of respiratory failure despite corticosteroid and cyclophosphamide therapy (81). Additional clinical review articles (82,83) of BOOP were written as well as a description (84) of 7 patients. There was also a report (85) of a 67-year-old patient with idiopathic BOOP who had migratory pulmonary infiltrates. The description of the clinical–histologic spectrum of bronchiolitis obliterans and BOOP was also published in 1992 (86,87).

The first International Congress on Bronchiolitis Obliterans Organizing Pneumonia was held at Kyoto University in Kyoto, Japan, in 1990. Professor Takateru Izumi was the Chairman of the Congress, and the proceedings were published in 1992 (88). During the symposium, the findings of 13 patients with idiopathic BOOP from Essen, Germany, were described (89). In a report of 29 patients with BOOP from Japan (90), 21 were idiopathic, 4 with rheumatoid arthritis, 1 with Behcet's disease, 2 with chronic thyroiditis, and 1 with alcoholic liver cirrhosis. Patients who had idiopathic BOOP with a febrile illness, elevated sedimentation rate, and patchy infiltrates almost all responded to corticosteroid therapy; those with linear opacities at the bases did not do as well. The high-resolution CT findings (91) in patients with idiopathic BOOP consisted of a combination of areas showing either a marked increase in lung density (air-space consolidation) or a slight increase in lung density (ground-glass opacities). The bronchoalveolar lavage findings (92) of BOOP confirmed the earlier findings of lymphocytosis, especially in patients who responded to corticosteroid therapy.

In conclusion, the first reference to obliteration of small airways was in 1835. The description of two patients with bronchiolitis obliterans in 1901 established the beginning of the study and understanding of bronchiolar diseases. Much was written during the first decade of the century about the causes of bronchiolitis obliterans. In the 1980s, triggered by description of BOOP and obliterative bronchiolitis associated with organ transplantation, an explosion of reports and new scientific investigation began a new understanding of the bronchiolar diseases that has established the bronchiolar disorders as an important aspect of clinical care.

REFERENCES

1. Reynaud AC. Memoire sur l'obliteration des bronches. *Mem Acad Med, Paris* 1835;4:117–167.
2. Lange W. Ueber eine eigenthumliche Erkrankung der kleinen Bronchien und Bronchiolen (Bronchitis et Bronchiolitis obliterans). *Dtsch Arch Klin Med* 1901;70:342–364.
3. Fraenkel A. Ueber Bronchiolitis fibrosa obliterans, nebst Bemerkungen uber Lungenhyperamie und indurirende Pneumonia. *Dtsch Arch Klin Med* 1902;73:484–512.
4. Galdi F. Pneumonia desquamative obliterans nebst Bemerkungen uber die Histologie der Lungeninduration. *Dtsch Arch F Klin Med* 1903; 75:239.
5. Hart C. Anatomische Untersuchungen uber die bei Masern vorkommenden Lungenerkrankungen. *Dtsch Arch Klin Med* 1904;79:108–128.
6. Jochmann G, Moltrecht, Uber seltenere Erkrankungsformen der Bronchien nach Masern und Keuchhusten. *Beitrage zur Path Anat zur Allgemeinen Path* 1904;36:340–352.
7. Edens. Uber bronchiolitis obliterans. *Dtsch Arch Klin Med* 1906;85:598–618.
8. Wegelin C. Uber Bronchitis obliterans nach Fremdkorperaspiration. *Beitrage zur Path Anat zur Allgemeinen Path* 1908;43:438–454.
9. Fraenkel A. Ein weiterer Beitrag zur Lehre von der Bronchiolitis obliterans fibrosa acuta. *Berl Klin Wochenschr* 1909;46(1):6–9.
10. Wagner JH. Bronchiolitis obliterans following the inhalation of acrid fumes. *Am J Med Sci* 1917;154:511–522.
11. Hubschmann P. Uber Inthienzaerkrankungen der Lunge und ihre Bezie-hungen zur Bronchiolitis obliterans. *Beitrage zur Path Anat zur Allgemeinen Path* 1918;63:202–253.
12. Blumgart HL, MacMahon HE. Bronchiolitis fibrosa obliterans: a clinical and pathologic study. *Med Clin North Am* 1929;13:197–214.
13. Leifer VP, Winkler W. Zur Diagnose der Bronchiolitis obliterans. *Wiener Klin Wochenshr* 1938; 51:1331–1332.
14. LaDue JS. Bronchiolitis fibrosa obliterans. *Arch Intern Med* 1941;68:663–673.
15. McAdams AJ. Bronchiolitis obliterans. *Am J Med* 1955;19:314–322.
16. Lowry T, Schuman LM. Silo-filler's disease: a syndrome caused by nitrogen dioxide. *JAMA* 1956;162:153–160.
17. McLean KH. The pathology of acute bronchiolitis: a study of its evolution. I: The exudative phase. *Australas Ann Med* 1956;5:254–267.
18. McLean KH. The pathology of acute bronchiolitis: a study of its evolution. II: The repair phase. *Australas Ann Med* 1957;6:29–43.
19. McLean KH. Bronchiolitis and chronic lung disease. *Br J Tuberc Dis Chest* 1958;52:104–113.
20. Davies GM. Fog bronchiolitis. *Lancet* 1963; i:580–581.
21. Ham JC. Acute infectious obstructing bronchiolitis: a potentially fatal disease in the adult. *Ann Intern Med* 1964;60:47–60.
22. Baar HS, Galindo J. Bronchiolitis fibrosa obliterans. *Thorax* 1966;21:209–214.
23. Dines DE. Acute bronchiolitis as a cause of chronic obstructive lung disease in adults. *Lancet* 1967;87:281–282.
24. Liebow AA, Carrington CB. The interstitial pneumonias. In: Simon M, Potchen EJ, LeMay M, eds. *Frontiers of pulmonary radiology*. New York: Grune & Stratton; 1969:102–141.
25. Macklem PT, Thurlbeck WM, Fraser RG. Chronic obstructive disease of small airways. *Ann Intern Med* 1971;74:167–177.
26. Gosink BB, Friedman PJ, Liebow AA. Bronchiolitis obliterans. *Am J Roentgenol* 1973; 117:816–832.
27. Niewoehner DE, Kleinerman J, Rice DB. Pathologic changes in the peripheral airways of young

cigarette smokers. *N Engl J Med* 1974;291:755–758.
28. Dale RC, Auchincloss JH, Gilbert R, Markarian B. Bronchiolitis obliterans: long-term follow-up. *NY State J Med* 1977;77:1485–1488.
29. Geddes DM, Corrin B, Brewerton DA, et al. Progressive airway obliteration in adults and its association with rheumatoid disease. *Q J Med* 1977;46:427–444.
30. Epler GR, Snider GL, Gaensler EA, et al. Bronchiolitis and bronchitis in connective tissue disease: a possible relationship to the use of penicillamine. *JAMA* 1979;242:528–532.
31. Turton CE, Williams G, Green M. Cryptogenic obliterative bronchiolitis in adults. *Thorax* 1981; 36:805–810.
32. Murphy KC, Atkins CJ, Offer RC, et al. Obliterative bronchiolitis in two rheumatoid arthritis patients treated with penicillamine. *Arth Rheum* 1981;24:557–560.
33. Roca J, Granena A, Rodriguez-Roisin R, et al. Fatal airway disease in an adult with chronic graft-versus-host disease. *Thorax* 1982;37:77–78.
34. Breatnach E, Kerr I. The radiology of cryptogenic obliterative bronchiolitis. *Clin Radiol* 1982; 33:657–661.
35. Williams T, Eidus L, Thomas P. Fibrosing alveolitis, bronchiolitis obliterans, and sulfasalaxine therapy. *Chest* 1982;81:766–768.
36. Homma H, Yamanaka A, Shinichi T, et al. Diffuse panbronchiolitis: a disease of the transitional zone of the lung. *Chest* 1983;83:63–69.
37. Churg A, Wright JL. Small-airway lesions in patients exposed to nonasbestos mineral dusts. *Hum Pathol* 1983;14:688–693.
38. Holness L, Tenenbaum J, Cooter NBE, Grossman RF. Fatal bronchiolitis obliterans associated with chrysotherapy. *Ann Rheum Dis* 1983; 42:593–596.
39. Burke CM, Theodore J, Dawkins KD, et al. Post-transplant obliterative bronchiolitis and other late lung sequelae in human heart–lung transplantation. *Chest* 1984;86:824–829.
40. Epler GR, Colby TV, McLoud TC, et al. Bronchiolitis obliterans organizing pneumonia. *N Engl J Med* 1985;312:152–158.
41. Epler GR, Mark EJ. A 65-year-old woman with bilateral pulmonary infiltrates. *N Engl J Med* 1986;314:1627–1635.
42. Coultas DB, Samet JM, Butler C. Bronchiolitis obliterans due to mycoplasma pneumoniae. *West J Med* 1986;144:471–474.
43. O'Duffy JD, Luthra HS, Unni KK, Hyate RE. Bronchiolitis in a rheumatoid arthritis patient receiving auranofin. *Arth Rheum* 1986;29:556–559.
44. Myers JL, Veal CF, Shin MS, Katzenstein AA. Respiratory bronchiolitis causing interstitial lung disease. *Am Rev Resp Dis* 1987;135:880–884.
45. Patel RC, Dutta D, Schonfeld SA. Free-base cocaine use associated with bronchiolitis obliterans organizing pneumonia. *Ann Intern Med* 1987;107:186–187.
46. Guerry-Force ML, Muller NL, Wright JL, et al. A comparison of bronchiolitis obliterans with organizing pneumonia, using interstitial pneumonia and small airways disease. *Am Rev Respir Dis* 1987;135:705–712.
47. Muller NL, Guerry-Force ML, Staples CA. Differential diagnosis of bronchiolitis obliterans with organizing pneumonia and usual interstitial pneumonia: clinical, functional, and radiologic findings. *Radiology* 1987;162:151–156.
48. Swinburn CR, Jackson GJ, Cobden I, et al. Bronchiolitis obliterans organizing pneumonia in a patient with ulcerative colitis. *Thorax* 1988; 43:735–736.
49. Myers JL, Katzenstein AA. Ultrastructural evidence of alveolar epithelial injury in idiopathic bronchiolitis obliterans-organizing pneumonia. *Am J Pathol* 1988;132:102–109.
50. McGregor CGA, Dark JH, Hilton CJ, et al. Early results of single lung transplantation in patients with end-stage pulmonary fibrosis. *J Thorac Cardiovasc Surg* 1989;98:350–354.
51. Kindt GC, Weiland JE, Davis WB, et al. Bronchiolitis in adults: a reversible cause of airway obstruction associated with airway neutrophils and neutrophil products. *Am Rev Respir Dis* 1989;140:483–492.
52. Sweatman MC, Pantin CFA, Lawrence R, Turner-Warwick M. Lung permeability in adult obliterative bronchiolitis. *Respir Med* 1989,83: 323–327.
53. Elliott CG, Colby TV, Kelly TM, et al. Charcoal lung: bronchiolitis obliterans after aspiration of activated charcoal. *Chest* 1989;96:672–674.
54. Cooper JD, Patterson GA, Grossman R, Maurer J. Double-lung transplant for advanced chronic obstructive lung disease. *Am Rev Respir Dis* 1989;139:303–307.
55. Bartter T, Irwin RS, Nash G, et al. Idiopathic bronchiolitis obliterans organizing pneumonia with peripheral infiltrates on chest roentgenogram. *Arch Intern Med* 1989;149:273–279.
56. Patel U, Jenkins PF. Bronchiolitis obliterans organizing pneumonia. *Respir Med* 1989;83:241–244.
57. Cordier JF, Louire R, Brune J. Idiopathic bronchiolitis obliterans organizing pneumonia: Definition of characteristic clinical profiles in a series of 16 patients. *Chest* 1989;96:999–1004.
58. Allen JN, Wewers MD. HIV-associated bronchiolitis obliterans organizing pneumonia. *Chest* 1989;96:197–198.
59. Santrach PJ, Askin FB, Wells RJ, et al. Nodular form of bleomycin-related pulmonary injury in patients with osteogenic sarcoma. *Cancer* 1989; 64:806–811.
60. Camus P, Lombard JN, Perrichon M, et al. Bronchiolitis obliterans organizing pneumonia in patients taking acebutolol or amiodarone. *Thorax* 1989;44:711–715.
61. King TE. Bronchiolitis obliterans. *Lung* 1989; 167:69–93.
62. Mehta PS, Mehta AS, Mehta SJ, Makhijani AB. Bhopal tragedy's health effects: a review of methyl isocyanate toxicity. *JAMA* 1990;264: 2781–2787.

63. Tsunoda N, Iwanaga T, Saito T, et al. Rapidly progressive bronchiolitis obliterans associated with Stevens-Johnson syndrome. *Chest* 1990;98: 243–245.
64. Tan WC, Chan RKT, Sinniah R. Idiopathic bronchiolitis obliterans with organizing pneumonia in Singapore. *Singapore Med J* 1990;31:493–496.
65. Sweatman MC, Millar AB, Strickland B, Turner-Warwick M. CT in adult obliterative bronchiolitis. *Clin Radiol* 1990;41:116–119.
66. Muller NL, Staples CA, Miller RR. Bronchiolitis obliterans organizing pneumonia: CT features in 14 patients. *AJR* 1990;154:983–987.
67. Tazelaar HD, Viggiano RW, Pickersgill J, Colby TV. Interstitial lung disease in polymyositis and dermatomyositis. *Am Rev Respir Dis* 1990;141: 727–733.
68. Matteson, EL, Ike RW. Bronchiolitis obliterans organizing pneumonia and Sjogren's syndrome. *J. Rheumatol* 1990;17:676–679.
69. Chien J, Chan CK, Chamberlain D, et al. Cytomegalovirus pneumonia in allogeneic bone marrow transplantation. *Chest* 1990;98:1034–1937.
70. Kaufman J, Komorowski R. Bronchiolitis obliterans: a new clinical–pathologic complication of irradiation pneumonitis. *Chest* 1990;97:1243–1244.
71. Tenholder MF, Becker GL, Cervoni MI. The myelodysplastic syndrome and bronchiolitis obliterans. *Ann Intern Med* 1990;112:714–715.
72. Peyrol S, Cordier JF, Grimaud JA. Intra-alveolar fibrosis of idiopathic bronchiolitis obliterans-organizing pneumonia. *Am J Pathol* 1990;137: 155–170.
73. Alegre-Martin J, De Sevilla TF, Garcia F, et al. Three cases of idiopathic bronchiolitis obliterans with organizing pneumonia. *Eur Respir J* 1991;4:902–904.
74. Abernathy EC, Hruban RH, Baumgartner WA, et al. The two forms of bronchiolitis obliterans in heart–lung transplant recipients. *Hum Pathol* 1991;22:1102–1110.
75. Cordier JF, Loire R, Peyrol S. Bronchiolitis obliterans organizing pneumonia (BOOP). *Rev Mal Respir* 1991;8:139–152.
76. Neagos GR, Lynch JP. Making sense of bronchiolitis obliterans and related disorders. *J Respir Dis* 1991;12:789–814.
77. van Thiel RJ, van der Burg S, Groote AD, et al. Bronchiolitis obliterans organizing pneumonia and rheumatoid arthritis. *Eur Respir J* 1991;4: 905–911.
78. Kaufman J, Komorowski R. Bronchiolitis obliterans organizing pneumonia in common variable immunodeficiency syndrome. *Chest* 1991;100: 552–553.
79. Cohen AJ, King TE, Downey GP. Rapidly progressive bronchiolitis obliterans organizing pneumonia (BOOP). *Chest* 1991;100[suppl]:6S.
80. de Hoyos AL, Patterson GA, Maurer JR, et al. Pulmonary transplantation. *J Thorac Cardiovasc Surg* 1992;103:295–306.
81. Gammon RB, Bridges TA, Al-Nezir H, et al. Bronchiolitis obliterans organizing pneumonia associated with systemic lupus erythematosus. *Chest* 1992;102:1171–1174.
82. Swinburn C. Bronchiolitis obliterans organizing pneumonia. *Br J Hosp Med* 1992;48:492–495.
83. Sharma OP. Bronchiolitis obliterans organizing pneumonia. *West J Med* 1992;157:172–173.
84. Flowers JR, Clunie G, Burke M, Constant O. Bronchiolitis obliterans organizing pneumonia. *Clin Radiol* 1992;45:371–377.
85. Epstein DM, Bennett MR. Bronchiolitis obliterans organizing pneumonia with migratory pulmonary infiltrates. *AJR* 1992;158:515–517.
86. Colby TV, Myers JL. Clinical and histologic spectrum of bronchiolitis obliterans, including bronchiolitis obliterans organizing pneumonia. Semin *Respir Med* 1992;13:119–133.
87. Wright JL, Cagle P, Churg A, et al. Diseases of the small airways. *Am Rev Respir Dis* 1992; 146:240–262.
88. Izumi T, ed. Proceedings of the International Congress on Bronchiolitis Obliterans Organizing Pneumonia. *Chest* 1992;102(1)[Suppl]:1S–50S.
89. Costabel U, Teschler H, Schoenfeld B, et al. BOOP in Europe. *Chest* 1992;102:14S–20S.
90. Yamamoto M, Ina Y, Kitaichi M, et al. Clinical features of BOOP in Japan. *Chest* 1992;102:21S–25S.
91. Nishimura K, Itoh H. High-resolution computed tomographic features of bronchiolitis obliterans organizing pneumonia. *Chest* 1992;102:26S–31S.
92. Nagai S, Aung H, Tanaka S, et al. Bronchoalveolar lavage cell findings in patients with BOOP and related diseases. *Chest* 1992;102: 32S–37S.

Diseases of the Bronchioles, edited by
Gary R. Epler. Raven Press, Ltd.,
New York © 1994.

2

Anatomical and Histological Classification of the Bronchioles

Charles G. Plopper* and Ank A. W. Ten Have-Opbroek†

**Department of Anatomy and Cell Biology, School of Veterinary Medicine, University of California, Davis, CA.*
†Department of Surgery, School of Medicine, University of California, Davis, CA; and Department of Pulmonology, School of Medicine, University of Leiden, P.O. Box 9602, 2300 R.C., Leiden, The Netherlands.

GENERAL DEFINITIONS AND TERMINOLOGY

In the respiratory system, air moves between the oral and nasal cavities and gas-exchange areas of the lungs through a series of branching tubes termed the *conducting*, or *tracheobronchial, airways*. As illustrated in Fig. 1, the tracheobronchial airways begin distal to the larynx and the *trachea,* which divides into two *primary bronchi*. The next generations of branching vary by species, but in general the primary bronchi give rise to the *lobar bronchi,* which enter individual lung lobes and branch further to become *intrapulmonary bronchi*. The distal portions of these bronchi consist of smaller branches called *bronchioles*. *Terminal bronchioles,* the most distal of these branches, occur at the beginning of the alveolar gas-exchange area. In humans, there is a *transitional zone* between the terminal bronchiole and the gas-exchange region in which cells characteristic of conducting airways and cells characteristic of the gas-exchange area intermix. This zone is characterized by *respiratory bronchioles,* which contain a number of alveoli and other characteristics of the gas-exchange area. The *pulmonary acinus* is generally defined as the entire gas-exchange area supplied by a single terminal bronchiole. An *alveolus* is a terminal air space or pocket whose wall is composed of gas-exchange tissue, called *interalveolar septa,* and which has only one outlet. The ducting system formed by the openings of adjacent alveoli is called an *alveolar duct*. The ducts end in *alveolar sacs*. Distances and position within the respiratory system are often indicated by *generations*. Each time an air passage branches, this is considered another *generation* of branching.

ARCHITECTURAL POSITION OF BRONCHIOLES

In the human lung, terminal bronchioles are found between the sixth and twenty-third generations of branching from the trachea; the average position seems to range somewhere between the thirteenth and the sixteenth. Table 1 summarizes some of the variations in human terminal bronchioles; measurements are based on casts produced by filling air passages to total lung capacity. The number of terminal bronchioles in the human lung has been estimated to be as few as 25,000 to over 65,000 (1,2). Terminal bronchioles vary in length from 0.8 to 2.5

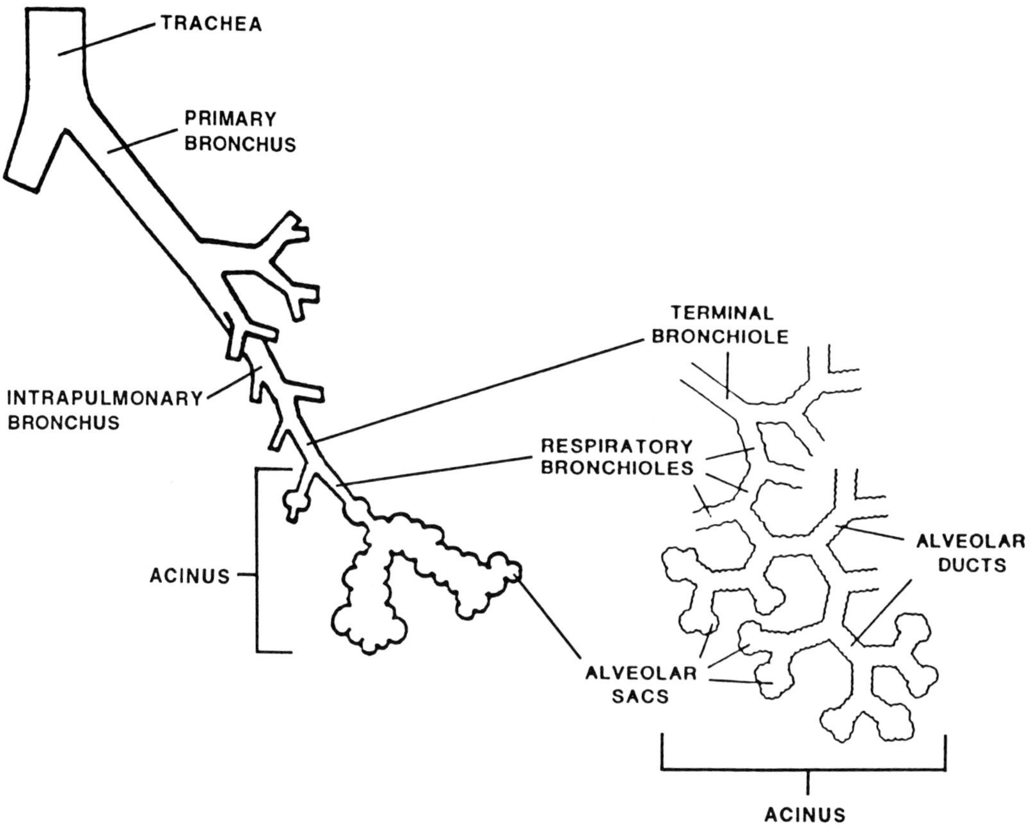

FIG. 1. The tracheobronchial airway tree: the trachea, primary bronchi, intrapulmonary bronchi, terminal bronchioles, and air passages of the pulmonary acinus.

mm and have an average luminal diameter of approximately 0.6 mm. The number of alveoli supplied by one terminal bronchiole ranges from 20,000 to 71,000 (3,4). Terminal bronchioles typically branch into two or three respiratory bronchioles (3,5). The human lung averages 3 generations of respiratory bronchioles (3,4); however, as many as 12 have been reported in some acini (6). Unlike terminal bronchioles, which appear to have a relatively uniform diameter from end to end, the lumina of respiratory bronchioles tend to get smaller in more distal generations (4,6). Likewise, the number of

TABLE 1. *Summary of variations in characteristics of terminal bronchioles in human lung among five studies measuring casts filling airways to total by capacity*

Estimated number	Number of generations to trachea	Diameter (mm)	Length (mm)	Reference
33,000	28	0.6	1.68	(34,2)
65,000	6–23 Mean = 13	0.6	1.65	(2)
27,000	15–16	0.5–0.66	1.18–1.25	(35)
25,000	Mean = 11	0.48–0.76	1.05–2.50	(1)
Not estimated	Not estimated	0.42–0.47	0.79–0.85	(4)

alveoli per respiratory bronchiole also changes with generational distance, increasing from one or two in the most proximal respiratory bronchioles to many more in the most distal ones (4,5,6). An overview of the architectural organization of the human tracheobronchial tree in relation to other species has been recently summarized by McBride (7).

One important characteristic of the relationship of terminal and respiratory bronchioles to the gas-exchange area is the high variation in acinar volume. This variability has been summarized by Mercer and Crapo (8). Estimates of acinar volume range from as low as 15.6 mm^3 to as high as 187 mm^3 (9,6). These authors emphasize that individual gas-exchange units supplied by either terminal or respiratory bronchioles can vary tremendously; consequently, any injury response detected in individual bronchioles within the same lung can also be expected to vary considerably. The assumption is that the higher the volume of air passing through an individual bronchiole, the more likely that bronchiole is to be injured by airborne toxicants, whether they be particles, reactive gases, or infectious microbes. Additional variability in injury can be expected due to differences in the number of airway generations between the trachea and a particular terminal or respiratory bronchiole if deposition of the agent is affected by alterations in the direction of the airway path and by increases in turbulence at branching points.

A critical step in defining a pathological response in distal bronchioles is the identification of the terminal bronchiole. This undertaking is problematic in lungs of any species, especially if they are not fixed at standard inflation pressure. The use of total diameter or luminal diameter to identify terminal bronchioles histologically is relatively inexact because reported diameters are based on casting of the airway lumen at total lung capacity. These diameters are in the range of 0.5 mm. If the wall is considered to have a thickness of one-quarter the diameter of the airspace, then an estimate of 1 mm for a total diameter might be useful, except for the fact that more proximal generations of bronchioles also have an average luminal diameter in the same range as that of terminal bronchioles (7). However, terminal bronchioles can easily be identified in serial sections or by isolation of tissue samples using microdissection prior to embedding (10). Either of these approaches will facilitate identification of the conducting airways in which alveolarization occurs.

CELLULAR ORGANIZATION OF BRONCHIOLES

The histological appearance of the distal bronchiole in the human lung is illustrated in Fig. 2. Unlike bronchi, bronchioles in the human lung do not have submucosal glands or cartilage associated with their walls but rather have connective tissue and smooth muscle. The wall of the bronchiole from the lumen outward consists of epithelium, a small zone of fine connective tissue, the lamina propria, a band of smooth muscle in the muscularis, and a connective tissue band, the adventitia, which interconnects with the extracellular matrix of interalveolar septa.

The epithelium of terminal bronchioles in the human lung is composed of columnar to high cuboidal epithelial cells of at least three types (Table 2). The composition of this epithelial population in comparison to other generations of airways, bronchi and bronchioles, has been recently reviewed (11). The first cell type is the ciliated cell, which extends from the basal lamina to the luminal surface. The abundance of ciliated cells in this region can be readily appreciated when viewed with the scanning electron microscope (Fig. 3). The ultrastructural appearance of ciliated cells includes large numbers of cilia anchored in the apex of the cell by basal bodies, a central nucleus, and an abundance of mitochondria in the apical cytoplasm (Fig. 4). The second

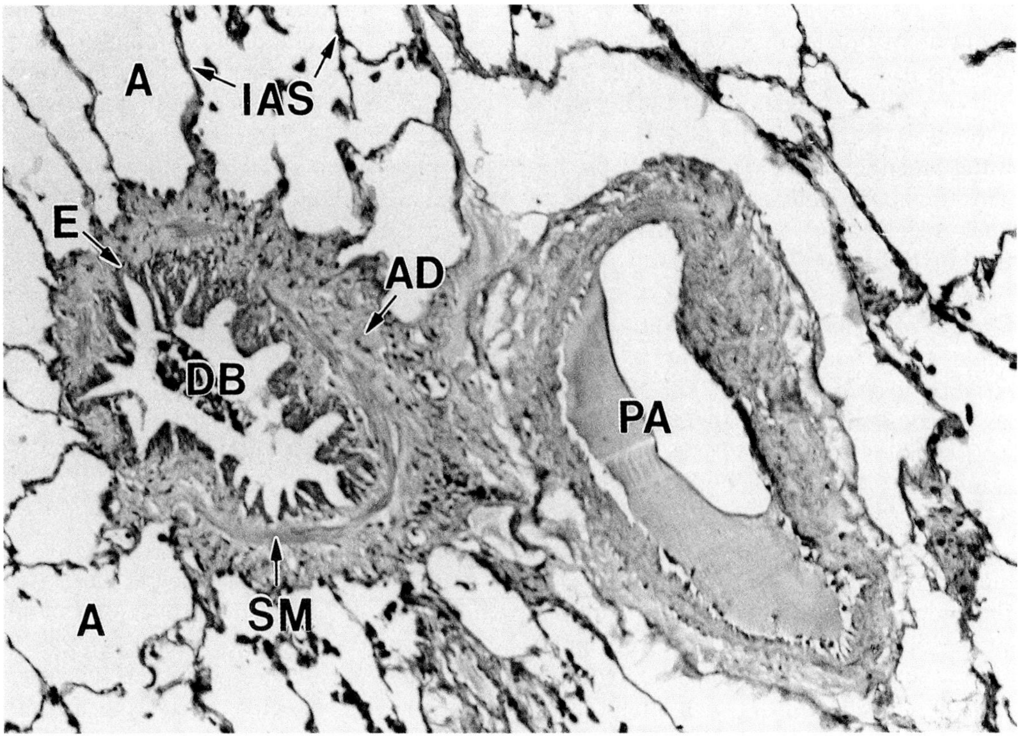

FIG. 2. Comparison of the histological organization of the distal bronchiole (*DB*) and a small pulmonary artery (*PA*). The luminal surface is lined by columnar epithelium (*E*). Bands of smooth muscle (*SM*) separate the lamina propria from the adventitia (*AD*) of the wall. Interalveolar septa (*IAS*) extend from the adventitia into the surrounding lung parenchyma. Alveolar airspace (*A*). Nuclear fast red. 140 ×.

type of epithelial cells is the nonciliated cells, which also extend from the basal lamina to the luminal surface (Fig. 4). The apical surface of these cells is often lined by short microvilli, and the cells are joined to neighboring ciliated or nonciliated cells by junctional complexes near the luminal surface. The lateral sides contain many cellular extensions and interdigitations with neighboring cells. In addition to a centrally

TABLE 2. *Cell types in epithelial populations of terminal and respiratory bronchioles*

Terminal bronchiole	Respiratory bronchiole
Cell types:	First population (near pulmonary arteriole)
Nonciliated columnar	Cell types:
Ciliated columnar	Noncilated columnar
Basal	Ciliated columnar
	Basal
	Second population (borders first population)
	Cell type:
	Nonciliated cuboidal
	Third population (opposite pulmonary arteriole)
	Cell types:
	Nonciliated cuboidal (type II cell)
	Squamous (type I cell)

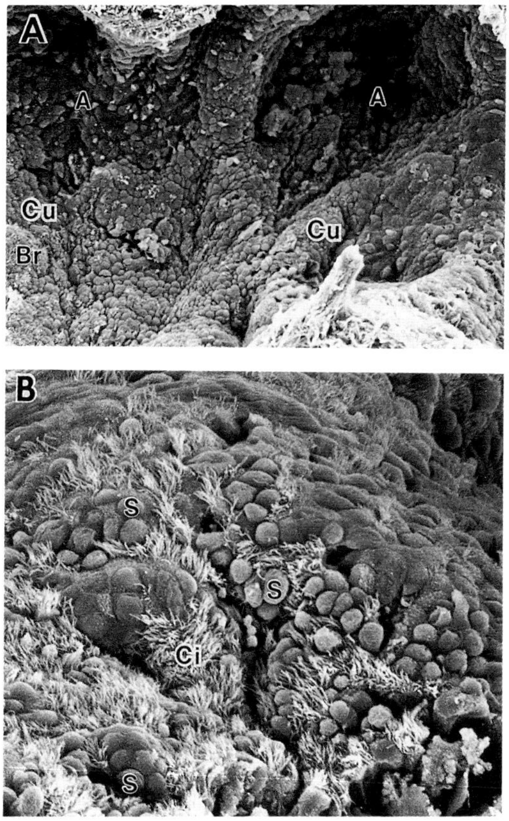

FIG. 3. Surface view of respiratory bronchiole and ciliated columnar epithelial cell population of respiratory bronchiole. **A,** The epithelial population characteristic of terminal broncioles (*Br*) extends into respiratory bronchioles in areas adjacent to the cuboidal population (*Cu*) and is associated with the opposite portions of the bronchiolar wall from the alveoli (*A*), which are lined by a combination of squamous and cuboidal epithelium. 570 ×. **B,** The bronchiolar columnar epithelial cells contain a mixture of ciliated cells with cilia projecting into the airway lumen (*Ci*) and nonciliated secretory cells (*S*). 1200 ×.

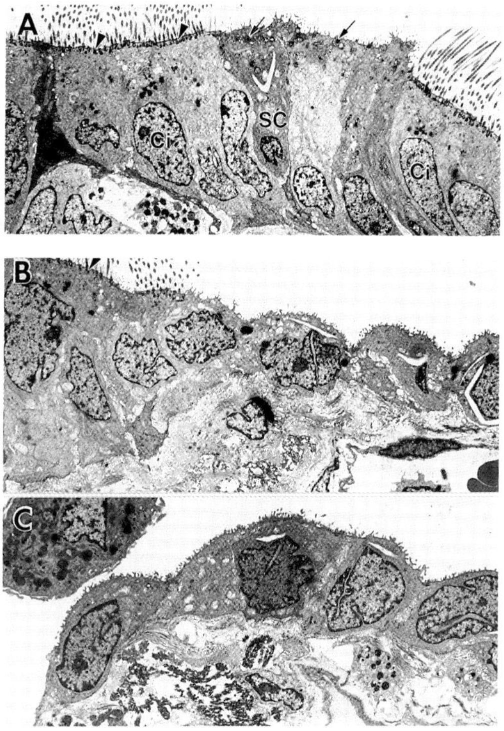

FIG. 4. Ultrastructural comparison of the columnar (A,B) and simple cuboidal (B,C) epithelial populations which line the respiratory bronchiole of human lung. **A,** The columnar epithelial population contains ciliated cells (*Ci*) with cilia anchored to the luminal aspect of the cell by basal bodies (*arrowheads*). The secretory cells (*SC*) extend from the basal lamina to the luminal surface. These cells contain secretory granules (*arrows*) 1700 ×. **B,** The simple cuboidal epithelial population joins tightly to the columnar population. These cells have extensive cytoplasmic extensions on their lateral surfaces and small numbers of secretory granules. 1800 ×. **C,** A capillary bed is not found immediately adjacent to this epithelium on their basal surfaces. 1900 ×.

placed nucleus, the other most characteristic feature of these cells is an abundance of membrane-bound secretory granules in the apical cytoplasm. These granules vary in appearance from those with a dense osmiophilic matrix, which is closely subtended by the membrane, to granules of somewhat larger size with a matrix of variable density that includes, in some cases, a small, dense central core. Another characteristic of these cells is abundant mitochondria and rough endoplasmic reticulum observed on the lateral and basal surfaces of the nucleus. The nucleus-to-cytoplasmic ratio varies considerably within these cells (12,13,14). Cells of the third type are also nonciliated but are more closely attached to the basal lamina than the other types in the population and do not extend to the airway surface. These cells, termed basal cells, are in very low abundance in the epithelium lining distal bronchioles.

The surface appearance of the respiratory bronchioles is illustrated in Fig. 3. By definition, the respiratory bronchiole comprises epithelial populations that are characteristic of more proximal conducting airways and of the gas-exchange area (Fig. 5). The epithelial lining of respiratory bronchioles appears to be composed of three populations (Table 2). The first of these populations resembles the terminal bronchiolar population and is generally found on the side closest to the pulmonary arteriole. This population has been estimated to occupy 65% of the luminal surface in the most proximal generation of the respiratory bronchioles and less than 5% of the bronchiolar lumen in the third and fourth generations of respiratory bronchioles (3). The second epithelial population lies adjacent to the first and consists of uniformly cuboidal nonciliated cells (Fig. 3 and 5). This population occupies a zone that is transitional between the taller ciliated population and the squamous/cuboidal cell mixture characteristic of alveolar gas-exchange areas (Fig. 3). This cell type is low cuboidal and contains a central nucleus that occupies a larger portion of the cell volume than is the case for any of the cell types in the first population (Fig. 4). These cuboidal cells contain small amounts of rough and smooth endoplasmic reticulum and a small number of mitochondria (12–16). They also contain electron-dense granules located throughout the cytoplasm. These cells are joined to neighbors by junctional complexes and have lateral cytoplasmic projections that interdigitate with neighboring cells. Other features include the presence of osmiophilic multivesicular bodies and lamellar bodies and a small scattering of other organelles. This cuboidal population varies in extent (Fig. 3) along the border of the first (columnar) epithelial population. The third population of respiratory bronchiolar epithelium has most of the phenotypic characteristics of alveolar epithelial lining (Fig. 5). The majority of cells are squamous and cover large areas of basal lamina (Fig. 3). Interdigitated between these cells are cuboidal cells with the ultrastructural features of alveolar type II cells. These squamous cells join the second cell population with tight junctions, and all three epithelial populations are continuous with each other along the basal lamina. Careful evaluation of airway casting has demonstrated that the third population, and a small alveolar outpocketings often associated with it, are polarized on the portions of the respiratory bronchiolar wall not occupied by the pulmonary arteriole and its accompanying adventitial connective tissue (Fig. 5) (4,6). Generally, the extracellular matrix below or outside of the third population contains a capillary bed, which lies very close to the squamous epithelial cells of this population.

BRONCHIOLAR SECRETORY CELLS AND SECRETORY PRODUCTS

All three of the nonciliated cuboidal or columnar cell types associated with the three epithelial populations found in respiratory bronchioles and the nonciliated columnar epithelial cell type associated with terminal bronchiolar epithelium have, as one of their functions, the biosynthesis and release of secretory products into the airway lumina. These secretory cells of distal airways synthesize a number of products including complex glycoproteins (or mucins), lysozyme, antileukoprotease, Clara cell 10-kD protein, and surfactant-associated proteins. In the human lung, the cellular sources of these proteins have been characterized primarily by glycoconjugate histochemistry and immunocytochemistry using antibodies raised specifically against the products.

The secretory cells of the proximal and distal conducting airways serve to keep the lining mucosa moist; to humidify inhaled air; and, in concert with beating cilia, to clean the air by removing dust particles, or-

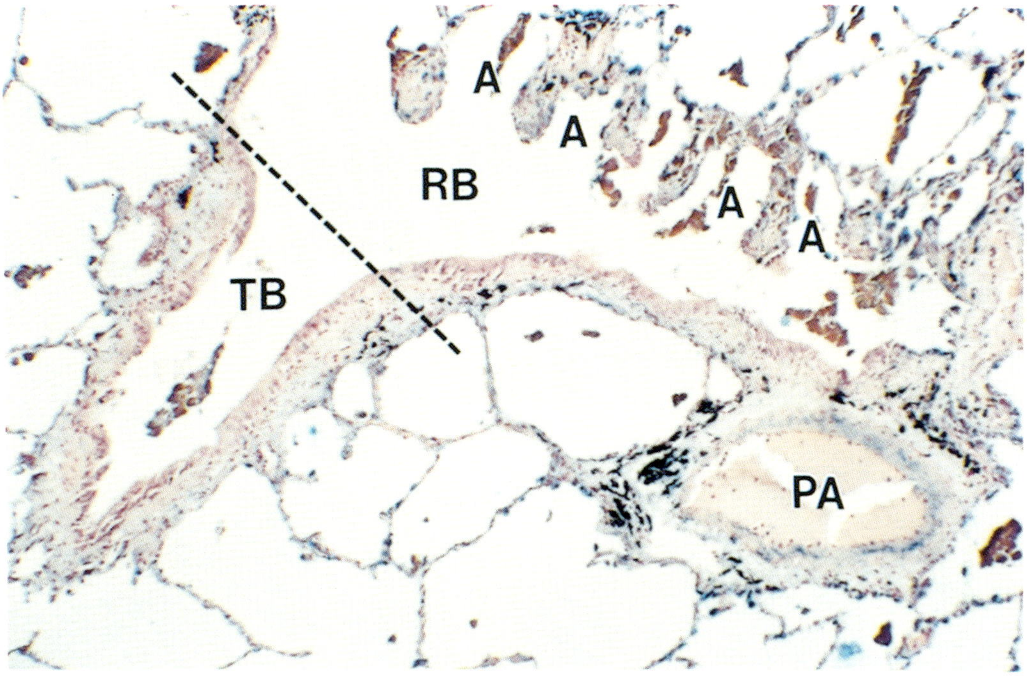

FIG. 5. Histological appearance of respiratory bronchiole (*RB*). The histological organization of the wall is similar to other distal bronchioles and the terminal bronchiole (*TB*). The respiratory bronchiole has bronchiolar epithelium on the side adjacent to the pulmonary arteriole (*PA*) and alveoli (*A*) opening into the lumen on the opposite side. Nuclear fast red. 85 ×.

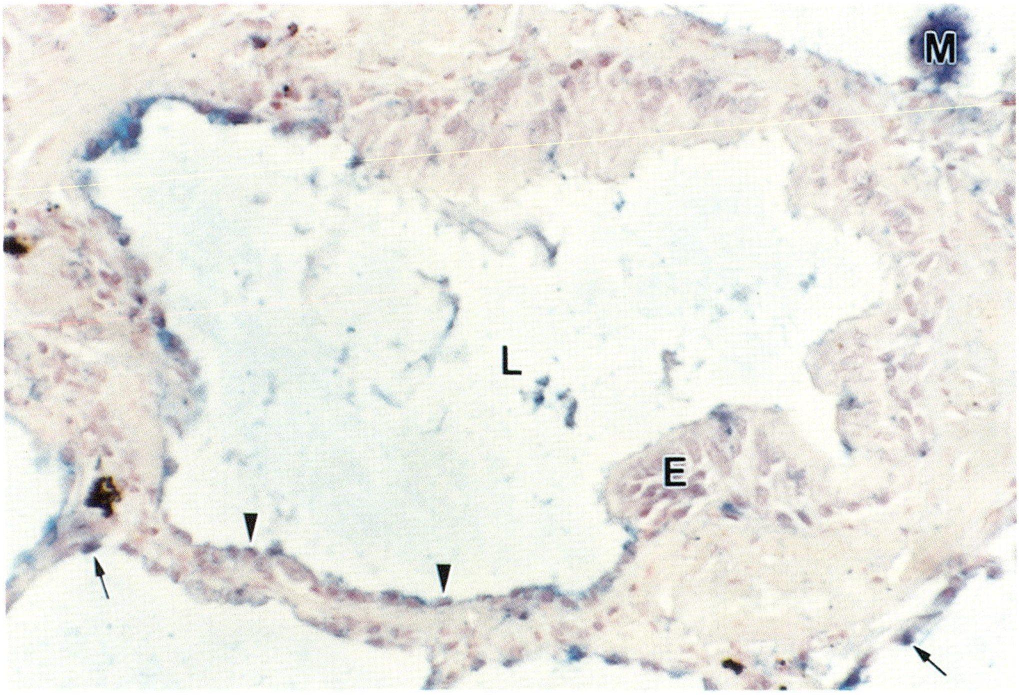

FIG. 6. Cross section of human respiratory bronchiole stained with a monoclonal antibody to human SP-A (Sals-Hu). Adjacent tissue section to that illustrated in Fig. 7 C, D. There is positive reaction for SP-A in the simple cuboidal epithelial population (*arrowheads*) that lines the respiratory bronchiolar epithelium both adjacent to the columnar epithelial population (*E*) and into alveolar airspaces. Type II alveolar epithelial cells (*arrows*) and alveolar macrophages (*M*) also react and are labeled positively with this antibody. Nuclear fast red counterstain. 360 ×.

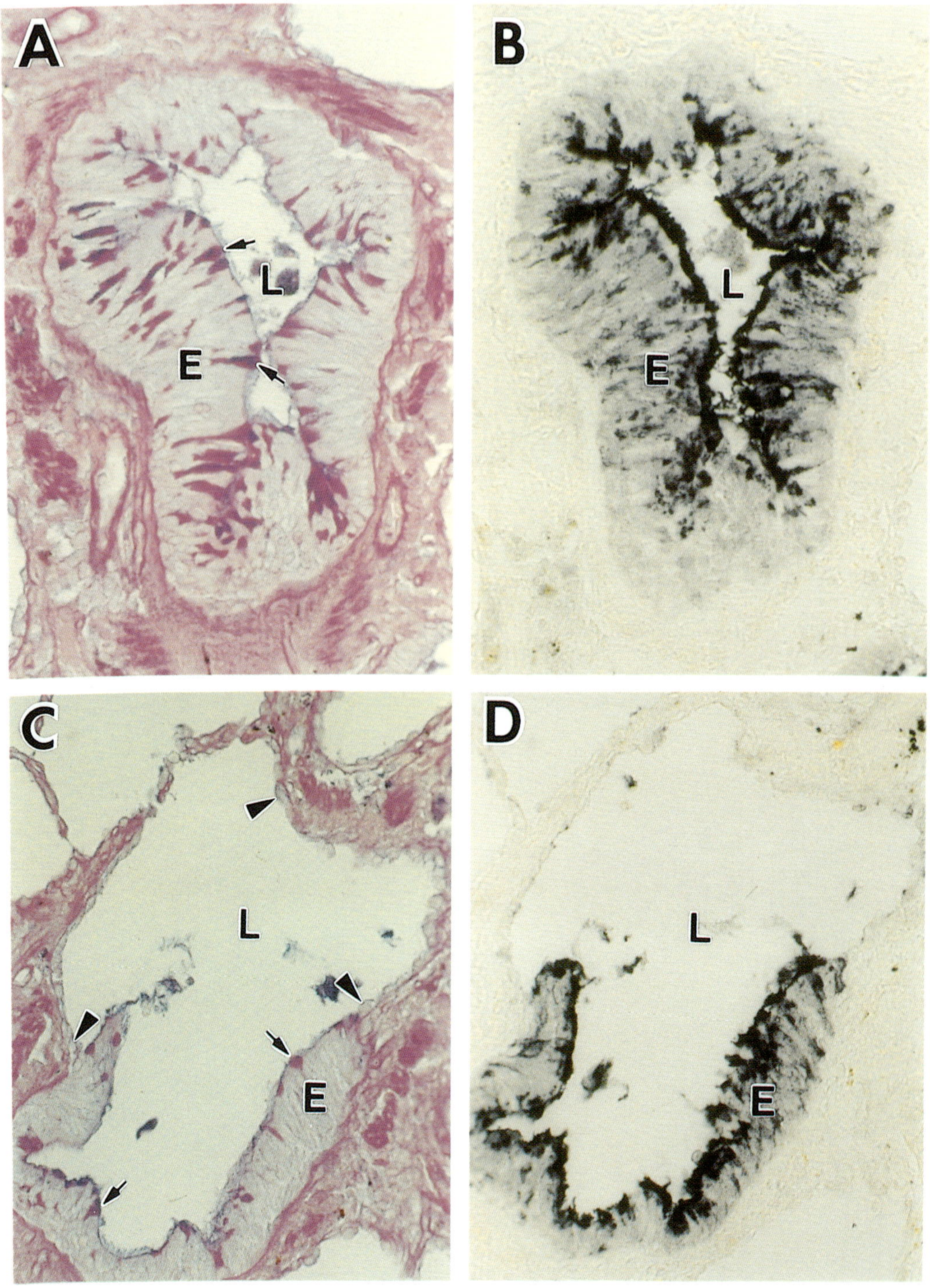

FIG. 7. Comparison of carbohydrate histochemistry and immunohistochemical detection of mucins in distal bronchiole and respiratory bronchiole. **A,** The epithelium (*E*) contains PAS/AB positive material (*arrows*), and there is positive material in the airway lumen (*L*). 360 ×. **B,** The columnar secretory cells also react with a monoclonal antibody (17B1) to large-molecular-weight glycoproteins. These antibodies label both the epithelial cells (*E*) and the ciliary surface projecting into the airway lumen (*L*). 360 ×. **C,** In the respiratory bronchiole, neutral and acidic mucins are present in the columnar secretory cells of the bronchiolar epithelium (*E*). The simple cuboidal epithelium (*arrowheads*) that lines the rest of the airway lumen (*L*) is not reactive. 240 ×. **D,** There is also a positive binding of the monoclonal antibody to secretory mucins in the columnar epithelial population (*E*) in the respiratory bronchiole. 240 ×.

16. ten Hav-Opbroek AAW, Otto-Verberne CJM, Dubbeldam JA, Dykman JH. The proximal border of the human respiratory unit, as shown by scanning and transmission electron microscopy and light microscopical cytochemistry. *Anat Rec* 1991;229:339–354.
17. Jeffery PK, Gaillard D, Moret S. Human airway secretory cells during development and in mature airway epithelium. *Eur Respir J* 1992;5:93–104.
18. Wolf RK. Mucociliary function. In: Parent RA, ed. *Comparative biology of the normal lung*. Boca Raton, FL: CRC Press; 1992:659–680.
19. Koren HS, Becker S. Antimicrobial defense mechanisms. In: Parent RA, ed. *Comparative biology of the normal lung*. Boca Raton, FL: CRC Press; 1992:747–769.
20. St. George JA, Wang S. Secretory glycoconjugates of trachea and bronchi. In: Parent RA, ed. *Treatise on pulmonary toxicology: comparative biology of the normal lung*. Boca Raton, FL: CRC Press; 1991:77–83.
21. Lamb D, Reid LM. Histochemical types of acidic glycoprotein produced by mucous cells of the tracheobronchial glands in man. *J Pathol* 1969;98:213–229.
22. Spicer SS, Chakrin L, Wardell J Jr, Kendrick W. Histochemistry of mucosubstances in the canine and human respiratory tract. *Lab Invest* 1971; 25:483–490.
23. Mariassy AT, McCray MN, Lauredo IT, Abraham WM, Wanner A. Lectin-detectable effects of localized pneumonia on airway mucous cell populations: role of cyclooxygenase metabolites. *Exp Lung Res* 1989;15:113–137.
24. St. George JA, Cranz DL, Zicker S, Etchison JR, Dungworth DL, Plopper CG. An immunohistochemical characterization of rhesus monkey respiratory secretions using monoclonal antibodies. *Am Rev Respir Dis* 1985;132:556–563.
25. Lin H, St. George JA, Plopper CG, Carlson DM, Wu R. An ELISA method for quantitation of tracheal mucins from humans and nonhuman primates. *Am Rev Respir Dis* 1988;
26. Kramps JA, Franken C. Low-molecular-weight protease inhibitor of the respiratory tract. *Surv Immunol Res* 1982;1:30–36.
27. Willems LNA, Kramps JA, Stijnen T, Sterk PJ, Weening JJ, Dijkman JH. Antileukorprotease-containing bronchiolar cells. *Am Rev Respir Dis* 1989;139(5):1244–1250.
28. Singh G, Singh J, Katyal SL, et al. Identification, cellular localization, isolation and characterization of human Clara cell specific 10 kDa protein. *J Histochem Cytochem* 1988;36:73–80.
29. Singh G, Katyal SK. Secretory proteins of Clara cells and type II cells. In: Parent RA, ed. *Comparative biology of the normal lung*. Boca Raton, FL: CRC Press; 1992:93–108.
30. Broers J, Jensen S, Travis W, et al. Expression of surfactant associated protein-A and Clara cell 10 kilodalton mRNA in neoplastic and non-neoplastic human lung tissue as detected by in situ hydribidation. *Lab Invest* 1992;66:337–346.
31. Singh G, Katyal SL, Brown WE, Phillips S, Kennedy AL, Anthony J. Amino-acid and cDNA nucleotide sequences of human Clara cell 10 kDa protein. *Biochim Biophys Acta* 1988;950: 329–337.
32. Andersson O, Nordlung-Moller L, Bronnegard M, Sireza F, Ripe E, Lund J. Purification and level of expression in bronchoalveolar lavage of a human polychlorinated biphenyl (PCB)-binding protein: evidence for a structural and functional kinship to the multihormonally regulated protein uteroglobin. *Am J Respir Cell Mol Biol* 1991;5:6–12.
33. Phelps DS, Floros J. Localization of surfactant protein synthesis in human lung by in situ hybridization. *Am Rev Respir Dis* 1988;137:939–942.
34. Horsfield K, Cumming G. Morphology of the bronchial tree in man. *J Appl Physiol* 1968; 24:373–383.
35. Yeh HC, Schum GM. Models of human lung airways and their application to inhaled particle deposition. *Bull Math Biol* 1980;42:461–480.

ganisms, and absorbed gases (17). The last process, called mucociliary clearance, is a process in which contaminants of inhaled air are trapped or dissolved in the mucous lining layer and then removed by ciliary transport. Mucociliary clearance is also responsible for removing alveolar macrophages from the respiratory tract (18). Secretory cell secretions contain substances that discourage bacterial colonization and growth or render them susceptible to neutralization by the host's immune system (17,19).

The epithelial mucins of the respiratory tract are polydisperse, high-molecular-weight glycoproteins (17,20). Several methods have been used to define mucous composition, including carbohydrate histochemistry and cytochemistry, autoradiography, immunohistochemistry, and biochemistry (20); all but the last have the advantage of localizing the constituents of mucus in situ. Carbohydrate histochemistry and cytochemistry using alcian blue (AB), periodic acid-Schiff (PAS), and high iron diamine (HID) allow distinction between neutral (PAS positive) and acidic (AB positive) mucins. The acidic mucins can be further characterized as sulfomucins or sialomucins based on presence or absence of sulfate esters (high iron diamine positive and negative, respectively). The distal columnar secretory cells present in human terminal and respiratory bronchioles contain both neutral and acidic mucins (Fig. 7) (16), as do most epithelial and glandular mucous cells of human bronchi and trachea (21,22). The predominance of either sulfomucin or sialomucin varies with airway level (20). Serous cells of human tracheobronchial glands contain neutral mucins (21). Additional information about the composition of glycoproteins in mucous and serous cells of human bronchi and submucosal glands has been provided by the use of lectins, which recognize specific sugars, primarily those that are in the terminal position in complex carbohydrates (20). These studies show the heterogeneity of content of both serous and mucous cells as well as species differences. The following sugars have been identified in the bronchial secretory cells of the human lung: fucose, galactose, N-acetyl glucosamine, and N-acetyl neuraminic acid (sialic acid). There is no information on sugar composition in distal bronchioles of humans. Based on lectin reactivity in airway cells of healthy animals, lectins have been used to detect shifts in secretory product with injury or disease (23). The presence of mucins in distal columnar secretory cells in humans has also been demonstrated by immunocytochemistry (16) using monoclonal antibodies to mucous glycoproteins (Fig. 7) (24,25). Studies in the Rhesus monkey using a panel of such monoclonal antibodies underscore the heterogeneity of respiratory secretory products and suggest variations in biophysical properties of secretion at different airway levels (24). The influence of mucin heterogeneity on the functional properties of the mucous blanket at different airway levels remains to be elucidated.

Antileukoprotease (ALP) is a low-molecular-weight proteinase inhibitor that accounts for at least 70% of the total inhibiting capacity of bronchial lavage fluid against neutrophil proteinases (26). Immunocytochemical studies in humans indicate that antileukoprotease is produced by serous cells of bronchial glands and columnar secretory cells of bronchioles. Studies of small airways disease and emphysema suggest that antileukoprotease may protect the lung tissue against inflammatory and destructive processes in distal human airways (27).

Another protective (antibacterial) agent in airway secretions, lysozyme, has been localized to alveolar type II cells and macrophages in the rat; in humans, it is found in serous cells of submucosal glands of major airways but not in type II cells (17,20,29). For more information about antimicrobial defense mechanisms of airway secretions, see the review written by Koren and Becker (19).

Clara cell-specific 10-kD protein (CCSP) constitutes about 0.15% of the soluble proteins in human lung lavage and has been localized to columnar secretory cells of human distal bronchioles (28). Recent observations in humans show that nonciliated columnar cells of both bronchial and bronchiolar epithelium may express the protein (30). Of interest, CCSP is not found in the cuboidal secretory cells of the respiratory bronchioles and the bronchioles immediately proximal to them. Data concerning the biochemical and functional properties of the 10-kD protein are available (31); however, its physiological role remains to be determined. Despite its similarity in size to antileukoprotease, CCSP does not appear to have the same function (29). Molecular studies suggest that human 10-kD protein (31) and a human polychlorinated biphenyl-binding protein purified from lavage fluid (32) are (partially) identical and homologous to rabbit uteroglobin, a small globular secretory protein present in the uterine and airway secretions (29).

Surfactant proteins (SP) form part of the pulmonary surfactant, a complex of lipids and proteins that lines the alveolar epithelial surface and stabilizes it during respiration. Knowledge of the composition, biosynthesis, and secretion of these phospholipids and proteins is extensive. To date, four types of surfactant proteins have been identified, namely, SP-A, SP-B, SP-C, and SP-D, which differ in molecular mass, composition, and physical properties. The surfactant proteins and lipids are definitely synthesized and secreted by alveolar type II cells and potentially by other bronchiolar secretory cell types. The major surfactant proteins, SP-A and SP-B, have also been localized to human bronchiolar epithelium using in situ hybridization (29,33). Immunocytochemical studies indicate that SP-A protein is restricted to the cuboidal secretory cells of the respiratory bronchioles and the bronchioles immediately proximal to them (Fig. 6, on page 21) (16). The bronchiolar localization of SP-B has not been further specified. In situ hybridization studies in rodents and rabbits suggest that SP-C synthesis is a property of parenchymal type II cells only. Although there are several putative functions of these proteins, especially for SP-A, the functional role of surfactant proteins is still largely unknown (31).

REFERENCES

1. Horsfield K, Gordon WI, Kemp W, Phillips S. Growth of the bronchial tree in man. *Thorax* 1987;42:383–388.
2. Weibel ER. *Morphometry of the human lung*. Berlin: Academic Press; 1963:1–151.
3. Hansen JE, Ampaya EP, Bryant GH, Navin JJ. Branching pattern of airways and air spaces of a single human terminal bronchiole. *J Appl Physiol* 1975;38:983–989.
4. Schreider JP, Raabe OG. Structure of the human respiratory acinus. *Am J Anat* 1981;162:221–232.
5. Berend N, Rynell AC, Ward HE. Structure of a human pulmonary acinus. *Thorax* 1991;46:117–121.
6. Haefeli-Bleuer B, Weibel ER. Morphometry of the human pulmonary acinus. *Anat Rec* 1988; 220:401–14.
7. McBride JT. Architecture of the tracheobronchial tree. In Parent RA, ed. *Treatise on pulmonary toxicology: comparative biology of the normal lung*. Boca Raton, FL: CRC Press; 1991: 49–61.
8. Mercer RR, Crapo JD. Architecture of the acinus. In Parent RA, ed. *Treatise on pulmonary toxicology: comparative biology of the normal lung*. Boca Raton, FL: CRC Press; 1991:109–119.
9. Boyden EA. The structure of the pulmonary acinus in a child of six years and eight months. *Am J Anat* 1972;132:275–300.
10. Plopper CG. Structural methods for studying bronchiolar epithelial cells. In: Gil J, ed. *Models of lung disease: microscopy and structural methods*. New York: Marcel Dekker; 1990:537–559.
11. Mariassy AT. Epithelial cells of trachea and bronchi. In: Parent RA, ed. *Treatise on pulmonary toxicology: comparative biology of the normal lung*. Boca Raton, FL: CRC Press; 1991:63–76.
12. Andre-Bougaran J, Pariente R, Legrand M, Cayrol E. Ultrastructure des grandes bronches normales. *Path Biol* 1975;23:629–38.
13. Basset F. Poirier J, Le Crom M, Turiaf J. Etude ultrastructural de l'epithelium bronchiolaire humain. *Z Zellvorschung* 1971;116:425–442.
14. Jarkovska D. Ultrastructure of the epithelium of the respiratory bronchioles in man. *Folia Morphol* 1970;18:352–358.
15. Plopper CG, Hill LH, Mariassy AT. Ultrastructure of the nonciliated bronchiolar epithelial (Clara) cell of mammalian lung. III: A study of man with comparison of 15 mammalian species. *Exp Lung Res* 1980;1:171–180.

16. ten Hav-Opbroek AAW, Otto-Verberne CJM, Dubbeldam JA, Dykman JH. The proximal border of the human respiratory unit, as shown by scanning and transmission electron microscopy and light microscopical cytochemistry. *Anat Rec* 1991;229:339–354.
17. Jeffery PK, Gaillard D, Moret S. Human airway secretory cells during development and in mature airway epithelium. *Eur Respir J* 1992;5:93–104.
18. Wolf RK. Mucociliary function. In: Parent RA, ed. *Comparative biology of the normal lung*. Boca Raton, FL: CRC Press; 1992:659–680.
19. Koren HS, Becker S. Antimicrobial defense mechanisms. In: Parent RA, ed. *Comparative biology of the normal lung*. Boca Raton, FL: CRC Press; 1992:747–769.
20. St. George JA, Wang S. Secretory glycoconjugates of trachea and bronchi. In: Parent RA, ed. *Treatise on pulmonary toxicology: comparative biology of the normal lung*. Boca Raton, FL: CRC Press; 1991:77–83.
21. Lamb D, Reid LM. Histochemical types of acidic glycoprotein produced by mucous cells of the tracheobronchial glands in man. *J Pathol* 1969;98:213–229.
22. Spicer SS, Chakrin L, Wardell J Jr, Kendrick W. Histochemistry of mucosubstances in the canine and human respiratory tract. *Lab Invest* 1971; 25:483–490.
23. Mariassy AT, McCray MN, Lauredo IT, Abraham WM, Wanner A. Lectin-detectable effects of localized pneumonia on airway mucous cell populations: role of cyclooxygenase metabolites. *Exp Lung Res* 1989;15:113–137.
24. St. George JA, Cranz DL, Zicker S, Etchison JR, Dungworth DL, Plopper CG. An immunohistochemical characterization of rhesus monkey respiratory secretions using monoclonal antibodies. *Am Rev Respir Dis* 1985;132:556–563.
25. Lin H, St. George JA, Plopper CG, Carlson DM, Wu R. An ELISA method for quantitation of tracheal mucins from humans and nonhuman primates. *Am Rev Respir Dis* 1988;
26. Kramps JA, Franken C. Low-molecular-weight protease inhibitor of the respiratory tract. *Surv Immunol Res* 1982;1:30–36.
27. Willems LNA, Kramps JA, Stijnen T, Sterk PJ, Weening JJ, Dijkman JH. Antileukorprotease-containing bronchiolar cells. *Am Rev Respir Dis* 1989;139(5):1244–1250.
28. Singh G, Singh J, Katyal SL, et al. Identification, cellular localization, isolation and characterization of human Clara cell specific 10 kDa protein. *J Histochem Cytochem* 1988;36:73–80.
29. Singh G, Katyal SK. Secretory proteins of Clara cells and type II cells. In: Parent RA, ed. *Comparative biology of the normal lung*. Boca Raton, FL: CRC Press; 1992:93–108.
30. Broers J, Jensen S, Travis W, et al. Expression of surfactant associated protein-A and Clara cell 10 kilodalton mRNA in neoplastic and non-neoplastic human lung tissue as detected by in situ hydribidation. *Lab Invest* 1992;66:337–346.
31. Singh G, Katyal SL, Brown WE, Phillips S, Kennedy AL, Anthony J. Amino-acid and cDNA nucleotide sequences of human Clara cell 10 kDa protein. *Biochim Biophys Acta* 1988;950: 329–337.
32. Andersson O, Nordlung-Moller L, Bronnegard M, Sireza F, Ripe E, Lund J. Purification and level of expression in bronchoalveolar lavage of a human polychlorinated biphenyl (PCB)-binding protein: evidence for a structural and functional kinship to the multihormonally regulated protein uteroglobin. *Am J Respir Cell Mol Biol* 1991;5:6–12.
33. Phelps DS, Floros J. Localization of surfactant protein synthesis in human lung by in situ hybridization. *Am Rev Respir Dis* 1988;137:939–942.
34. Horsfield K, Cumming G. Morphology of the bronchial tree in man. *J Appl Physiol* 1968; 24:373–383.
35. Yeh HC, Schum GM. Models of human lung airways and their application to inhaled particle deposition. *Bull Math Biol* 1980;42:461–480.

Diseases of the Bronchioles, edited by
Gary R. Epler. Raven Press, Ltd.,
New York © 1994.

3

Chest Radiographic Findings of the Healthy and Diseased Bronchioles

Theresa C. McLoud

Associate Professor of Radiology, Harvard Medical School, Boston, MA, and Chief of Thoracic Radiology, Massachusetts General Hospital, Boston, MA.

A bronchiole may be defined as an airway that does not contain cartilage in its wall. A bronchiole may be purely conducting (up to and including the terminal bronchiole) or transitory (the respiratory bronchioles that carry out both conduction and gas exchange). Imaging of the bronchioles and diseases related to the bronchioles has been quite limited because the bronchioles are radiologically invisible. Therefore, most of the radiologic manifestations of bronchiolar disease depend on indirect effects of airway obstruction, such as hyperinflation and air trapping. When pathologic changes associated with small airway disease extend into the pulmonary interstitium (respiratory bronchiolitis, mineral dust bronchiolitis) or into the alveoli (bronchiolitis obliterans organizing pneumonia, or BOOP), they may produce roentgenographically visible opacities. Both high-resolution computed tomography and ultrafast computed tomography, which permits functional imaging of the lung during respiration, hold promise for better definition and evaluation of bronchiolar disease. This chapter, however, deals with standard imaging techniques in the evaluation of bronchiolar diseases.

STANDARD RADIOGRAPHIC TECHNIQUES

The Standard Chest Roentgenogram

The bronchioles are radiographically invisible on the standard chest roentgenogram. In patients with bronchiolar disease, the radiographic findings are usually secondary to small airways obstruction and include hyperinflation, which may either be diffuse or focal, and air trapping. Roentgenographic signs of overinflation include changes in the diaphragm, the retrosternal space, and the cardiac silhouette (1) (Fig. 1). In the presence of overinflation, the diaphragm is depressed, usually below the level of the seventh rib anteriorly and the eleventh interspace or twelfth rib posteriorly (1). The normal "dome" configuration is flattened, particularly in the lateral view. The low position of the diaphragm increases the angle of the costophrenic sinuses so that they approach 90°. Costophrenic muscle slips, extending from the diaphragm to the posterior and posterolateral ribs, may be identified. The best criterion for the determination of overinflation

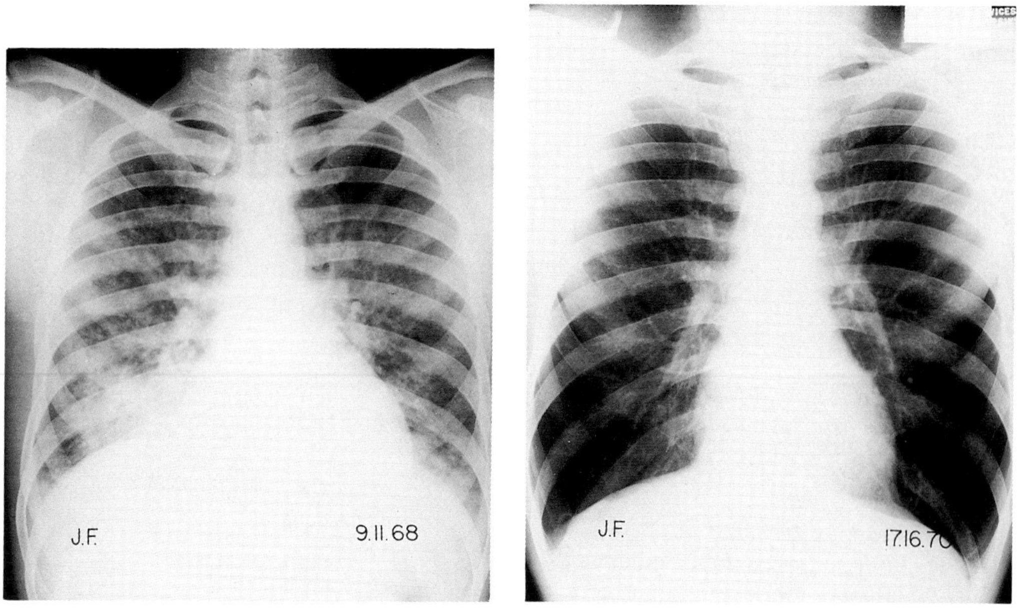

A B

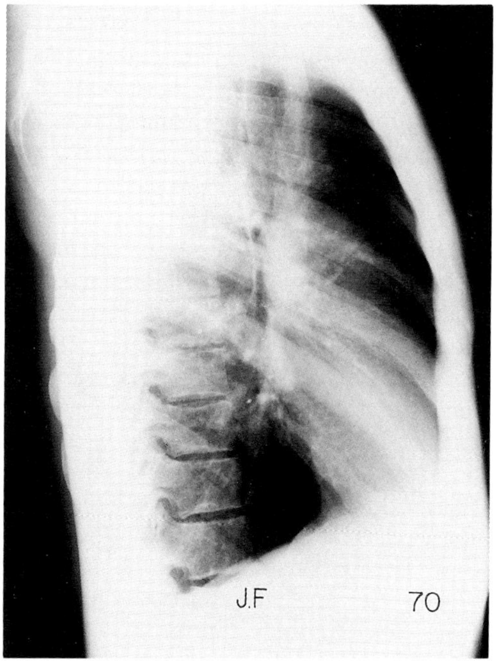

C

FIG. 1. Bronchiolitis obliterans secondary to noxious gas inhalation. A 25-year-old man sustained an intense exposure to sulfur dioxide. **A,** An initial chest radiograph showed nonspecific alveolar or "ground glass" opacities diffusely distributed throughout the lungs. The findings are consistent with noncardiogenic edema secondary to acute alveolar injury. **B,** Posteroanterior and **C,** lateral chest radiographs obtained 10 months after recovery from the initial illness. There is evidence of severe overinflation with flattening of the diaphragm and increase in the retrosternal clear space. Pulmonary function tests showed evidence of severe airflow obstruction. (Reprinted with permission from ref. 43.)

is a measurement of the sum of the height of each diaphragmatic dome measured in the posterior-anterior projection from a line extending from the costophrenic to the costovertebral angle and in the lateral projection from the posterior to the anterior costophrenic sulcus (2). Increase in the depth of the retrosternal air space, that is, the space separating the sternum from the anterior cardiovascular structures, is also a sign of overinflation. Changes in the size and contour of the thoracic cage are variable, and neither thoracic kyphosis nor anterior bowing of the sternum is a reliable sign of overinflation (3). When diaphragmatic depression occurs as a result of overinflation, the heart tends to be elongated, narrow, and central in position (1).

Local overinflation of a segment or a lobe may be a roentgenographic sign of focal bronchiolar disease. Such areas usually display several signs of abnormality. One sign is decrease in lung density, which is due both to an excess of air and to a decrease in blood flow secondary to hypoxic vasoconstriction. The volume of the affected lung may be normal, less than normal, or greater than normal depending on the disease process. If blood flow is reduced, the vessel caliber will be decreased (1) (Fig. 2).

A

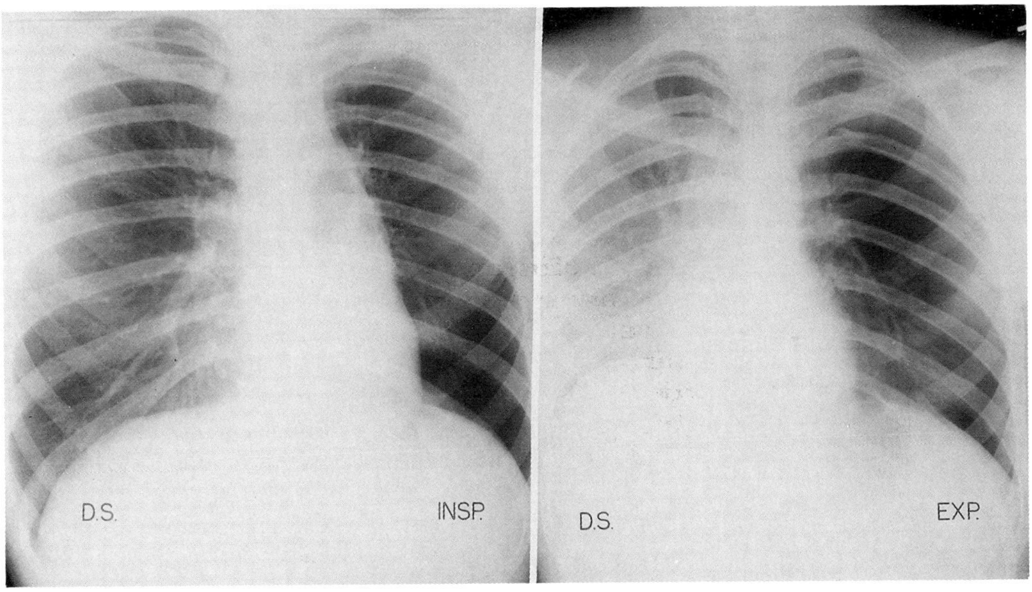

B

C

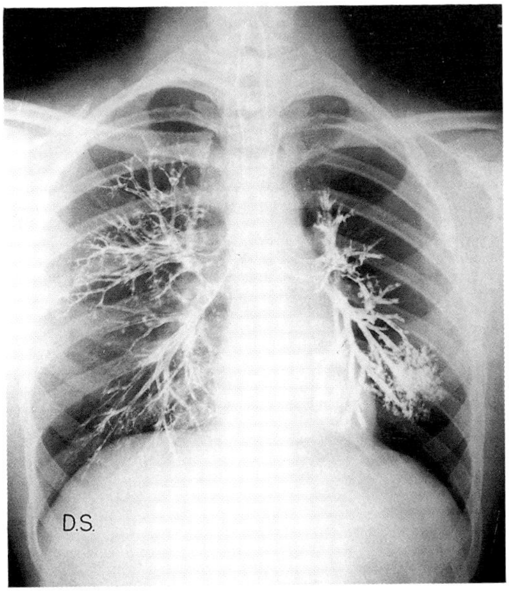

FIG. 2. Swyer-James syndrome. A 17-year-old male student was found to have a left hyperlucent lung on a routine chest radiograph obtained when he entered a university. At the age of 9 he had been hospitalized for 2 weeks for a bronchopneumonia of the left lung that was severe enough to necessitate the use of an oxygen tent. He recovered within 2 weeks. **A,** Inspiratory radiograph displays a small left lung with diminished vascularity and shift of the mediastinum toward that side. **B,** An expiratory film shows striking air trapping on the left and a swing of the mediastinum to the opposite side. **C,** A bronchogram shows normal filling of the largest airways on both sides and normal distal arborization on the right. On the left there is abrupt termination of the contrast material at the level of the smaller bronchi, giving a "pruned tree" appearance. Bronchoscopy was not performed because the bronchogram demonstrated the patency of the major bronchi. (Reprinted with permission from ref. 43.)

Radiographic features of bronchiolitis are variable. In a study of 52 patients with bronchiolitis of varied etiology, Gosink and her associates (4) described three main patterns of disease: (a) nodular opacities (18 patients), (b) alveolar opacities (39 patients), and (c) hyperinflation (2 patients); in several patients a combination of these patterns was shown. The nodules varied in size and included those less than or greater than 5 mm. The patient population in this study most likely contained a large number of patients who would now be classified as having BOOP. This disease is characterized by patchy areas of consolidation and may also have rounded opacities (4,5).

The Expiration Chest Radiograph and Fluoroscopy

It is possible with standard imaging to elicit dynamic signs of air trapping that may be seen with bronchiolar diseases. These changes occur during respiration. They can readily be seen on fluoroscopy, although many of the signs are seen equally clearly on radiographs exposed during full inspiration and maximal expiration (1). In regard to the assessment of diffuse air trapping, measurement of diaphragmatic excursion is considered a reliable sign. The normal diaphragmatic excursion is in the range of 3 to 4 cm; the range in diffuse air trapping may be no more than 1 to 2 cm (6).

When focal air trapping associated with bronchiolitis is present, air is trapped within the affected lung parenchyma during expiration and the volume changes little, whereas the remainder of the lung deflates normally (1) (Fig. 2). Radiographic signs depend on both the volume and the anatomic location of the affected lung; density during expiration of the affected area is not altered significantly, but contrast between the affected area and the normally deflated lung is maximally accentuated at residual volume (1). Contiguous structures are displaced away from the affected lobe or lung during expiration: the mediastinum shifts to its contralateral side and elevation of the hemidiaphragm is restricted (1). Such dynamic changes are particularly impressive fluoroscopically: the mediastinum may be seen to swing like a pendulum away from the lesion during expiration and back to the midline during inspiration.

In the assessment of local and general air trapping, Greenspan and his colleagues (7) used a 1-second forced expiratory volume (FEV_1) radiograph in addition to films exposed at total lung capacity and residual volume: in over 200 subjects studied, local air trapping was identified in 16, 12 of whom had a normal spirogram; in 9 patients air trapping was detectable only on the FEV_1 roentgenogram. FEV_1 radiography does not appear to be a clinically useful tool and has largely been abandoned.

Radiographic signs of diffuse or focal hyperinflation and air trapping may be very subtle on standard radiographs. Computed tomography, particularly ultrafast CT scanning and high-resolution computed tomography, offer an increased sensitivity in the detection of these phenomena. Computed tomography and its applications in bronchiolar disease are discussed in Chapter 4.

Bronchography

Bronchography has become an obsolete procedure. Its primary application in recent years has been in the diagnosis and determination of extent of bronchiectasis. This procedure has been replaced by computed tomography. However, it is important to know that abnormalities due to bronchiolar disease may be identified by bronchography. Bronchiolar diseases may be associated with bronchiectasis (Fig. 3). In bronchiolar disease, particularly bronchiolitis obliterans, the bronchi typically terminate in squared or tapered endings and filling of peripheral bronchiolar radicals is notably absent.

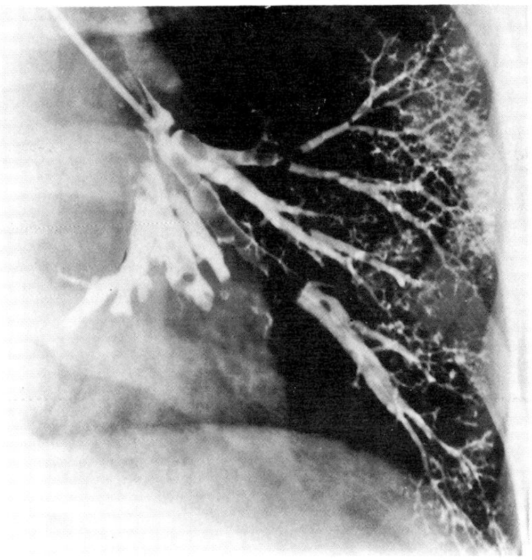

FIG. 3. Bronchiolitis obliterans associated with bronchiectasis. Left bronchogram shows bronchiectasis involving some of the basal segments of the left lower lobe. Note the abrupt termination of dilated bronchi with squared endings. There is lack of alveolar and peripheral bronchiolar filling.

BRONCHIOLAR DISEASES

Airway Disorders

Acute Infectious Bronchiolitis in Children

Acute infectious bronchiolitis results from diffuse inflammation of the small airways in children usually under the age of 3 years. It is usually secondary to viral infection, most commonly due to respiratory syncytial virus (RSV). The most common symptoms are wheezing, tachypnea, and occasionally cough. The radiographic findings typically consist of diffuse hyperinflation of the lungs (Fig. 4). This is frequently the only abnormality (8). Diffuse air trapping can be demonstrated with expiration films on fluoroscopy. Fine nodular opacities in the range of 1 to 2 mm may occasionally occur, and increased linear opacities may be identified in the perihilar areas (9,10). Pathologic correlation shows that the latter patterns are due to peribronchiolitis and to small focal areas of atelectasis and pneumonitis (1,10, 11). Usually the disease completely resolves, but in occasional cases bronchiolitis obliterans may occur as a late sequela.

Diffuse Panbronchiolitis

Diffuse panbronchiolitis is a disease of unknown etiology characterized by chronic inflammation exclusively located in the region of the respiratory bronchioles. Secondary obstructive effects occur. It has been recognized almost exclusively in Japan (12). The disease is typically diffusely disseminated throughout the lungs bilaterally, particularly in the lower lobes. The most typical radiographic pattern on standard chest radiography is that of a disseminated nodular pattern with lower zone predominance (12) (Fig. 5). Occasionally patients may show findings of lung hyperinflation in the early phase of the disease (12).

Bronchiolitis Obliterans

Bronchiolitis obliterans was first described by Lange in 1901 (13). Although it is a relatively rare disease, it has recently become the subject of renewed interest. Histologically, bronchiolitis obliterans is defined by (a) the presence of granulation tissue plugs within the lumina of small airways and occasionally alveolar ducts, and (b) the destruction of small airways with obliterative scarring (4,14). If granulation tissue within the small airways extends into the alveoli, the disease is called bronchiolar obliterans organizing pneumonia (BOOP).

The causes of bronchiolitis obliterans vary and include exposure to toxic fumes, infections, drugs, and connective tissue diseases. In addition to these major or widespread reactions, bronchiolitis obliterans may be seen distal to obstruction or bronchiectasis or as a secondary change in such

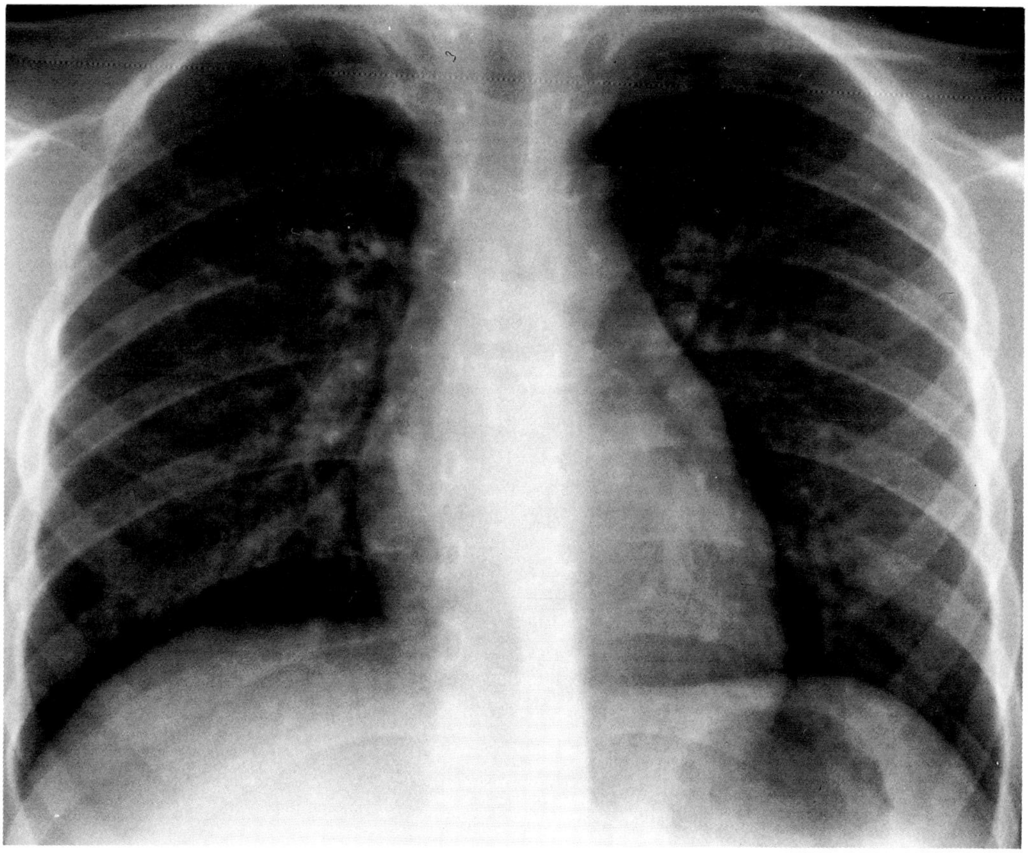

A

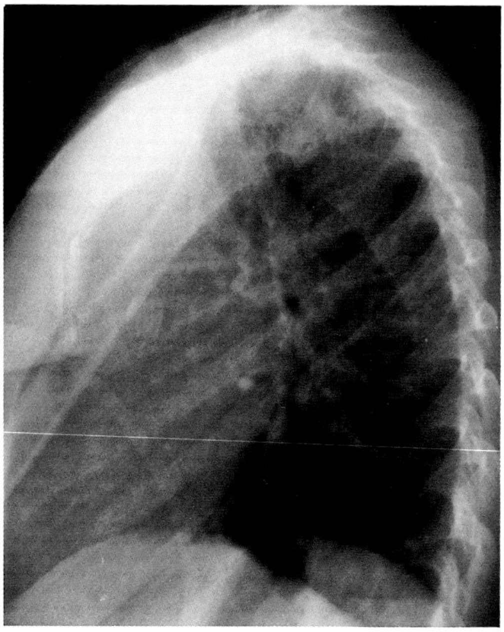

B

FIG. 4. Acute infectious bronchiolitis in a 2-year-old child. **A and B,** There is evidence of overinflation with increased anterior-posterior diameter on the lateral view. Peribronchial thickening and increased linear opacities can be identified in the perihilar areas.

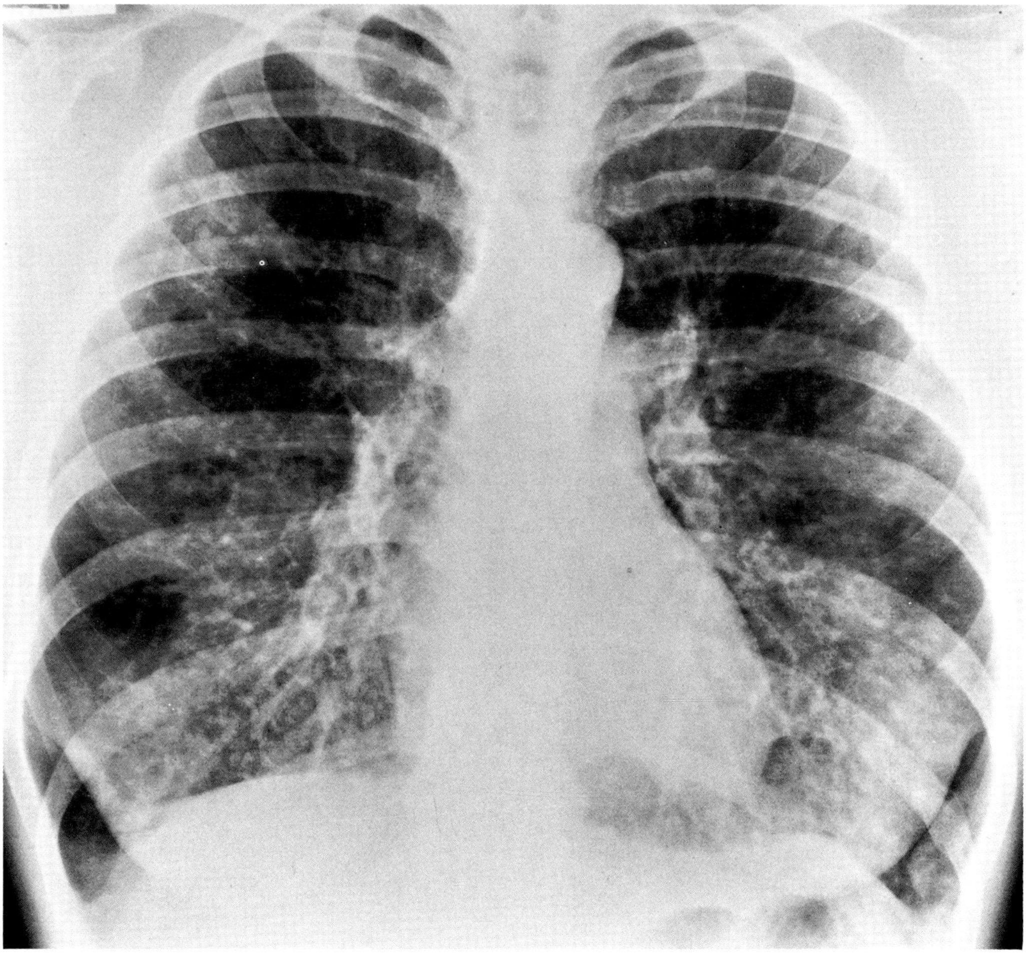

FIG. 5. A 45-year-old Japanese woman with proven panbronchiolitis. Radiographic abnormalities predominate in the lower lung zones. Bronchial wall thickening and nodular opacities can be identified.

diverse lesions as eosinophilic pneumonia, hypersensitivity pneumonitis, and malignant neoplasms. Epler and Colby (14) proposed the following clinical classification of bronchiolitis obliterans: (a) toxic fume bronchiolitis obliterans, (b) postinfectious bronchiolitis obliterans, (c) bronchiolitis obliterans associated with connective tissue disease and organ transplantation, and (d) localized lesion with bronchiolitis obliterans. This classification will serve as a framework for the present review of the radiographic features of bronchiolitis obliterans.

Toxic Fume Bronchiolitis Obliterans

Exposure to toxic fumes of such gases as sulfur dioxide, ammonia, chlorine, phosgene, oxides of nitrogen, and ozone may produce both acute and chronic damage to the airways and lung parenchyma. The acute or immediate reaction consists of acute alveolar injury and severe fibrinous bronchiolitis and peribronchiolitis, sometimes with denuding of the epithelium of the airways (1). The chest radiograph obtained at this stage reveals the nonspecific changes seen in the adult respiratory distress syndrome (ARDS), which consist of diffuse alveolar or "ground glass" opacities uniformly distributed throughout the lungs (Fig. 1). The heart size is usually normal, and pleural effusions are absent (1,15). If recovery from this phase of the disease occurs it is sometimes followed 1 to 3 weeks later by the development of irreversible airflow obstruction. Histologically, a relatively pure bronchiolitis obliterans can be identified. In mild cases the chest radiograph may appear normal, whereas in severe cases hyperinflation can be identified (15,16) (Fig. 1). Alternatively, this stage may be characterized radiographically by multiple discrete nodular opacities of various sizes distributed uniformly throughout both lungs (1,17,18).

Postinfectious Bronchiolitis Obliterans

Postinfectious bronchiolitis obliterans is usually seen in children but may occur in young adults after mycoplasma infection and in older adults after viral infection (19,20). Histologic findings are on a spectrum from relatively pure bronchiolitis obliterans, which correlates clinically with obstructive disease (14,19,20), to a lesion with more extensive organizing pneumonia and sometimes interstitial scarring (4,14,19). The radiographic pattern in children has been described above. In adults, the chest radiograph either is normal (14,21) or demonstrates a diffuse nodular or reticulonodular pattern (4,14). The nodular pattern appears to correlate with histologic evidence of pure bronchiolitis obliterans, while the reticulonodular pattern reflects additional interstitial fibrosis and scarring (4). Diffuse hyperinflation is rare.

Swyer-James syndrome (22) is an interesting clinical entity that appears to be the result of a localized or unilateral acute viral bronchiolitis in infancy or in early childhood (23,24). It is recognized by an abnormal chest radiograph that demonstrates a lobar or unilateral hyperlucent lung (Fig. 2). Additional radiologic features of the abnormal hyperlucent lung include normal or slightly reduced lung volume on inspiration, severe airway obstruction during expiration, greatly reduced circulation (oligemia), and a diminutive hilus (1,23). The volume of the affected lung in the adult is related to the age at which bronchiolar damage occurred (1). Radiographically Swyer-James syndrome must be distinguished from two entities: (a) an endobronchial lesion incompletely obstructing the lumen of a main or lobar bronchus, and (b) pulmonary artery agenesis. The former can be diagnosed readily by bronchoscopy, and in the latter expiratory air trapping does not occur. Pulmonary arteriography or computed tomography performed after injection of contrast media can be useful in differentiating the two entities.

Bronchiolitis Obliterans Associated with Connective Tissue Disease and Organ Transplantation

Bronchiolitis obliterans with or without organizing pneumonia is one of a number of diverse pulmonary lesions seen in the connective tissue disorders both as a de novo process (25,26,27) and as an apparent drug reaction (27,28,29). Bronchiolitis obliterans may be seen with any of the connective tissue disorders, but most cases have been reported in patients with rheumatoid arthritis (28) and after penicillamine treatment (27,28). The chest radiograph in bronchiolitis obliterans associated with connective tissue disease or penicillamine treatment is normal or occasionally shows hyperinflated lungs (Fig. 6). The histologic finding in such cases is that of a pure bronchiolitis obliterans.

Bronchiolitis obliterans has recently been reported as a complication of bone marrow (30,31) and heart–lung transplantation (32). Most of the cases described following allogenic bone marrow transplantation have developed in patients with some degree of

A
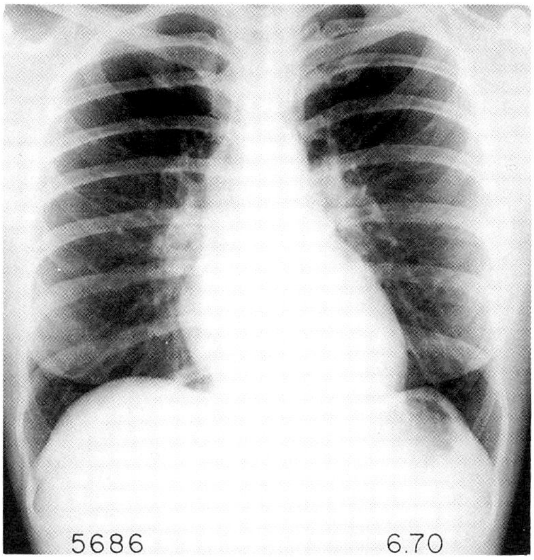

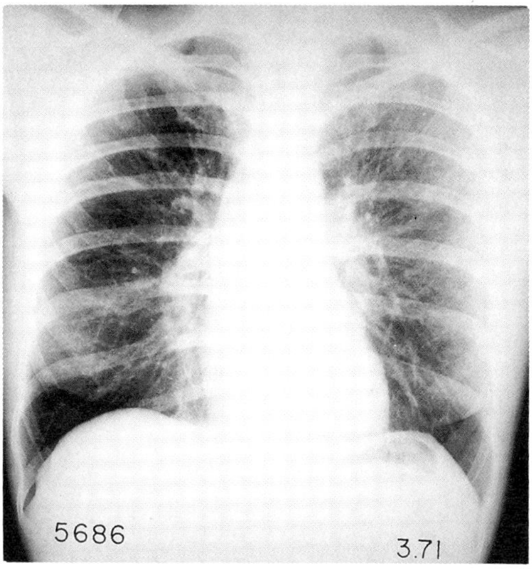

B

C
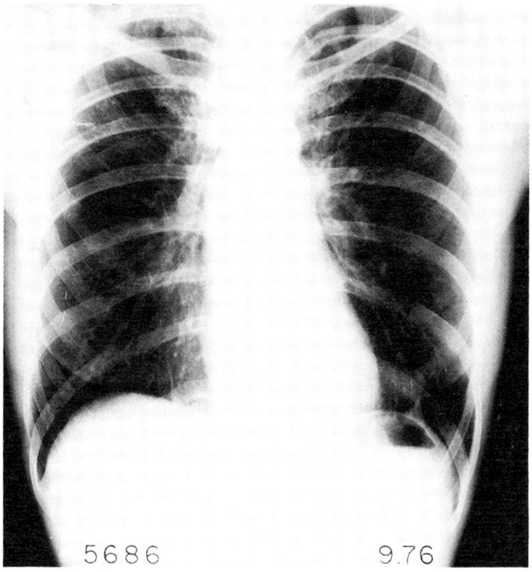

FIG. 6. Bronchiolitis obliterans associated with penicillamine treatment. A 43-year-old woman with known scleroderma had been treated with penicillamine for 8 months. She was admitted after 3 weeks of dyspnea and nonproductive cough. Pulmonary function tests showed evidence of severe airflow obstruction. A specimen obtained by open lung biopsy revealed bronchiolitis obliterans. **A,** Chest radiograph obtained prior to penicillamine treatment is normal. **B,** Another study obtained at the time of admission shows a few ill-defined nodules in the upper lobes. **C,** Despite withdrawal of penicillamine therapy, a chest radiograph obtained 5 years later shows progression of bronchiolitis obliterans with development of moderate hyperinflation. (Reprinted with permission from ref. 43.)

acute or chronic graft-versus-host disease. Predictably the chest radiograph is normal or the lungs appear hyperinflated. Bronchiolitis obliterans is a late complication of heart–lung and isolated lung transplantation. It is thought to represent primarily a form of chronic rejection (33,34). Morrish and others (35) reported the radiographic findings in 4 patients with bronchiolitis obliterans following single and double lung transplantations. These included slight to moderate decrease in the size of peripheral vessels in the lung parenchyma as well as slight to moderate volume loss and subsegmental atelectasis in the affected lung. In 2 of the 4 cases new thin linear irregular areas of increased opacity were also identified. High-resolution CT has been reported to show additional findings. Burke and colleagues (32) also described the chest radiographic findings in 5 of 14 long-term survivors of heart–lung transplantation. The findings were somewhat different and consisted of coarse nodular or reticulonodular opacities associated with peribronchial thickening.

Localized Lesion with Bronchiolitis Obliterans

Bronchiolitis obliterans may be associated with localized discrete radiographic opacities or nodules (4). Histologically such lesions are usually referred to as *focal organizing pneumonia*. They are frequently incidental radiographic findings in asymptomatic patients in whom lung biopsy specimens are obtained to exclude carcinoma. Detailed descriptions of the radiographic features are rare, but the appearances are usually that of an irregular sublobar area of air space consolidation or an irregular nodule (4) (Fig. 7). These lesions are thought to be the residue of previous pneumonias. However, a specific cause may not be demonstrated in individual cases.

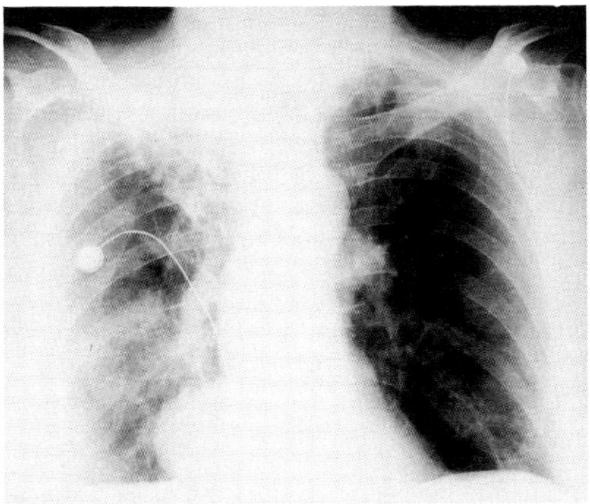

FIG. 7. Localized lesion with bronchiolitis obliterans. A 67-year-old man with a history of tuberculosis complained of a cough with occasional hemoptysis of 3 months' duration. A portable chest radiograph demonstrates fibrocalcific scarring in the right upper lobe secondary to previous tuberculosis. There is also a large mass in the right cardiophrenic angle. The lesion was removed at thoracotomy, and histologic examination showed a focal fibrotic organizing lesion with bronchiolitis obliterans. (Reprinted with permission from ref. 43.)

Interstitial Diseases

Respiratory Bronchiolitis

Respiratory bronchiolitis is a mild inflammatory reaction characterized by a distinct pathologic lesion in cigarette smokers. The lesion is characterized histologically by the accumulation of pigmented macrophages within respiratory bronchioles and adjacent air spaces associated with mild thickening of the peribronchiolar interstitium (36). Respiratory bronchiolitis may be associated with mild abnormalities of lung function that occur in cigarette smokers; however, it is usually not a cause of clinically significant disease (37). Pulmonary function tests may show evidence of restriction, although impaired diffusion is usually present in all patients (38). Severe obstruction with hyperinflation is rare (38).

The radiographic findings consist of a pattern usually associated with infiltrative lung disease. Reticular or reticulonodular opacities are the most frequent finding and were present in two-thirds of cases reported by Yousem and colleagues (38). The radiographic appearance may be identical to that of desquamative interstitial pneumonitis, although on occasion patients with desquamative interstitial pneumonia may show more "ground glass" or alveolar opacities.

Bronchiolitis Obliterans Organizing Pneumonia

BOOP is a disease entity proposed by Epler et al. (5) in 1985 to describe a group of 50 patients in whom there was a subacute illness characterized by cough, sometimes dyspnea, crackles in the lungs, and a restrictive defect with reduced diffusing capacity on pulmonary function testing. Lung biopsies from these patients showed involvement of distal airways, alveolar ducts, and alveoli by granulation tissue of uniform age. The condition was generally responsive to steroids. Although BOOP may be seen in association with connective tissue diseases such as rheumatoid arthritis as well as in association with drugs and HIV infection, the majority of cases remain idiopathic. The term *cryptogenic organizing pneumonia* has been used to describe the entity in the British literature (39). In the original series that we reported (5) the standard radiographic findings fell into one of three groups. The vast majority of patients (69%) had bilateral patchy "ground glass" or alveolar opacities (Fig. 8). There was no zonal or lobar predominance. These sometimes began as focal lesions and progressed bilaterally over time. A pattern more consistent with interstitial or infiltrative lung disease was seen in 20% of the subjects and usually consisted of small linear or nodular opacities (Fig. 9). Cavities, effusions, and hyperinflation were rare. The severity of the radiographic abnormalities correlated significantly with the extent of histologic disease in respiratory bronchioles and alveolar ducts, but not in the larger terminal bronchioles. However, Chandler and others (40), in a review of 24 patients with BOOP, found only 50% had alveolar opacities and 44% had predominantly interstitial changes. The consolidation may be peripheral in nature (41). However, the peripheral distribution may be much more easily recognized on computed tomography than on standard films (42).

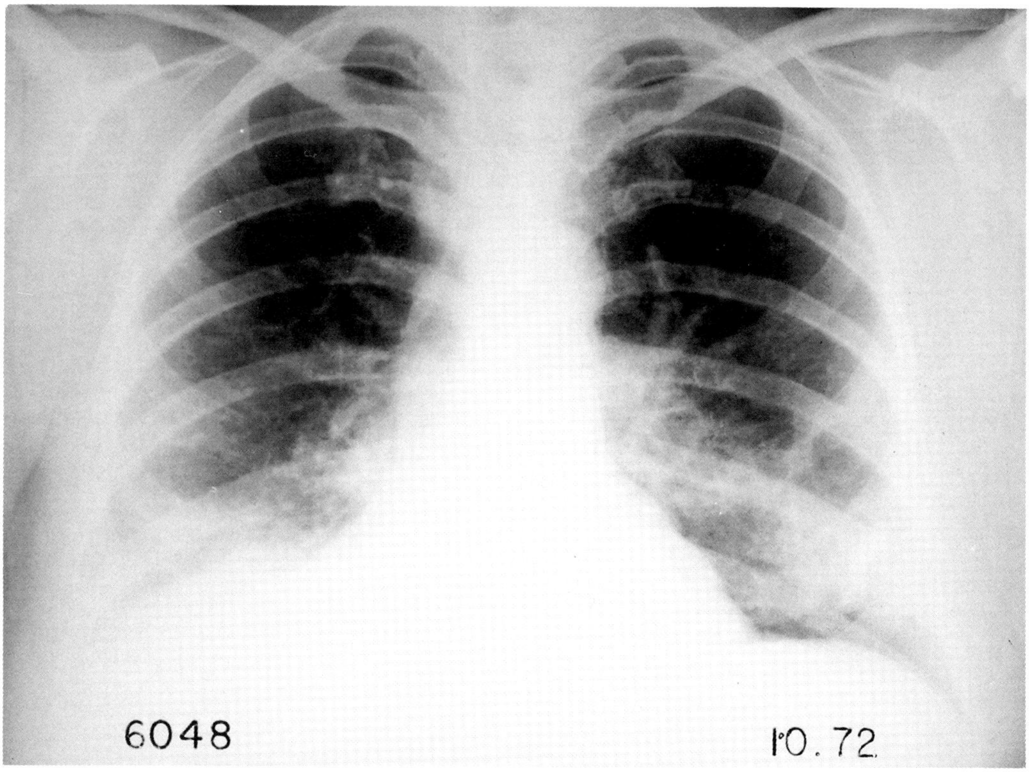

FIG. 8. BOOP. A 46-year-old woman had a fever and had experienced dyspnea during exertion for several months. Pulmonary function tests showed a restrictive pattern with no evidence of airflow obstruction. Specimen obtained at open lung biopsy revealed BOOP. The chest radiograph demonstrates bilateral basal patchy "ground glass" or alveolar opacities.

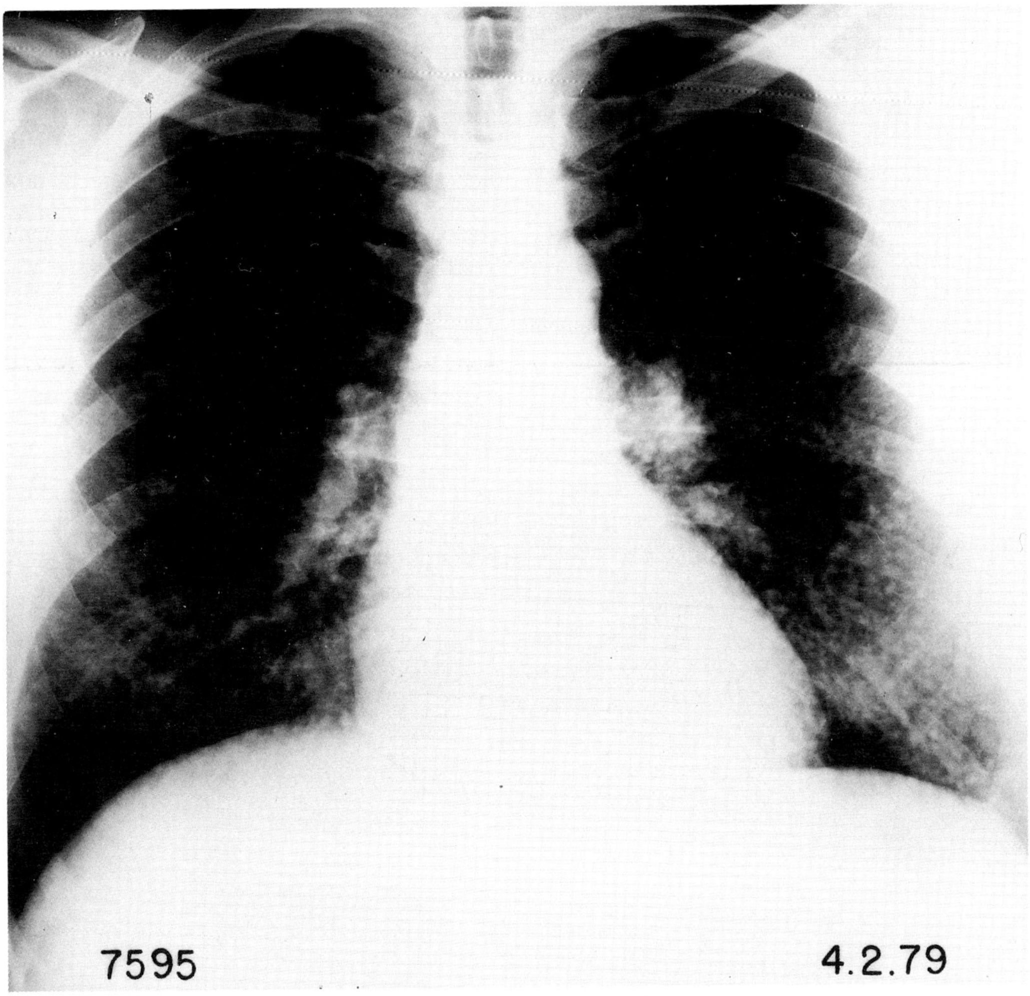

FIG. 9. BOOP. A 45-year-old man had a mild upper respiratory infection, followed by a high fever and respiratory distress. He was treated with antibiotics with no response. A specimen obtained at open lung biopsy showed BOOP. The chest radiograph reveals a diffuse pattern of small nodular opacities more marked in the lower lung zones. (Reprinted with permission from ref. 43.)

Comparisons of the radiology of BOOP and idiopathic pulmonary fibrosis have been made by Müller et al. (42) and Chandler et al. (40). These authors, as well as Epler and colleagues (5), conclude that the radiographic features are sufficiently different to allow differentiation of the two conditions in most cases on the basis of the radiographs alone. In BOOP, the nodular and linear opacities correspond to bronchiolar and peribronchiolar inflammation whereas the alveolar or "ground glass" opacities correspond to organizing pneumonia. More recently we have seen a number of patients who have presented with fairly diffuse uniform alveolar disease (Fig. 10). This pattern is frequently associated with extremely low lung volumes, reflecting the restrictive nature of the process. The majority of patients with this disorder respond to corticosteroid therapy. Clinical improvement is seen within several days, and the response may be dramatic. As many as one-third of the patients may experience a relapse with return of radiographic opacities when corticosteroid therapy is discontinued (5).

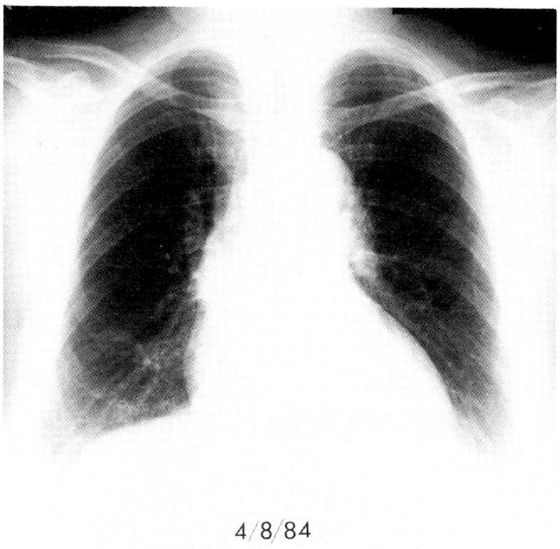

A

FIG. 10. BOOP. A 65-year-old woman had been treated intermittently with prednisone for polymyalgia rheumatica. Two months before admission, corticosteroid administration was gradually decreased and then discontinued. One month later, she developed a nonproductive cough and exertional dyspnea. Pulmonary function tests revealed marked restriction. A specimen obtained by open lung biopsy revealed the diagnosis of BOOP. **A,** In this chest radiograph obtained several months prior to admission, the lungs are normal. **B,** Chest radiograph obtained at admission shows evidence of extensive patchy "ground glass" opacities in both upper and middle lung zones. **C,** Less than a week after intensive corticosteroid therapy, dramatic improvement is noted. (Reprinted with permission from ref. 43.)

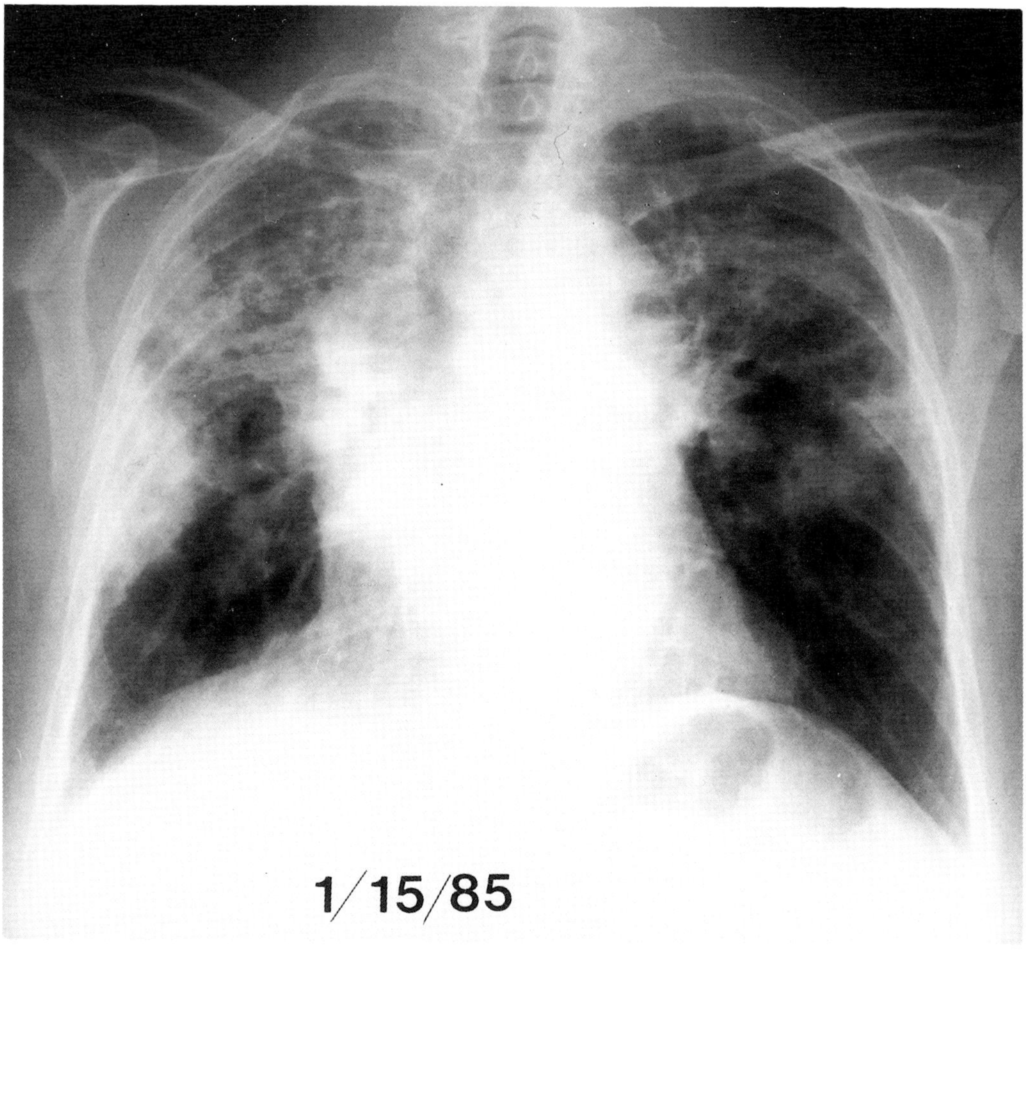

B

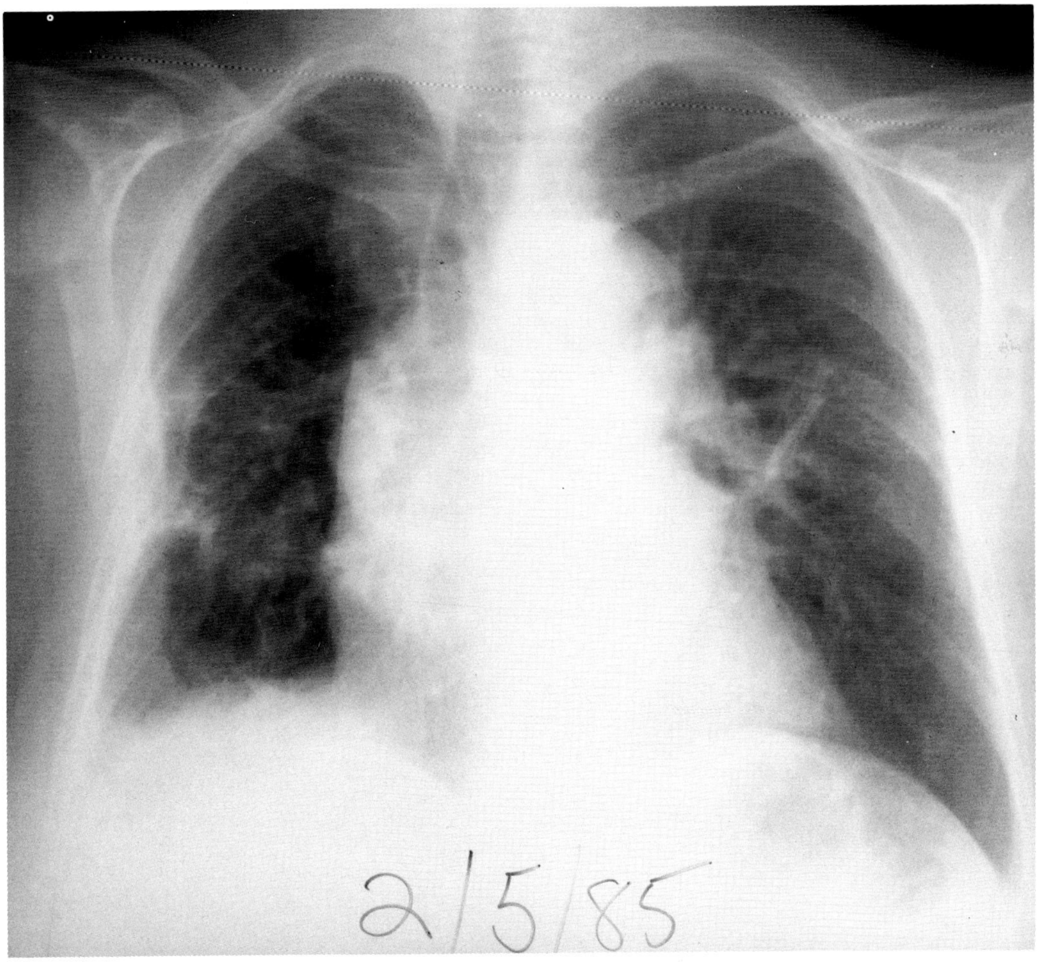

C

FIG. 10. Continued. **C,** Less than a week after intensive corticosteroid therapy, dramatic improvement is noted. (Reprinted with permission from ref. 43.)

CONCLUSION

There is a wide spectrum of radiographic changes in patients with bronchiolar diseases. Frequently the chest radiographs may be normal or show hyperinflation. When inflammatory changes occur around peripheral bronchioles, a pattern suggestive of infiltrative or interstitial lung disease may occur with a typical nodular or reticulonodular pattern. In patients with BOOP, usually the predominant radiographic feature is that of the extensive pneumonia. This entity can often be readily recognized or at least distinguished from infiltrative lung diseases such as idiopathic pulmonary fibrosis by the patchy or diffuse alveolar opacities. Computed tomography, particularly high-resolution computed tomography, has improved imaging of bronchiolar diseases.

REFERENCES

1. Fraser RG, Paré JA, Paré PD, Fraser RS. *Diagnosis of diseases of the chest.* Philadelphia: WB Saunders; 1990.
2. Thomson KR, Eyssen GE, Fraser RG. Discrimination of normal and overinflated lungs and prediction of total lung capacity based on chest film measurements. *Radiology* 1976;119:721–726.

3. Christie RV. Emphysema of the lungs. *Br Med J* 1944;1:105–110.
4. Gosink BB, Friedman PJ, Liebow AA. Bronchitis obliterans: roentgenographic-pathologic correlation. *AJR* 1973;117:816–832.
5. Epler GR, Colby TV, McLoud TC, et al. Bronchiolitis obliterans organizing pneumonia. *N Engl J Med* 1985;312:152–158.
6. Clark TJH. Inspiratory obstruction. *Br Med J* 1970;3:682–686.
7. Greenspan RH, Sagel S, McMahon J, et al. Timed expiratory chest films in the detection of air trapping. *Invest Radiol* 1973;8:264.
8. Koch DA. Roentgenologic consideration of capillary bronchiolitis. *AJR* 1959;82:433–438.
9. Engel S. Bronchiolitis. *Br J Dis Chest* 1959; 53:125–129.
10. Sawazaki H, Watabe S, Onoki S, et al. Two cases of bronchiolitis obliterans. *Jpn J Chest Dis* 1962;21:635–637.
11. Felson B, Felson H. Acute diffuse pneumonia of asthmatics. *AJR* 1955;74:235–240.
12. Homma H, Yamanaka A, Tanimoto S, et al. Diffuse panbronchiolitis: a disease of the transitional zone of the lung. *Chest* 1983;83:63–69.
13. Lange W. Uber eine eigenthumliche: Erkrankung der kleinen bronchien und bronchiolen. *Dtsh Arch Klin Med* 1901;70:342–364.
14. Epler GR, Colby TV. The spectrum of bronchiolitis obliterans. *Chest* 1983;83:161–162.
15. Charan NB, Meyers CG, Lakshimorayan S, et al. Pulmonary injuries associated with acute sulfur dioxide inhalation. *Am Rev Respir Dis* 1979; 119:555–560.
16. Yockey CC, Eden BM, Byrd RB. The McConnell missile accident: clinical spectrum of nitrogen dioxide exposure. *JAMA* 1980;244:1221–1223.
17. Cornelius EA, Betlach EH. Silo-filler's disease. *Radiology* 1960;74:232–235.
18. Lowry T, Schuman LM. "Silo-filler's disease": a syndrome caused by nitrogen dioxide. *JAMA* 1956;162:153–158.
19. Laraya-Cuasay LR, DeForest A, Huff D, Lischner H, Huang NN. Chronic pulmonary complications of early influenza virus infection in children. *Am Rev Respir Dis* 1977;116:617–625.
20. Nikke P, Meretoja O, Valtonen V, et al. Severe bronchiolitis probably caused by varicella-zoster virus. *Crit Care Med* 1982;10:344–346.
21. Seggev JS, Mason UG III, Worthen S, et al. Bronchiolitis obliterans: report of three cases with detailed physiologic studies. *Chest* 1983; 83:169–174.
22. Swyer PR, James GCW. A case of unilateral pulmonary emphysema. *Thorax* 1953;8:133–143.
23. MacLeod WM. Abnormal transradiancy of one lung. *Thorax* 1962;9:147–152.
24. Reid L, Simon G. Unilateral lung transradiancy. *Thorax* 1962;17:230–239.
25. Herzog CA, Miller RR, Hoidal JR. Bronchiolitis and rheumatoid arthritis. *Am Rev Respir Dis* 1979;119:555–560.
26. Schwartz MI, Matthay RA, Sahn SA, et al. Interstitial lung disease in polymyositis and dermatomyositis: an analysis of six cases and review of the literature. *Medicine* 1976;55:89–104.
27. Epler GR, Snider GL, Gaensler EA, et al. Bronchiolitis and bronchitis in connective tissue disease. *JAMA* 1979;242:528–532.
28. Geddes DM, Corrin B, Brewerton DA, et al. Progressive airway obliteration in adults and its association with rheumatoid disease. *Q J Med* 1977;46:427–444.
29. Murphy KC, Atkins CJ, Offer RC, et al. Obliterative bronchiolitis in two rheumatoid arthritis patients treated with penicillamine. *Arthritis Rheum* 1981;24:557–560.
30. Ostrow D, Buskard N, Hill RS, et al. Bronchiolitis obliterans complicating bone marrow transplantation. *Chest* 1985;87:828–830.
31. Stein-Streilen J, Lipscomb MF, Hart DA, et al. Graft-versus-host reaction in the lung. *Transplantation* 1981;32:38–44.
32. Burke CM, Theodore J, Dawkins KD, et al. Post transplant obliterative bronchiolitis and other late lung sequellae in human heart–lung transplantation. *Chest* 1984;86:824–829.
33. Glanville AR, Baldwin JC, Burke CM, et al. Obliterative bronchiolitis after heart–lung transplantation: apparent arrest by augmented immunosuppression. *Ann Intern Med* 1987;107: 300–304.
34. Burke CM, Glanville AR, Theodore J, et al. Lung immunogenicity rejection, and obliterative bronchiolitis. *Chest* 1987;92:547–549.
35. Morrish WF, Herman SJ, Weisbrod GL, et al. Bronchiolitis obliterans after lung transplant: findings at chest radiography and high-resolution CT. *Radiology* 1991;179:487–490.
36. Niewoehner D, Kleinerman J, Rue D, et al. Pathologic changes in the peripheral airways of young cigarette smokers. *N Engl J Med* 1974; 291:755–758.
37. Cosio M, Hale K, Niewoehner D. Morphologic and morphometric effects of prolonged cigarette smoking on the small airways. *Am Rev Respir Dis* 1980;122:265–271.
38. Yousem SA, Colby TV, Gaensler EA. Respiratory bronchiolitis associated interstitial lung disease and its relationship to desquamative interstitial pneumonia. *Mayo Clin Proc* 1989;64: 1373–1380.
39. Davison AG, Heard BE, McAllister WAC, et al. Cryptogenic organizing pneumonitis. *Q J Med* 1983;207:382–394.
40. Chandler PW, Shin MS, Friedman SE, et al. Radiographic manifestations of bronchiolitis obliterans with organizing pneumonia vs. usual interstitial pneumonia. *AJR* 1986;147:899–906.
41. Barter T, Irwin RS, Nash G, et al. Idiopathic bronchiolitis obliterans organizing pneumonia with peripheral infiltrates on chest roentgenogram. *Arch Intern Med* 1989;149:273–279.
42. Müller NL, Guerry Force ML, Staples C, et al. Differential diagnosis of bronchiolitis obliterans with organizing pneumonia and usual interstitial pneumonia: clinical, functional and radiologic findings. *Radiology* 1987;162:151–156.
43. McLoud TC, et al. Bronchiolitis obliterans. *Radiology* 1986;159:1–8.

Diseases of the Bronchioles, edited by
Gary R. Epler. Raven Press, Ltd.,
New York © 1994.

4

Bronchiolar Diseases: Computed Tomography

Thomas E. Hartman,* Stephen J. Swensen,† and Nestor L. Müller*

**Department of Radiology, University of British Columbia and Vancouver General Hospital, 855 W. 12th Ave., Vancouver, British Columbia V5Z 1M9, Canada.*
†Department of Diagnostic Radiology, Mayo Clinic, Rochester, MN.

Computed tomography (CT) is currently the best imaging modality to assess the pulmonary parenchyma and airways (1–4). It allows identification of airways 1 to 2 mm in diameter and vessels 0.1 to 0.2 mm in diameter and assessment of abnormalities down to the level of the secondary pulmonary lobule (5). The secondary pulmonary lobule, the unit of lung supplied by three to five terminal bronchioles (Reid lobule) (6), constitutes the basic unit of lung anatomy and physiology. The terminal bronchioles supplying the secondary lobule measure approximately 1 mm in diameter and cannot be distinguished on CT from the adjacent pulmonary artery of similar size. The terminal bronchiole and artery supplying the lobule are located in the center of the lobule and give off smaller branches at intervals along their course. On CT the vessels can be seen as linear, branching, or dot-like structures near the center of the secondary pulmonary lobule (7). The normal intralobular bronchioles cannot be identified because the thickness of their wall is less than or equal to 0.15 mm. However, bronchiolar abnormalities may be detected when there is thickening of the bronchiolar wall, peribronchiolar inflammation or fibrosis, bronchiolectasis, or, indirectly, by evidence of decreased perfusion and air trapping (1–5,7,8).

Several studies have described the CT findings of various abnormalities of the bronchioles including bronchiolitis obliterans, bronchiolitis obliterans with organizing pneumonia (BOOP), panbronchiolitis, and respiratory bronchiolitis. Because optimal assessment of bronchiolar abnormalities requires the use of high-resolution CT, we first briefly summarize the optimal technique for performance of CT in these patients.

HIGH-RESOLUTION CT TECHNIQUE

The CT image is a two-dimensional representation of a three-dimensional cross-sectional slice with the third dimension being slice thickness. The slice thickness ranges from 1 to 10 mm, depending on the width of the x-ray beam (collimation). All structures within a unit volume of the slice (voxel) are represented as a single unit (pixel) on the image. The x-ray characteristics of the structures within a given voxel are therefore averaged to produce the image. This volume averaging results in loss of spatial resolution. Therefore, the thicker the slice, the lower the ability of CT to resolve small structures. Detailed analysis of the lung parenchyma requires the use of 1- to 2-mm collimation scans.

Standard CT reconstruction algorithms improve contrast resolution but decrease spatial resolution. To increase spatial resolution, thus optimizing visualization of fine parenchymal detail, high-spatial-frequency reconstruction algorithms are required. These are available in all current CT scanners.

The combination of thin-section CT (1- to 2-mm collimation) and the use of a high-spatial-frequency reconstruction algorithm is referred to as *high-resolution CT*. Further improvement in image quality can be obtained by targeting the image to one lung or portion of lung.

In the authors' opinion, the optimal technique for airway assessment uses high-resolution CT sections taken at 10-mm intervals through the chest. Since many of the findings in airways diseases may have a patchy distribution, wider spacing of high-resolution CT sections risks missing diagnostic information. Narrower spacing increases scanning time and radiation dose to the patient.

Recent studies suggest a potential role for the use of dynamic CT in the diagnosis of airways diseases. With the acquisition of several images per second, dynamic CT enables the assessment of parenchymal changes during a vital capacity maneuver. This should facilitate the detection of dynamic abnormalities and air trapping (9,10). The presence of air trapping can also be demonstrated by comparing CT images obtained at end-expiration with end-inspiration images.

BRONCHIOLITIS OBLITERANS

The high-resolution CT findings in bronchiolitis obliterans are a combination of direct and indirect signs resulting from the thickening of the bronchiolar wall by inflammation and fibrosis and from obstruc-

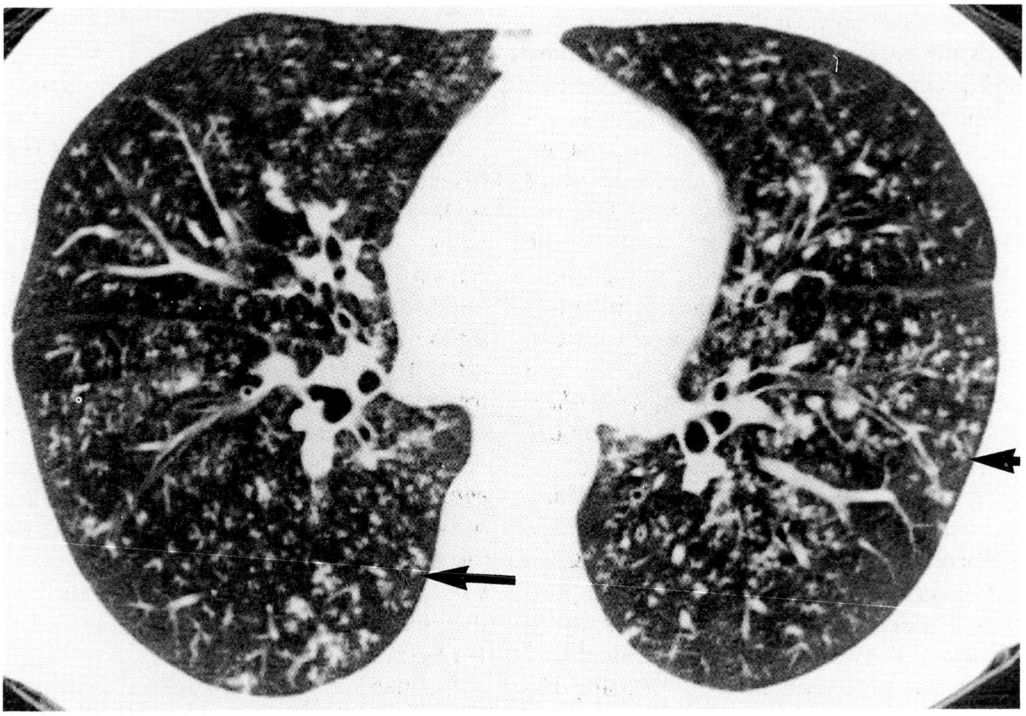

FIG. 1. A 28-year-old man with bronchiolitis obliterans. High-resolution CT section through the level of the superior segmental bronchi demonstrates small branching structures within the secondary lobule (*arrows*).

tion of the bronchiolar lumen (11,12). Thickening of the bronchiolar wall in bronchiolitis obliterans may be identified on high-resolution CT by the visualization of centrilobular branching structures distinct from pulmonary vessels (Fig. 1). Although this is a direct sign of bronchiolitis obliterans that may be demonstrated in patients with marked thickening of the bronchiolar walls, it is present in only a minority of cases.

Bronchiolitis obliterans is often associated with dilatation of the proximal bronchioles and bronchi. The presence of bronchial dilatation with or without thickening of the bronchial wall (bronchiectasis) is a common, albeit indirect and nonspecific, sign of bronchiolitis obliterans on high-resolution CT (Fig. 2).

Other common indirect signs of bronchiolitis obliterans are the presence of decreased perfusion and air trapping. The inability to ventilate directly a portion of lung leads to local hypoxia and reflex vasoconstriction of the pulmonary arteries or arterioles supplying that region. This variance in perfusion between involved and uninvolved regions of lung, called *mosaic perfusion,* is a common finding in bronchiolitis obliterans. On CT, mosaic perfusion is identified by the presence of areas of relatively decreased attenuation and areas of increased attenuation in a patchy distribution (Fig. 3). The areas with decreased attenuation are due to reflex vasoconstriction. The vessels in these areas are reduced in size compared to normal lung. The areas of relatively increased attenuation correspond to more normal lung, which is receiving preferential perfusion. Another finding in bronchiolitis obliterans is the presence of air trapping. This can be most readily identified by comparing inspiratory with expiratory CT sections (Fig. 4).

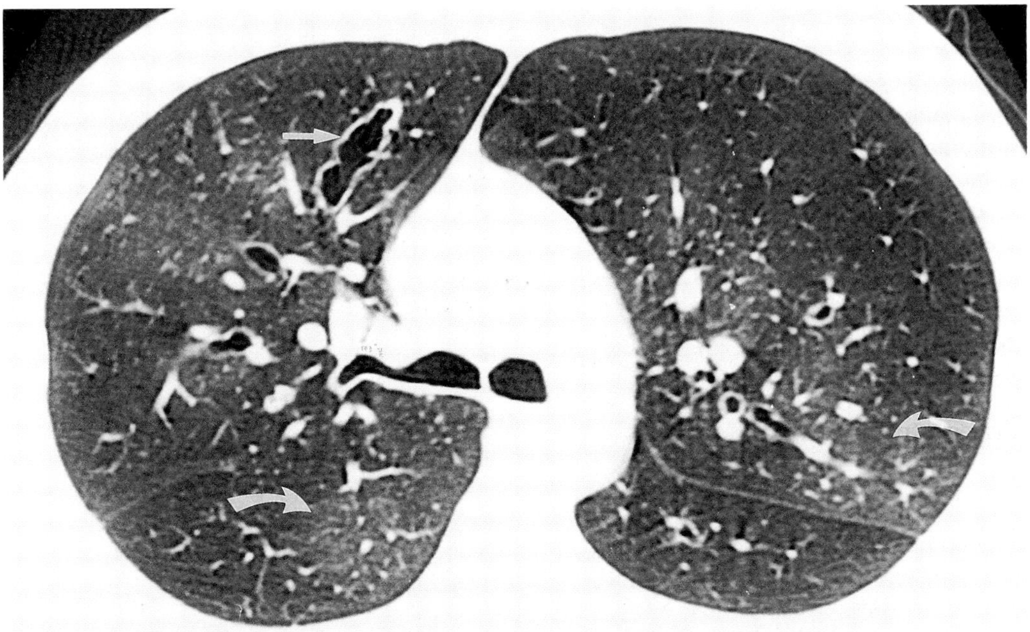

FIG. 2. A 23-year-old man with bronchiolitis obliterans presumably due to previous viral infection. High-resolution CT section at the level of the tracheal carina demonstrates areas of cylindrical and varicose bronchiectasis (*arrow*). Also seen are patchy areas of increased (*curved arrows*) and decreased attenuation characteristic of mosaic perfusion.

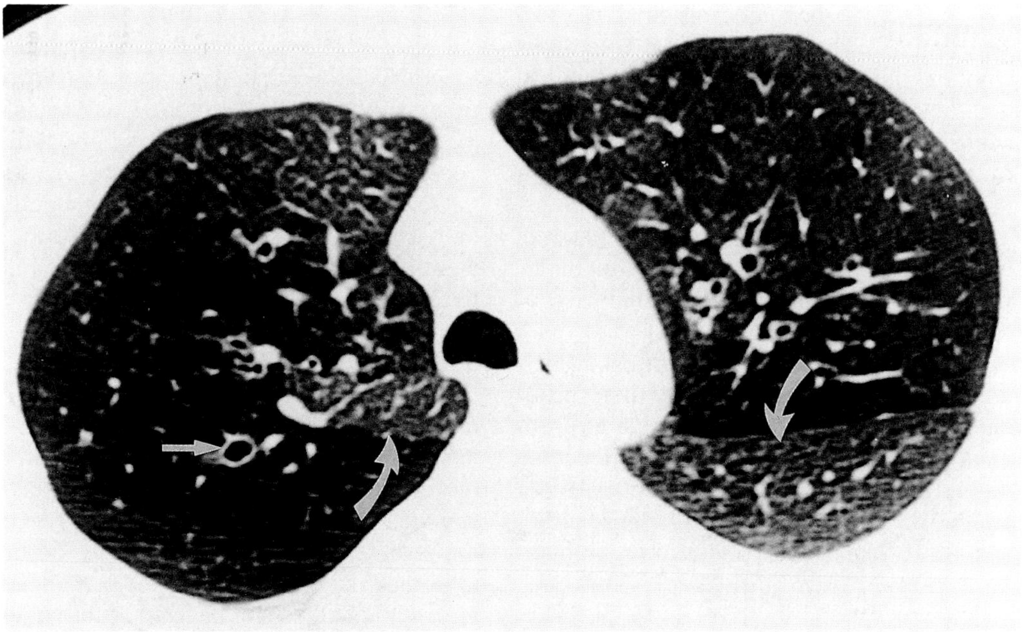

FIG. 3. A 37-year-old man with bronchiolitis obliterans due to viral infection. High-resolution CT section through the level of the aortic arch demonstrates patchy areas of increased (*curved arrows*) and decreased parenchymal attenuation consistent with mosaic perfusion. Also noted are several dilated bronchi (*arrow*).

Centrilobular branching structures, bronchial dilatation, mosaic perfusion, and air trapping may be demonstrated singly or in combination in individual cases of bronchiolitis obliterans. The various causes of bronchiolitis obliterans result in a similar appearance on CT; however, on occasion, associated findings may help to identify specific etiologies. The CT findings have been described in bronchiolitis obliterans secondary to infection, collagen vascular disease, transplants, and drugs.

Infection

Numerous infectious agents have been demonstrated to cause bronchiolitis obliterans. The most common causes are viruses (respiratory syncytial virus in infants and adenovirus) and *Mycoplasma pneumoniae* (13,14). Mosaic perfusion and bronchial dilatation are the most commonly seen abnormalities on high-resolution CT, whereas centrilobular branching structures are demonstrated only rarely (Fig. 5).

FIG. 4. A 7-year-old girl with bronchiolitis obliterans due to anhydrous ammonia inhalation. **A,** CT scan through the level of the lower lobe bronchi taken in inspiration. Areas of increased and decreased parenchymal attenuation, which represent mosaic perfusion, are demonstrated. **B,** CT scan of the same patient at the same level taken in expiration demonstrates no change in the attenuation in the medial segment of the right middle lobe, the anterior and medial segments of the right lower lobe, and the majority of the left lower lobe, consistent with air trapping. Normally ventilated lungs are seen to increase in attenuation on the expiratory films. Also note difference in caliber between the vessels in the normal lung and in the lung with air trapping (*arrows*).

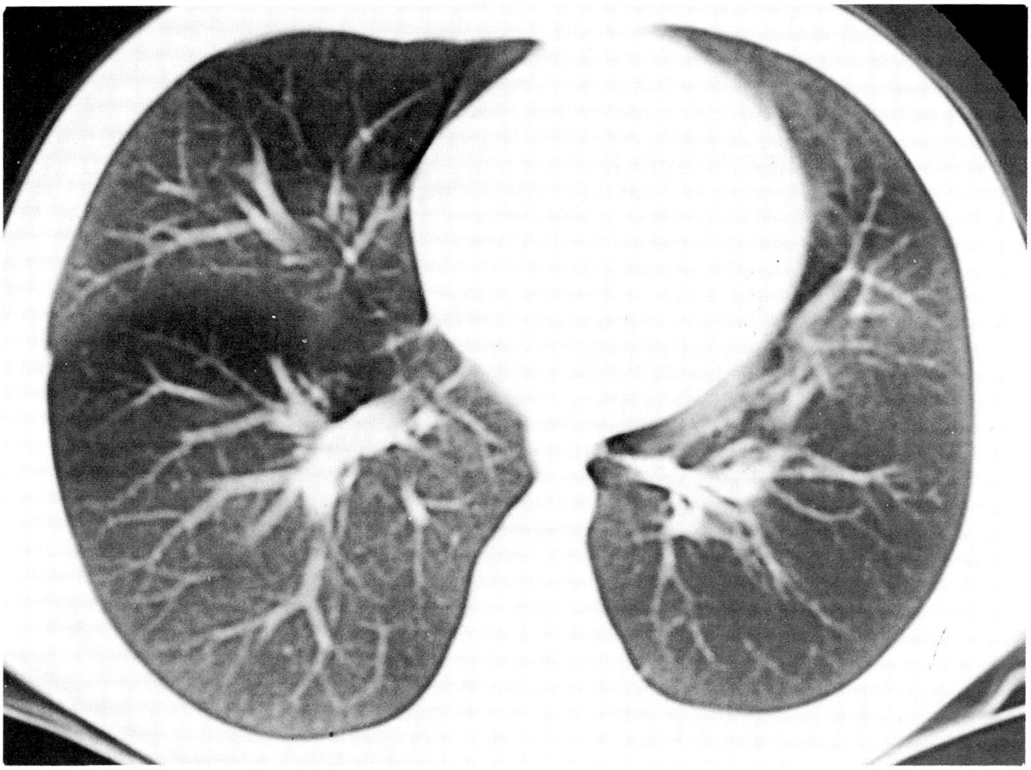

A

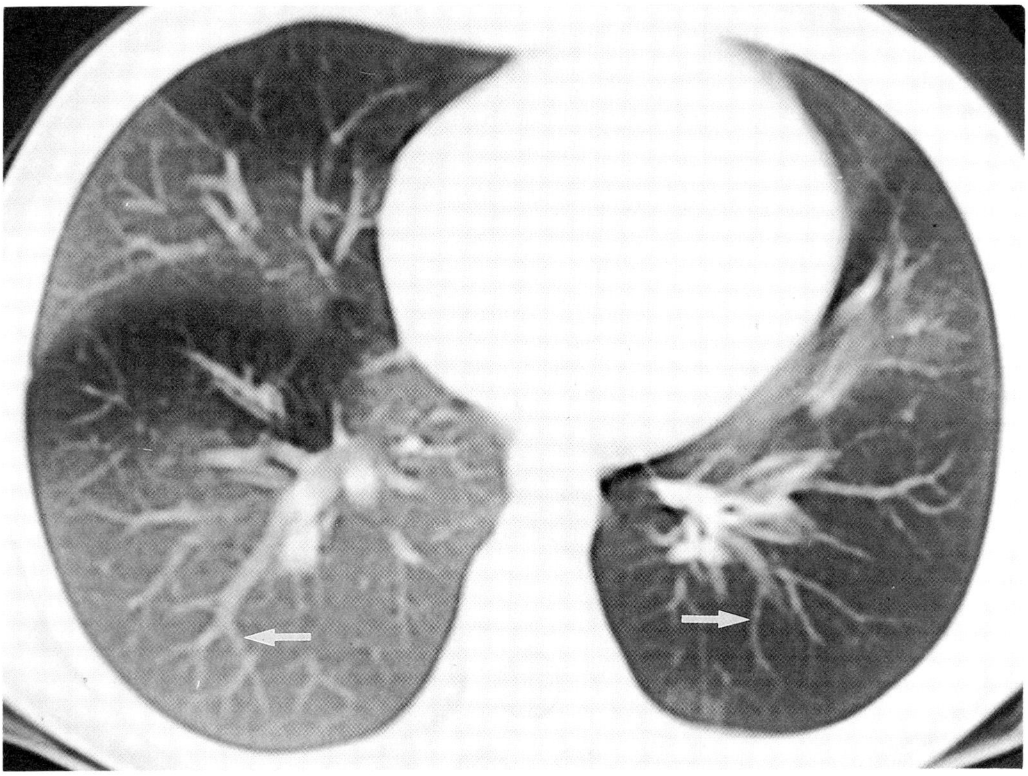

B

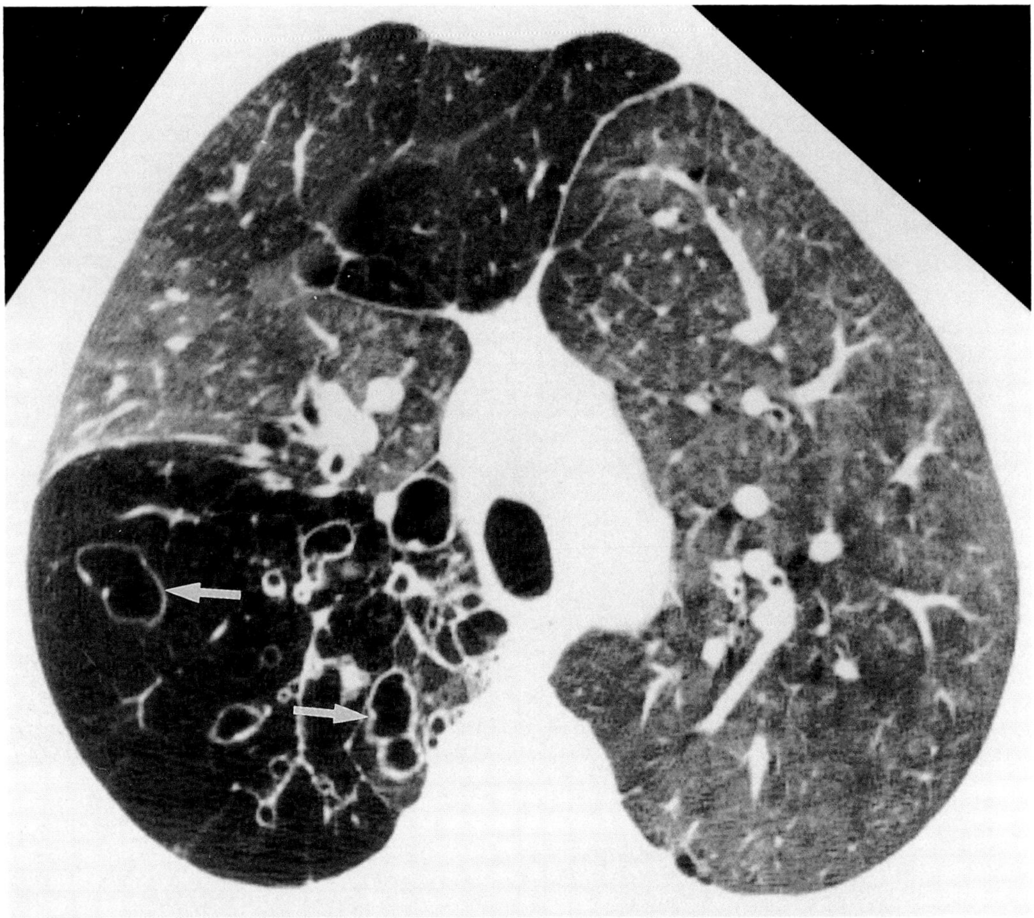

FIG. 5. A 32-year-old man with bronchiolitis obliterans due to infection. High-resolution CT section at the level of the aortic arch shows areas of mosaic perfusion and bronchiectasis (*arrows*). Note the asymmetric distribution of the abnormalities, being most severe in the right lower lobe, consistent with an infectious etiology.

A particular subset of asymmetric bronchiolitis obliterans is seen in patients with Swyer-James syndrome (Fig. 6). In these patients, the findings of bronchiolitis obliterans are confined to a single lung or a single lobe. In a group of nine patients studied with high-resolution CT (15) bronchiectasis and diminished pulmonary artery size were seen in all nine and hyperlucent lung consistent with decreased perfusion in eight.

Connective Tissue Disease

Bronchiolitis obliterans may be seen in association with connective tissue diseases, most commonly rheumatoid arthritis (16). The findings described on high-resolution CT include centrilobular branching structures, bronchial dilatation, and areas of mosaic perfusion (17) (Fig. 7).

Lung and Heart–Lung Transplant

Bronchiolitis obliterans is a relatively common manifestation of chronic rejection in patients who have undergone lung or heart–lung transplant. Morrish and others (18) reported the high-resolution CT findings of four single lung transplant patients who developed bronchiolitis obliterans. Pe-

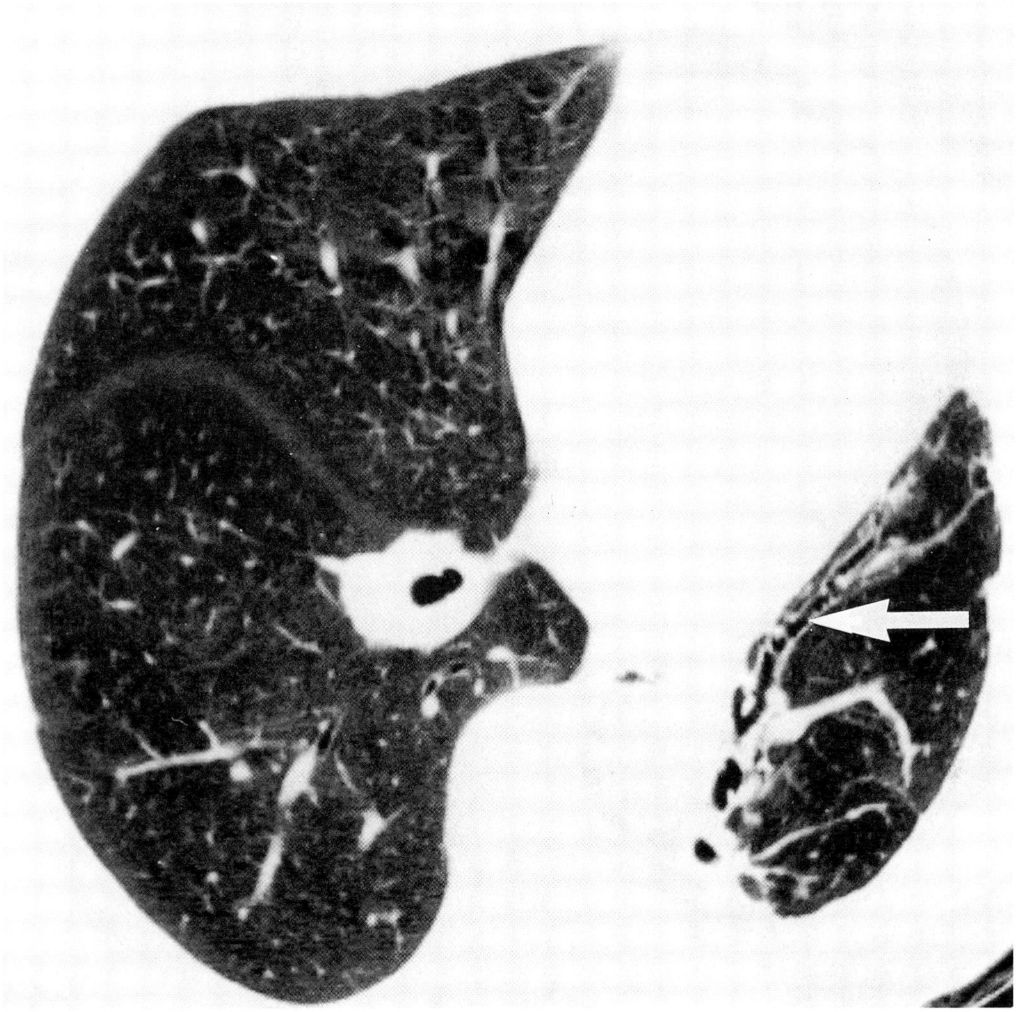

FIG. 6. A 63-year-old woman with bronchiolitis obliterans. High-resolution CT section through the level of the lower lobe bronchi shows that the left lung is smaller than the right. Note also the bronchiectasis (*arrow*) in the involved left lung. Findings are consistent with Swyer-James syndrome.

ripheral bronchiectasis was present in all four patients and decreased areas of perfusion in three. In two patients studied by Padley and colleagues (17), one had bronchiectasis and one had areas of decreased perfusion on high-resolution CT. Lentz and others (19) recently reported that dilatation of lower lobe bronchi as shown by high-resolution CT is a good indicator of bronchiolitis obliterans in heart–lung transplant patients and that increased bronchial dilatation on subsequent scans correlated with impairment in pulmonary function.

Graft-versus-Host Disease

Bronchiolitis obliterans is a well recognized manifestation of chronic graft-versus-host disease in patients who have undergone bone marrow transplant (Fig. 8). The findings on high-resolution CT reported by

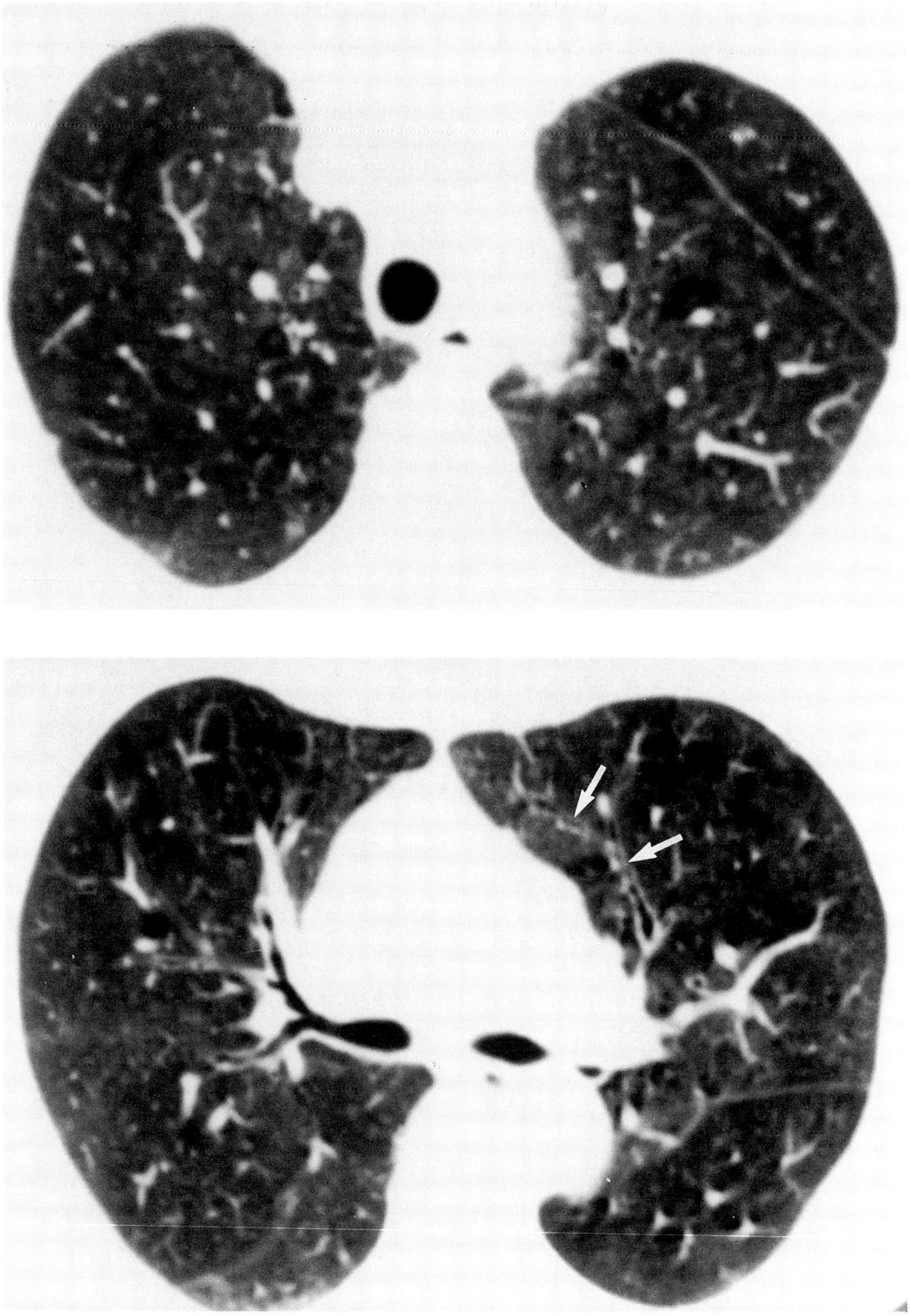

A

B

FIG. 7. A 49-year-old woman with rheumatoid arthritis and bronchiolitis obliterans. **A,** High-resolution CT section through the level of the aortic arch demonstrates areas of mosaic perfusion. **B,** High-resolution CT section through the level of the middle lobe bronchus demonstrates areas of bronchiectasis (*arrows*).

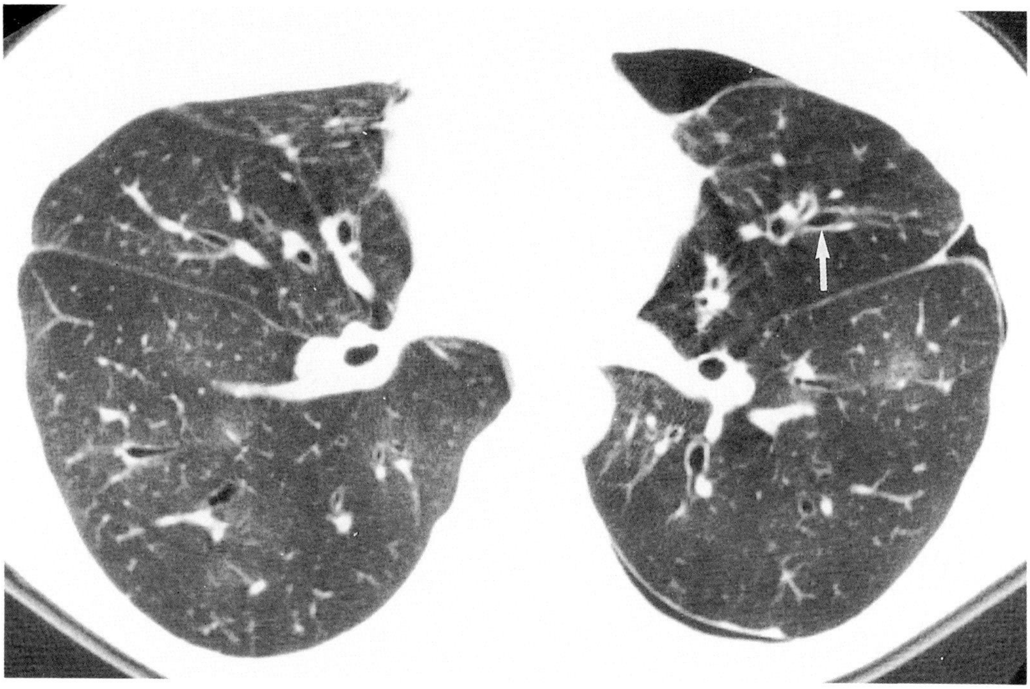

FIG. 8. A 29-year-old woman with bone marrow transplant. High-resolution CT section at the level of the bronchus intermedius demonstrates bronchiectasis (*arrow*) and mosaic perfusion consistent with bronchiolitis obliterans in this patient with graft-versus-host disease. Incidental note is made of a small left pneumothorax.

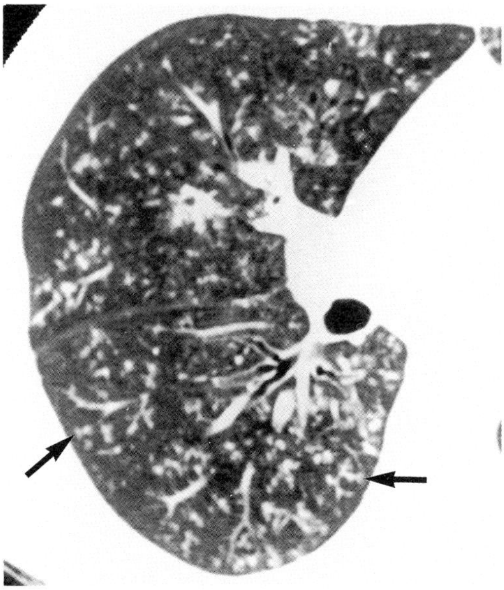

FIG. 9. A 28-year-old man with bronchiolitis obliterans secondary to foreign body related to amyl nitrate inhalation. High-resolution CT section at the level of the superior segmental bronchus of the right lower lobe demonstrates small branching structures (*arrows*) near the center of the secondary lobule consistent with bronchiolitis obliterans.

Padley and others (17) included centrilobular branching structures, bronchial dilatation, and mosaic perfusion.

Drugs

Drugs, both therapeutic and illicit, can induce bronchiolitis obliterans. Penicillamine is one of the better known causes. High-resolution CT findings that have been described include centrilobular branching structures, bronchial dilatation, mosaic perfusion, and air trapping (17,20,21). A single case of bronchiolitis obliterans associated with inhalation of amyl nitrate reported by Padley and colleagues (17) demonstrated all of the findings on high-resolution CT (Fig. 9).

BRONCHIOLITIS OBLITERANS ORGANIZING PNEUMONIA

In 1985, Epler and colleagues (22) described 50 patients who had bronchiolitis obliterans associated with patchy organizing pneumonia. This disorder differed from bronchiolitis obliterans in that it was potentially completely reversible with corticosteroid therapy. Although in North America this condition is usually referred to as bronchiolitis obliterans organizing pneumonia (BOOP), the clinical, functional, and radiographic manifestations are primarily due to the organizing pneumonia (23–25).

Müller and others (26) described the CT findings in 14 patients with BOOP. The predominant findings included areas of air space consolidation in 10 patients and nod-

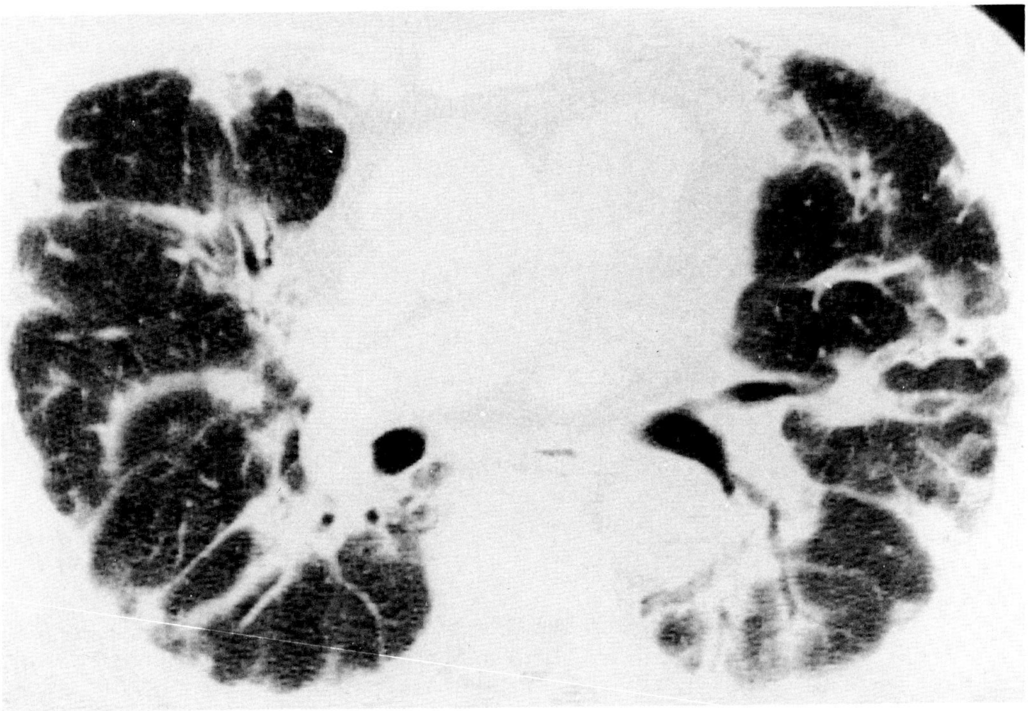

FIG. 10. A 72-year-old woman with idiopathic bronchiolitis obliterans organizing pneumonia. High-resolution CT through the level of the right pulmonary artery shows areas of consolidation along the bronchovascular bundles (*arrows*) and in a subpleural distribution. Bronchial dilatation is seen in the areas surrounded by consolidation.

ules in 7. All the patients had areas of air space consolidation, small nodules, or both on CT exam (Fig. 10). In 6 of 14 patients the consolidation had a subpleural distribution (Fig. 11). In addition, bronchial dilatation was present in 6 patients and pleural effusions in 4. The bronchial dilatation was demonstrated only in areas with air space consolidation (Fig. 12).

Nishimura and Itoh (27) compared open lung biopsy specimens with high-resolution CT images obtained prior to biopsy in eight patients with idiopathic BOOP. Regions of dense consolidation were due to organized pneumonia within peripheral air spaces. Regions of ground-glass attenuation corresponded to alveolitis. All eight patients had either consolidation or nodules on high-resolution CT. Bronchiolitis obliterans did not contribute to the high-resolution CT findings in their patients.

On occasion, differentiation of BOOP and usual interstitial pneumonia can be difficult on the chest radiograph. The presence or absence of honeycombing on high-resolution CT may be helpful in these cases. Honeycombing is present in over 90% of patients with usual interstitial pneumonia (28) but has not been reported in BOOP (26,27).

DIFFUSE PANBRONCHIOLITIS

Diffuse panbronchiolitis is an inflammatory lung disease prevalent in Orientals but rare in Europeans and North Americans. Akira and others (29) reported the high-

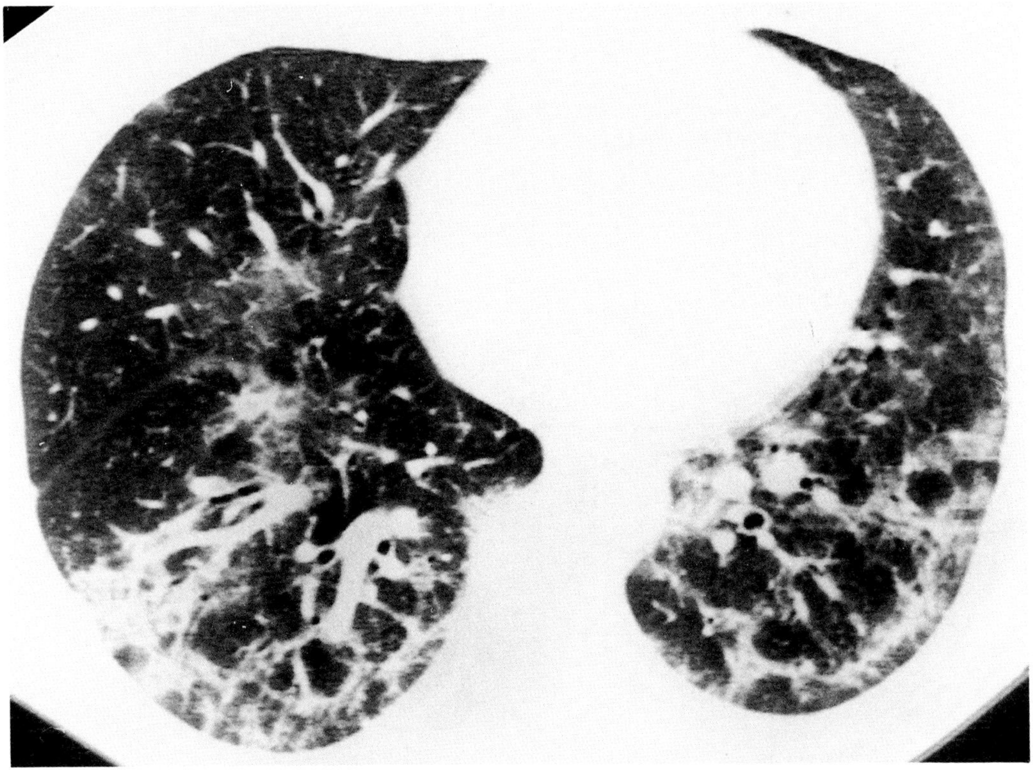

FIG. 11. A 36-year-old woman with idiopathic BOOP. High-resolution CT section 1 cm above the diaphragm. Areas of consolidation are seen in a subpleural distribution predominantly in the posterior lower lobes. Bronchial dilatation can be seen in the areas of consolidation.

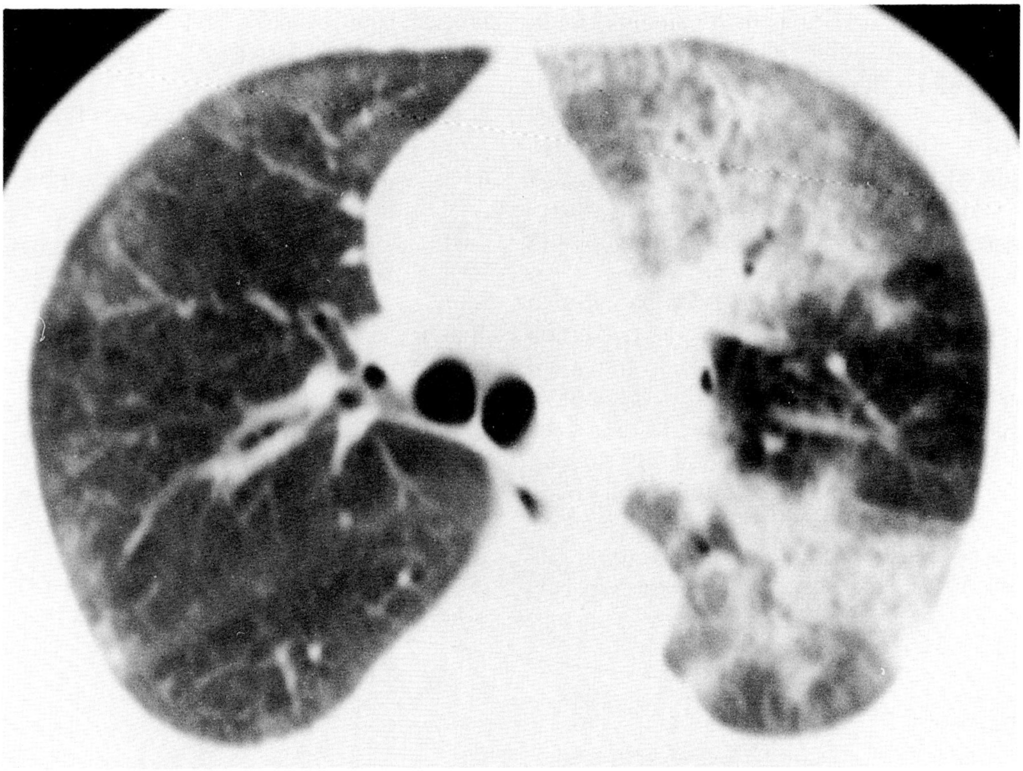

FIG. 12. A 77-year-old man with idiopathic BOOP. High-resolution CT section through the level of the right upper lobe bronchus shows patchy areas of consolidation in both lungs, more marked on the left.

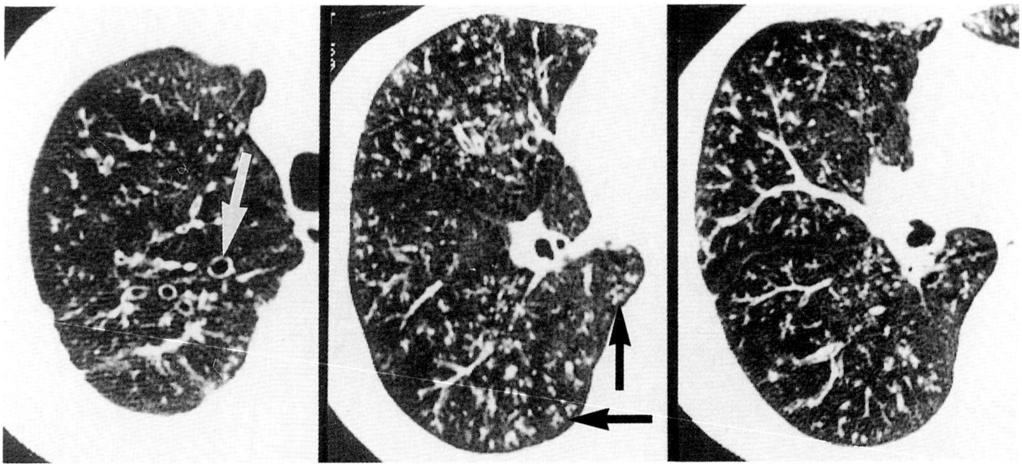

FIG. 13. Japanese patient with panbronchiolitis. High-resolution CT sections of the right lung at three levels demonstrate centrilobular branching structures (*black arrows*), centrilobular nodules and bronchiectasis (*white arrow*). (Case courtesy of Dr. Masanori Akira, Osaka, Japan.)

resolution CT findings in 20 patients. As in bronchiolitis obliterans, the high-resolution CT findings in panbronchiolitis include centrilobular branching structures, mosaic perfusion, air trapping, and bronchial dilatation. However, in panbronchiolitis, nodules 1 to 3 mm in diameter with a centrilobular distribution are frequently present in addition to the centrilobular branching structures and bronchiolar dilatation (29,30) (Fig. 13). The centrilobular branching structures have been shown to represent segments of bronchiolectasis filled with secretions while the centrilobular nodules surrounded the respiratory bronchioles within the secondary pulmonary lobule (30). This combination of high-resolution CT findings in an Oriental patient is virtually diagnostic of panbronchiolitis.

RESPIRATORY BRONCHIOLITIS

Most cigarette smokers have pathologic evidence of respiratory bronchiolitis; however, very few individuals become symptomatic (31). The high-resolution CT findings in respiratory bronchiolitis were recently described by Remy and colleagues (32) and Karg (33). Although most patients with respiratory bronchiolitis have normal high-resolution CT scans, abnormalities that

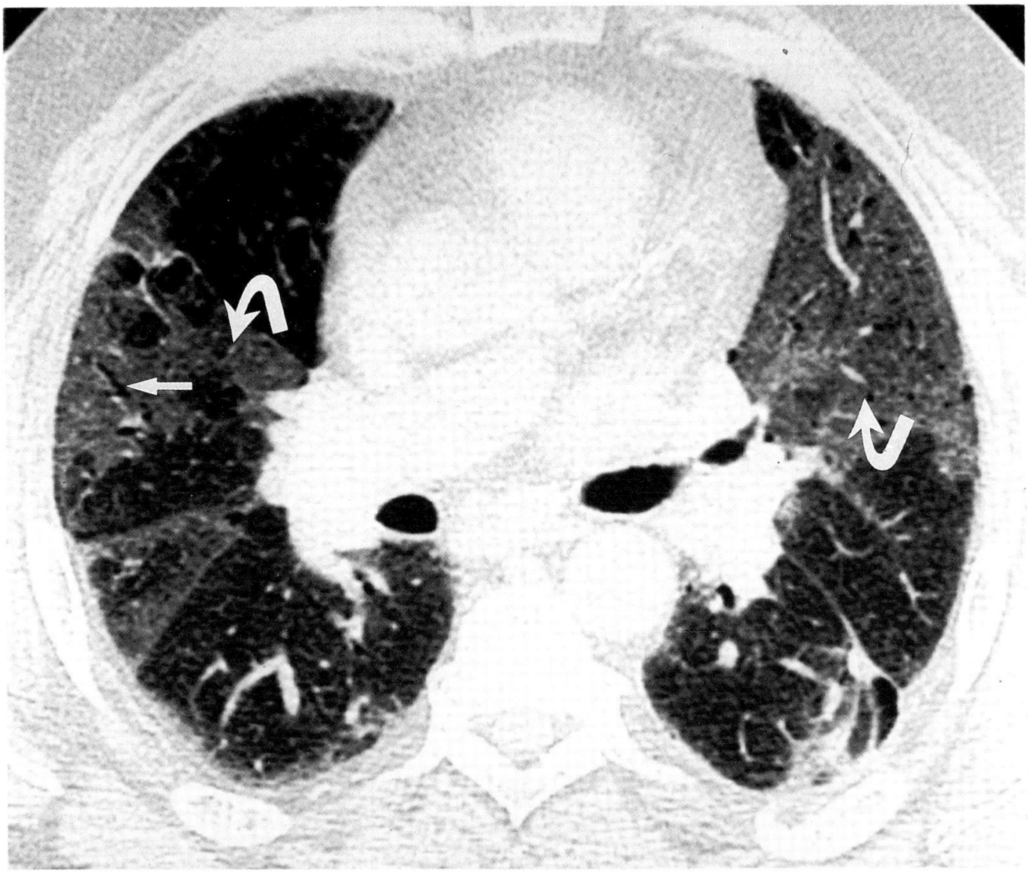

FIG. 14. A 52-year-old male smoker with respiratory bronchiolitis. High-resolution CT section at the level of the lingular bronchus demonstrates areas of "ground-glass" attenuation in a patchy distribution (*curved arrows*). Localized bronchial dilatation is seen in the right middle lobe (*arrow*).

may be seen include parenchymal micronodules and areas of ground-glass attenuation in a patchy distribution with or without associated bronchial dilatation (Fig. 14).

CONCLUSION

The predominant diagnostic CT findings in bronchiolitis obliterans regardless of cause include branching centrilobular structures, bronchial dilatation (bronchiectasis), mosaic perfusion, and air trapping. However, these findings are nonspecific and a careful clinical history is essential in distinguishing the various potential etiologies.

The literature on the CT findings in bronchiolitis obliterans organizing pneumonia is limited. Although subpleural areas of consolidation with associated bronchial dilatation and lack of honeycombing may be suggestive, the CT findings are not diagnostic and lung biopsy is required for definitive diagnosis.

REFERENCES

1. Müller NL, Miller RR. Computed tomography of chronic diffuse infiltrative lung disease. I. *Am Rev Respir Dis* 1990;142:1206–1215.
2. Müller NL, Miller RR. Computed tomography of chronic diffuse infiltrative lung disease. II. *Am Rev Respir Dis* 1990;142:1440–1448.
3. Müller NL. Clinical value of high-resolution CT in chronic diffuse lung disease. *AJR* 1991;157: 1163–.
4. Grenier P, Maurice F, Musset D, Menu Y, Nahum H. Bronchiectasis: assessment by thin-section CT. *Radiology* 1986;161:95–99.
5. Webb WR. High-resolution lung CT: normal anatomy and pathologic findings. *J Thorac Imaging* 1993 (*in press*).
6. Reid L. The secondary lobule in the adult human lung with special reference to its appearance in bronchograms. *Thorax* 1958;13:110–115.
7. Murata K, Itoh H, Todo G, et al. Centrilobular lesions of the lung: demonstration by high-resolution CT and pathologic correlation. *Radiology* 1986;161:641–645.
8. Murata K, Khan A, Herman PG. Pulmonary parenchymal disease: evaluation with high-resolution CT. *Radiology* 1989; 170:629–635.
9. Webb WR, Stern ET, Kanth N, Gamsu G. Dynamic pulmonary CT: findings in healthy adult men. *Radiology* 1993;186:117–124.
10. Stern EJ, Webb WR, Golden JA, Gamsu G. Cystic lung disease associated with eosinophilic granuloma and tuberous sclerosis: air trapping at dynamic ultrafast high-resolution CT. *Radiology* 1992;182:325–329.
11. Sweatman MC, Millar AB, Strickland B, Turner-Warwick M. Computed tomography in adult obliterative bronchiolitis. *Clin Radiol* 1990; 41:116–119.
12. Lynch DA, Brasch RC, Hardy KA, Webb WR. Pediatric pulmonary disease: assessment with high-resolution ultrafast CT. *Radiology* 1990; 176:243–248.
13. King TE Jr. Bronchiolitis obliterans. *Lung* 1989; 167:69–93.
14. Yousem SA. Small airways disease. *Pathol Ann* 1991;26(Pt 2):109–143.
15. Marti-Monmati L, Perales FR, Catala F. CT findings in Swyer-James syndrome. *Radiology* 1989;172:477–480.
16. Geddes DM, Corrin B, Brewerton DA, et al. Progressive airway obliteration in adults and its association with rheumatoid disease. *Q J Med* 1977;46:427–444.
17. Padley SPG, Adler BD, Hansell DM, Müller NL. Bronchiolitis obliterans: high-resolution CT findings and correlation with pulmonary function tests. *Clin Radiol* 1993;47:236–240.
18. Morrish WF, Herman SJ, Weisbord GL, Chamberlain DW. Bronchiolitis obliterans after lung transplantation: findings at chest radiography and high-resolution CT. *Radiology* 1991;179: 487–490.
19. Lentz D, Bergin CJ, Berry GJ, Stoehr C, Theodore J. Diagnosis of bronchiolitis obliterans in heart–lung transplant patients: importance of bronchial dilatation on CT. *AJR* 1992;159:463–467.
20. Padley SPG, Adler B, Hansell DM, Müller NL. High-resolution computed tomography of drug-induced lung disease. *Clin Radiol* 1992;46:232–236.
21. Kuhlman JE. The role of chest computed tomography in the diagnosis of drug-related reactions. *J Thorac Imaging* 1991;6:52–61.
22. Epler GR, Colby TV, McLoud TC, Carrington CB, Gaensler EA. Bronchiolitis obliterans organizing pneumonia. *N Engl J Med* 1985;312: 152–158.
23. Geddes DM. BOOP and COP [Editorial]. *Thorax* 1991;46:545–547.
24. Woodhead MA, Du Bois RM. Bronchiolitis obliterans, cryptogenic organizing pneumonitis and BOOP [Editorial]. *Respir Med* 1991;85:177–178.
25. Davison AG, Heard BE, McAllister WAC, Turner-Warwick MEH. Cryptogenic organizing pneumonitis. *Q J Med* 1983;52 (new series), No. 207:382–393.
26. Müller NL, Staples CA, Miller RR. Bronchiolitis obliterans organizing pneumonia: CT features in 14 patients. *AJR* 1990;154:983–987.
27. Nishimura K, Itoh H. High-resolution computed tomographic features of bronchiolitis obliterans organizing pneumonia. *Chest* 1992;102[Suppl]: 26–31.

28. Staples CA, Müller NL, Vedal S, Abboud R, Ostrow D, Miller RR. Usual interstitial pneumonia: correlation of CT with clinical, functional and radiologic findings. *Radiology* 1987;162:377–381.
29. Akira M, Kitakani F, Yong-Sik L, et al. Diffuse panbronchiolitis: evaluation with high-resolution CT. *Radiology* 1988;168:433–438.
30. Nishimura K, Kitaichi M, Izumi T, Itoh H. Diffuse panbronchiolitis: correlation of high-resolution CT and pathologic findings. *Radiology* 1992;184:779–785.
31. Myers JL, Veal CF Jr, Shin MS, Katzenstein AA. Respiratory bronchiolitis causing interstitial lung disease: a clinicopathologic study of six cases. *Am Rev Respir Dis* 1987;135:880–884.
32. Remy-Jardin M, Remy J, Boulenquez C, Sobaszek A, Edme J-L, Furon D. Morphologic effects of cigarette smoking on airways and pulmonary parenchyma in healthy adult volunteers: CT evaluation and correlation with pulmonary function tests. *Radiology* 1993;186:107–115.
33. Karg K. Small airways disease: classification and clinical, radiologic and pathologic features. *Radiology* 1992;185:354 (abst).

Diseases of the Bronchioles, edited by Gary R. Epler. Raven Press, Ltd., New York © 1994.

5

Bronchoalveolar Lavage Characteristics of the Bronchiolar Diseases

Ulrich Costabel

Ruhrlandklinik, Tüschener Weg 40, D-45239 Essen, Germany.

In the past decade, bronchoalveolar lavage (BAL) has become an increasingly used tool not only for research purposes in pulmonary interstitial and airway disorders but also for clinical applications. BAL recovers cells and noncellular components from the lower respiratory tract and the alveolar spaces. It is thought that alterations in lavage fluid and cells reflect pathologic changes in the corresponding parenchymal constituents. A number of studies have shown a good correlation between the type and number of inflammatory cells obtained by BAL and those observed in histologic sections of lung biopsy specimen or derived from mechanically disaggregated lung tissue in several interstitial lung disorders, such as idiopathic pulmonary fibrosis, sarcoidosis, and hypersensitivity pneumonitis (1–5). For the diseases of the bronchioles, such correlation studies are not available.

BAL has several advantages over biopsy procedures. It is safe, minimally invasive, and associated with virtually no morbidity, even in severely thrombocytopenic patients. Lethal complications directly attributable to BAL have not been reported (6). Thus, it can be used repeatedly to investigate serial changes. Furthermore, lavage samples a much larger area of the lungs than can be obtained by the small tissue fragments of transbronchial biopsy or by open biopsy specimens. Therefore it presumably gives a better representative average picture of the inflammatory and immunologic changes in the lung than biopsies. Nevertheless, the results of BAL should not be used esoterically but should be considered in the context of other information from conventional investigative methods. In this chapter, first some technical aspects of BAL are considered, then an overview is given of established clinical applications. The chapter concludes with detailed descriptions of lavage characteristics of bronchiolar diseases, a field that has gained attention in the literature during the past 5 years.

TECHNICAL CONSIDERATIONS

Detailed guidelines and recommendations regarding the technical aspect of BAL have been published by scientific societies (6–8), setting up a framework that defines the performance of BAL as well as the laboratory processing and analysis of the recovered constituents. The guidelines are based on the principle of the so-called smallest common denominator, hence allowing a number of technical variations in the different steps of the BAL procedure. It has to be realized that the BAL method is incompletely standardized (9). When the guidelines are followed, however, the results of lavage are sufficiently valid for practical diagnostic purposes. For example, the correct information on cell differentials is important for clinical purposes. In this respect, the total volume of instilled fluid can range from 100 to 250 ml without affecting the results of cell differentials (10).

Bronchoscopic Procedure

In brief, BAL is performed by fiberoptic bronchoscopy with topical anesthesia. It involves the instillation of 100 to 300 ml total volume of sterile saline in 20 to 50 ml aliquots into a subsegment of the lung, while the bronchoscope is placed in a wedge position occluding the lumen of the subsegmental bronchus. In diffuse lung disease, the middle or lingular lobe is used as a standard site of BAL. Localized shadowing naturally requires lavage of the radiographically involved area. Several studies have evaluated the interlobar variation of lavage cell differentials, lymphocyte subpopulations, and asbestos body counts by performing a bilateral lavage and analyzing the right and the left sides independently (11–14). In general, these studies have shown a good interlobar correlation in patients with nonfocal disease on the chest radiogram. These observations indicate that in patients with diffuse lung disease BAL at one site should yield representative information on the whole lung.

Usually, 50 to 70% of the instilled volume is recovered. In obstructive airway disease and emphysema the recovery rate is significantly lower and may be less than 30%. Differential evaluation of the "bronchial" (first aliquot) and "alveolar" (subsequent aliquots) samples may be useful in airway diseases (15).

Adverse Effects

Fever some hours after BAL is by far the most frequent adverse effect, occurring in 3 to 30% of patients, depending on the instilled volume. If a total volume below 150 ml is used, fever is seen in less than 3% of patients. Larger volumes will increase the frequency to 30% or more (16,17).

Rarely, patients with hyperreactive airways develop bronchospasm. In addition, BAL may cause transient alveolar infiltration and a short-lasting decrease in lung volumes and arterial oxygen (6).

Laboratory Processing

Routine processing in the laboratory includes the analysis of total and differential cell counts, and when possible the determination of lymphocyte subsets by monoclonal antibody techniques. Dependent on the clinical situation, in addition to the usual May-Grünwald-Giemsa stains, special stains, such as iron, PAS, silver, or touidine blue stains, may be required for the identification of alveolar bleeding, tumor cells, or certain infective agents. If infection is suspected, a complete microbiologic assessment including cultures can be performed. Quantitative measurements of asbestos bodies by the vacuum filtration method can be used to document suspected asbestos exposure (18,19).

A large number of soluble components have been measured in lavage fluid (7). Currently, none of them has proven to be useful in clinical decisions. They are too nonspecific to be of diagnostic value. The hope that some of them may be predictive of prognosis has also been in vain.

The most recent possibilities in this respect were such extracellular matrix proteins as procollagen-III-peptide, hyaluronate, fibronectin, and vitronectin, as biochemical markers of connective tissue metabolism (20–23). The prognostic significance of these molecules is still uncertain, however. One follow-up study (24) of 84 patients with sarcoidosis monitored for 12 months failed to demonstrate any relationship between initial lavage procollagen-III-peptide and subsequent functional deterioration. The same was found for fibronectin (25). For vitronectin, follow-up data are not yet available. Most likely, increased lavage levels of any of these substances reflect ongoing inflammation associated with increased turnover of extracellular matrix proteins, but not necessarily a progressively fibrosing process.

BAL collagenase may be a suitable indicator of prognosis. In a follow-up study (26) of patients with sarcoidosis during a 1- to 4-year period, 55% of those with detectable lavage collagenase required subsequent treatment, compared with only 26% of those without. The finding needs confirmation by other studies.

In general, the quantitative expression of noncellular lavage constituents is hampered by the lack of satisfactory reference standards to correct for the variable and unpredictable dilutional effects of the epithelial lining fluid during the procedure (9). The fluid dynamics are complex and not well understood (27). Whether the soluble substance of interest originates from secretion by cells located in the alveolar lumen or in the interstitial tissue, or from systemic sources via passive or active transport from plasma, is unknown in many instances. This lack of knowledge adds to the difficulties in interpreting the results of solute measurements.

BRONCHOALVEOLAR LAVAGE AS A CLINICAL DIAGNOSTIC TOOL

BAL is broadly indicated in every patient with unclear interstitial lung disease or unclear pulmonary shadowing, no matter what cause is suspected. The underlying disorders may be of infectious, noninfectious immunologic, or malignant etiology (Table 1). BAL may also be indicated in patients with normal chest radiograms when clinical and lung-function tests are abnormal and point toward a diffuse lung disease. In some diseases, both infectious and noninfectious, lavage findings are diagnostic and may obviate the need for biopsy (Table 2). In others, the findings are not diagnostic but may contribute to the diagnosis and management of these diseases (Table 3). For example, even a normal lavage may be useful to exclude some disorders with high probability.

TABLE 1. *Indications for bronchoalveolar lavage*

Interstitial infiltrates
Sarcoidosis
Hypersensitivity pneumonitis
Drug-induced pneumonitis
Idiopathic pulmonary fibrosis
Connective-tissue disorders
Pulmonary eosinophilic granuloma
Pneumoconioses
Lymphangitic carcinomatosis
Alveolar infiltrates
Pneumonia
Alveolar hemorrhage syndromes
Alveolar proteinosis
Eosinophilic pneumonia
BOOP
Pulmonary infiltrates in the immunocompromised patient
HIV infection
Cytostatic treatment, irradiation
Immunosuppressive treatment
Transplant recipients
Occupational dust exposure

Diagnostic Bronchoalveolar Lavage Findings

Increasing numbers of patients who are immunocompromised, either by HIV infection or by receiving immunosuppressive treatment for malignancy or organ transplantation, are prone to develop pulmonary infections. In this setting, lavage has probably achieved the greatest practical value in diagnosing such infections and differentiating them from alveolar hemorrhage, pulmonary involvement by the underlying malignancy, and drug-induced pneumonitis (28). The sensitivity of BAL in the diagnosis of bacterial infections ranges from 60 to 90%; in mycobacterial, fungal, and most viral infections from 70 to 80%; and in pneumocystis carinii pneumonia 90 to 95% or higher (6).

TABLE 2. *Diagnostic BAL findings*

BAL finding	Diagnosis
Pneumocystis carinii, fungi, CMV transformed cells	Opportunistic infection
Milky fluid, noncellular oval bodies, amorphous debris	Alveolar proteinosis
Hemosiderin-laden macrophages, intracytoplasmic fragments of red blood cells in macrophages, free red blood cells	Alveolar hemorrhage syndrome
Malignant cells of solid tumors, lymphoma, leukemia	Malignant infiltrate
Dust particles in macrophages, quantifying asbestos bodies	Dust exposure
Eosinophils greater than 25%	Eosinophilic pneumonia
Positive lymphocyte transformation test to beryllium salts	Chronic beryllium disease

TABLE 3. *Nonspecific BAL findings*

Normal finding
No active sarcoidosis
No active hypersensitivity pneumonitis
No beryllium disease
No eosinophilic pneumonia
No alveolar proteinosis
No alveolar hemorrhage syndrome
Lymphocytosis
Sarcoidosis
Hypersensitivity pneumonitis
Chronic beryllium disease
Tuberculosis
BOOP
Drug-induced pneumonitis
Malignant infiltrates
Alveolar proteinosis
Pneumoconioses
Connective-tissue disorders
Crohn's disease
Primary biliary cirrhosis
HIV infection
Viral pneumonia
Neutrophilia
Idiopathic pulmonary fibrosis
Acute respiratory distress syndrome
Bacterial pneumonia
Connective-tissue disorders
Wegener's granulomatosis
Pneumoconioses
Bronchitis
Diffuse panbronchiolitis
Transplant bronchiolitis obliterans
Idiopathic bronchiolitis obliterans
Eosinophilia
Eosinophilic pneumonia
Churg-Strauss syndrome
Hypereosinophilic syndrome
Allergic bronchopulmonary aspergillosis
Idiopathic pulmonary fibrosis
Drug-induced reaction
Asthma bronchiale

In pulmonary alveolar proteinosis, BAL analysis may obviate the need of biopsy in almost all patients. The gross appearance of the fluid is milky and turbid. Light microscopy reveals (a) acellular oval bodies, (b) few and foamy macrophages, and (c) a dirty background due to large amounts of amorphous debris (6,29).

Diffuse alveolar hemorrhage can be diagnosed by BAL in all patients, even if the bleeding is occult, by the demonstration of numerous hemosiderin-laden macrophages and, in patients with fresh bleeding episodes, free red blood cells in the fluid and fragments of red blood cells in the cytoplasm of macrophages. Since many syndromes are part of this group of disorders, other clinical and laboratory findings have to establish the cause of the bleeding (6).

Malignant infiltrates, if diffuse, can be reliably diagnosed in 60 to 90% of cases (6).

Eosinophilic infiltrates usually show more than 25% eosinophils in the cell differentials if the lavage is performed in the involved segment (6,30).

Bronchoalveolar Lavage as a Valuable Adjunct to Diagnosis

Using monoclonal antibody techniques, sarcoidosis (CD4/CD8 greater than 5.0 in 60% of patients), eosinophilic granuloma (histiocytosis X) ($CD1^+$ Langerhans cells greater than 4% in 50% of patients), and hypersensitivity pneumonitis (CD4/CD8 below 1.3 and lymphocytes greater than 50%

TABLE 4. *CD4/CD8 ratio in diseases with lymphocytic alveolitis*

CD4/CD8 increased	CD4/CD8 normal	CD4/CD8 decreased
Sarcoidosis	Tuberculosis	Hypersensitivity pneumonitis
Beryllium disease	Lymphangitic carcinomatosis	Drug-induced pneumonitis
Asbestos-induced alveolitis		BOOP
Alveolar proteinosis		Silicosis
Crohn's disease		HIV infection
Connective-tissue disorders		

in more than 90% of patients) can be diagnosed in the appropriate clinical setting (6,31). Diseases with an increase in lavage lymphocytes can be further differentiated into those with an elevated, normal, or decreased CD4/CD8 ratio (Table 4).

In idiopathic pulmonary fibrosis the lavage profile alone is nonspecific, with an increase in neutrophils in 70 to 90%, an associated increase in eosinophils in 40 to 60%, and an additional increase in lymphocytes in 10 to 20% of patients (6,32). A lone increase in lymphocytes is rare in idiopathic fibrosis, and other diseases should then be thoroughly excluded. However, although lavage cytology is nonspecific, it can be helpful in certain clinical circumstances. For example, given a patient with slowly progressive interstitial lung disease, finger clubbing, and subpleural fibrosis with honeycombing found on CT examination, lavage cytology with an increase in neutrophils with or without eosinophils is highly suggestive of idiopathic pulmonary fibrosis and may obviate the need of open biopsy, especially in patients with higher age or increased risk for open biopsy.

Assessment of Disease Activity

BAL has the potential to be useful also for assessment of disease activity and prognosis. This is, however, the most critically discussed topic in the field of BAL. In sarcoidosis, although differences were observed for several lavage findings between clinically active and inactive patient groups, the range of overlap between groups is large, and none of the investigated findings has been proved clinically useful to indicate prognosis reliably enough in a given individual patient (33). In idiopathic pulmonary fibrosis, a marked increase in neutrophils and/or eosinophils was reported to adversely affect prognosis, whereas elevated lymphocyte counts were found to be more likely associated with a good response to corticosteroid treatment (6,32). Repeated lavage measurements may be the more suitable approach than a single study to assess the evolution of disease activity and natural history. Larger prospective studies are required to clarify this issue before BAL should be routinely used for this purpose.

BRONCHOALVEOLAR LAVAGE IN DISEASES OF THE BRONCHIOLES

Before the lavage fluid reaches the alveolar spaces, it has to pass through the airways. Thus, material from the airways will undoubtedly be included in the recovered fluid. The proportional contribution from the airways will depend on the inflammatory status of bronchi and bronchioles. More inflamed airways with increased cellular shedding into the lumen will contribute to a larger extent. It is evident that immunologic and inflammatory events not only in the alveolar interstitium but also in the airways can be assessed by BAL. The characteristic changes in the various bronchiolar diseases are summarized in Table 5.

TABLE 5. *BAL profile in bronchiolar diseases.*

	Macrophages	Lymphocytes	Neutrophils	Eosinophils	CD4/CD8 ratio
Cigarette-related bronchiolitis	↑↑↑		↑	(↑)	↓
Diffuse panbronchiolitis			↑↑↑		n.d.[a]
Idiopathic bronchiolitis obliterans			↑↑↑	↑	n.d.
Transplant bronchiolitis obliterans			↑↑	↑	↓
Idiopathic BOOP		↑↑↑	↑↑	↑	↓

[a]Not determined.

Smoking-Related Diseases of the Bronchioles

Cigarette-Related Bronchiolitis

Cigarette smoking has a major impact on the integrity of the pulmonary structure and function. There is increasing evidence that cigarette smoke initiates an early inflammatory response in the airways. The lesion is predominantly located in the membranous and respiratory bronchioles, which are also designated as small airways (34, 35). Hence, the concept of small airways disease has emerged. Small airways disease is thought to represent an early manifestation in the clinical spectrum of chronic obstructive pulmonary disease, which ranges from chronic bronchitis with or without airflow obstruction to severe disabling emphysema. Since available literature regarding BAL on smoking-related chronic airways inflammation does not specifically address small airways disease but rather reports the findings in asymptomatic smokers and chronic bronchitis patients, in the following the lavage characteristics of these groups are reviewed.

Asymptomatic Smokers

Even in healthy, asymptomatic smokers the changes in BAL fluid and cells are remarkable (36–38). On gross examination, the recovered fluid has a light to dark brown and turbid appearance caused by the color of the tar-laden alveolar macrophages. The total number of cells is drastically increased, approximately fourfold compared to healthy nonsmokers. This increase is almost entirely caused by an expansion of alveolar macrophages. Although the proportion of neutrophils is low, with average values of 1 to 2% in both nonsmokers and smokers, there is a tenfold increase in the absolute number of neutrophils in smokers' lavage. The eosinophil number is also increased but to a lesser extent (36,37). The proportion of lavage lymphocytes is rather low in smokers, and their absolute number is unchanged. Morphologically, smokers' macrophages show impressive changes, being larger in size and laden with blackish-blue pigmented cytoplasmic inclusions in the May-Grünwald-Giemsa stain.

When taking into account changes in the functional status of cells and in the soluble components, several pathophysiologic consequences are emerging from BAL studies. Alveolar macrophages from smokers, chronically activated by inhaled particles in cigarette smoke, display increased motility, including enhanced responsiveness to chemotactic stimuli, increased metabolic activity, and increased content and releasability of lysosomal enzymes, such as elastase and other proteases, which may contribute to tissue damage in the lungs (39,40).

The neutrophil accumulation in the lower respiratory tract of smokers may be caused by at least two mechanisms. First, neutrophils may be attracted to this site by chemotactic factors spontaneously released by smokers' macrophages (41). Second, a cigarette smoke–induced loss of the functional activity of a chemotactic factor inactivator may play a role, as recently reported in lavage fluid of smokers (42).

Neutrophils may contribute to the chronic inflammation associated with small airways disease of smokers in two ways. First, they increase the local protease burden through the release of a neutrophil elastase, which is elevated in BAL of smokers (43). Second, they increase the oxidant burden by the spontaneous release of oxidants. Another source of oxidants is the cigarette smoke itself. Oxidants contribute to tissue destruction by oxidizing and thereby inactivating important defensive proteins such as alpha-1-proteinase inhibitor. At present, however, it remains controversial whether this occurs in human smokers. Deficient functional alpha-1-proteinase inhibitor activity has been reported in lavage fluid of smokers in some studies, though not in others (44,45). Even a compensatory increase of this inhibitor in lavage fluid of smokers has been demonstrated (46).

Immunologic functions of cells in the lower respiratory tract appear also to be influenced by cigarette smoking (for review see 38). Most likely smoking has a suppressive effect on the pulmonary immune system. The accessory function of alveolar macrophages is diminished in smokers, and the interleukin-1 production by lipopolysaccharide-stimulated macrophages and the mitogenic response of lung lymphocytes are reduced. In parallel, the CD4/CD8 ratio of T cells is decreased and the percentage of $CD57^+$ natural killer subset, as well as the functional natural killer activity, is low in smokers' BAL (47–49). This suppression of the local immune system may be a cofactor for the higher incidence of infections and pulmonary malignancies in smokers.

Chronic Bronchitis

Smokers with chronic bronchitis, defined clinically by the symptoms of chronic cough and sputum production, have increased neutrophils in bronchial and BAL fluid. This increase is much more pronounced in the bronchial than in the bronchoalveolar sample, as demonstrated by Martin and colleagues (50), who separately analyzed the first instilled 50 ml of lavage fluid, and later by Thompson and associates (51), who employed 20-ml aliquots to sample the airways contents. In the proximal "bronchial" sample, smokers with chronic bronchitis have more neutrophils than asymptomatic smokers, both in terms of relative proportions and in terms of absolute numbers. In the distal "alveolar" samples, the difference is seen only in relative proportions but not in absolute numbers, due to the fact that patients with chronic bronchitis tend to have a lower percentage recovery of BAL fluid and a less pronounced increase in total cell counts than asymptomatic smokers (37,48, 51). The mean percentage of neutrophils in lavage fluid of patients with chronic bronchitis ranges from 5 to 15% (37,50,51).

Several studies (48,50,51) indicate that the increase in neutrophils seems to correlate with the functional degree of airflow obstruction. Thompson and coworkers (51) additionally reported an association between airway neutrophilia and sputum production, as well as pack years of cigarettes smoked. A separate study (52) showed that the proportion of goblet cells in the bronchial sample was increased both in asymptomatic smokers and in patients with chronic bronchitis, and correlated with the percent neutrophils.

In a group of patients with chronic bronchitis and pulmonary emphysema, the degree of emphysema was assessed by both computed tomography and diffusing capacity, and elastase burden and antielastase capacity were measured in BAL fluid. Most interestingly, the severity of emphysema correlated directly with the elastase burden and inversely with the elastase inhibitory capacity (53). These data support the protease–antiprotease theory for the pathogenesis of cigarette smoke induced human emphysema.

In agreement with recent recommendations (6), at present there is no indication for the clinical use of BAL in the diagnosis and monitoring of chronic bronchitis because of the lack of specificity of these findings. However, BAL can be safely applied for the investigation of the mechanisms involved in the development of the disease.

Respiratory Bronchiolitis With Interstitial Lung Disease

Respiratory bronchiolitis with interstitial lung disease is caused by cigarette smoking. The pathologic findings include inflammation of the respiratory bronchioles, filling of the bronchiolar lumen and neighbouring alveoli with pigmented macrophages, and associated mild interstitial inflammation and fibrosis (54,55). The clinical course is benign. All patients remain stable or improve after cessation of smoking.

BAL findings are unremarkable and do not differ from asymptomatic healthy smokers. In three patients in whom a BAL was performed, the total cell count was smoker-specifically increased. The cell differentials were normal, with 96, 97, and 94% macrophages; 2, 2, and 3% lymphocytes; and 2, 1, and 3% neutrophils, respectively (54).

Mineral Dust Bronchiolitis

The major pulmonary lesion caused by inhalation of mineral dust is parenchymal fibrosis, either interstitial, as in asbestosis, or nodular, as in silicosis. There is increasing evidence, however, that exposure to inorganic dust can also cause small airways disease, the morphologic appearance of which is fibrotic thickening of the walls of the membranes and respiratory bronchioles (56).

There is a lack of reports that specifically address BAL findings in bronchiolitis due to mineral dust. Therefore, in the following, the lavage findings in interstitial lung disease caused by mineral dust exposure is reviewed. In general, BAL can be used to document mineral dust exposure by the detection of dust particles or fibers, either in the cytoplasm of alveolar macrophages or by quantitative asbestos body counting of filtered fluid (6,14). The demonstration of dust in BAL is indicative of exposure but is not evidence of disease. There is currently no known lavage level of particles above which development of disease is inevitable.

Asbestos Dust

Individuals with known exposure to asbestos, but without radiographic or functional signs of interstitial fibrosis, may have abnormal BAL cell differentials. This situation, probably reflecting the early preclinical inflammatory response to asbestos, is termed subclinical alveolitis and occurs in 30 to 50% of asbestos-exposed workers (6,57,58). The predominant finding is a lymphocytic alveolitis, with reported mean values of lavage lymphocytes ranging from 17 to 30% (58–61). Usually, the lymphocyte percentages in asbestos-exposed subjects without interstitial lung disease are higher than in those suffering from manifest asbestosis (6). An additional mild increase in lavage neutrophils is also seen in this subclinical alveolitis.

In patients with asbestosis, a mild neutrophilic alveolitis (neutrophils ranging from 4 to 17% in average) is the characteristic lavage finding, with or without an additional increase in eosinophils and/or lymphocytes. The incidence of an abnormal lavage cell differential is 50 to 80% in asbestosis (57,62–65). The CD4/CD8 ratio is elevated in some subjects with asbestosis or with asbestos exposure (59,66,67). Since the cellular lavage findings are nonspecific, they do not contribute to the diagnosis of asbestosis. Whether they have a prognostic significance is unclear at present.

The quantitative assessment of counting BAL asbestos bodies by vacuum filtration, however, can give useful clinical information in patients with radiographic changes suggestive of asbestos-related disorders and a history of uncertain exposure. A lavage asbestos body count of 1/ml fluid roughly corresponds to a lung asbestos body concentration of 1000/g tissue (18,19). A negative lavage asbestos body count does not exclude asbestos-related disease, however.

A variety of functional studies have been performed with lavage cells to elucidate the pathogenesis of human asbestosis (68). The phagocytosis of asbestos stimulates alveolar macrophages to release chemotactic factors for neutrophils, attracting them to the alveolar spaces (69,70). Activated macrophages play a central role in the progression from asbestos-induced alveolitis to fibrosis by the release of modulators of the extracellular matrix such as plasminogen activator (71), products that mediate injury to parenchymal cells such as oxygen radicals (64), and, finally, mediators that stimulate fibroblast proliferation such as fibronectin and insulin-like growth factor-1 (61,64). The clinical relevance of these interesting insights into the immunopathology remains to be determined, however.

Silica Dust

In coal worker's pneumoconiosis the number of total cells in BAL is increased, and a mild increase in neutrophils with mean percentages of 3 to 6% is seen in about 40% of patients (6,64,72,73). The increase is more pronounced in progressive massive fibrosis than in simple pneumoconiosis (73).

In other forms of silica exposure or disease, mainly mixed-dust pneumoconiosis, or in granite workers, a moderate increase in lymphocytes with mean values ranging from 12 to 26% has been found (6,58,64,74–76). The CD4/CD8 ratio is decreased in silicotic disease (67,76).

Quantification of the alveolar silica-dust burden showed a significantly higher silica level in the BAL of silica-exposed subjects than in unexposed individuals, but there was no difference between subjects with silicosis and those with exposure only and no evidence of disease (77).

Regarding the local immunology of human silicosis, lavage studies in individuals exposed to silica dust revealed that silica-activated macrophages are focal to the pathogenesis of this disease (6). They release neutrophil chemotactic activity, thereby recruiting neutrophils to the alveoli, which in turn release free elastolytic activity (72). In addition, macrophages generate oxygen radicals and toxic enzymes such as proteases and glycosidases, which may mediate injury to lung parenchymal cells (72,73). Furthermore, they secrete fibronectin and other growth factors that are important for fibroblast proliferation and progression of the disease to massive fibrosis (64,75). Finally, alveolar macrophages release proinflammatory cytokines such as interleukin-1, interleukin-6, and tumor necrosis factor (78). Some of these effects may be counterbalanced by the increase in $CD8^+$ suppressor T cells observed in BAL of human silicosis (67,76). As in asbestosis, the clinical impact of these findings for the management of patients with silicosis has yet to be clarified.

Diffuse Panbronchiolitis

Diffuse panbronchiolitis is a chronic diffuse bilateral lung disease that is rare outside Japan (79). Pathologically, it is characterized by a centrilobular lesion with chronic inflammation and accumulation of foamy histiocytes in the walls of respiratory bronchioles and the adjacent alveolar ducts and alveoli (80). An infectious etiology is possible, since patients respond to erythromycin.

Ichikawa and associates (81) performed BAL in 11 patients with this disease and found a very high percentage of neutrophils (mean of 55 ± 24%) with a corresponding decrease in the macrophage portion and no change in other cell types. This finding is similar to acute purulent bronchitis, where the mean proportion of neutrophils is 68 ± 8% (37), and contrasts to chronic bronchitis, where the neutrophils are only moderately increased to mean values of 5 to 15% (37,50,51,81).

Furthermore, neutrophil-derived elastolytic-like activity was found in 9 of 11 patients with diffuse panbronchiolitis, but in only 1 of 11 patients with chronic bronchitis (82). These findings suggest an important role for neutrophils through the release of proteolytic enzymes, such as elastase, in the pathogenesis of diffuse panbronchiolitis. Finally, treatment with erythromycin, but not with ampicillin, significantly reduced the number of neutrophils and elastase activity in lavage fluid and led to a significant improvement in lung function (82).

Bronchiolitis Obliterans (Constrictive Bronchiolitis)

The term bronchiolitis obliterans (without organization) refers to a rare clinical syndrome characterized by progressive airflow obstruction (83–85). The chest radiogram is normal or shows hyperinflation. The most common histologic finding is constrictive bronchiolitis with bronchiolar inflammation, fibrosis, scarring, and stenosis but without the intraluminal plugs or polyps that are found in bronchiolitis obliterans organizing pneumonia (BOOP).

Bronchiolitis obliterans occurs in a variety of settings. It may be idiopathic or seen after fume inhalation, bone marrow or heart–lung transplantation, and in association with connective tissue disorders (86,87).

Reports on BAL findings in constrictive bronchiolitis are limited to idiopathic bronchiolitis and to bronchiolitis obliterans after heart–lung or lung transplantation.

Idiopathic Bronchiolitis Obliterans

Dorinsky and colleagues (88) were the first to report the BAL results in four adults with idiopathic bronchiolitis obliterans. They found that neutrophils comprised 53 ± 13% of the lavage cells, eosinophils 3 ± 3%, and lymphocytes 5 ± 4%. Thus a marked increase in neutrophils, to a similar extent as found in diffuse panbronchiolitis (81), was the characteristic finding. The relevant control groups had far less neutrophils in their lavage fluid, e.g., patients with chronic bronchitis have only 3% and asymptomatic smokers only 1.5%.

In a subsequent paper, the same group of authors (89) extended their study population to 16 adult patients with idiopathic bronchiolitis obliterans. They confirmed the high percentage of lavage neutrophils. In addition, they were able to detect the neutrophil products collagenase and myeloperoxidase in the lavage fluid of these patients, underscoring the possible pathophysiologic role of neutrophils in this disorder.

These authors concluded that in patients who are clinically suspected to have bronchiolitis obliterans, i.e., patients with an accelerated onset of severe obstructive disease with failure to improve after bronchodilators, the findings of a high percentage, greater than 25% of neutrophils in lavage fluid, may be sufficient for a presumptive diagnosis.

Transplant Bronchiolitis Obliterans

Bronchiolitis obliterans after heart–lung or single-lung transplantation is thought to represent chronic transplant rejection. It has emerged as the major complication in long-term lung transplant recipients, developing in as many as 30 to 50% of patients (90,91). Early detection by transbronchial biopsy and aggressive treatment have reduced the incidence to only 8% at Papworth Hospital (92).

BAL in lung transplant recipients has been extensively performed by the Pittsburgh group. Results of lavage cell differentials are not specific for the various kinds of pulmonary complications, and thus have to be interpreted in the context of other data. Bronchiolitis obliterans, or late rejection, as designated by Dauber and coworkers (93), shows as major lavage finding an elevation in the proportion and number of neutrophils (mean 20%), occasionally also of eosinophils. Toronto investigators (94) also observed lavage neutrophilia in progressive bronchiolitis obliterans after heart–lung transplantation. Neutrophilia is also seen in bacterial pneumonia and in acute rejection (93). The presence of lavage neutrophilia without detectable infection is highly suggestive of bronchiolitis obliterans. Cytomegalovirus pneumonia and *Pneumocystis carinii* pneumonia are associated with a lymphocytic alveolitis (93).

A positive primed lymphocyte test (PLT) is strongly associated with bronchiolitis obliterans. In this test, lavage lymphocytes are cultured with donor cells harvested from the spleen or lymph nodes at the time of organ procurement. The test is positive when a brisk proliferative response of lavage lymphocytes occurs. A positive PLT was found at time of diagnosis of bronchiolitis obliterans in 23 of 27 patients (95). In the absence of clinically manifest pulmonary disease, a positive PLT is strongly predictive of the subsequent development of bronchiolitis obliterans. In this regard, PLT was positive in 9 of 23 lavages from clinically stable patients with a negative transbronchial biopsy. About 100 days later, follow-up biopsies showed bronchiolitis obliterans in 7 of the 9 patients who initially were PLT positive (96).

A recent study demonstrated that the donor-specific alloreactivity of lavage lymphocytes in the PLT is directed against donor class I antigens in patients with bronchiolitis obliterans, but against donor class II antigens in those with episodes of acute rejection (97). Most interestingly, during periods of acute infection, donor antigen-specific PLT reactivity was not observed.

The CD4/CD8 ratios of lavage lymphocytes do not correlate with the presence of bronchiolitis obliterans. They tend to decline over time in long-term survivors of lung transplantation, probably as the result of the immunosuppressive treatment (94).

In about 2 to 10% of allogeneic bone marrow transplant recipients, bronchiolitis obliterans may occur and is thought to be related to graft-versus-host disease and to methotrexate therapy (83). BAL studies, however, have not been reported yet in this disorder.

Bronchiolitis Obliterans Organizing Pneumonia

BOOP is a distinct clinicopathologic entity in the spectrum of infiltrative lung diseases. Clinically, the disease is characterized by a preceding flu-like illness and a short history of progressive dyspnea. Radiographically, the typical findings are bilateral patchy peripheral infiltrates. Pathohistologically, the characteristic pattern consists of buds of organization tissue within the lumina of distal bronchioles, alveolar ducts, and adjacent alveoli (98–101). Most cases are idiopathic. The entity is also seen in association with connective-tissue disorders, drug reactions, cocaine inhalation, virus infections, and other conditions (102).

Idiopathic Bronchiolitis Obliterans Organizing Pneumonia

The profile of the BAL cell differentials in idiopathic BOOP has recently been reported by several groups (103–105), with remarkably similar results (Table 6). BAL cytology usually shows a mixed cellularity, with an increase in all cell types, most markedly of lymphocytes, but also of neutrophils and eosinophils. Other features are the frequent presence of foamy macro-

TABLE 6. *BAL features of idiopathic BOOP: comparison of three studies*

	Costabel et al. (103), *n* = 10, mean ± SD	Nagai et al. (104), *n* = 12, alveolar pattern,[a] mean ± SD	King and Mortenson (105), *n* = 11, mean ± SEM
Macrophages, %	39 ± 19	51 ± 27	
Lymphocytes, %	44 ± 19	41 ± 26	23 ± 6
Neutrophils, %	10 ± 13	4 ± 3	14 ± 4
Eosinophils, %	6 ± 8	3 ± 6	5 ± 2
CD4/CD8, ratio	0.6 ± 0.5	1.1 ± 1.1	
$CD57^+$ natural killer cells, %	6 ± 4		
$HLA\text{-}DR^+$ activated T cells, %	16 ± 12		

[a]Nagai et al. analyzed BAL data in different chest radiographic patterns (alveolar, mixed, and interstitial) and found no significant differences among the groups.

phages, mast cells, and plasma cells. In our own study (103), lymphocytosis was present in all patients (Fig. 1), neutrophils were elevated in 4, eosinophils in 8, mast cells in 6, and plasma cells were found in 4 of 10 patients.

Though direct correlation studies between lavage and histology have not been performed, the lavage cytology seems to reflect the histologic and ultrastructural descriptions of the cellular infiltrate in BOOP. The intra-alveolar organizing buds are composed of numerous alveolar macrophages, constantly associated with lymphocytes and plasma cells, and in some cases also with neutrophils, eosinophils, and mast cells (101). The same inflammatory cells are present in the alveolar septa (100,101). The foamy macrophages, as seen in lavage cytology, are also observed in histologic sections (101).

Regarding the lavage lymphocyte subsets in BOOP, the most consistent finding is a decrease in the CD4/CD8 ratio (103,104). Only 1 of our patients had a normal ratio (see Fig. 2). Increased proportions of activated T cells, as evidenced by HLA-DR antigen expression, were seen in 8 of our 10 patients. $CD57^+$ natural killer cells were within the normal range in all our patients (103).

BAL may be of value to distinguish between BOOP and other interstitial lung diseases. The lavage findings in BOOP are most similar to those in hypersensitivity pneumonitis (103,104), with the exception that the $CD57^+$ cell type, characteristically elevated in hypersensitivity pneumonitis (106), is not increased in BOOP. An increase in this cell type favors the diagnosis of hypersensitivity pneumonitis against that of BOOP.

In comparison with idiopathic pulmonary fibrosis, patients with BOOP have higher lymphocyte proportions (103–105). A normal lymphocyte count and a lone increase in neutrophils and/or eosinophils was not seen in any of our patients with BOOP but occurs frequently in those with idiopathic pulmonary fibrosis. The CD4/CD8 ratio is usually not decreased (103,104), and plasma cells are not observed in idiopathic fibrosis.

Chronic eosinophilic pneumonia is another disorder that has to be considered in the differential diagnosis of BOOP. In this regard, the eosinophils in BAL have a higher discriminative value. In our nine cases with chronic eosinophilic pneumonia, lavage eosinophils always exceeded 20%. This was true in only one patient with BOOP. In addition, patients with eosinophilic pneumonia usually have higher eosin-

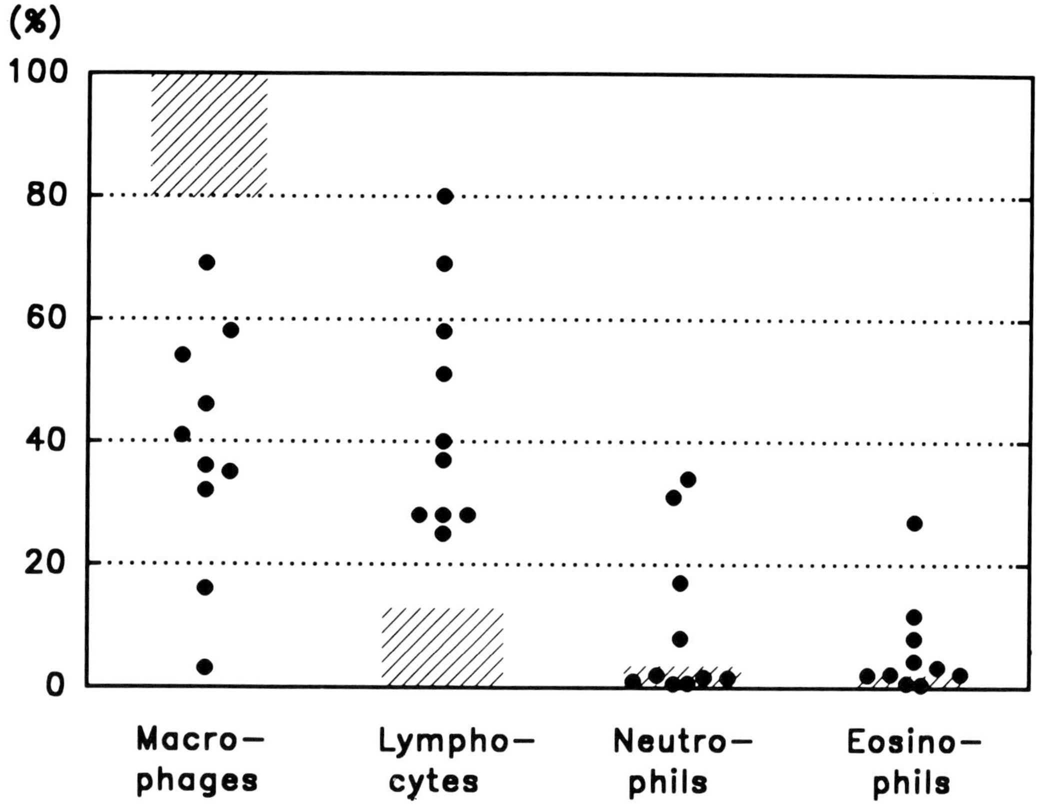

FIG. 1. BAL cell differentials in BOOP. The hatched area represents the normal range. (Reprinted with permission from ref. 103.)

ophil than lymphocyte percentages, whereas in BOOP the lymphocyte percentages are higher than the eosinophil counts (103,104).

Sarcoidosis represents no problem in the lavage differential diagnosis versus BOOP, since active patients with symptomatic sarcoidosis have high CD4/CD8 ratios, whereas this ratio is decreased in those with BOOP.

Thus, BAL may be of considerable value in the clinical evaluation of patients with BOOP. In a patient presenting with typical symptoms and clinical findings and with patchy peripheral infiltrates, after infection has been excluded by a sterile lavage fluid, a lavage cell profile with more than 20% lymphocytes, between 2 and 25% eosinophils, a CD4/CD8 ratio less than 1.0, and $CD57^+$ cells in the normal range, is highly suggestive of idiopathic BOOP and may warrant a therapeutical trial of corticosteroid therapy.

Serial lavage performed in seven patients with idiopathic BOOP revealed that, after 3 to 6 months of corticosteroid treatment, only two patients had achieved completely normal lavage findings, whereas all showed complete radiographic clearing, and three had mild residual restriction (107). The most consistent BAL pathology after this follow-up period was the constant decrease in the CD4/CD8 ratio. The results of this study give support to the idea that corticosteroid therapy should be given for longer than 6 months to prevent early relapse of the disease.

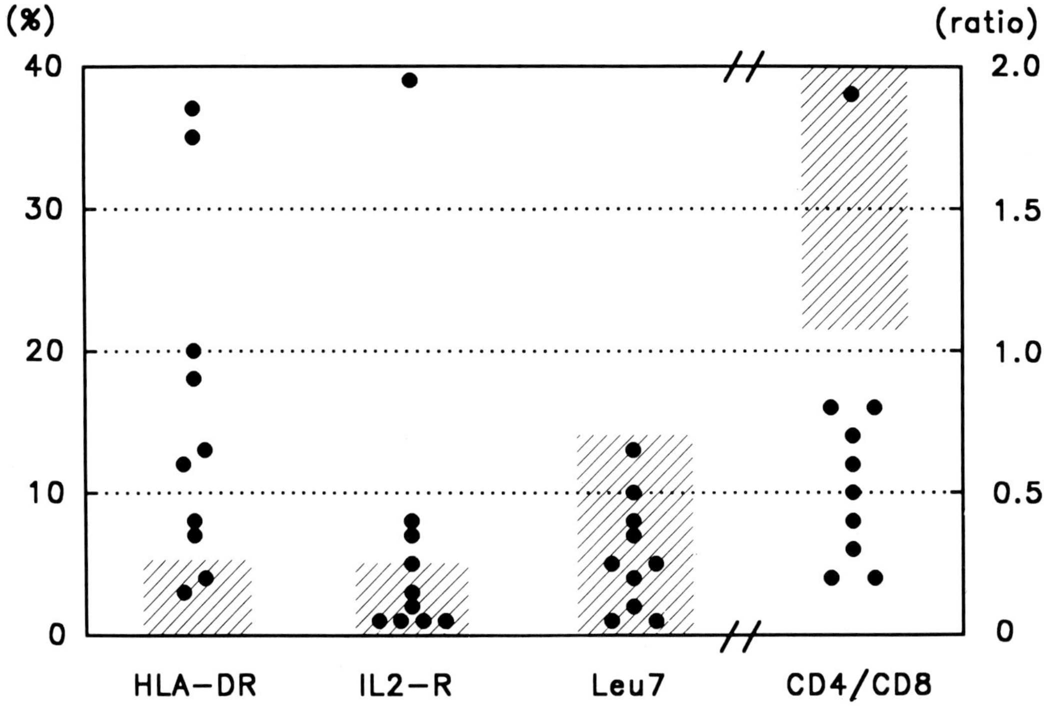

FIG. 2. BAL lymphocyte subsets in BOOP. The hatched area represent the normal range. Shown is the surface marker expression as percentage of lymphocytes and the CD4/CD8 ratio. HLA-DR, activated T cells; IL2-R, interleukin-2 receptor (CD25) positive T cells; Leu7 (CD57), natural killer cells. (Reprinted with permission from ref. 103.)

Bronchiolitis Obliterans Organizing Pneumonia in Association with Other Conditions

Reports on BAL cytology in nonidiopathic BOOP are rare. Camus and associates (108) found an increase in neutrophils in two patients with drug-associated BOOP. A patient with acebutolol intake had 15% neutrophils, and another with amiodarone toxicity had 80% neutrophils. This is clearly different from idiopathic BOOP and resembles more the lavage findings seen in patients with constrictive bronchiolitis obliterans.

BAL cell differentials in a patient with BOOP and HIV infection showed 48% lymphocytes, 5% neutrophils, and 1% eosinophils (109), and in a patient with BOOP after bone marrow transplantation and cytomegalovirus pneumonia, 45% lymphocytes and 15% neutrophils (110). Thus, in these two cases there was a lymphocytic predominance similar to that in idiopathic BOOP.

REFERENCES

1. Hunninghake GW, Kawanami O, Ferrans VJ, et al. Characterization of the inflammatory and immune effector cells in the lung parenchyma of patients with interstitial lung disease. *Am Rev Respir Dis* 1981;123:407–412.
2. Abe S, Munakata M, Nishimura M, et al. Gallium-67 scintigraphy, bronchoalveolar lavage, and pathologic changes in patients with pulmonary sarcoidosis. *Chest* 1984;85:650–655.
3. Semenzato G, Chilosi M, Ossi E, et al. Bronchoalveolar lavage and lung histology: comparative analysis of inflammatory and immunocompetent cells in patients with sarcoidosis and hypersensitivity pneumonitis. *Am Rev Respir Dis* 1985;132:400–404.
4. Campbell DA, Poulter LW, duBois RM. Immunocompetent cells in bronchoalveolar la-

vage reflect the cell populations in transbronchial biopsies in pulmonary sarcoidosis. *Am Rev Respir Dis* 1985;132:1300–1306.
5. Paradis IL, Dauber JH, Rabin BS. Lymphocyte phenotypes in bronchoalveolar lavage and lung tissue in sarcoidosis and idiopathic pulmonary fibrosis. *Am Rev Respir Dis* 1986;133:855–860.
6. Klech H, Hutter C, Costabel U, eds. Clinical guidelines and indications for bronchoalveolar lavage: report of the European Society of Pneumology Task Group on BAL. *Eur Respir Rev* 1992;2:47–127.
7. Klech H, Pohl W, eds. Technical recommendations and guidelines for bronchoalveolar lavage: report of the European Society of Pneumology Task Group on BAL. *Eur Respir J* 1989;2:561–585.
8. American Thoracic Society. Clinical role of bronchoalveolar lavage in adults with pulmonary disease. *Am Rev Respir Dis* 1990;142:481–486.
9. Costabel U. Bronchoalveolar lavage: a standardized procedure or a technical dilemma? *Eur Respir J* 1991;4:776–777.
10. Helmers RA, Dayton CS, Floerchinger C, Hunninghake GW. Bronchoalveolar lavage in interstitial lung disease: effect of volume of fluid infused. *J Appl Physiol* 1989;67:1443–1446.
11. Garcia JGN, Wolven RG, Garcia PL, Keogh BA. Assessment of interlobar variation of bronchoalveolar lavage cellular differentials in interstitial lung diseases. *Am Rev Respir Dis* 1986;133:444–449.
12. Peterson MW, Nugent KM, Jolles H, Monick M, Hunninghake GW. Uniformity of bronchoalveolar lavage in patients with sarcoidosis. *Am Rev Respir Dis* 1988;137:799–784.
13. Schmekel B, Blom-Bülow B, Hörnblad Y, Laitinen LA, Linden M, Venge P. Granulocytes and their secretory products, myeloperoxidase and eosinophil cationic protein, in bronchoalveolar lavage fluid from two lung lobes in normal subjects. *Eur Respir J* 1991;4:867–871.
14. Teschler H, Konietzko N, Schoenfeld B, Ramin C, Schraps T, Costabel U. Distribution of asbestos bodies in the human lung as determined by bronchoalveolar lavage. *Am Rev Respir Dis* 1993;147:1211–1215.
15. Rennard SI, Ghafouri M, Thompson AB, et al. Fractional processing of sequential bronchoalveolar lavage to separate bronchial and alveolar samples. *Am Rev Respir Dis* 1990;141:208–217.
16. Strumpf IJ, Feld MK, Cornelius MJ, Keogh BA, Crystal RG. Safety of fiberoptic bronchoalveolar lavage in evaluation of interstitial lung disease. *Chest* 1981;80:268–271.
17. Dhillon DP, Haslam PL, Townsend PJ, Primett Z, Collins JV, Turner-Warwick M. Bronchoalveolar lavage in patients with interstitial lung diseases: side effects and factors affecting fluid recovery. *Eur J Respir Dis* 1986;68:342–350.
18. Sebastian P, Armstrong B, Monchaux G, Bignon J. Asbestos bodies in bronchoalveolar lavage fluid and in lung parenchyma. *Am Rev Respir Dis* 1988;137:75–78.
19. De Vuyst P, Dumortier P, Moulin E, et al. Asbestos bodies in bronchoalveolar lavage reflect lung asbestos body concentration. *Eur Respir J* 1988;1:362–367.
20. Low RB, Cutroneo KR, Davis GS, Giancola MS. Lavage type III procollagen N-terminal peptides in human pulmonary fibrosis and sarcoidosis. *Lab Invest* 1983;48:755–759.
21. Hällgren R, Eklund A, Engström-Laurent A, Schmekel B. Hyaluronate in bronchoalveolar lavage fluid: a new marker in sarcoidosis reflecting pulmonary disease. *Br Med J* 1985; 290:1778–1781.
22. Rennard SI, Crystal RG. Fibronectin in bronchopulmonary lavage fluid: elevation in patients with interstitial lung disease. *J Clin Invest* 1981;69:113–122.
23. Pohl WR, Conlan MG, Thompson AB, et al. Vitronectin in bronchoalveolar lavage fluid is increased in patients with interstitial lung disease. *Am Rev Respir Dis* 1991;143:1369–1375.
24. O'Connor C, Ward K, van Breda A, McIlgorm A, FitzGerald MX. Type 3 procollagen peptide in bronchoalveolar lavage fluid: poor indicator of course and prognosis in sarcoidosis. *Chest* 1989;96:339–344.
25. O'Connor C, Odlum C, van Breda A, Power C, FitzGerald MX. Collagenase and fibronectin in bronchoalveolar lavage fluid of patients with sarcoidosis. *Thorax* 1988;43:393–400.
26. Ward K, O'Connor CM, Odlum C, Power C, Fitzgerlad MX. Pulmonary disease progress in sarcoid patients with and without bronchoalveolar lavage collagenase. *Am Rev Respir Dis* 1990;142:636–641.
27. Walters EH, Gardiner PV. Bronchoalveolar lavage as a research tool. *Thorax* 1991;46:613–618.
28. Stover DE, Zaman MB, Hajdu SI, et al. Bronchoalveolar lavage in the diagnosis of diffuse pulmonary infiltrates in the immunosuppressed host. *Ann Intern Med* 1984;101:1–7.
29. Milleron BJ, Costabel U, Teschler H, et al. Bronchoalveolar lavage cell data in alveolar proteinosis. *Am Rev Respir Dis* 1991;144:1330–1332.
30. Allen JN, Davis WB, Pacht ER. Diagnostic significance of increased bronchoalveolar lavage fluid eosinophils. *Am Rev Respir Dis* 1990; 142:642–647.
31. Costabel U, Zaiss AW, Guzman J. Sensitivity and specificity of BAL findings in sarcoidosis. *Sarcoidosis* 1992;9[Suppl 1]:211–214.
32. Haslam PL, Turton CWG, Lukoszek A, et al. Bronchoalveolar lavage fluid cell counts in cryptogenic fibrosing alveolitis and their relation to therapy. *Thorax* 1980;35:328–339.
33. Gilbert SR, Hunninghake GW. Sarcoidosis. In: Baughman RP, ed. *Bronchoalveolar lavage*. St. Louis: Mosby–Year Book; 1992:93–115.
34. Hogg JC, Macklem PT, Thurlbeck WM. Site and nature of airway obstruction in chronic obstructive lung disease. *N Engl J Med* 1968; 278:1355–1360.
35. Cosio M, Ghezzo H, Hogg JC, et al. The rela-

tions between structural changes in small airways and pulmonary-function tests. *N Engl J Med* 1977;298:1277–1281.
36. BAL Cooperative Group. Bronchoalveolar lavage constituents in healthy individuals, idiopathic pulmonary fibrosis, and selected comparison groups. *Am Rev Respir Dis* 1990;141: S169–202.
37. Maier KL, Leuschel L, Costabel U. Increased oxidized methionine residues in BAL fluid proteins in acute or chronic bronchitis. *Eur Respir J* 1992;5:651–658.
38. Costabel U, Guzman J. Effect of smoking on bronchoalveolar lavage constituents. *Eur Respir J* 1992;5:776–779.
39. Fels AOS, Cohn ZA. The alveolar macrophage. *J Appl Physiol* 1986;60:353–369.
40. Holt PG. Immune and inflammatory function in cigarette smokers. *Thorax* 1987;42:241–249.
41. Hunninghake GW, Crystal RG. Cigarette smoking and lung destruction. *Am Rev Respir Dis* 1983;128:833–838.
42. Robbins RA, Gossman GL, Nelson KJ, Koyama S, Thompson AB, Rennard SI. Inactivation of chemotactic factor inactivator by cigarette smoke. *Am Rev Respir Dis* 1990;142: 763–768.
43. Janoff A, Raju L, Dearing R. Levels of elastase activity in bronchoalveolar lavage fluid of healthy smokers and nonsmokers. *Am Rev Respir Dis* 1983;127:540–544.
44. Gadek JE, Fells GA, Crystal RG. Cigarette smoking induces functional antiprotease deficiency in the lower respiratory tract of humans. *Science* 1979;206:1315–1316.
45. Stone PJ, Calore JD, McGowen SE, Bernardo J, Snider GL, Franzblau C. Functional alpha-1-protease inhibitor in the lower respiratory tract of cigarette smokers is not decreased. *Science* 1983;221:1187–1189.
46. Stockley RA, Morrison HM. Elastase inhibitors of the respiratory tract. *Eur Respir J* 1990;3[Suppl 9]:9s–15s.
47. Costabel U, Bross KJ, Reuter C, Rühle KH, Matthys H. Alterations in immunoregulatory T-cell subsets in cigarette smokers. *Chest* 1986; 90:39–44.
48. Costabel U, Maier K. Teschler H, Wang YM. Local immune components in chronic obstructive pulmonary disease. *Respiration* 1992;59 [Suppl 1]:17–19.
49. Takeuchi M, Nagai S, Izumi T. Effect of smoking on natural killer cell activity in the lung. *Chest* 1988;94:688–693.
50. Martin TR, Raghu G, Maunder RJ, Springmeyer SC. The effects of chronic bronchitis and chronic air-flow obstruction on lung cell populations recovered by bronchoalveolar lavage. *Am Rev Respir Dis* 1985;132:254–260.
51. Thompson AB, Daughton D, Robbins RA, Ghafouri MA, Oehlerking M, Rennard SI. Intraluminal airway inflammation in chronic bronchitis. *Am Rev Respir Dis* 1989;140:1527–1537.
52. Spurzem JR, Thompson AB, Daughton DM, Mueller M, Linder J, Rennard SI. Chronic inflammation is associated with an increased proportion of goblet cells recovered by bronchial lavage. *Chest* 1991;100:389–393.
53. Fujita J, Nelson NL, Daughton DM, et al. Evaluation of elastase and antielastase balance in patients with chronic bronchitis and pulmonary emphysema. *Am Rev Respir Dis* 1990; 142:57–62.
54. Myers JL, Veal CF, Shin MS, Katzenstein AA. Respiratory bronchiolitis causing interstitial lung disease. *Am Rev Respir Dis* 1987;135:880–884.
55. Yousem SA, Colby TV, Gaensler EA. Respiratory bronchiolitis-associated interstitial lung disease and its relationship to desquamative interstitial pneumonia. *Mayo Clin Proc* 1989; 64:1373–1380.
56. Churg A, Wright JL. Small airways disease and mineral dust exposure. *Pathol Annu* 1983;18: 233–251.
57. Hayes AA, Mullan B, Lovegrove FT, Rose AH, Musk AW, Robinson BW. Gallium lung scanning and bronchoalveolar lavage in crocidolite-exposed workers. *Chest* 1989;96:22–26.
58. Costabel U, Teschler H. Inflammation and immune reactions in interstitial lung disease associated with inorganic dust exposure. *Eur Respir J* 1990;3:363–364.
59. Wallace JM, Oishi JS, Barbers RG, Batra P, Aberle DR. Bronchoalveolar lavage cell and lymphocyte phenotype profiles in healthy asbestos-exposed shipyard workers. *Am Rev Respir Dis* 1989;139:33–38.
60. Spurzem JR, Saltini C, Rom W, Winchester RJ, Crystal RG. Mechanisms of macrophage accumulation in the lungs of asbestos exposed subjects. *Am Rev Respir Dis* 1987;136:276–280.
61. Begin R, Martel M, Desmarais Y, et al. Fibronectin and procollagen 3 levels in bronchoalveolar lavage of asbestos-exposed human subjects and sheep. *Chest* 1986;89:237–243.
62. Gellert AR, Langford JA, Winter RJD, Uthayakumar S, Sinha G, Rudd RM. Asbestosis: assessment by bronchoalveolar lavage and measurement of pulmonary epithelial permeability. *Thorax* 1985;40:508–514.
63. Robinson BWS, Rose AH, James A, Whitaker D, Musk AW. Alveolitis of pulmonary asbestosis. *Chest* 1986;90:396–402.
64. Rom WN, Bitterman PB, Rennard SI, Cantin A, Crystal RG. Characterization of the lower respiratory tract inflammation of nonsmoking individuals with interstitial lung disease associated with chronic inhalation of inorganic dusts. *Am Rev Respir Dis* 1987;136:1429–1434.
65. Haslam PL, Dewar A, Butchers P, Primett ZS, Newman-Taylor A, Turner-Warwick M. Mast cells, atypical lymphocytes, and neutrophils in bronchoalveolar lavage in extrinsic allergic alveolitis. *Am Rev Respir Dis* 1987;135:353–47.
66. Delclos GL, Flitcraft DG, Brousseau KP, et al. Bronchoalveolar lavage analysis, gallium-67

lung scanning and soluble interleukin-2 receptors in asbestos exposure. *Environ Res* 1989; 48:164–178.
67. Costabel U, Bross KJ, Huck E, Guzman J, Matthys H. Lung and blood lymphocyte subsets in asbestosis and in mixed dust pneumoconiosis. *Chest* 1987;91:110–112.
68. Rom WN, Travis WD, Brody AR. Cellular and molecular basis of the asbestos-related diseases. *Am Rev Respir Dis* 1991;143:408–422.
69. Hayes AA, Rose AH, Musk AW, Robinson BWS. Neutrophil chemotactic factor release and neutrophil alveolitis in asbestos-exposed individuals. *Chest* 1988;94:521–525.
70. Garcia JGN, Griffith DE, Cohen AB, Callan KS. Alveolar macrophages from patients with asbestos exposure release increased levels of leukotriene B4. *Am Rev Respir Dis* 1989; 139:1494–1501.
71. Cantin A, Allard C, Begin R. Increased alveolar plasminogen activator in early asbestosis. *Am Rev Respir Dis* 1989;139:604–609.
72. Scharfman A, Hayem A, Davril M, Hannothiaux MH, Lafitte JJ. Special neutrophil elastase inhibitory activity in BAL fluid from patients with silicosis and asbestosis. *Eur Respir J* 1989;2:751–757.
73. Wallaert B, Lassalle Ph, Fortin F, et al. Superoxide anion generation by alveolar inflammatory cells in simple pneumoconiosis and progressive massive fibrosis of nonsmoking coal workers. *Am Rev Respir Dis* 1990;141:129–133.
74. Christman JW, Emerson RJ, Graham WGB, Davis GS. Mineral dust and cell recovery from the bronchoalveolar lavage of healthy Vermont granite workers. *Am Rev Respir Dis* 1985;132: 393–399.
75. Begin R, Cantin A, Boileau RD, Bisson GY. Spectrum of alveolitis in quartz-exposed human subjects. *Chest* 1987;92:1061–1076.
76. Araujo AT, Alfarrabo E, Freitas e Costa M. The role of monoclonal antibodies in the study of chronic inflammatory respiratory diseases induced by dust inhalation. *Eur J Respir Dis* 1986;69[Suppl 146]:203–210.
77. Lusuardi M, Capelli A, Donner CF, Capelli O, Velluti G. Semi-quantitative x-ray microanalysis of bronchoalveolar lavage samples from silica-exposed and nonexposed subjects. *Eur Respir J* 1992;5:798–803.
78. Gosset P, Lasalle P, Vanhée D, et al. Production of tumor necrosis factor-alpha and interleukin-6 by human alveolar macrophages exposed *in vitro* to coal mine dust. *Am J Respir Cell Mol Biol* 1991;5:431–436.
79. Homma H, Yamanaka A, Tanimoto S, et al. Diffuse panbronchiolitis: a disease of the transitional zone of the lung. *Chest* 1983;83:63–69.
80. Kitaichi M. Pathology of diffuse panbronchiolitis from the viewpoint of differential diagnosis. In: Grassi C, Rizzato G, Pozzi E, eds. *Sarcoidosis and other granulomatous disorders*. Amsterdam: Elsevier Science Publishers; 1988: 741–746.
81. Ichikawa Y, Koga H, Tanaka M, Nakamura M, Tokunaga N, Kaji M. Neutrophilia in bronchoalveolar lavage fluid of diffuse panbronchiolitis. *Chest* 1990;98:917–923.
82. Ichikawa Y, Ninomiya H, Koga H, et al. Erythromycin reduces neutrophils and neutrophil-derived elastolytic-like activity in the lower respiratory tract of bronchiolitis patients. *Am Rev Respir Dis* 1992;146:196–203.
83. Wright JL, Cagle P, Churg A, Colby TV, Myers J. State of the art: diseases of the small airways. *Am Rev Respir Dis* 1992;146:240–262.
84. Geddes DM, Corrin B, Brewerton DA, Davies RJ, Turner-Warwick M. Progressive airway obliteration in adults and its association with rheumatoid disease. *Q J Med* 1977;46:427–444.
85. Turton CW, Williams G, Green M. Cryptogenic obliterative bronchiolitis in adults. *Thorax* 1981; 36:805–810.
86. King TE. Bronchiolitis obliterans. *Lung* 1989; 167:69–93.
87. du Bois RM, Geddes DM. Obliterative bronchiolitis, cryptogenic organising pneumonitis and bronchiolitis obliterans organizing pneumonia: three names for two different conditions. *Eur Respir J* 1991;4:774–775.
88. Dorinsky PM, Davis WB, Lucas JG, Weiland JE, Gadek JE. Adult bronchiolitis: evaluation by bronchoalveolar lavage and response to prednisone therapy. *Chest* 1985;88:58–63.
89. Kindt GC, Weiland JE, Davis WB, Gadek JE, Dorinsky PM. Bronchiolitis in adults: a reversible cause of airway obstruction associated with airway neutrophils and neutrophil products. *Am Rev Respir Dis* 1989;140:483–492.
90. Burke CM, Theodore J, Dawkins KD, et al. Post-transplant obliterative bronchiolitis and other late lung sequelae in human heart–lung transplantation. *Chest* 1984;86:824–829.
91. Griffith BP, Hardesty RL, Trento A, et al. Heart–lung transplantation: lessons learned and future hopes. *Ann Thorac Surg* 1987;43:6–16.
92. Higenbottam TW. Lung rejection after transplantation. *Eur Respir J* 1989;2:1–2.
93. Dauber JH, Paradis IL, Duncan SR, Yousem SA. Pulmonary transplantation. In: Baughman RP, ed. *Bronchoalveolar lavage*. St. Louis: Mosby–Year Book; 1992:64–89.
94. Maurer JR, Gough E, Chamberlain DW, Patterson GA, Grossman RF. Sequential bronchoalveolar lavage studies from patients undergoing double lung and heart–lung transplant. *Transplant Proc* 1989;21:2585–2587.
95. Keenan RJ, Lega ME, Dummer JS, et al. Cytomegalovirus serologic status and postoperative infection correlated with risk of developing chronic rejection after pulmonary transplantation. *Transplantation* 1991;51:433–438.
96. Rabinowich H, Zeevi A, Yousem SA, et al. Alloreactivity of lung biopsy and bronchoalveolar lavage-derived lymphocytes from pulmonary transplant recipients: correlation with acute re-

jection and bronchiolitis obliterans. *Clin Transplant* 1990;4:376.
97. Reinsmoen NL, Bolman RM, Savik K, Butters K, Hertz M. Differentiation of class I- and class II-directed donor-specific alloreactivity in bronchoalveolar lavage lymphocytes from lung transplant recipients. *Transplantation* 1992;53:181–189.
98. Epler GR, Colby TV, McLoud TC, Carrington CB, Gaensler EA. Bronchiolitis obliterans organizing pneumonia. *N Engl J Med* 1985; 312:152–158.
99. Cordier JF, Loire R, Brune J. Idiopathic bronchiolitis obliterans organizing pneumonia. *Chest* 1989;96:999–1004.
100. Myers JL, Katzenstein AA. Ultrastructural evidence of alveolar epithelial injury in idiopathic bronchiolitis obliterans organizing pneumonia. *Am J Pathol* 1988;132:102–109.
101. Peyrol S, Cordier JF, Grimaud JA. Intra-alveolar fibrosis of idiopathic bronchiolitis obliterans organizing pneumonia. *Am J Pathol* 1990; 137:155–170.
102. Costabel U, Guzman J. BOOP: what is old, what is new? *Eur Respir J* 1991;4:771–773.
103. Costabel U, Teschler H, Guzman J. Bronchiolitis obliterans organizing pneumonia (BOOP): the cytological and immunocytological profile of bronchoalveolar lavage. *Eur Respir J* 1992; 5:791–797.
104. Nagai S, Aung H, Tanaka S, et al. Bronchoalveolar lavage cell findings in patients with BOOP and related diseases. *Chest* 1992;102: 32S–37S.
105. King TE, Mortenson RL. Cryptogenic organizing pneumonitis: the North American experience. *Chest* 1992;102:8S–13S.
106. Semenzato G, Agostini C, Zambello R, et al. Lung T-cells in hypersensitivity pneumonitis: phenotypic and functional analyses. *J Immunol* 1986;137:1164–1172.
107. Teschler H, Nusch A, Schoenfeld B, Hartung W, Konietzko N, Costabel U. Bronchiolitis obliterans organizing pneumonia (BOOP): BAL cytology and immunocytology before and during corticosteroid treatment. *Am Rev Respir Dis* 1991;143:A53.
108. Camus P, Lombard JN, Perrichon M, Piard F, Guerin JCI, Thivolet FB. Bronchiolitis obliterans organizing pneumonia in patients taking acebutolol or amiodarone. *Thorax* 1989;44: 711–715.
109. Allen JN, Wewers MD. HIV-associated bronchiolitis obliterans organizing pneumonia. *Chest* 1989;96:197–198.
110. Chien J, Chan CK, Chamberlain D, et al. Cytomegalovirus pneumonia in allogeneic bone marrow transplantation: an immunopathologic process? *Chest* 1990;98:1034–1037.

Diseases of the Bronchioles, edited by
Gary R. Epler. Raven Press, Ltd.,
New York © 1994.

6

Bronchiolar Pathology

Thomas V. Colby

Department of Surgical Pathology, Mayo Clinic, 200 First St., Rochester, MN.

Pathologic changes in the bronchioles, including bronchiolitis and related lesions, are inextricably tied to the clinical circumstances with which they are associated. Any discussion of these conditions requires clinicopathologic correlation, and the chapters in this book take such an approach. In some cases a given pathologic finding is unique (or nearly so) to a specific condition, such as respiratory bronchiolitis in cigarette smokers, but in most cases a given pathologic change in the bronchioles is associated with many conditions, and ascribing etiology and pathogenesis requires clinical correlation. This is because the number and pattern of bronchiolar responses to injury are limited.

This chapter reviews pathologic patterns of bronchiolar injury and repair. Because of the scope of this book, some patterns, though extremely important clinically, such as asthma and chronic bronchitis/emphysema, are not discussed in great detail.

Bronchiolar pathology can be grouped as in Table 1. There is considerable overlap among the groups in Table 1, and for convenience some of the patterns listed are defined clinicopathologically, whereas others are primarily histologic patterns.

Each of the groups in Table 1 includes a spectrum of changes and at the ends of the spectrum in each group there may be overlap with other groups; for example, cellular infiltrates involving bronchioles (cellular bronchiolitis) are seen in asthma and chronic bronchitis/emphysema, and mucostasis is found in asthma, chronic bronchitis/emphysema, and the airways in constrictive bronchiolitis. The groupings in Table 1 are also not static; there may be evolution from one group to another, for example, cellular bronchiolitis, which may be associated with slow progression to bronchiolitis obliterans with intraluminal polyps or constrictive bronchiolitis.

The groupings in Table 1 are based on the morphologically dominant changes. Asthma and chronic bronchitis/emphysema are well recognized and characterized and are kept as separate groups rather than under the generic heading of cellular bronchiolitis, which includes a variety of less common conditions.

The histologic terminology of bronchiolar disease is confusing, and similar terms have often been used for different lesions. The approach used in this chapter is primarily descriptive and based on the morphologic changes, which are put into clinicopathologic focus in later chapters.

ASTHMATIC-TYPE CHANGES

The histologic changes of asthma are well known and derived primarily from studies of fatal asthma (status asthmaticus) (1,2). The changes described include mucus stasis and plugging, bronchiolar epithelial sloughing, luminal and mural eosinophils, eosino-

TABLE 1. *Spectrum of bronchiolar pathology*

Asthmatic-type changes
Chronic bronchitis/emphysema-associated bronchiolar changes
Cellular bronchiolitis (acute, chronic, with or without fibrosis)
Subtypes: follicular bronchiolitis, diffuse panbronchiolitis
Respiratory bronchiolitis
Bronchiolitis obliterans
Subtypes: bronchiolitis obliterans with intraluminal polyps, constrictive bronchiolitis
Mineral dust associated airway disease
Peribronchiolar fibrosis and bronchiolar metaplasia

phil debris, submucosal edema, smooth muscle hypertrophy, goblet cell hyperplasia, bronchial gland hypertrophy, and hyaline thickening of the basement membrane region. Other inflammatory cells, including lymphocytes and neutrophils, may be part of the infiltrate of asthma. The net effect of all these changes is luminal narrowing and airflow obstruction.

In patients with nonfatal asthma or in tissue that becomes available between asthmatic attacks, the above changes may be considerably muted or even lacking. This is not surprising since asthma is a reversible condition. The spectrum of histologic changes seen in nonfatal asthma include entirely normal bronchiolar histology, subtle increases in the smooth muscle and basement membrane layer, goblet cell hyperplasia, and mild inflammatory infiltrates occasionally with mucus stasis in small airways. A small percentage of patients show chronic changes including bronchiolar and peribronchiolar scarring. Although there is some overlap of the changes of asthma with other conditions, the most distinctive his-

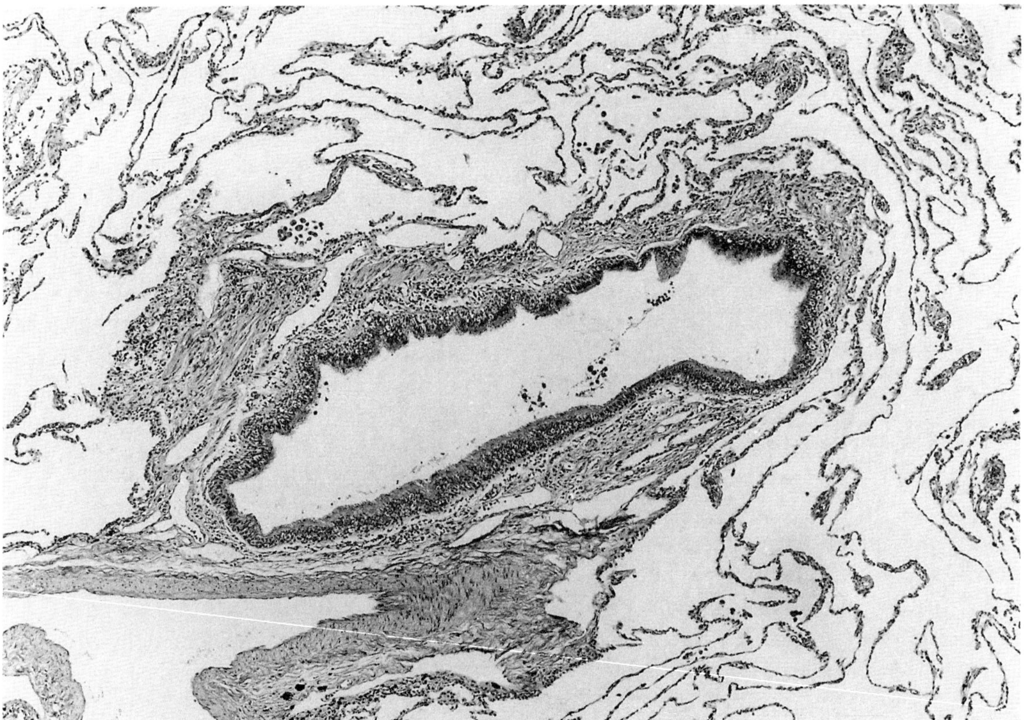

FIG. 1. Emphysema. Mild bronchiolar inflammation and ectasia are seen in this membranous bronchiole from a patient with emphysema associated $alpha_1$ antitrypsin deficiency. There is a mild cellular bronchiolitis with bronchiolectasis.

tologic features are the eosinophils, the thickening of the basement membrane zone, and hypertrophy of the smooth muscle.

CHRONIC BRONCHITIS/EMPHYSEMA ASSOCIATED BRONCHIOLAR CHANGES

The functional changes associated with chronic bronchitis and emphysema are much better known, more extensively studied, and much more dramatic than the morphologic changes in the small airways (Fig. 1). Collectively, the term "small airways disease" has been used for the functional changes ascribed to the bronchioles in this setting. The histologic changes have recently been the subject of study, and grading systems have been developed (3).

The morphologic changes in the small airways of patients with chronic bronchitis and emphysema can be broadly grouped as follows:

1. *Inflammatory changes:* chronic inflammatory infiltrate in the walls of small bronchioles; these changes overlap with respiratory bronchiolitis.
2. *Fibrotic changes:* fibrosis of the bronchiolar wall may be subtle, but it is partly responsible for the liminal changes.
3. *Luminal changes:* the small airways in chronic bronchitis/emphysema frequently show mucus plugging and luminal distortion. Bronchioles may be ectatic or narrowed and constricted with an apparent rigidity to their walls; in this regard there is overlap with constrictive bronchiolitis.

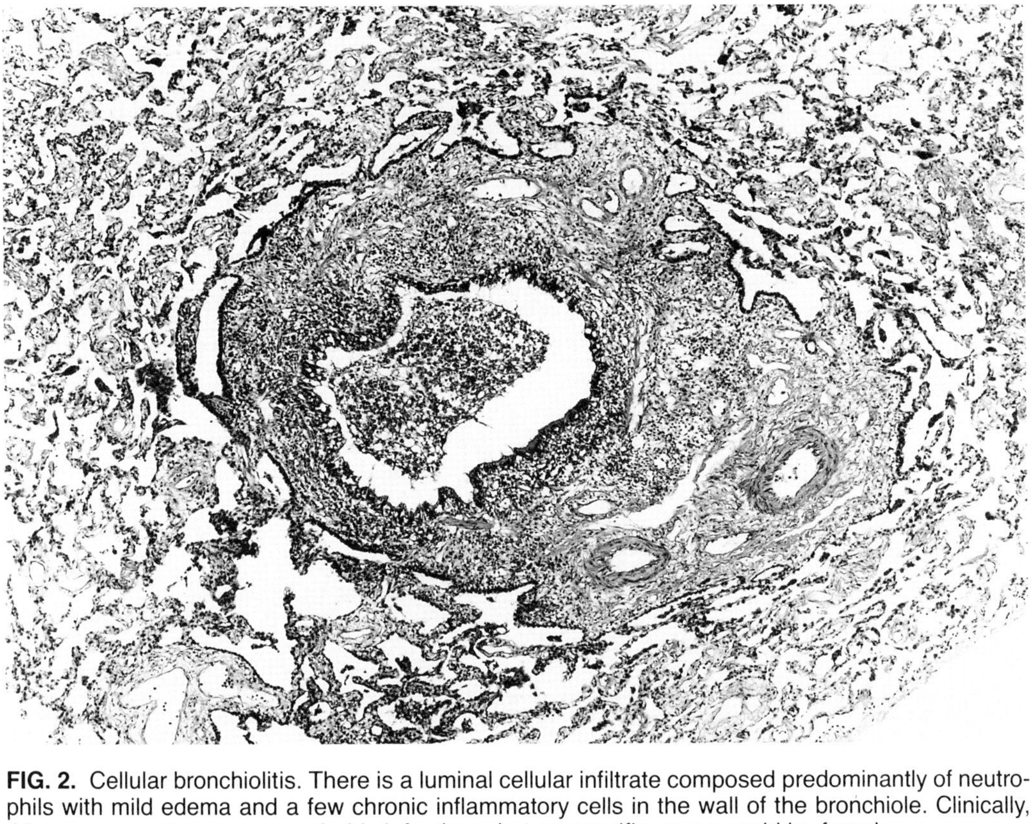

FIG. 2. Cellular bronchiolitis. There is a luminal cellular infiltrate composed predominantly of neutrophils with mild edema and a few chronic inflammatory cells in the wall of the bronchiole. Clinically, this was an acute process, probably infectious, but no specific cause could be found.

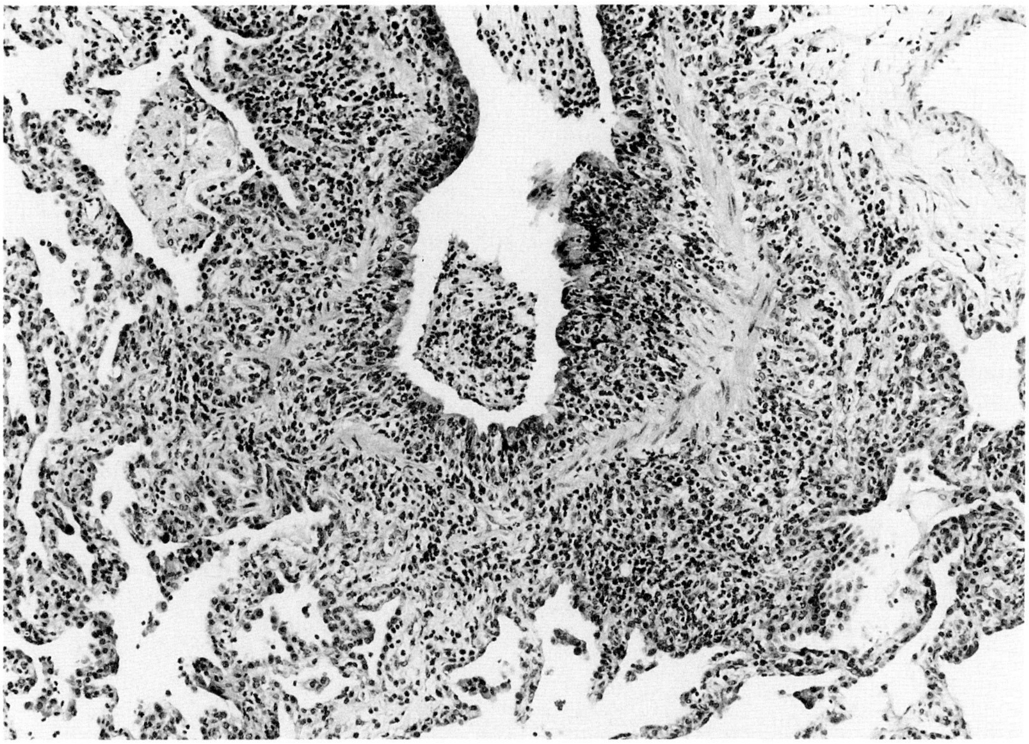

FIG. 3. Acute and chronic cellular bronchiolitis caused by mycoplasma infection. There is a luminal exudate of neutrophils and a chronic inflammatory infiltrate in the submucosa and wall of the bronchiole. The infiltrate is composed of lymphocytes and plasma cells. The normal bronchiolar epithelium has been sloughed and replaced by a low cuboidal metaplastic epithelium.

4. *Loss of radial attachments:* the loss of radial tethering of small airways also causes luminal distortion narrowing and is thought to be one of the explanations why bronchioles collapse and cause airflow obstruction during expiration.

CELLULAR BRONCHIOLITIS

Cellular bronchiolitis (4) is a useful morphologic descriptor for the spectrum of changes seen with inflammatory cellular infiltrates of bronchioles, either luminal or mural or both, particularly in a setting in which an obvious clinical diagnosis is not apparent (Figs. 2–7). Further descriptive modifiers are often helpful: acute or chronic depending on the cell type present, necrotizing if there is evidence of epithelial or mural necrosis of the bronchiole, and follicular if there is associated germinal center hyperplasia. Some degree of mural or peribronchiolar fibrosis is common in cellular

FIG. 4. Cellular bronchiolitis. Necrotizing acute bronchiolitis caused by adenovirus infection. **A,** There is complete necrosis and sloughing of a portion of the bronchiolar epithelium and a luminal exudate rich in neutrophils. The wall shows chronic inflammation with lymphocytes and plasma cells. **B,** Within the exudate where the mucosa has been lost, dark smudge cells, characteristic of adenovirus infection, are apparent.

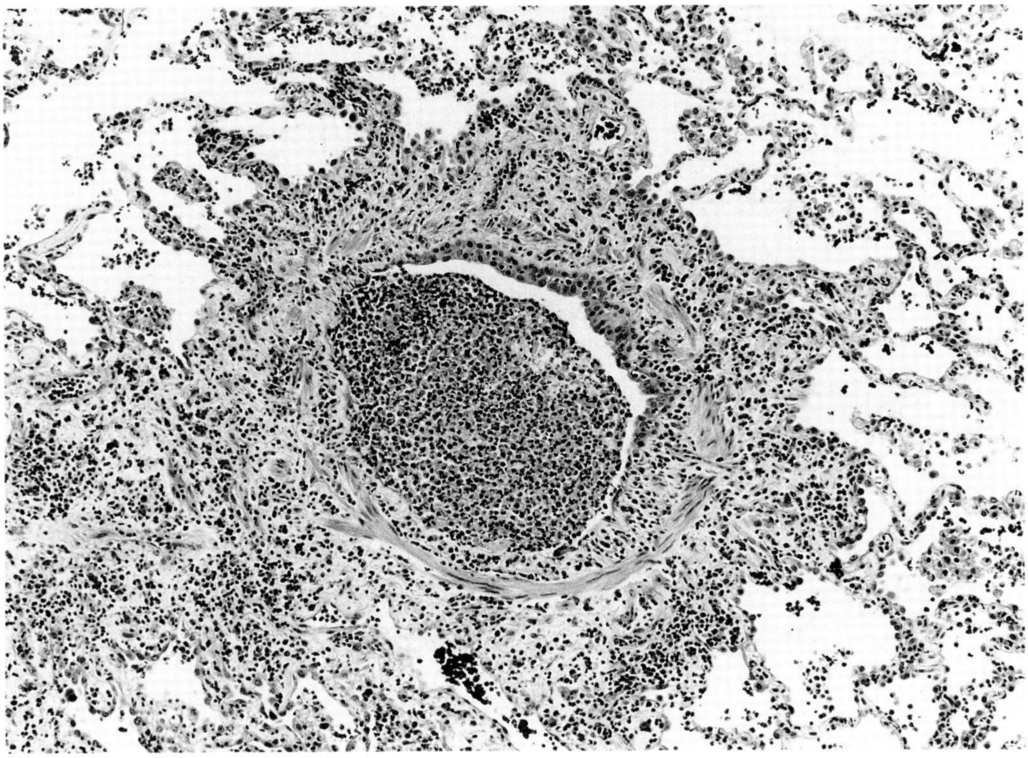

A

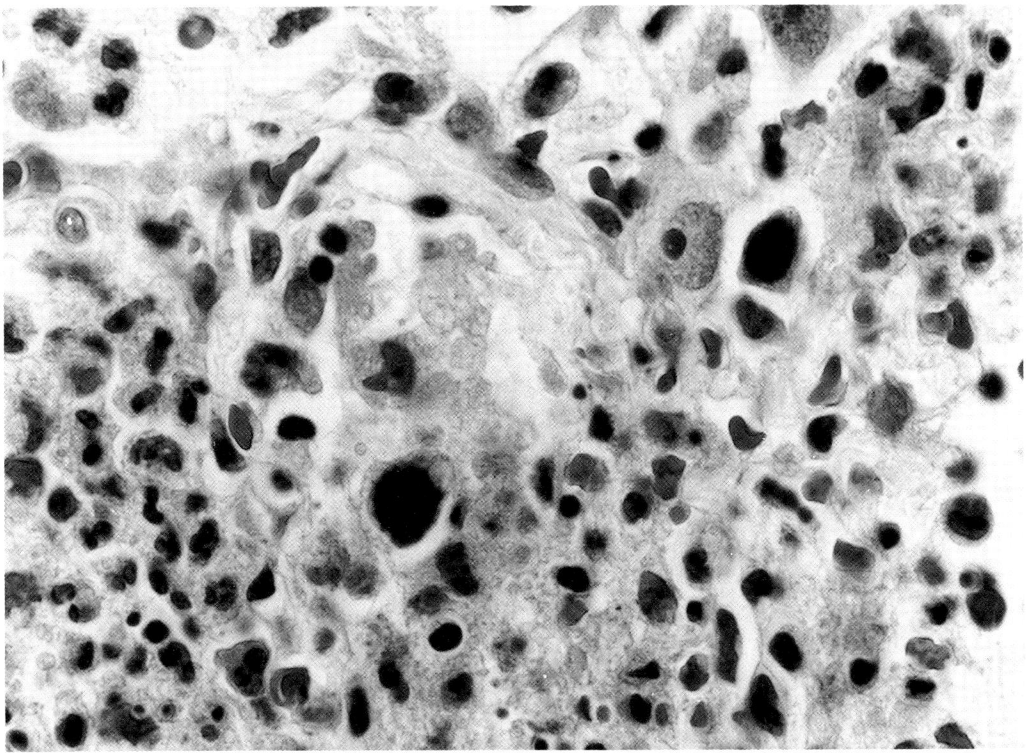

B

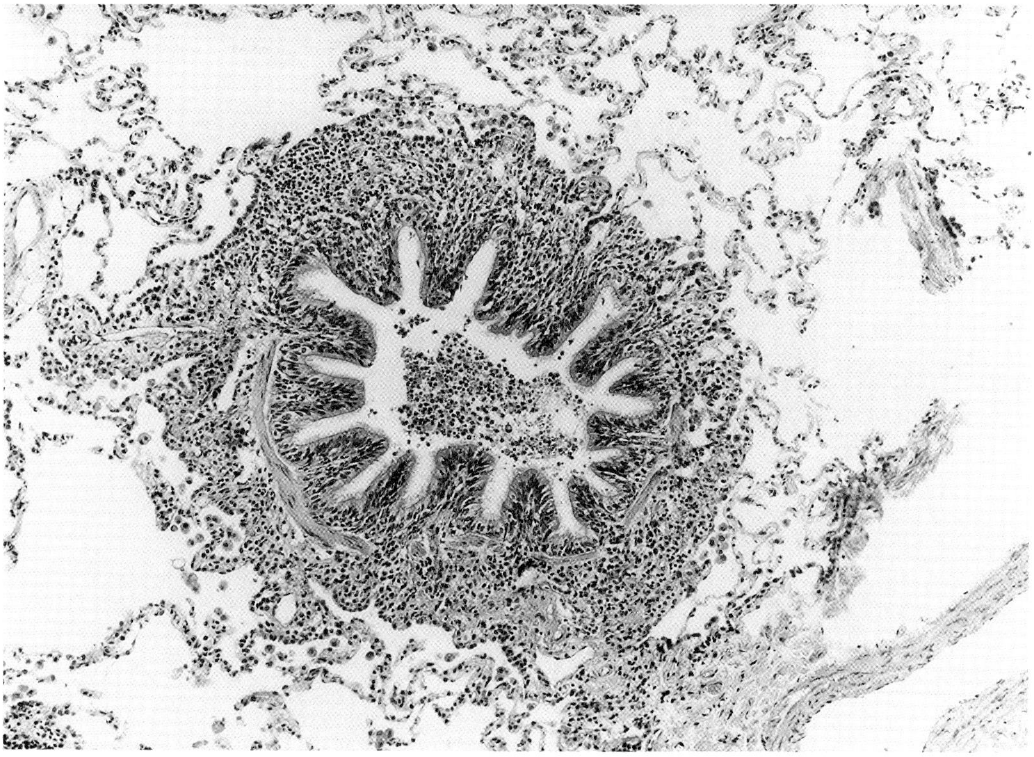

FIG. 5. Acute and chronic cellular bronchiolitis with neutrophils in the lumen and chronic inflammation in the wall. The patient had a history of progressive cough with occasional hemoptysis. Pulmonary functions showed obstruction, and x-ray examination showed reticulonodular infiltrates. The symptoms improved with antibiotics. Such an appearance could be seen with bronchiectasis, acquired immunodeficiencies, connective-tissue diseases, and other conditions.

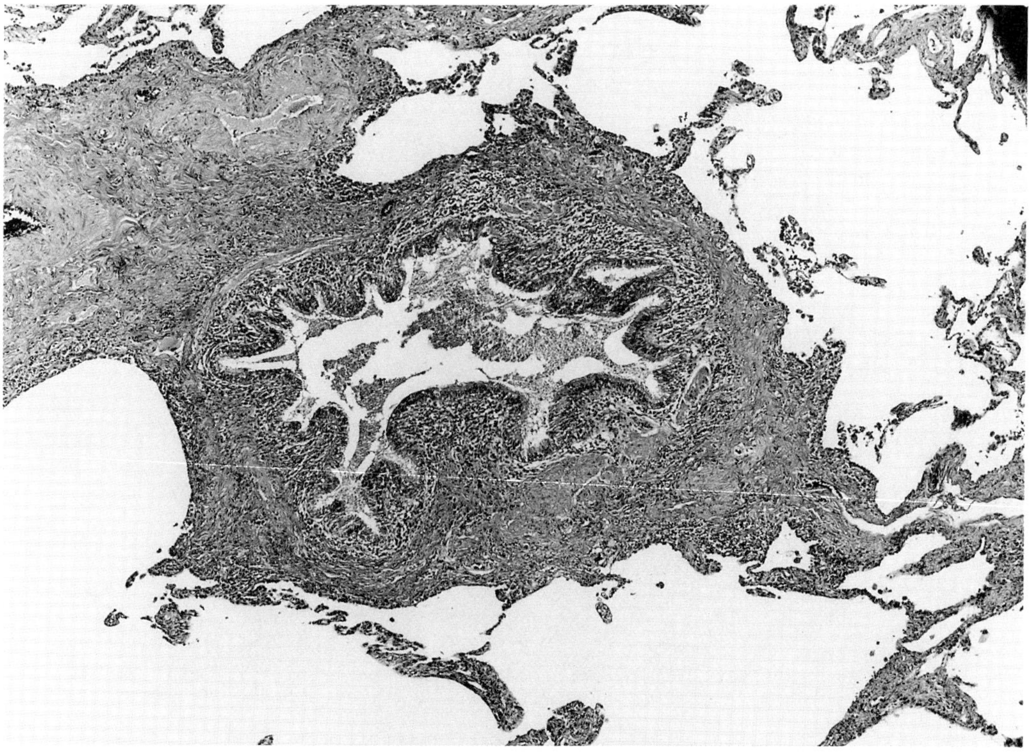

FIG. 6. Cellular bronchiolitis. Chronic bronchiolitis and chronic inflammation peribronchiolar fibrosis in a patient with well-established bronchiectasis.

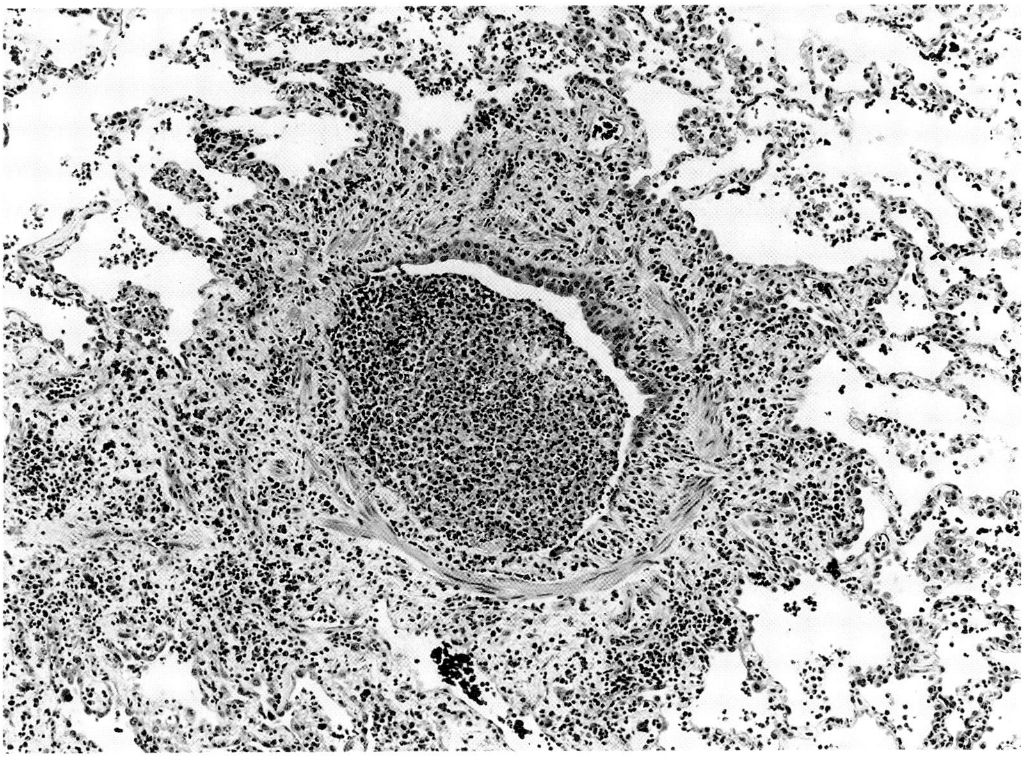

A

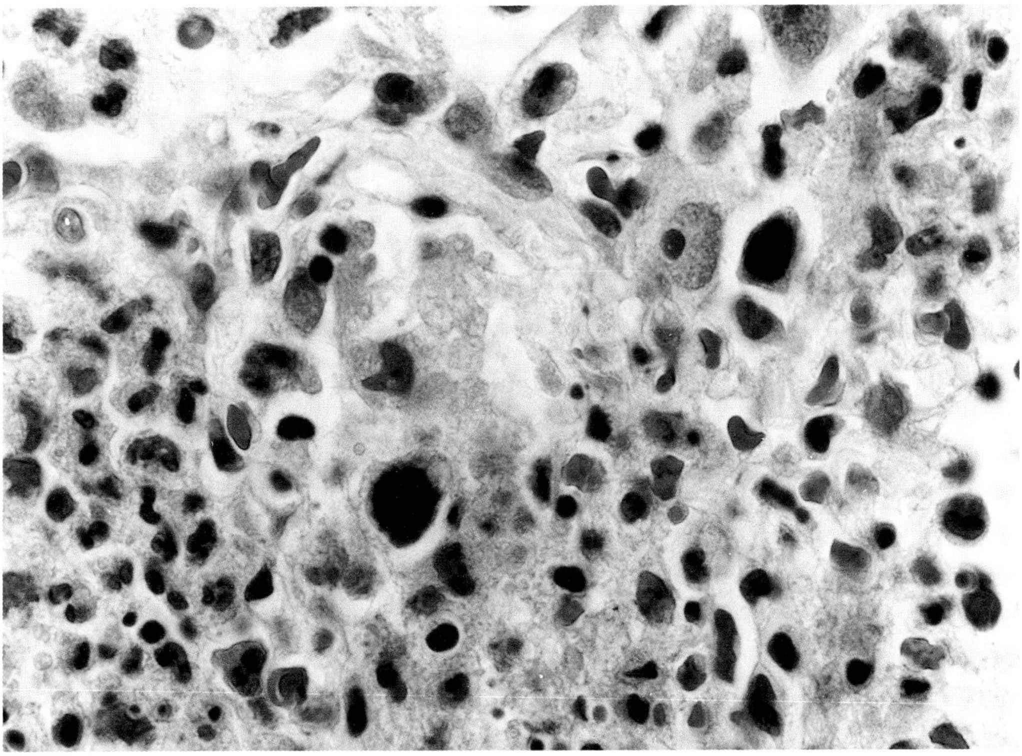

B

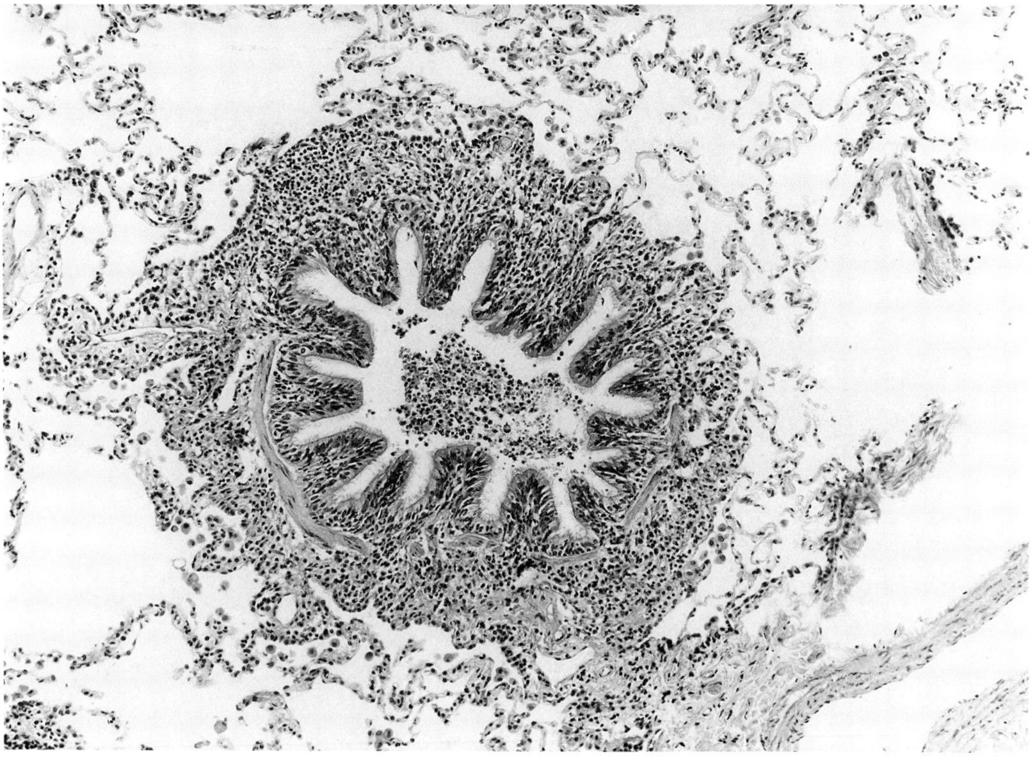

FIG. 5. Acute and chronic cellular bronchiolitis with neutrophils in the lumen and chronic inflammation in the wall. The patient had a history of progressive cough with occasional hemoptysis. Pulmonary functions showed obstruction, and x-ray examination showed reticulonodular infiltrates. The symptoms improved with antibiotics. Such an appearance could be seen with bronchiectasis, acquired immunodeficiencies, connective-tissue diseases, and other conditions.

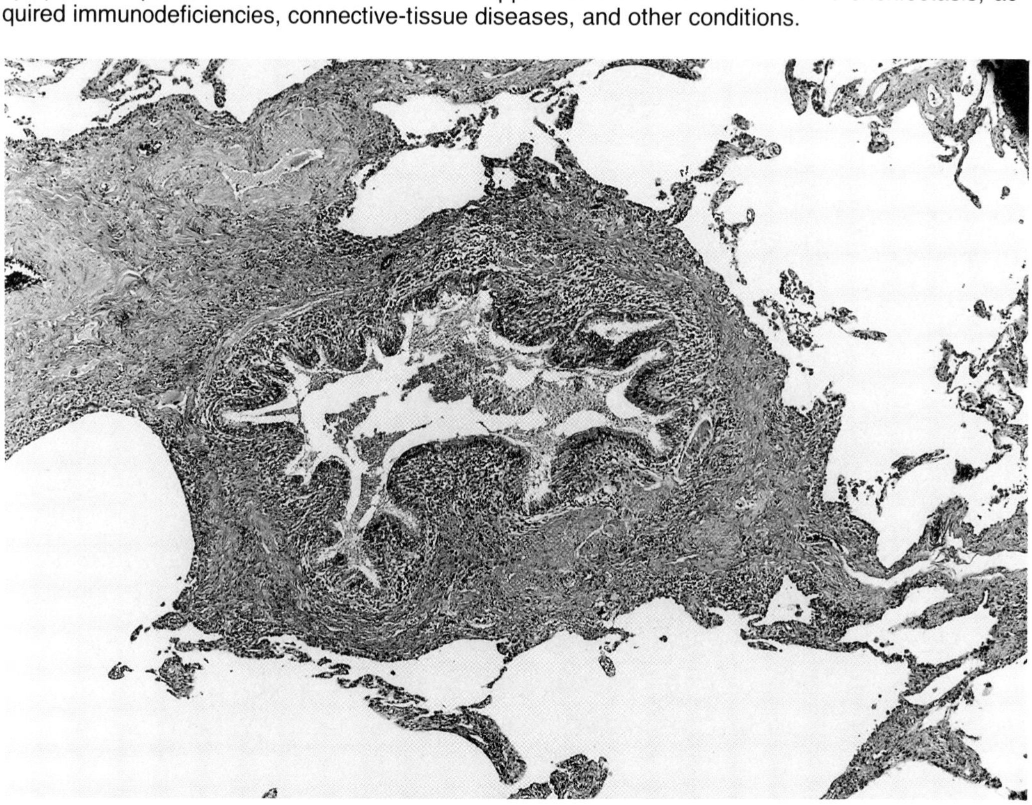

FIG. 6. Cellular bronchiolitis. Chronic bronchiolitis and chronic inflammation peribronchiolar fibrosis in a patient with well-established bronchiectasis.

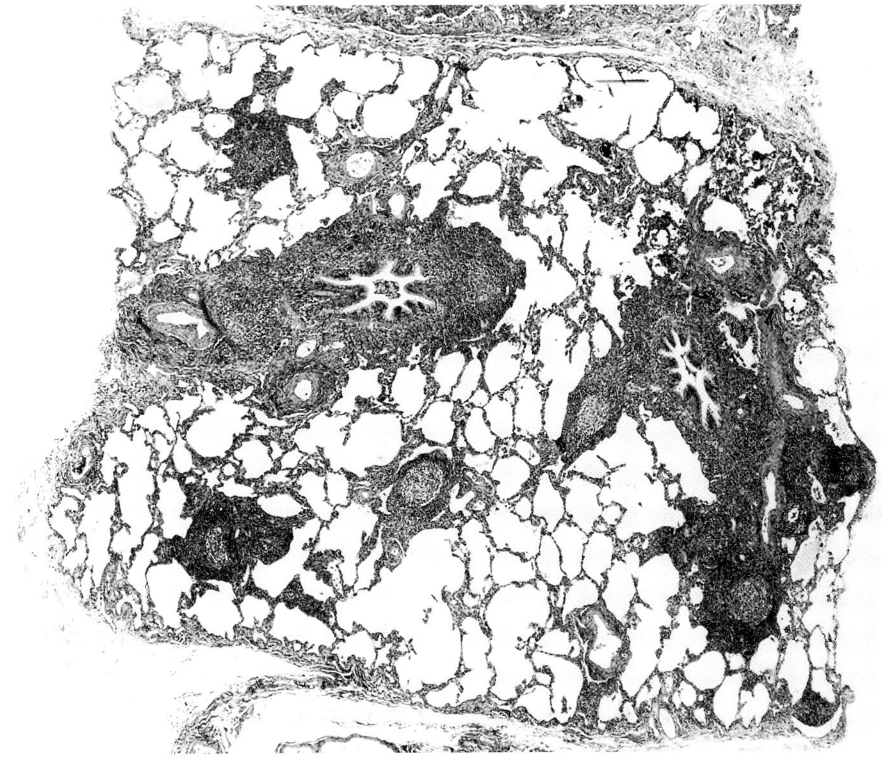

A

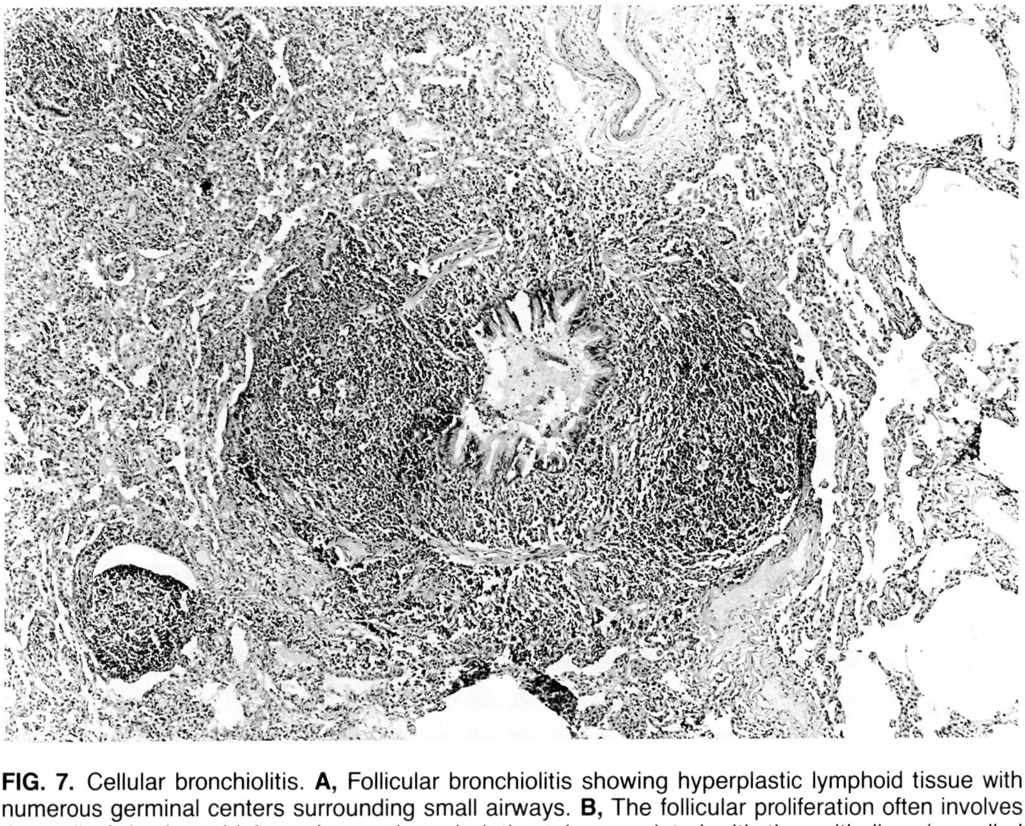

B

FIG. 7. Cellular bronchiolitis. **A,** Follicular bronchiolitis showing hyperplastic lymphoid tissue with numerous germinal centers surrounding small airways. **B,** The follicular proliferation often involves the wall of the bronchiole and sometimes is intimately associated with the epithelium (so-called lymphoepithelium).

bronchiolitis, particularly examples that are chronic, such as those associated with bronchiectasis.

The histologic changes seen in diffuse panbronchiolitis (DPB) are very distinctive (Fig. 8) and in some cases are virtually diagnostic of the condition (5). There is dense chronic inflammatory infiltrate of bronchioles, sometimes with luminal neutrophils, with preferential involvement of the respiratory bronchioles associated with an interstitial accumulation of foamy histiocytes. The last feature is extremely unusual in other conditions but may occasionally be seen in bronchiectasis. The respiratory bronchiolar lesion with its accompanying changes has been termed the "unit lesion of DPB" (5).

Conditions showing a cellular bronchiolitis are many and varied (4) and include diseases generally considered airway diseases as well as some that are considered interstitial diseases:

1. Acute viral infections in children and adults
2. *Mycoplasma pneumoniae* pneumonia
3. Acute fume or toxic exposures
4. Transplant-associated airway injury
5. Bronchiectasis
6. Associated with connective-tissue diseases (especially Sjögren's and rheumatoid arthritis)
7. Extrinsic allergic alveolitis
8. Aspiration
9. Distal to an obstructing lesion
10. Asthma, chronic bronchitis/emphysema

RESPIRATORY BRONCHIOLITIS

Respiratory bronchiolitis is a sufficiently distinct lesion to warrant segregation in its own right. Respiratory bronchiolitis was first described by Niewoehner and colleagues (6) as an incidental finding at autopsy usually, but not always, in young male smokers. We now recognize respiratory bronchiolitis as an extremely common incidental finding in cigarette smokers, and the term "smokers' bronchiolitis" often seems appropriate.

Respiratory bronchiolitis primarily affects respiratory bronchioles, but some inflammatory changes are also seen in the terminal bronchioles. There is a mild chronic inflammatory infiltrate in the wall of the respiratory bronchiole associated with slight fibrosis and smooth muscle thickening and widening of the surrounding alveolar walls, which show a mild chronic inflammatory infiltrate. The most distinctive feature of respiratory bronchiolitis is the prominent accumulation of macrophages in the lumina of respiratory bronchioles and the immediately adjacent alveoli (Fig. 9). The macrophages generally show tan-brown pigmentation of the cytoplasm and positivity with digested PAS and iron stains. They often contain small, dark flecks of material typical of cigarette smokers.

Respiratory bronchiolitis is usually an incidental finding in lobectomy specimens for bronchogenic carcinoma and at autopsy in patients with a history of cigarette smoking. Rarely, respiratory bronchiolitis may be sufficiently extensive in its involvement of lung parenchyma to produce a mild form of interstitial lung disease: respiratory bronchiolitis associated interstitial lung disease (7,8) (Fig. 10).

The term "respiratory bronchiolitis" has sometimes been used in a generic sense for any inflammatory condition affecting the respiratory bronchiole, and thus many of

FIG. 8. A, Diffuse panbronchiolitis associated with chronic inflammation of membranous bronchioles with prominent accumulations of foam cells in the surrounding interstitium. **B,** The major site of injury in diffuse panbronchiolitis (the "unit lesion") is in the respiratory bronchiole, where similar chronic inflammatory infiltrate and the distinctive accumulations of interstitial foam cells are found.

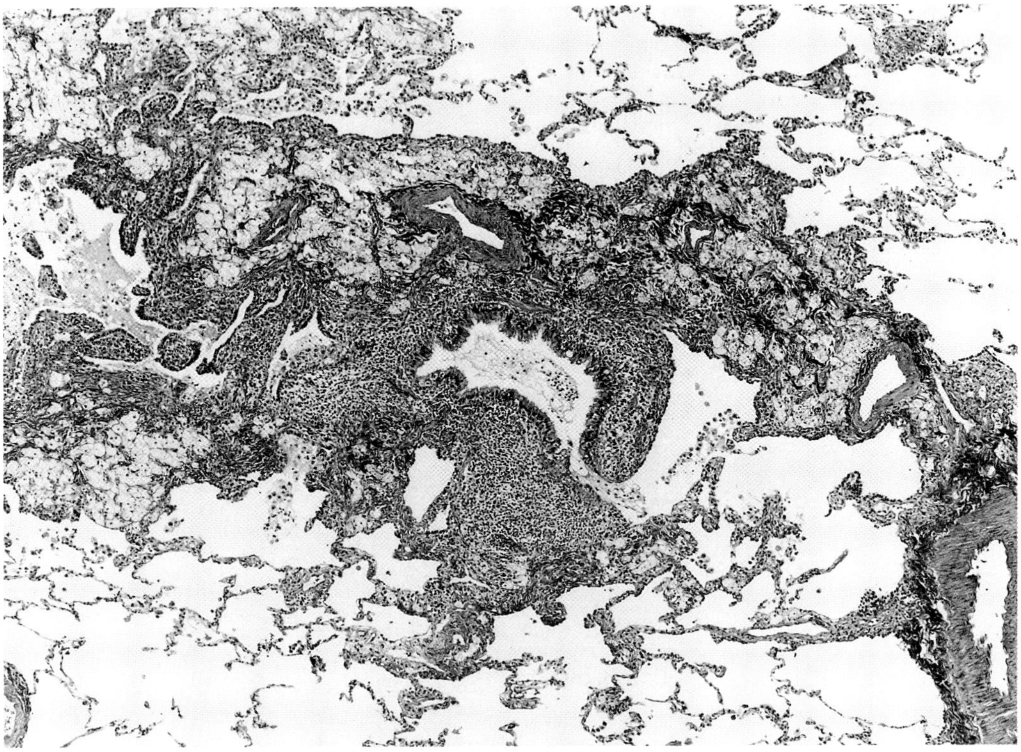

A

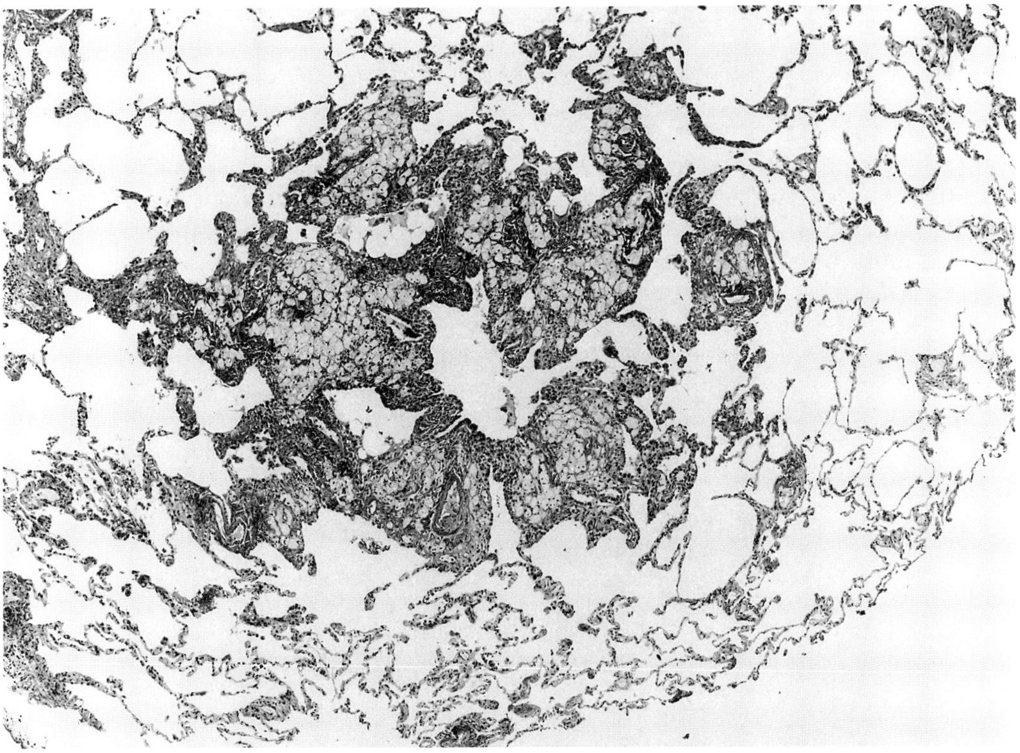

B

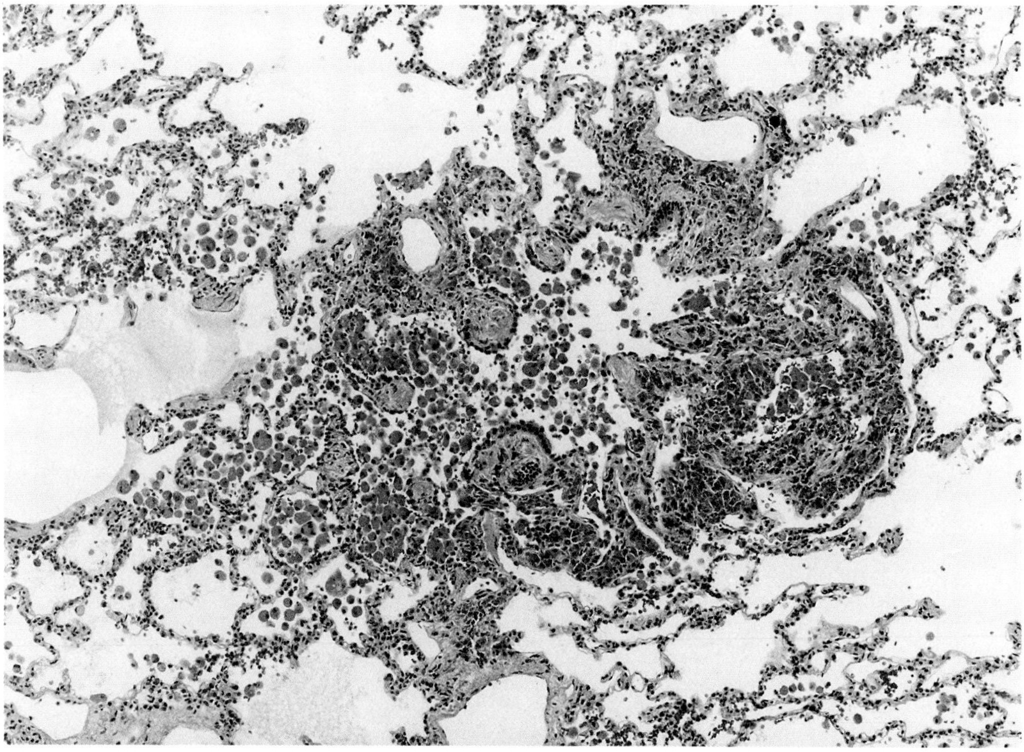

FIG. 9. Respiratory bronchiolitis associated with cigarette smoking from an unused donor lung harvested for lung transplantation. This lesion was clinically and histologically an incidental finding; it manifests as mild thickening and interstitial infiltrate involving a respiratory bronchiole associated with increased macrophages within the bronchiolar lumen and the immediately surrounding alveoli.

the conditions described as cellular bronchiolitis might have a component of respiratory bronchiolitis when the term is used in this fashion. Thus it is important to know the context in which the term "respiratory bronchiolitis" is used.

BRONCHIOLITIS OBLITERANS

The term "bronchiolitis obliterans" has probably been the one term describing bronchiolar pathology that has been associated with the most confusion. This is because bronchiolitis obliterans has been used to describe both a clinical syndrome and two subsets of histologic findings herein described as classic bronchiolitis obliterans with intraluminal polyps and constrictive bronchiolitis (3,4).

Broadly speaking, bronchiolitis obliterans in the clinical sense refers to a syndrome of chronic airflow obstruction usually associated with radiographic hyperinflation that

FIG. 10. Respiratory bronchiolitis associated interstitial lung disease. **A,** There is marked interstitial and air space cellular infiltrates around a small bronchiole in an architecturally normal lung biopsy showing no significant fibrosis. **B,** Higher power shows features remarkably similar to desquamative interstitial pneumonia. This patient had signs, symptoms, and functional findings of interstitial lung disease thought to be related to cigarette smoking.

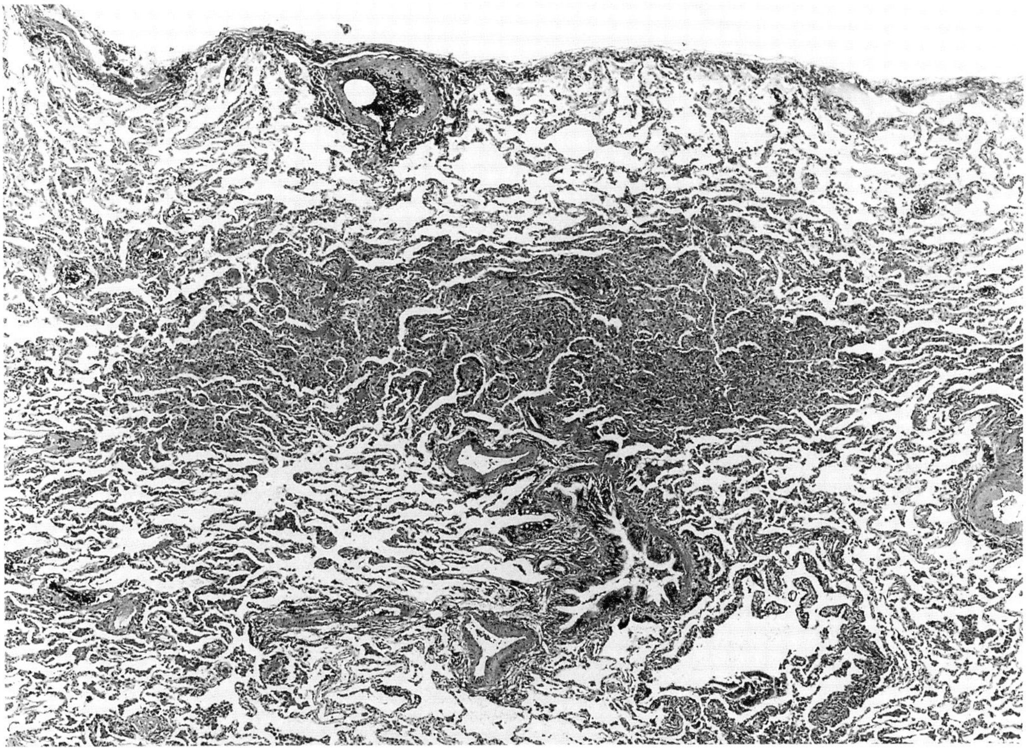

A

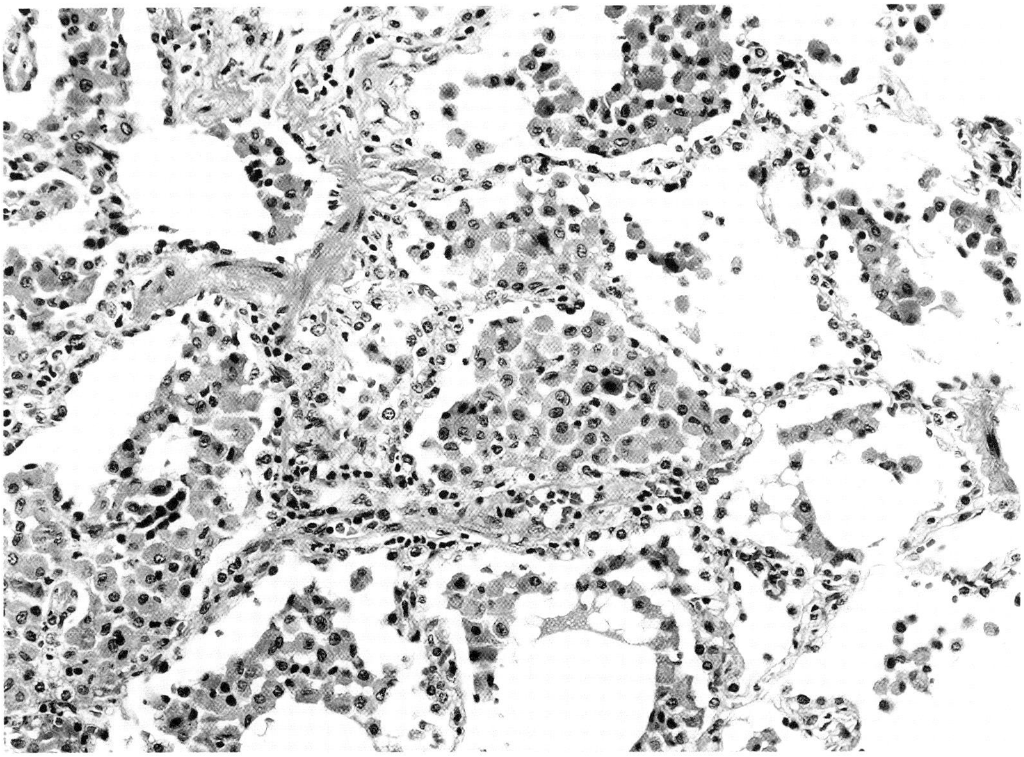

B

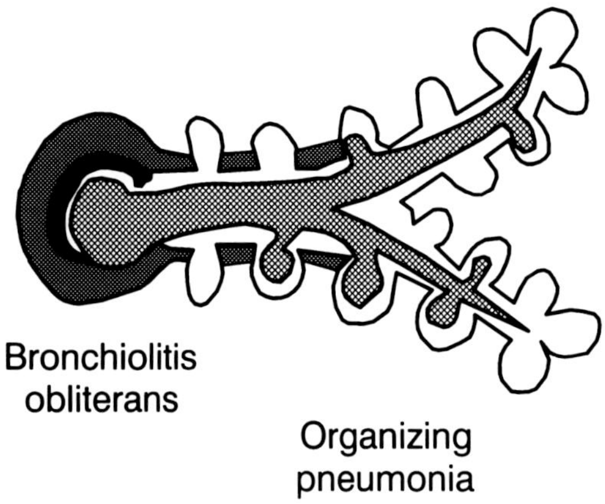

FIG. 11. Diagramatic representation of classic bronchiolitis obliterans with intraluminal polypoid tissue continuous with organizing pneumonia in the more distal parenchyma.

is due to pathologic changes in the small airways. Pathologically, bronchiolitis obliterans has referred to two groups of lesions, and it was initially thought that the two were temporally related; i.e., one necessarily lead to the other. It is now clear that practically speaking these two groups show relatively little overlap clinically or histologically and generally occur in different clinicopathologic settings (4,9).

Classic Bronchiolitis Obliterans with Intraluminal Polyps

Bronchiolitis obliterans with intraluminal polyps was first described and thus represents classic bronchiolitis obliterans. Bron-

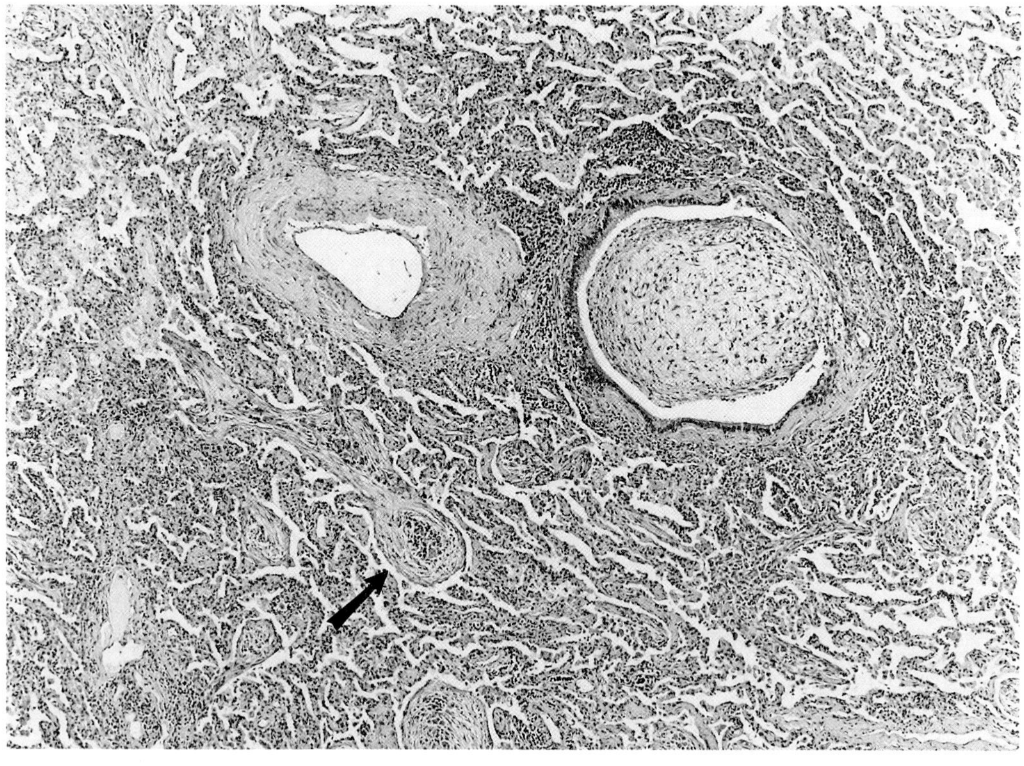

FIG. 12. Bronchiolitis obliterans with intraluminal polyps. A bronchiole with an edematous polyp of connective tissue occupying much of the lumen can be seen. The surrounding tissue shows inflammation in alveolar walls and some organizing connective tissue (similar to the endobronchial polyp) involving alveolar ducts (*arrow*). This illustration is taken from the reactive tissue around a lung abscess.

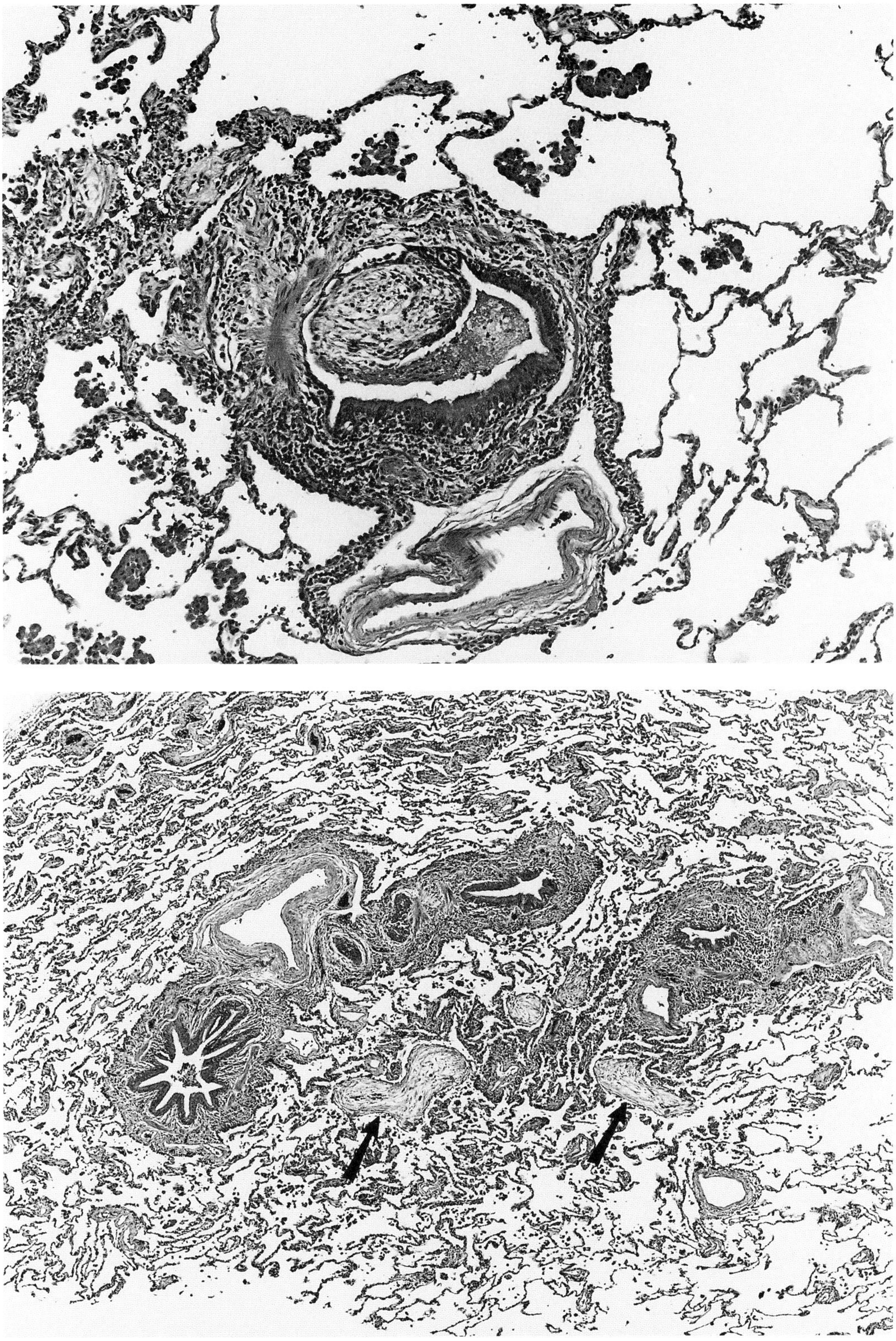

A

B

FIG. 13. Bronchiolitis obliterans with intraluminal polyps. **A,** A small endobronchial polyp of myxoid connective tissue is shown partially occupying the bronchiolar lumen attached at a region of epithelial loss and ulceration. The immediately surrounding lung tissue shows minimal changes. **B,** Foci of chronic cellular bronchiolitis and organization (*arrows*) within alveolar ducts are also seen. This specimen is from a patient with idiopathic BOOP.

chiolitis obliterans with intraluminal polyps is a common, nonspecific, reparative reaction seen in a number of localized and diffuse conditions of the lung; it is usually accompanied by organizing pneumonia in the more distal parenchyma; and, despite the implications of two different names, the two are usually part of the same reparative process (Fig. 11).

Histologically, bronchiolitis obliterans with intraluminal polyps is associated with proliferations of polypoid endobronchial connective tissue composed of myxoid fibroblastic tissue occasionally with central clusters of mononuclear inflammatory cells (Figs. 12 and 13). The polyps may appear to flow free within a bronchiole or to be attached to the wall at a site of mucosal ulceration, depending on the level of the section. These polypoid proliferations are usually continuous with a similar proliferation in the more distal airways, especially the alveolar ducts (i.e., organizing pneumonia, as shown in Fig. 11). The surrounding alveolar walls usually show a mild to moderate chronic inflammatory infiltrate with some reactive type II alveolar lining cells lining their walls. Foamy macrophages may be seen in the alveoli. This constellation of changes has been called bronchiolitis obliterans with organizing pneumonia (BOOP).

BOOP may be part of other pathologic changes and as such may be seen in a wide variety of conditions, such as with Wegener's granulomatosis, around metastatic neoplasms, or in the wall of an abscess. Bronchiolitis obliterans with patchy organizing pneumonia may also be the only histologic change present. In either case, there are many conditions in the differential diagnosis, and only a minority of cases showing BOOP represent the idiopathic syndrome (idiopathic BOOP) as described by Epler and colleagues (10).

Conditions that show BOOP include (3, 4,9):

1. Organizing diffuse alveolar damage
2. Organizing infections: viral, mycoplasma, bacterial, fungal, pneumocystis, those associated with chronic bronchitis, bronchiectasis, and cystic fibrosis
3. Organizing pneumonia distal to obstruction
4. Organizing aspiration pneumonia
5. Drug, fume, or toxic exposure (organizing phase)
6. Connective-tissue diseases
7. Extrinsic allergic alveolitis
8. Eosinophilic pneumonia
9. Secondary reaction associated with diffuse panbronchiolitis
10. Idiopathic BOOP
11. As part of a localized process (focal organizing pneumonia) or associated with other lesions such as tumors or abscesses

It is apparent from the above list that many conditions show BOOP. Idiopathic BOOP is probably the best known member in this group, and it is the lesion for which the term BOOP was coined. Idiopathic BOOP has purposely been put near the bottom of this list to emphasize that many other conditions may show a similar pattern and enter into the differential diagnosis of idiopathic BOOP. Based on the above list, idiopathic BOOP should be considered a diagnosis of exclusion.

Constrictive Bronchiolitis

Constrictive bronchiolitis (Figs. 14–20) is a considerably less common pattern than

FIG. 14. Constrictive bronchiolitis occurring after mycoplasma infection with **A** foci of complete luminal obliteration (*arrows*) and **B** foci of cellular bronchiolitis with distorted and scarred bronchiolar wall showing chronic inflammation and luminal mucostasis.

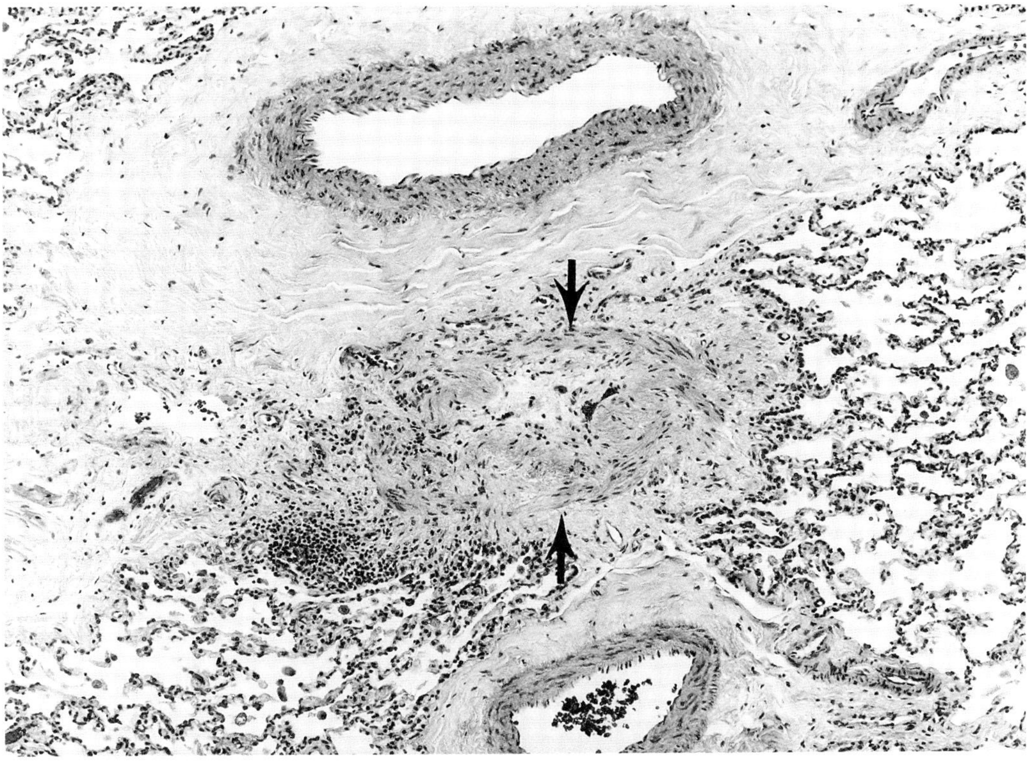

A

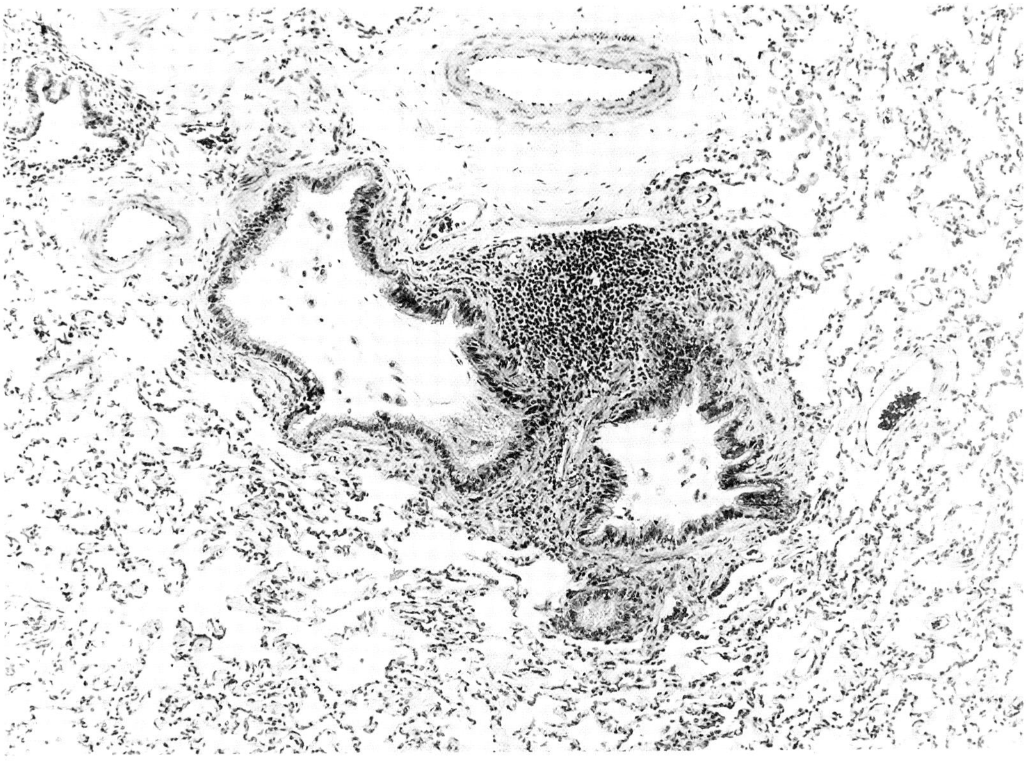

B

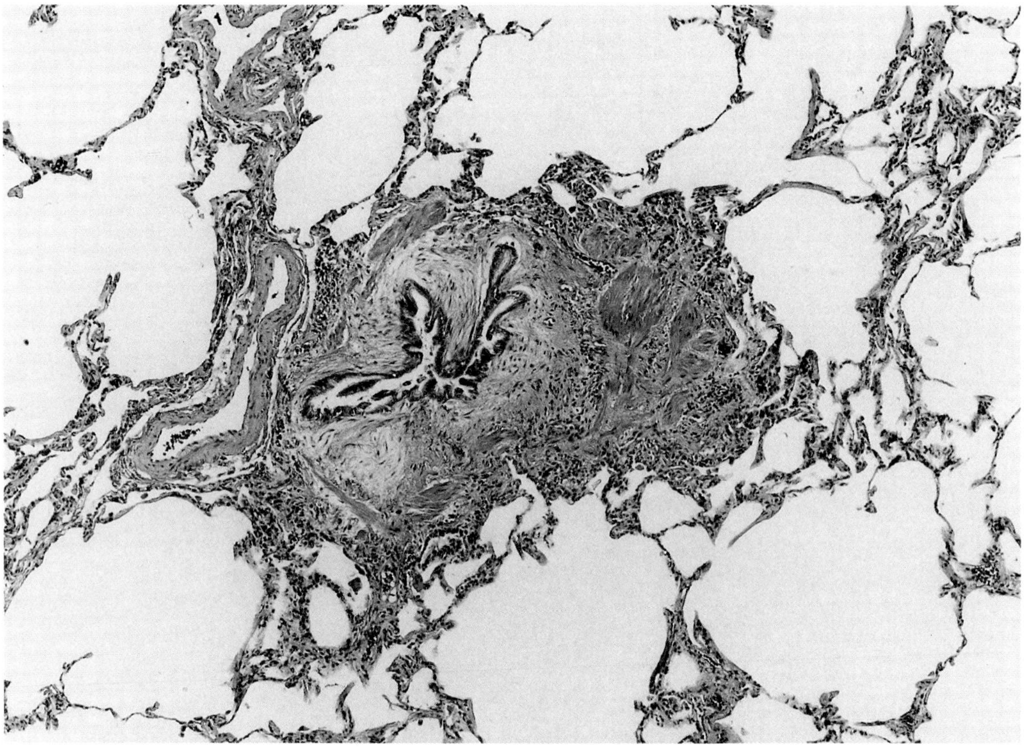

A

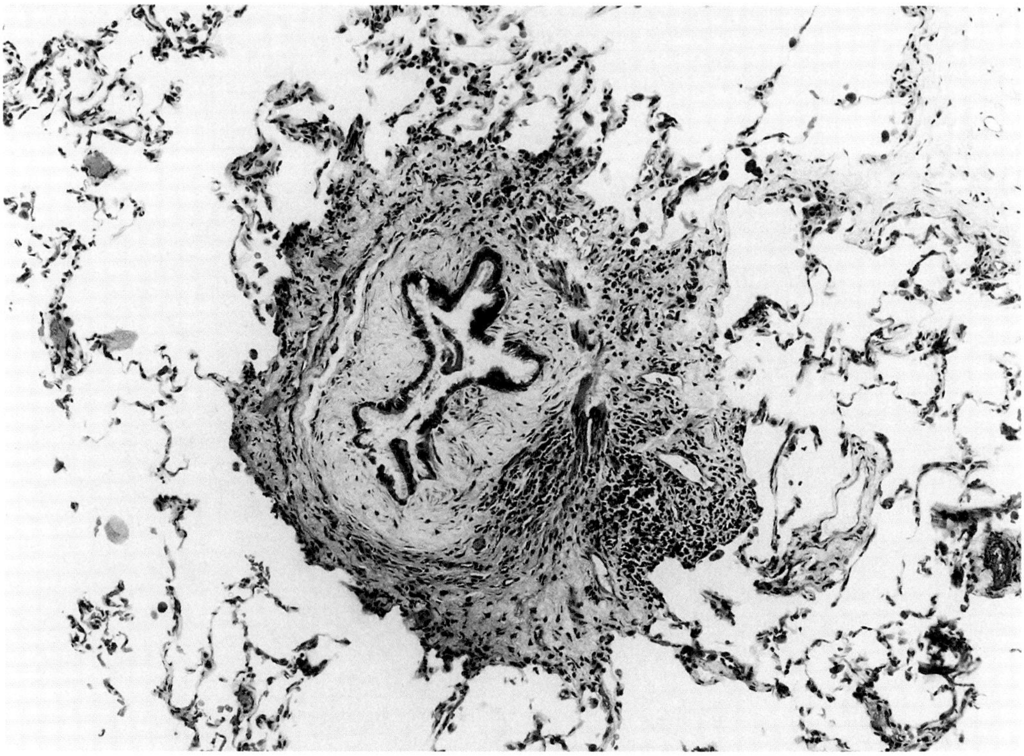

B

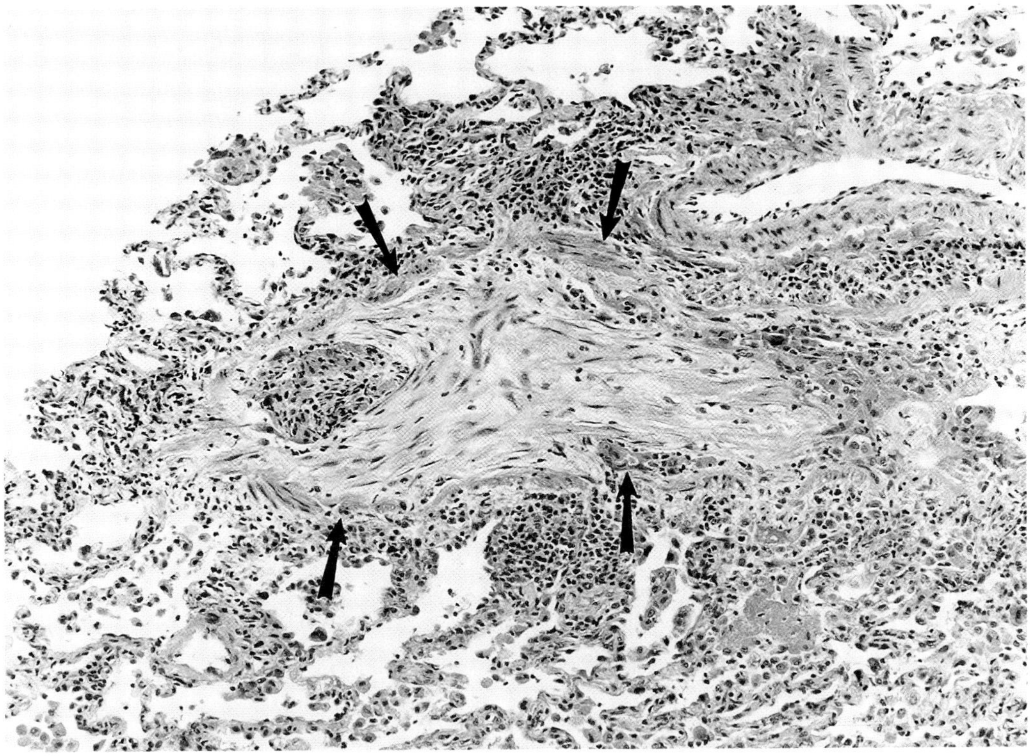

FIG. 16. Constrictive bronchiolitis (*arrows*) in a patient who had a prior bone marrow transplantation and developed progressive cough and shortness of breath with obstructive pulmonary function tests.

bronchiolitis obliterans with intraluminal polyps. The term "constrictive bronchiolitis" is preferable since complete luminal obliteration is relatively uncommon when compared with the spectrum of less than obliterative changes (3,4). Constrictive bronchiolitis is usually a pure bronchiolar lesion, primarily affecting membranous bronchioles, with relatively little change in the respiratory bronchioles and more distal parenchyma.

The histologic changes of constrictive bronchiolitis include a spectrum from subtle minor abnormalities of the airways to complete obliteration. Early changes are seen as mural thickening of the bronchiole due to submucosal collagenization. Concentric narrowing increases with severity and is commonly associated with distortion of the lumen, mucostasis, and chronic inflammation in the wall (cellular bronchiolitis). Sometimes bronchiolar dilatation with mucus stasis is seen, and some cases have bronchiolar smooth-muscle hyperplasia. Subtle changes can be better appreciated with an elastic tissue stain, which highlights the

FIG. 15. Constrictive bronchiolitis with severe and progressive airflow obstruction in two patients with rheumatoid arthritis. **A,** A patient who had not taken penicillamine and later died from progressive airflow obstruction. **B,** A patient who was receiving penicillamine. The disease stabilized when the penicillamine was stopped and a course of corticosteroid therapy was given.

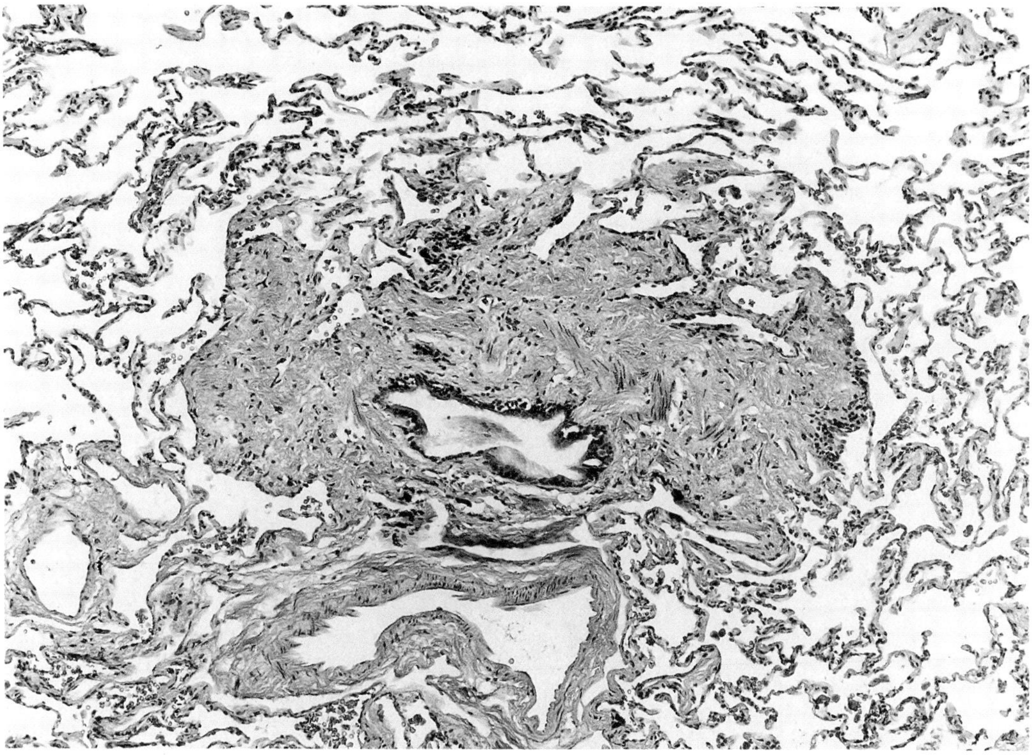

FIG. 17. Constrictive bronchiolitis. Peribronchiolar scarring and luminal narrowing associated with severe airflow obstruction appearing after a toxic exposure to ammonia gas in a young man.

submucosal collagen deposition. Adventitial scarring is an occasional finding in constrictive bronchiolitis (Fig. 17).

Constrictive bronchiolitis is the usual histologic correlate of the clinical syndrome of bronchiolitis obliterans. Clinicopathologic conditions in which constrictive bronchiolitis may be seen include:

1. Healed infections (especially viral and mycoplasma)
2. Healed toxin or fume exposure
3. As a component of chronic bronchitis/emphysema, cystic fibrosis, bronchiectasis
4. Connective-tissue diseases
5. Bone marrow or heart–lung transplantation
6. Drug reactions
7. Idiopathic

While many of the causes of a BOOP pattern are similar to those that cause constrictive bronchiolitis, one rarely actually observes the former evolving into the latter,

FIG. 18. Idiopathic constrictive bronchiolitis in a 49-year-old woman with progressive cough, shortness of breath, and obstructive changes demonstrated by pulmonary function tests. **A,** The biopsy shows luminal narrowing caused by increase in submucosal scarring and chronic inflammatory cells. **B,** As evidence of the lack of air flow, some of the bronchioles show luminal mucus and histiocytes.

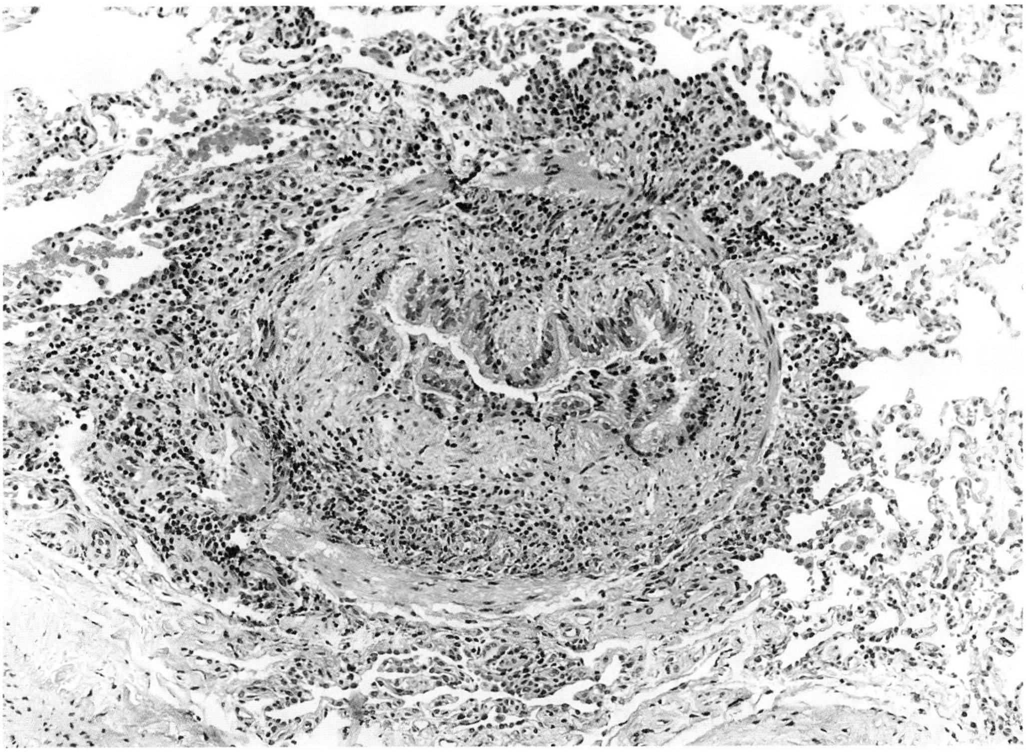

A

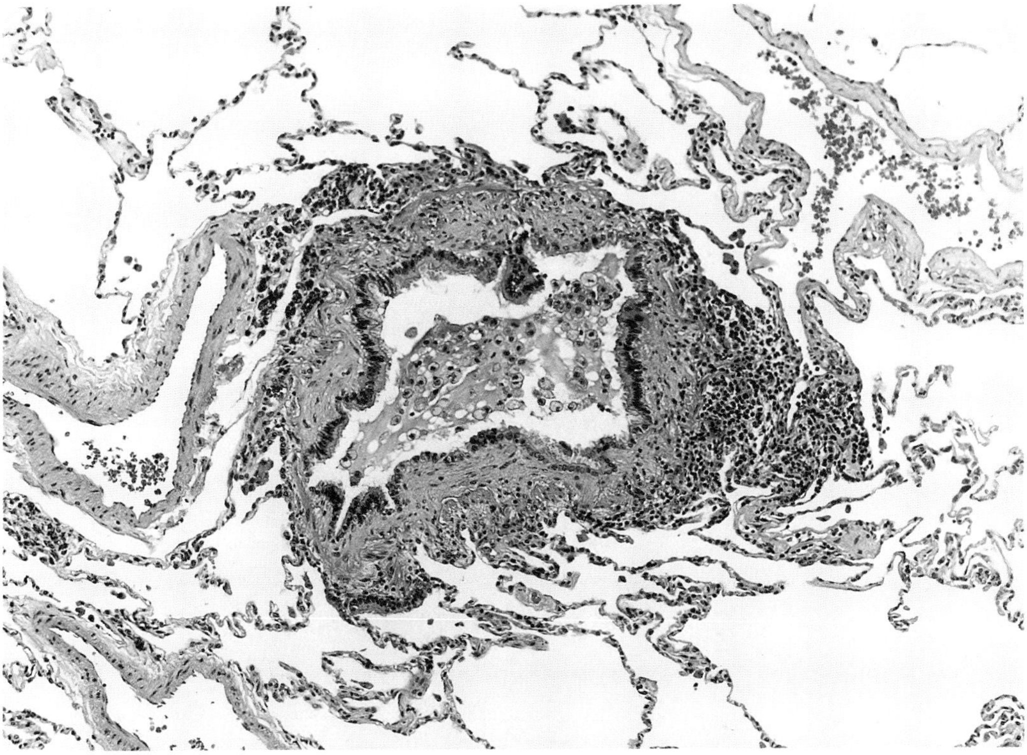

B

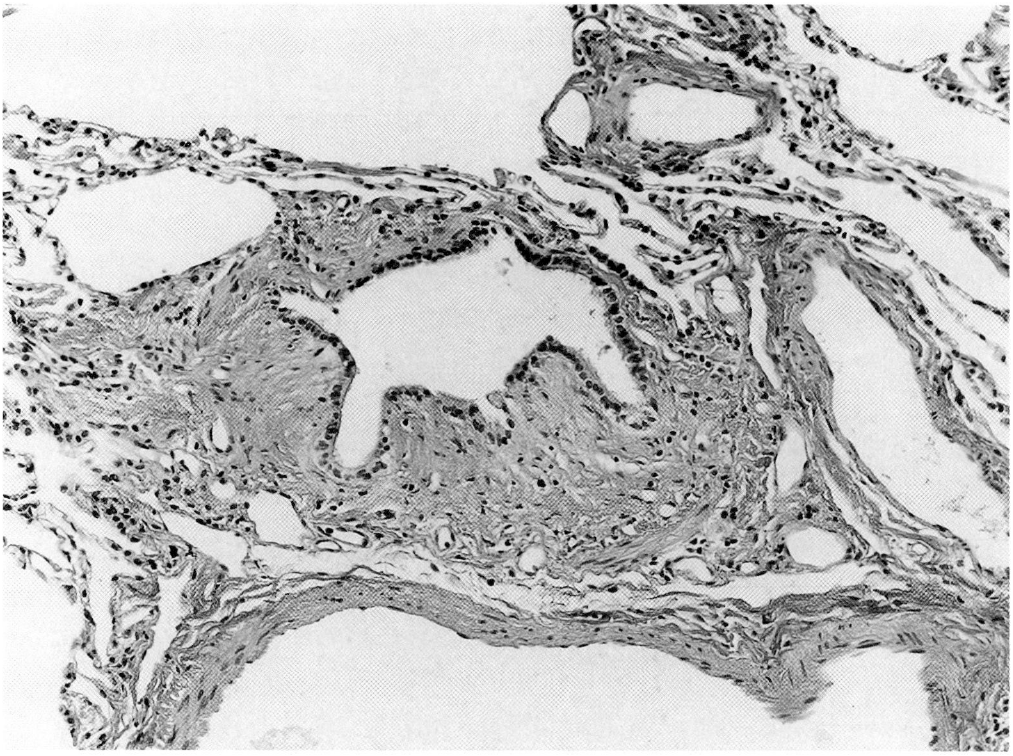

A

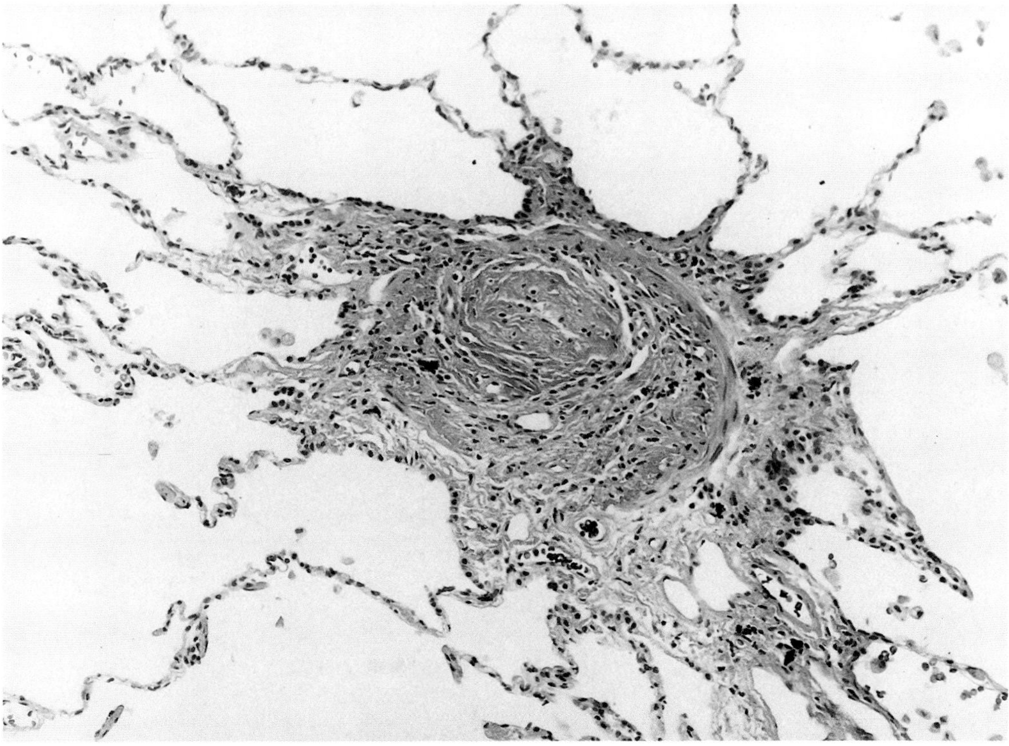

B

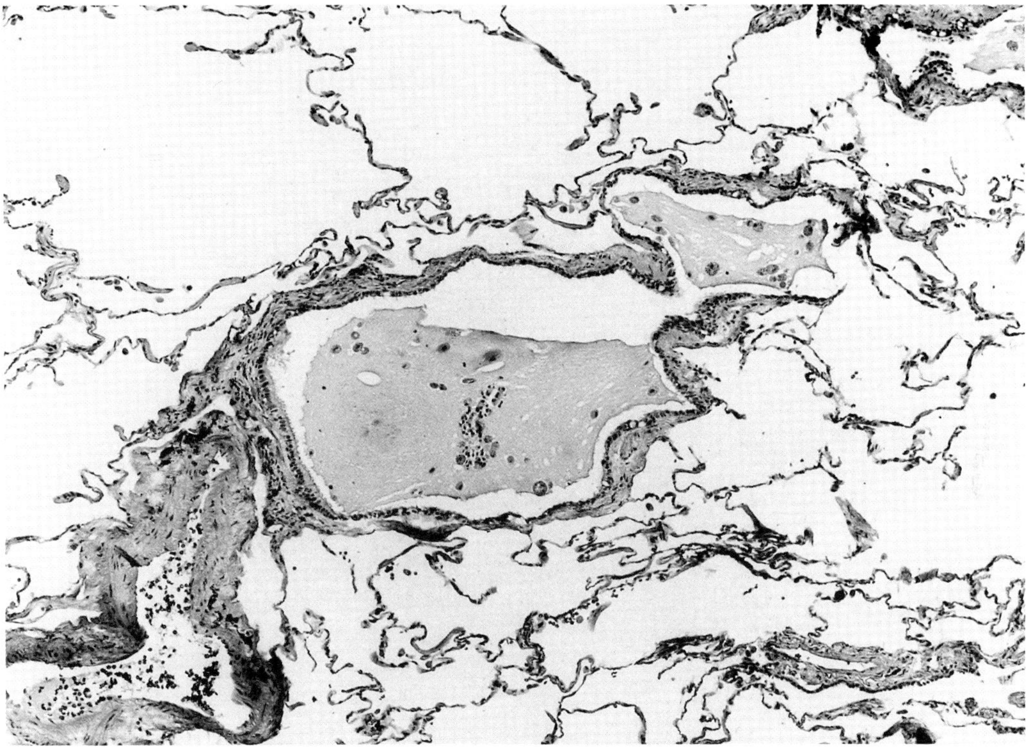

FIG. 20. Abnormal bronchioles with luminal mucostasis. This 67-year-old woman had severe obstructive lung disease of unknown etiology. The small airways show marked ectasia and mucostasis, and they were presumed to be the cause of her problem. Such an appearance is quite commonly seen in smokers with chronic bronchitis and emphysema, although these changes may be seen in nonsmokers with constrictive bronchiolitis. This patient had never smoked cigarettes.

and practically speaking they comprise separate and distinct clinicopathologic groups.

DUST-ASSOCIATED BRONCHIOLAR PATHOLOGY

Inhalation of dust may be associated with its deposition around small airways: mineral dust airways disease (3). This condition primarily affects respiratory bronchioles and alveolar ducts with increased fibrous tissue associated with the dust in the airway wall. The chronic inflammatory response is usually minimal. A number of dusts may produce this reaction, including asbestos, iron oxide, aluminum oxide, silica, silicate, and coal. Mineral dust airways disease is probably best considered a form of pneumoconiosis.

FIG. 19. Constrictive bronchiolitis. This 59-year-old woman developed idiopathic airflow obstruction (presumably postviral, but no specific diagnosis was ever made) that led to lung transplantation after 9 months of progressive disease. **A,** The explanted lung shows scarring of the small airways primarily in the form of submucosal thickening with luminal narrowing. **B,** Only a few bronchioles (less than 10%) show complete luminal obliteration.

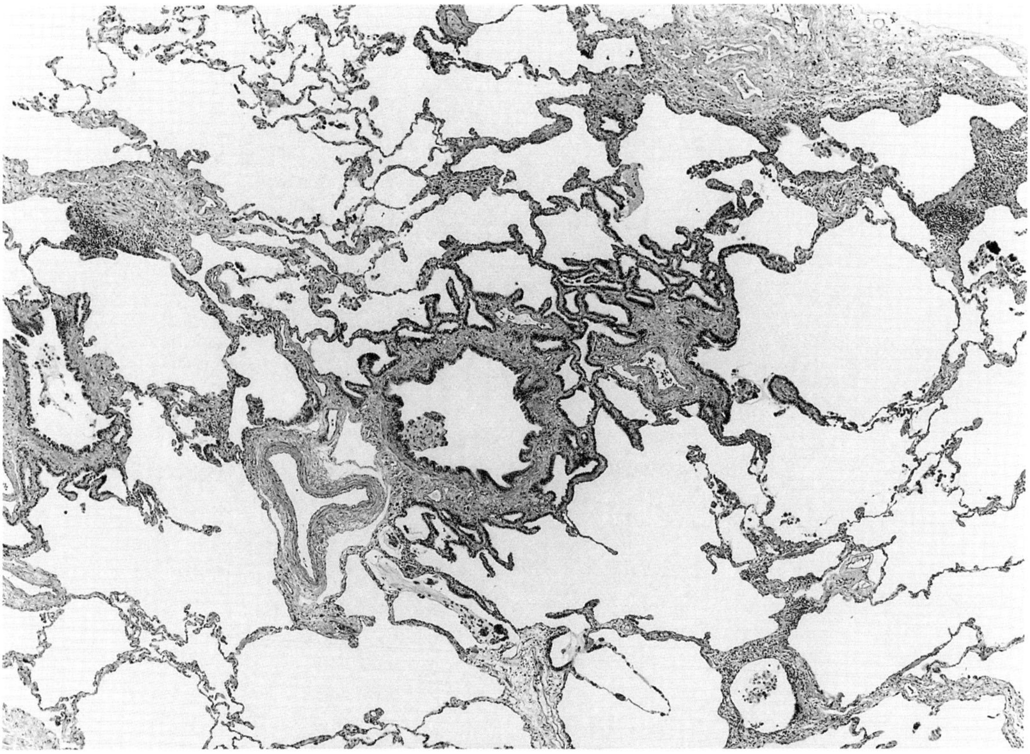

A

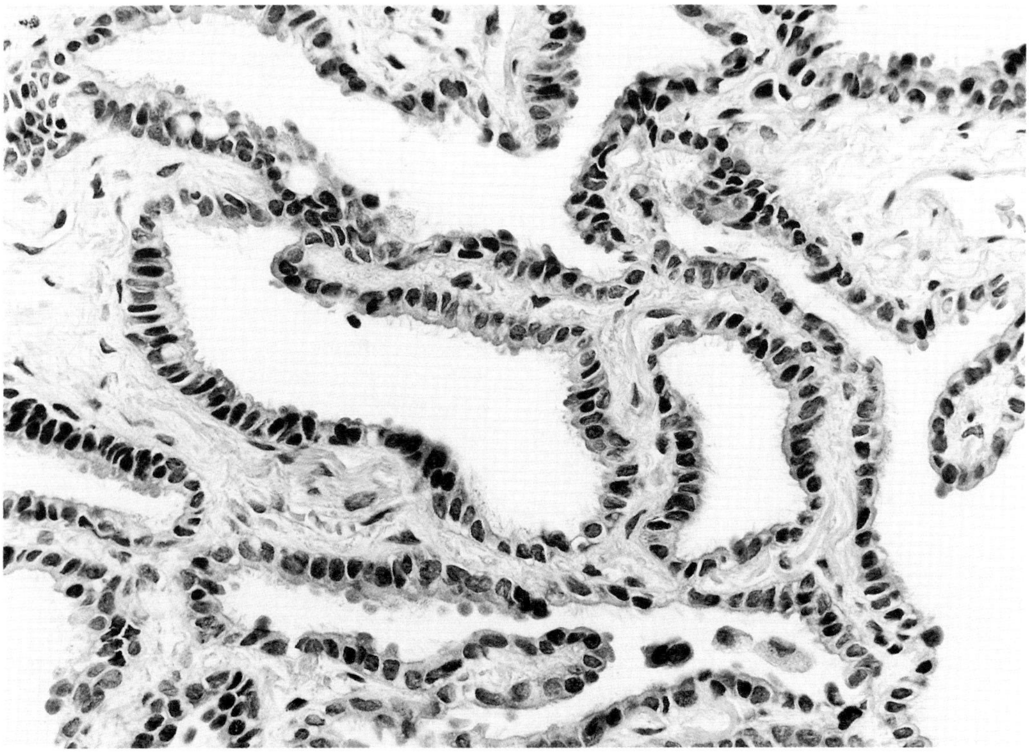

B

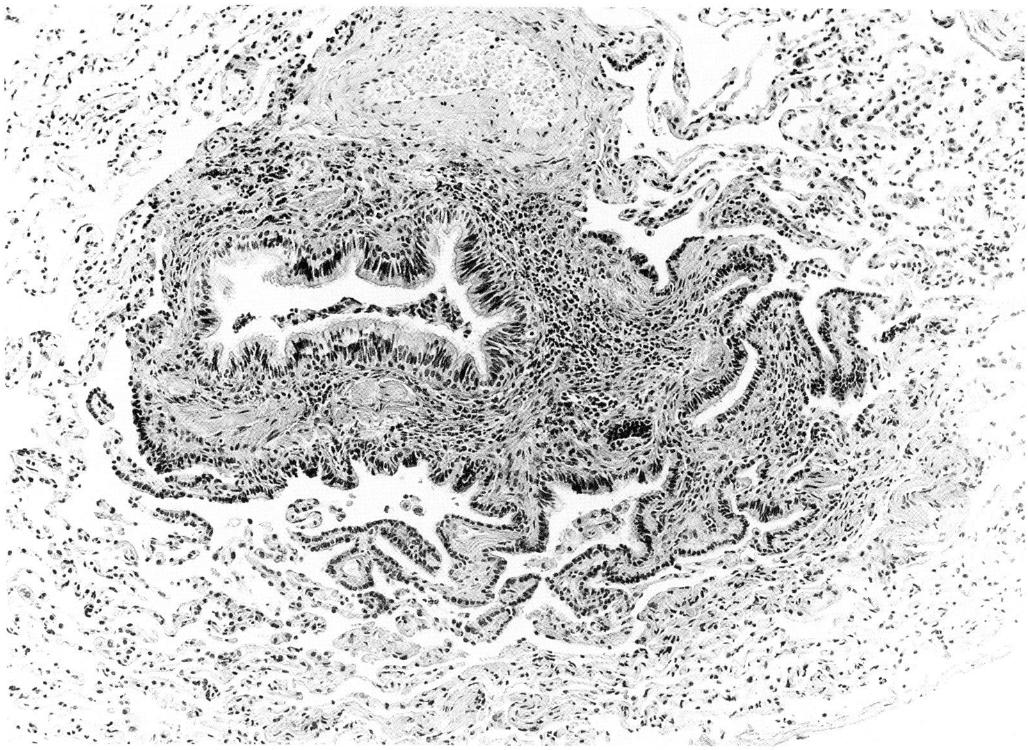

FIG. 22. Cellular bronchiolitis with postinflammatory scarring. Mild chronic inflammation is seen in the wall of the bronchiole, which is also thickened. Peribronchiolar scarring and bronchiolar metaplasia involve the scarred alveolar walls. This 40-year-old woman had shortness of breath and stable interstitial infiltrates for 2 years, which were ultimately interpreted as the residue of a prior (undiagnosed) bronchiolitis.

PERIBRONCHIOLAR FIBROSIS AND BRONCHIOLAR METAPLASIA

A poorly understood group of cases are associated with pathologic changes of the bronchioles and the surrounding alveolar tissue (9). Histologically, one sees distorted bronchioles with thickened walls usually with smooth muscle hyperplasia and mild chronic inflammation (Figs. 21 and 22). The most distinctive feature is the extension of metaplastic bronchiolar epithelium onto surrounding fibrotic alveolar walls (bronchiolarization). In some patients, there is a history of a prior inflammatory event (for example, viral bronchiolitis or extrinsic allergic alveolitis), but this is not true in all. Clinically, the cases usually manifest as

FIG. 21. Postinflammatory bronchiolar and peribronchiolar scarring. **A,** Some thickening and slight scarring of the bronchiolar wall and scarring of the surrounding alveoli, which are lined by metaplastic bronchiolar epithelium. **B,** High-power evaluation shows that many of the cells are ciliated; that feature, plus the fact that the scarring shows a predilection for involvement of bronchioles, is helpful in excluding bronchioalveolar carcinoma. This biopsy was from a patient with radiographically stable interstitial lung disease. The changes probably represent the residue of some prior inflammatory process that, at the time of biopsy, could not be diagnosed.

interstitial lung disease, which may be misdiagnosed histologically as idiopathic pulmonary fibrosis or as bronchioloalveolar carcinoma. Because of the clinical features and the fibrosis that is present, constrictive bronchiolitis is rarely considered, even though there is histological overlap with features seen in constrictive bronchiolitis as well as asthma and chronic bronchitis/emphysema.

REFERENCES

1. Dunnill MS. The pathology of asthma with special reference to changes in the bronchial mucosa. *J Clin Pathol* 1960;13:27–33.
2. Hogg JC. Asthma as a bronchiolitis. *Semin Respir Med* 1992;13:114–118.
3. Wright JL, Cagle P, Churg A, Colby TV, Myers JL. Diseases of the small airways. *Am Rev Respir Dis* 1992;146:240–262.
4. Colby TV, Myers JL. Clinical and histologic spectrum of bronchiolitis obliterans including bronchiolitis obliterans organizing pneumonia. *Semin Respir Med* 1992;13:119–133.
5. Kitaichi M, Nishimura K, Izumi T. Diffuse panbronchiolitis. In: Sharma OP, ed. *Lung disease in the tropics*. New York: Marcel Dekker; 1991: 479–509.
6. Niewoehner D, Kleinerman J, Rice D. Pathologic changes in the peripheral airways of young cigarette smokers. *N Engl J Med* 1974;291:755–758.
7. Myers J, Veal C Jr, Shin M, Katzenstein A-L. Respiratory bronchiolitis causing interstitial lung disease: a clinicopathologic study of six cases. *Am Rev Respir Dis* 1987;135:880–884.
8. Yousem S, Colby T, Gaensler E. Respiratory bronchiolitis–associated interstitial lung disease and its relationship to desquamative interstitial pneumonia. *Mayo Clin Proc* 1989;64:1373–1380.
9. Colby TV, Lombard CL, Yousem SA, Kitaichi M. *Atlas of pulmonary surgical pathology*. Philadelphia: WB Saunders; 1991.
10. Epler GR, Colby TV, McCloud TC, Carrington CB, Gaensler EA. Bronchiolitis obliterans organizing pneumonia. *New Engl J Med* 1985;312: 152–158.

Diseases of the Bronchioles, edited by
Gary R. Epler. Raven Press, Ltd.,
New York © 1994.

7

The Clinician's Classification of the Diseases of the Bronchioles

Gary R. Epler

Associate Clinical Professor, Boston University School of Medicine. Chairman, Department of Medicine, New England Baptist Hospital, 125 Parker Hill Avenue, Boston MA.

The classification of the bronchiolar disorders in the early 1900s was limited to three categories of bronchiolitis obliterans. During the past two decades, the classification has become much more complex as new entities and new associated syndromes have been described. In addition, the complexity is increased because there are distinct but nonspecific pathological lesions, each with several different clinical settings. This could result in two separate classifications, one for the pathologist (1–3) and one for the clinician (4–7). The classification in this chapter has been developed from the historic review of the terminology used in both the clinical and pathological descriptions and represents the result of the combination of these two perspectives.

HISTORIC PERSPECTIVE OF BRONCHIOLAR TERMINOLOGY

Specific terms of the bronchiolar disorders began to appear in 1901 when Dr. Wilhelm Lange (8) described an idiopathic respiratory illness that resulted in the death of two patients; he used the term *bronchiolitis obliterans*. Autopsy revealed lungs studded with diffuse small nodules that represented lesions involving the small terminal airways, the bronchioles. Microscopically, the lumina of these bronchioles were narrowed or obliterated by a mushroom or cone-shaped granulation tissue plug that reached into the airway from the bronchiolar wall. The next year, a fatal case related to inhalation of nitric acid fumes was described, and the term *bronchiolitis fibrosa obliterans* was used (9). In 1904, measles (10,11) and pertussis (11) infections were implicated as a cause of bronchiolitis obliterans; although this term did not appear in the titles of the reports, the pathological description was consistent with a bronchiolar obliterative lesion.

Thus, in less than 5 years, the classification of bronchiolitis obliterans consisted of three categories, idiopathic, post toxic fume inhalation, and post infectious (Table 1). In 1906, the term *bronchiolitis obliterans* was used in a report about three patients with a fume-related lesion as a result of nitric acid, sulfuric acid, and ammonia fume inhalation (12). Two years later the term *bronchitis obliterans* was used in the description of the findings in a 3-year-old child who died after aspirating a prune pit (13). Microscopically, the bronchioles showed plugs of connective tissue growing into the lumen from the bronchiolar wall. The next year, *bronchiolitis obliterans fibrosa acuta* appeared in a report about four patients; in two it was idiopathic, and in the

TABLE 1. *The 1904 classification of bronchiolitis obliterans*

Idiopathic
Post fume exposure
Post respiratory infection

From refs. 4, 8–11.

two others it resulted from nitric acid fume exposure (14).

The term *bronchiolitis obliterans* was used in a 1917 report implicating fumes from trinitrotoluene as a cause (15). In the same report, the term *fibrosing obliterative bronchiolitis* was noted in the discussion section. The term *bronchiolitis obliterans* also appeared in a report regarding an influenza-related illness 1 year later (16). In a 1929 report, the term *bronchiolitis fibrosa obliterans* described five patients who died from the illness (17). The cause was unknown for most of these patients, while some had related infections. The lesion was characterized by bronchioles obliterated or partially obliterated by organizing granulation tissue.

In 1941, LaDue (4) used the term *bronchiolitis fibrosa obliterans* in the title of an updated review of this disorder and discussed a classification of three categories (Table 1). In the first, the disease occurs after inhalation of irritant and damaging substances such as nitric or sulfuric acid, poison gases, or vapors of solvents, or after ingestion of foreign bodies. In the second, the illness is a complication of acute infectious diseases such as measles, influenza, or scarlet fever, or occurs in the course of chronic bronchitis or asthma. In the third, the cause is idiopathic.

About the same time, there were several reports of bronchiolar disorders among infants. The term *bronchiolitis* was used when Engel and Newns (18) used the term *proliferative mural bronchiolitis* to describe a disease entity in infancy and differentiated three bronchiolar lesions: simple mural bronchiolitis, proliferative mural bronchiolitis, and destructive mural bronchiolitis. The authors described the clinical and histologic findings of the proliferative bronchiolitis type in five infants aged 2 to 13 months. The clinical features were consistent with bronchopneumonia, while the histologic findings showed thickening of the bronchiolar wall, especially of the medium bronchioles, while larger bronchioles and bronchi were much less affected, and the proliferative part of the lesion affected the basal cells. They further noted that the proliferative lesion had been described in large epidemics of measles and influenza, but the illness described in this report was of unknown cause. The term *acute bronchiolitis (capillary bronchitis)* appeared the next year in a 1941 report (19) of the roentgenographic description of four infants aged 8 weeks to 3 years. Within the next 10 years, the term *bronchiolitis* became generally accepted by pediatricians. Much was published about the epidemiology, pathology, physiology, and treatment of the disease in infants during the next 40 years (20). Respiratory syncytial virus is the most common cause. Other viral agents, such as adenovirus, rhinovirus, parainfluenza virus, mumps, influenza virus, and Mycoplasma, have been associated with bronchiolitis in infants and children.

In 1955, the term *bronchiolitis obliterans* was used in an updated review of the literature (21). This report also included a description of a 38-year-old man who died with extensive bronchiolitis obliterans after exposure to nitrogen dioxide. The characteristic lesion showed the bronchiolar lumen virtually obliterated by organizing exudate, which often projected in a polypoid fashion. In 1956, the term *bronchiolitis fibrosa obliterans* appeared in the breakthrough report (22) that established nitrogen dioxide as a cause of this lesion in silo-filler's disease. The autopsy findings showed that the lungs were filled throughout with small, discrete palpable nodules. Microscopically, these nodules were typical lesions of bronchiolitis fibrosa obliterans. The photomicrographs showed bronchiole lumens filled by partially organizing fibrin plug. The later stage of organization of the bronchial plug showed that the muscular coat was destroyed, permitting free ingrowth of fibroblastic tissue obliterating the lumen, and no epithelium remained.

In the late 1950s, McLean (23–25) used the term *acute bronchiolitis* in a two-part description of the pathology of this lesion. He examined 27 selected blocks of lung tissue from 70 adult patients and about 20,000 cut sections (23–25). In the first part (23) the lesions of acute viral bronchiolitis, acute bacterial bronchiolitis, and bacterial bronchiolitis secondary to viral infection were described. In second part (24), the morphology of the damaged bronchiole was described in terms of the structural components of the wall, changes within the bronchiolar lumen, bronchiolar collapse, and obliteration of the bronchioles. These findings were summarized in a 1958 report (25) regarding bronchiolitis and chronic lung disease.

In the early 1960s, the term *fog bronchiolitis* described the respiratory illness in nine patients as a result of the 1962 London fog; all patients recovered as the fog cleared (26). The next year, the term *acute infectious obstructing bronchiolitis* appeared in a report (27) of a febrile illness in seven adult patients, aged 29 to 64 years. In 1966, *bronchiolitis fibrosa obliterans* described the lesion that occurred in a 56-year-old man who first developed an abnormal radiograph of bilateral fine mottling, then symptoms 9 months later, and died from this illness of unknown cause (28). The histological findings at autopsy showed concentric rings of fibrosis typical of constrictive bronchiolitis. The interstitium was spared. The next year, the term *acute bronchiolitis* described the cause of chronic obstructive lung disease in two adults as a result of an acute upper respiratory tract infection (29).

In the 1970s, the classification of the bronchiolar disorders began to emerge as much more complex than the three-category classification of 1904. In 1971, the term *small airways disease* described seven patients with chronic air-flow obstruction, all with reticular pattern on their chest roentgenograms and four with chronic hypercapnia. The investigators (30) preferred the term *disease* in this description rather than *bronchitis* or *bronchiolitis* because the last two terms were thought to be used variably.

In 1974, *respiratory bronchiolitis* appeared in a report (31) of the pathologic changes in the peripheral airways of 19 cigarette smokers with a mean age of 26 seen at autopsy as a result of nonhospital sudden deaths. A similar study of 97 patients (32) showed that in smokers and ex-smokers, the membranous bronchioles showed increased goblet cell metaplasia while the respiratory bronchioles showed increased intraluminal and airway wall inflammatory cells, wall fibrosis, and pigment deposition. Almost 10 years later, small airway lesions were reported (33) in the lungs of seven workers exposed to nonasbestos mineral dust. The lesions were seen in the walls of membranous and respiratory bronchioles and alveolar ducts, with the last two being significantly different compared to a matched population of persons with no dust exposure. Churg (33) termed this lesion *mineral dust airways disease* and noted it as a nonspecific reaction of the small airways to inorganic particulates.

In 1973, Gosink and colleagues (34) described two subdivisions for the infection-related category for a description of 52 patients with bronchiolitis obliterans. The first included patients categorized as *postpneumonic:* the lesions appeared to be a residual from an incompletely resolved pneumonia. The second, designated *chronic pulmonary infection,* consisted of patients with chronic bronchitis or recurrent respiratory tract infection, including three with asthma. Toxic fume inhalation was found in eight patients, although three cases arose from aspiration, and 21 cases were in the idiopathic classification. Among the idiopathic group, ten patients had coexisting diseases such as congestive heart failure, lymphoma, leukemia, pulmonary alveolar proteinosis, myasthenia gravis, scleroderma, and rheumatoid arthritis. Two types of bronchiolitis obliterans were described pathologically; most commonly the respiratory bronchioles were filled with characteristic polypoid masses of organized exudate. Less frequently, peribronchial and mural infiltration by mononuclear cells and granulation tissue resulted in a constrictive bronchiolitis with luminal narrowing.

Connective tissue-related bronchiolitis obliterans became the fourth general category in 1977 when Geddes and colleagues (35) used the term *progressive airway obliteration* in the title of a report for an association of bronchiolitis obliterans with rheumatoid arthritis (Table 2). The term *obliterative bronchiolitis* was used in the histological description of the lesion. In addition, a new category or subcategory of *drug-related obliterative bronchiolitis* was also considered a possibility in those patients who had received penicillamine. The lesion occurs most commonly in rheumatoid arthritis, although it has been reported in virtually all of the rheumatological and connective-tissue disorders. On ausculatory examination of the chest, a midinspiratory squeak and early inspiratory crackles (36) were often heard. The chest radiograph is usually normal. The prognosis is poor and may be fatal in as high as 50% of patients with rheumatoid arthritis.

Terms appearing in several additional reports of bronchiolar disorders during these years included *bronchiolitis obliterans* (37, 41), *cryptogenic obliterative bronchiolitis* (38,40), and *bronchiolitis fibrosa obliterans* (39). During this time, the term *bronchiolitis* appeared in the title of a review (20) of the bronchiolar disorders in infants and adults.

TABLE 2. *A 1983 expanded classification of bronchiolitis obliterans*

Idiopathic
Fume-related
Postinfection
Connective-tissue related
Post-transplantation
BOOP

From ref. 5.

Post transplantation obliterative bronchiolitis was an additional category added in 1982 when airflow obstruction was established as a complication of bone marrow transplantation (42). The term *necrotizing obliterative bronchiolitis* appeared in this report, and the lesion has been reported in 10% of patients who develop graft-versus-host disease. Virtually only recipients of allogeneic bone marrow transplants are at risk. In 1984, the term *obliterative bronchiolitis* was used for the same lesion occurring as a complication in heart–lung transplantation (43), and emerged as the most life-threatening complication occurring in heart–lung recipients. The incidence may be as high as 50% in long-term recipients. In 1989, the term *obliterative bronchiolitis* appeared in a report (44) of this process as a complication of single lung transplantation, and the same term was used in the reports of double lung transplantation as well (45,46). Therefore, in all of these reports, the term *obliterative bronchiolitis* described the clinical and pathological process in patients with this post-transplant complication. However, the term *post transplantation bronchiolitis obliterans* appeared in one sentence in a report (47) about the chest radiographic findings after bilateral lung transplantation. In a report (48) regarding the working formulation for the standardization of nomenclature in the diagnosis of heart and lung rejection, the term *bronchiolitis obliterans,* not obliterative bronchiolitis, was categorized as *subtotal* or *total,* and *active* or *inactive*.

A separate and single category of *diffuse panbronchiolitis* was described by Japanese investigators in 1983 (49). The disorder may be related to the HLA antigen Bw54 (50). Chronic sinusitis is a unique finding and occurs in 75% of patients. Pseudomonas infection is a late and bad prognostic sign. The prognosis is poor, 30% survival at 10 years.

In 1989, the term *bronchiolitis obliterans* appeared in a report (5) of a patient who died from this lesion after charcoal aspiration. The next year, *rapidly progressive bronchiolitis obliterans* described this process associated with Stevens-Johnson syndrome (52). During this time, the term *bronchiolitis obliterans* was used in an updated review, and the classification of bronchiolitis obliterans was divided into two categories of known etiology and unknown etiology (53).

THE INTERSTITIAL BRONCHIOLAR DISORDERS

For the most part, the terms and associated bronchiolar disorders have been related to airway abnormalities and can be classified as airway disorders either with or without airflow obstruction. However, over the years, there has been mention of alveolar involvement in the descriptions of bronchiolitis obliterans, but it was not noted to be of sufficient importance to be classified as a separate entity. For example, in the 1901 microscopic description, Lange (8) noted foci of alveoli filled with a cellular exudate similar to the bronchiolar plugs that obliterated the airway. When bronchioles were cut lengthwise, the connective tissue could be followed from the bronchiole into the alveoli, but growth of the connective tissue plugs originating from the alveolar walls into the alveoli was not seen. In the 1929 description (17) of five patients with bronchiolitis obliterans, the findings of an 18-year-old who died after an acute, fulminant, febrile illness showed the lumina of the bronchioles partially or completely obliterated by organizing granulation tissue, and in a few areas a dense fibrinous exudate filling the alveolar spaces bordering the bronchioles showed beginning organization. During a 1967 symposium in Boston, Liebow and Carrington (54) discussed a lesion that was more consistent with an interstitial process when they wrote about bronchiolitis obliterans and diffuse alveolar damage and used the term *bronchiolitis interstitial pneumonia (BIP)*. In this disorder, the changes in the bronchioles appeared to be the same as those of the alveoli. The clinical course was rapidly progressive to respiratory insufficiency. The authors suggested that it was possible that the viral or Mycoplasma agent responsible for the diffuse alveolar damage could also affect the more proximal respiratory passages.

In 1985, *bronchiolitis obliterans organizing pneumonia (BOOP)* was used in a description of 50 patients with an idiopathic illness responsive to corticosteroid therapy (55). It was defined as granulation tissue plugs within lumina of small airways, sometimes with complete obstruction of small airways, and granulation tissue extending into alveolar ducts and alveoli. Additional pathological features included (a) proliferation of connective tissue that forms intraluminal polyps (proliferative bronchiolitis obliterans), (b) fibrinous exudates, (c) alveolar accumulations of foamy macrophages, (d) inflamed alveolar walls, and (e) evenly spaced, rounded balls of myxomatous connective tissue (1,2,56). The architecture was maintained. The bronchiolitis obliterans component of bronchiolitis obliterans organizing pneumonia is the proliferative bronchiolitis obliterans lesion (1,2).

Idiopathic BOOP is distinctly different from the airway lesion of constrictive bronchiolitis obliterans because it is an interstitial process with crackles on examination, patchy infiltrates radiographically, abnormal diffusing capacity, and is responsive to steroid therapy (Table 3). It is different from idiopathic pulmonary fibrosis (IPF) and usual interstitial pneumonia (UIP) because of the flu-like illness, the patchy nature of the infiltrates (which are not linear opacities with honeycombing), and favorable response to steroid therapy (57).

TABLE 3. *Idiopathic bronchiolitis obliterans compared to idiopathic BOOP*

Description	Bronchiolitis obliterans (obliterative bronchiolitis)	BOOP
Pathology	Constrictive lesion	Proliferative lesion
General	Airflow disorder	Interstitial disorder
Chest exam	Early crackles	Late crackles
Chest radiograph	Normal	Patchy infiltrates
Pulmonary function	Abnormal FEV_1 and $FEV_1/FVC\%$	Abnormal vital capacity and diffusion
Therapy response	Poor	Good
Prognosis	Poor	Good

BOOP is an inflammatory lesion; UIP is a progressively fibrotic lesion.

Post infectious BOOP may occur as the result of several types of viruses; for example, adenovirus DNA has been detected in lung tissue of such patients (58). The pathological lesion is the same as the idiopathic type. Generally, the clinical syndrome is corticosteroid responsive. The process has also been reported as a result of cytomegalovirus (CMV) infection (59).

Connective tissue disease related BOOP has been reported for polymyalgia rheumatica (60), polymyositis and dermatomyositis (61), Sjogren's syndrome (62), Bichet's disease (63), chronic thyroiditis (63), and rheumatoid arthritis (63). The lesion is the same as the idiopathic type. The treatment is usually favorable, but because of the underlying systemic illness, complete resolution is less frequent.

Drug-related BOOP has been increasingly reported as a result of a variety of agents including acebutolol (64), amiodarone (64,65), and bleomycin (66). Patients usually have a favorable response to corticosteroid therapy.

Focal BOOP has been reported as a lesion excised for neoplastic exploration (67). Naming a separate category for this process remains questionable. These lesions may be curative by excision, but they may represent a spectrum of idiopathic BOOP that eventually develops into typical bilateral patchy infiltrates requiring steroid therapy for resolution.

Miscellaneous causes and systemic syndromes associated with BOOP have been described, including free-base cocaine use (68), ulcerative colitis (69), HIV infection (70), myelodysplastic syndrome (71), radiation therapy (72), and common variable immunodeficiency syndrome (73).

Several editorials (74–77) have been written about the two terms *idiopathic bronchiolitis obliterans organizing pneumonia* and *cryptogenic organizing pneumonia* (74). These lesions can be separated by the pathologists; therefore the term BOOP is used for the classification in this chapter. There are several other reasons for using this term (78). First, it is a distinct pathological and clinical entity. Second, the term is preferable to the short version *bronchiolitis obliterans* because of the clear distinction between the two disorders (Table 3). Third, the term is specific; it includes the bronchioles and alveolar spaces: the process occurs simultaneously in the bronchioles and alveoli. Fourth, the term is recognized throughout the world (57,63,65,67,79–85).

Respiratory bronchiolitis-interstitial lung disease is a term used by Myers and colleagues (86) for a distinctive syndrome occurring in smokers. It is the second bronchiolar disorder occurring in smokers. Histologically, the lesion is characterized by pigmented macrophages within respiratory bronchioles and neighboring alveolar ducts. The alveolar septa show a chronic inflammatory cellular infiltrate. Ultra structural examination may show needle-like electron-lucent particles within phagolysosomes. The illness is reversible if patients stop smoking; some patients may require corticosteroid therapy.

ADDITIONAL PATHOLOGICAL TERMS FOR BRONCHIOLAR ABNORMALITIES

In addition to the terms discussed above, pathologists use other descriptive terms. Some of these may apply to the clinical setting and eventually prove useful to the clinician and in the clinical classification. The term *cellular bronchiolitis* has been used to characterize acute or chronic inflammation sometimes with mural or peribronchiolar fibrosis and purulent exudate in the lumen (1). The term *follicular bronchiolitis* is appropriate if germinal centers are present (1). The clinical findings associated with follicular bronchiolitis in the adult have been somewhat characterized but not sufficiently to classify this lesion as a separate entity; however, the clinical category is appropriate for the pediatric disorder as described in Chapter 28.

The constrictive bronchiolitis pattern described by pathologists often correlates clinically with a nonsteroidal responsive scar. Constrictive bronchiolitis is also seen as a secondary lesion in several primary lung disorders, such as asthma, chronic bronchitis, and hypersensitivity pneumonitis (Table 4) (1,2).

The proliferative bronchiolitis obliterans pattern often correlates clinically with a steroid-responsive inflammatory lesion. The distinction between these two patterns is important for the clinician because of the therapeutic and prognostic implications. The proliferative pattern is seen as a primary lesion as a cause of the pulmonary process in several clinical settings including idiopathic, post infection, and drug reactions, and as a complication of transplantation (Table 5) (1,2). Proliferative bronchiolitis obliterans is also seen as a secondary lesion in several primary lung disorders, such as eosinophilic pneumonia, hypersensitivity pneumonia, or lung cancers (1,2) (Table 6).

TABLE 4. *Constrictive bronchiolitis as a secondary lesion*

Chronic asthma
Chronic bronchitis
Bronchiectasis
Cystic fibrosis
Chronic hypersensitivity pneumonitis

From refs. 1,2.

TABLE 5. *Proliferative bronchiolitis obliterans as a primary lesion*

Idiopathic
Fume and toxin exposure
Organizing infections
Connective-tissue disorders
Drug reaction
Bone marrow and heart–lung transplantation
Organizing diffuse alveolar damage (organizing ARDS)
Organizing aspiration pneumonia
Distal to obstruction
Focal reaction

From refs. 1,2.

THE CLINICAL CLASSIFICATION OF THE BRONCHIOLAR DISORDERS

The clinical classification in Table 7 is a result of considering the historic perspective of the bronchiolar terminology, review of the terminology of interstitial disorders, and consideration of the additional pathological terms. The airway disorders have been divided into two categories much the same as chronic bronchitis with and without airflow obstruction. The interstitial disorders are classified separately as a third category.

Bronchiolitis without airflow obstruction is a category with the least amount of systematic clinical information available and the most difficult to classify. The frequency of bronchiolitis in adults is unknown and

TABLE 6. *Proliferative bronchiolitis obliterans as a secondary lesion*

Chronic bronchitis
Bronchiectasis
Cystic fibrosis
Acute and chronic eosinophilic pneumonia
Hypersensitivity pneumonitis
Lung abscess
Lung cancer
Wegener's granulomatous

From refs. 1,2.

TABLE 7. *Clinical classification of diseases affecting the bronchioles*

I. Bronchiolitis without airflow obstruction
II. Bronchiolar disorders with airflow obstruction
  Bronchiolitis (membranous bronchiolitis)
    Acute bronchiolitis
    Chronic bronchiolitis
  Smokers' respiratory bronchiolitis and bronchiolitis
  Mineral-dust bronchiolitis
  Diffuse panbronchiolitis
  Bronchiolitis obliterans (constrictive bronchiolitis)
    Idiopathic
    Fume-related
    Postinfection
    Rheumatologic disorders (connective-tissue diseases)
    Drug reaction
    Post-transplantation obliterative bronchiolitis
    Miscellaneous
III. Interstitial bronchiolar disorders
  Respiratory bronchiolitis–interstitial lung disease
  BOOP
    Idiopathic
    Postinfection
    Rheumatological disorders (connective-tissue diseases)
    Drug-related
    Focal lesion
    Immunological disorders
    Miscellaneous

difficult to establish because biopsies are not obtained, the illnesses are probably too mild to report to physicians, and no large-scale epidemiological studies have been performed. The pathologist describes these lesions as an acute or chronic inflammatory process of the bronchioles, commonly seen alone in such conditions as viral infections, or as part of chronic bronchitis, an infectious process, or lung cancer (1). Yet, even though bronchiolitis is probably also clinically common in the adult, the clinician has difficulty separating the symptoms and findings of inflamed bronchi from those of inflamed bronchioles. Most likely, the most common type of bronchiolitis in the adult represents the post-viral and nonproductive hacking cough that occurs several days after a winter viral illness and persists for a minimum of 3 weeks and often 1 to 3 months. The cough is not associated with sputum production. The chest physical examination is usually normal, especially in bronchiolitis without clinically important airflow obstruction. The chest radiograph is normal, and pulmonary function is normal. Treatment consists of a cough suppressant, hydration, reassurance, and a short course of corticosteroid therapy for prolonged and severe episodes.

Bronchiolar disorders with airflow obstruction are classified into five categories. The category of *acute and chronic bronchiolitis* is the most difficult to classify clinically because the clinical findings are similar to those of acute and chronic bronchitis. The pathologist notes the same findings in bronchiolitis with or without airflow obstruction, except that the inflammatory process may be more severe in patients without airflow obstruction. The clinician has the same difficulty separating clinically inflamed bronchi from inflamed bronchioles. The clinical process is the same as bronchiolitis without airflow obstruction with a nonproductive cough as the most common finding; however, dyspnea may develop 2 to 4 weeks after the cough in patients with airflow obstruction. The chest physical examination is usually normal, but wheezing or early inspiratory crackles may be heard. The chest radiograph is normal or shows hyperinflation. Pulmonary function testing shows airflow obstruction with abnormalities in the FEV1, which may or may not improve after bronchodilator inhalation. The diffusing capacity is variable, either normal or slightly decreased, but usually not the increased level associated with asthma. Treatment also consists of a cough suppressant and hydration. A short course of corticosteroid therapy may often be necessary for eventual resolution.

Respiratory bronchiolitis and bronchiolitis occurring in cigarette smokers is primarily a pathologic diagnosis; however, because of important clinical and prognostic consequences, the lesion has been classified as a separate clinical category. Mineral dust bronchiolitis is also primarily a pathologic diagnosis but may have important clinical implications and is therefore appropriate for a clinical classification. Diffuse panbronchiolitis is a distinct clinical entity. *Bronchiolitis obliterans* is a distinct clinical entity with several specific clinical settings and in general is the most commonly used term; however, the term *obliterative bronchiolitis* appears to be preferred in the literature regarding post-transplantation complications with the exception of the lung rejection study group (48). The pathologic term *constrictive bronchiolitis* is also an excellent clinical term because it can differentiate patients with a nonsteroid responsive, disabling airflow disease from patients with proliferative bronchiolitis obliterans, a steroid-responsive inflammatory process. Both these terms would be useful for a clinical classification because of these important therapeutic and prognostic distinctions; however, they have not yet gained sufficient use in the clinical setting. In addition, the clinically useful terms *obliterative* or *obliterans* are not used in the term *constrictive bronchiolitis*.

Interstitial bronchiolar disorders includes two major categories. Respiratory bronchiolitis-interstitial lung disease is a distinct clinical entity and appropriate for the clinical classification. BOOP is also a distinct clinical disorder appropriate for a clinical classification. In addition to the idiopathic type, several specific clinical settings and systemic illnesses that are associated with BOOP have been classified as subcategories.

TABLE 8. *The bronchiolar diseases in children*

Acute bronchiolitis
Respiratory syncytial virus
Adenovirus
Influenza
Chronic bronchiolitis
Follicular bronchiolitis
Bronchiolitis obliterans
Idiopathic
Post-viral infection
Rheumatological disorders

PEDIATRIC CLASSIFICATION OF THE BRONCHIOLAR DISORDERS

The classification for the pediatric bronchiolar disorders is similar to the adult classification, except fewer reports of specific syndromes have been published (Table 8). Categories include acute bronchiolitis (20) and bronchiolitis obliterans (87). Follicular bronchiolitis has a separate pediatric classification.

CONCLUSION

The classification of the bronchiolar disorders continues to evolve as new causes and associated systemic disorders are described and additional clinical and epidemiological data emerge. The classification given in this chapter is based on the historic development of these disorders; the pathological findings are used as major categories and clinical setting as subcategories. The classification is adaptable to new insights and discoveries.

REFERENCES

1. Colby TV, Lombard C. Yousem SA, Kitaichi M. Interstitial diseases. In *Atlas of pulmonary surgical pathology*. Philadelphia: WB Saunders; 1991:205–306.
2. Colby TV, Myers JL. Clinical and histologic spectrum of bronchiolitis obliterans, including

bronchiolitis obliterans organizing pneumonia. *Semin Respir Med* 1992;13:119–133.
3. Wright JL, Cagle P, Churg A, et al. Diseases of the small airways. *Am Rev Respir Dis* 1992; 146:240–262.
4. LaDue JS. Bronchiolitis fibrosa obliterans. *Arch Intern Med* 1941;68:663–673.
5. Epler GR, Colby TV. The spectrum of bronchiolitis obliterans. *Chest* 1983;83:161–162.
6. Bignon J, Jaubert F, Laurent Ph. Les bronchilites obstructives. *Rev Mal Respir 1987;4:199–215.*
7. Meier-Sydow J. Klassifikation und Synopsis der Bronchiolitis und der Atemwegserkrankungen bei Alveolitis und Fibrose. *Atemw Lungenkrkh Jahrgang* 1989;15:273–276.
8. Lange W. Ueber eine eigenthumliche Erkrankung der kleinen Bronchien und Bronchilen (Bronchitis et Bronchiolitis obliterans). *Dtsch Arch Klin Med* 1901;70:324–364.
9. Frankel A. Ueber bronchiolitis fibrosa obliterans, nebst Bemerkungen uber Lungenhyperamie und indurirende Pneumonie. *Dtsch Arch Klin Med* 1902;73:484–512.
10. Hart C. Anatomische untersuchungen uber die bei Masern vorkommenden Lungenerkrankungen. *Dtsch Arch Klin Med* 1904;79:108–128.
11. Jochmann G, Moltrecht. Uber seltenere Erkrankungsformen der bronchien nach masern und keuchhusten. *Beitr Pathol Anat Allg pathol* 1904;36:340–352.
12. Edens. Uber bronchiolitis obliterans. *Dtsch Arch Klin Med* 1906;85:598–618.
13. Wegelin C. Uber bronchitis obliterans nach Fremdkorperaspiration. Beit Pathol Anat 1908; 43:438–454.
14. Frankel A. Ein weiterer Beitrag zur Lehre von der bronchiolitis obliterans fibrosa acuta. *Berl Klin Wochenschr* 1909;1:6–9.
15. Wagner JH. Bronchiolitis obliterans following the inhalation of acrid fumes. *Am J Med Sci* 1917;154:511–523.
16. Hubschmann P. Ueber Inthienzaerkrankungen der Lunge und ihre Beziehungen zur Bronchiolitis obliterans. *Beitr Pathol Anat Allg Pathol* 1918;63:202–252.
17. Blumgart HL, MacMahon HE. Bronchiolitis fibrosa obliterans: a clinical and pathologic study. *Med Clin North Am* 1929;13:197–214.
18. Engle S, Newns GH. Proliferative mural bronchiolitis. *Arch Dis Child* 1940;15:219–229.
19. Paul LW. Roentgenologic diagnosis of acute bronchiolitis (capillary bronchitis) in infants. *Am J Roentgenol* 1941;51:41–49.
20. Wohl MEB, Chernick V. Bronchiolitis. *Am Rev Respir Dis* 1978;118:759–781.
21. McAdams AJ. Bronchiolitis obliterans. *Am J Med* 1955;19:314–322.
22. Lowry T, Schuman LM. Silo-filler's disease: a syndrome caused by nitrogen dioxide. *JAMA* 1956;162:153–160.
23. McLean KH. The pathology of acute bronchiolitis: a study of its evolution. I: The exudative phase. *Australas Ann Med* 1956;5:254–267.
24. McLean KH. The pathology of acute bronchiolitis: a study of its evolution. II: The repair phase. *Australas Ann Med* 1957;6:29–43.
25. McLean KH. Bronchiolitis and chronic lung disease. *Br J Tuberculosis Dis Chest* 1958;52:104–113.
26. Davies GM. Fog bronchiolitis. *Lancet* 1963; March 16:580–581.
27. Ham JC. Acute infectious obstructing bronchiolitis: a potentially fatal disease in the adult. *Ann Intern Med* 1964;60:47–60.
28. Baar HS, Galindo J. Bronchiolitis fibrosa obliterans. *Thorax* 1966;21:209–214.
29. Dines DE. Acute bronchiolitis as a cause of chronic obstructive lung disease in adults. *Lancet* 1967;87:281–282.
30. Macklem PT, Thurlbeck WM, Fraser RG. Chronic obstructive disease of small airways. *Ann Intern Med* 1971;74:167–177.
31. Niewoehner DE, Kleinerman J, Rice DB. Pathologic changes in the peripheral airways of young cigarette smokers. *N Engl J Med* 1974;291:755–758.
32. Wright JL, Lawson LM, Pare PD, et al. Morphology of peripheral airways in current smokers and ex-smokers. *Am Rev Respir Dis* 1983; 127:474–477.
33. Churg A, Wright JL. Small-airway lesions in patients exposed to nonasbestos mineral dusts. *Hum Pathol* 1983;14:688–693.
34. Gosink BB, Friedman PJ, Liebow AA. Bronchiolitis obliterans. *A J R* 1973;117:816–832.
35. Geddes DM, Corrin B, Brewerton DA, et al. Progressive airway obliteration in adults and its association with rheumatoid disease. *Q J Med* 1977;46:427–444.
36. Epler GR, Snider GL, Gaensler EA, et al. Bronchiolitis and bronchitis in connective tissue disease. *JAMA* 1979;242:528–532.
37. Dale RC, Auchincloss JH, Gilbert R, Markarian B. Bronchiolitis obliterans. *NY State J Med* 1977;77:1485–1488.
38. Turton CW, Williams G, Green M. Cryptogenic obliterative bronchiolitis in adults. *Thorax* 1981; 36:805–810.
39. Hawley PC, Whitcomb ME. Bronchiolitis fibrosa obliterans in adults. *Arch Intern Med* 1981;141:1324–1327.
40. Breatnach E, Kerr I. The radiology of cryptogenic obliterative bronchiolitis. *Clin Radiol* 1982; 33:657–661.
41. Seggev JS, Mason UG, Worthen S, et al. Bronchiolitis obliterans: report of three cases with detailed physiologic studies. *Chest* 1983;83:169–174.
42. Roca J, Granena A, Rodriguez-Roisin R, et al. Fatal airway disease in an adult with chronic graft-versus-host disease. *Thorax* 1982;37:77–78.
43. Burke CM, Theodore J, Dawkins KD, et al. Post-transplant obliterative bronchiolitis and other late lung sequelae in human heart–lung transplantation. *Chest* 1984;86:824–829.
44. McGregor CGA, Dark JH, Hilton CJ, et al.

Early results of single lung transplantation in patients with end-stage pulmonary fibrosis. *J Thorac Cardiovasc Surg* 1989;98:350–354.
45. DeHoyos A, Snell G, Miller J, Winton T, Maurer J. Long term outcome after lung transplantation. *Chest* 1992[Suppl];102:199S.
46. Colt HG, Janssen JP, Dumon JF, Noirclerc MJ. Endoscopic management of bronchial stenosis after double lung transplantation. *Chest* 1992; 102:10–16.
47. Herman SJ, Weisbrod GL, Weisbrod L. Chest radiographic findings after bilateral lung transplantation. *AJR* 1989;153:1181–1185.
48. Yousem SA, Berry GJ, Brunt EM, et al. A working formulation for the standardization of nomenclature in the diagnosis of heart and lung rejection: lung rejection study group. *J Heart Transplant* 1990;9:593–601.
49. Homma H, Yamanaka A, Shinichi T, et al. Diffuse panbronchiolitis: a disease of the transitional zone of the lung. *Chest* 1983;83:63–69.
50. Sugiyama Y, Kudoh S, Maeda H, et al. Analysis of HLA antigens in patients with diffuse panbronchiolitis. *Am Rev Respir Dis* 1990;141: 1459–1462.
51. Elliott CG, Colby TV, Kelly TM, et al. Charcoal lung: bronchiolitis obliterans after aspiration of activated charcoal. *Chest* 1989;96:672–674.
52. Tsunoda N, Iwanaga T, Saito T, et al. Rapidly progressive bronchiolitis obliterans associated with Stevens-Johnson syndrome. *Chest* 1990;98: 243–245.
53. King TE. Bronchiolitis obliterans. *Lung* 1989; 167:69–93.
54. Liebow AA, Carrington CB. The interstitial pneumonias. In: Simon M, Potchen EJ, LeMay M, eds. *Frontiers of pulmonary radiology*. New York: Grune & Stratton; 1969:102–141.
55. Epler GR, Colby TV, McLoud TC, et al. Bronchiolitis obliterans organizing pneumonia. N Engl J Med 1985; 312:152–158.
56. Kitaichi M. Pathologic features and the classification of interstitial pneumonia of unknown etiology. *Bull Chest Dis Res Inst Kyoto Univ* 1990; 23:1–18.
57. Guerry-Force ML, Muller NL, Wright JL, et al. A comparison of bronchiolitis obliterans with organizing pneumonia, usual interstitial pneumonia and small airways disease. *Am Rev Respir Dis* 1987;135:705–712.
58. Kuwano K, Hayashi S, MacKenzie A, Hogg JC. Detection of adenovirus DNA in paraffin-embedded lung tissues from patients with bronchiolitis obliterans and organizing pneumonia (BOOP) using in situ hybridization. *Am Rev Respir Dis* 1990;141:A319.
59. Chien J, Chan CK, Chamberlain D, et al. Cytomegalovirus pneumonia in allogeneic bone marrow transplantation. *Chest* 1990;98:1034–1037.
60. Epler GR, Mark EJ. A 65-year-old woman with bilateral pulmonary infiltrates. *N Engl J Med* 1986;314:1627–1635.
61. Tazelaar HD, Viggiano RW, Pickersgill J, Colby TV. Interstitial lung disease in polymyositis and dermatomyositis. *Am Rev Respir Dis* 1990;141: 727–733.
62. Matteson EL, Ike RW. Bronchiolitis obliterans organizing pneumonia and Sjogren's syndrome. *J Rheumatol* 1990;17:676–679.
63. Yamamoto M, Kitaichi M, Tamura M. Clinical features of BOOP in Japan. *Chest* 1992;102:21S.
64. Camus P, Lombard JN, Perrichon M, et al. Bronchiolitis obliterans organizing pneumonia in patients taking acebutolol or amiodarone. *Thorax* 1989;44:711–715.
65. Costabel U, Teschler H, Schoenfeld B, et al. BOOP in Europe. *Chest* 1992;102:14S.
66. Santrach PJ, Askin FB, Wells RJ, Azizkhan RG, Merten DF. Nodular form of bleomycin-related pulmonary injury in patients with osteogenic sarcoma. *Cancer* 1989;64:806–811.
67. Cordier JF, Loire R, Brune J. Idiopathic bronchiolitis obliterans organizing pneumonia: definition of characteristic clinical profiles in a series of 16 patients. *Chest* 1989;96:999–1004.
68. Patel RC, Dutta D, Schonfeld SA. Free-base cocaine use associated with bronchiolitis obliterans organizing pneumonia. *Ann Intern Med* 1987;107:186–187.
69. Swineburne CR, Jackson GJ, Cobden I, et al. Bronchiolitis obliterans organizing pneumonia in a patient with ulcerative colitis. *Thorax* 1988; 43:735–736.
70. Allen JN, Wewers MD. HIV-associated bronchiolitis obliterans organizing pneumonia. *Chest* 1989;96:197–198.
71. Tenholder MF, Becker GL, Cervoni MI. The myelodysplastic syndrome and bronchiolitis obliterans. *Ann Intern Med* 1990;112:714–715.
72. Kaufman J, Komorowski R. Bronchiolitis obliterans: a new clinical-pathologic complication of irradiation pneumonitis. *Chest* 1990;97:1243–1244.
73. Kaufman J, Komorowski R. Bronchiolitis obliterans organizing pneumonia in common variable immunodeficiency syndrome. *Chest* 1991;100: 552–553.
74. Costabel U, Guzman J. BOOP: what is old, what is new? *Eur Respir J* 1991;4:771–773.
75. Geddes DM. BOOP and COP. *Thorax* 1991; 46:545–547.
76. [Anonymous]. Organising pneumonia: COP/ BOOP and SOP [Editorial]. *Lancet* 1992;340: 699–700.
77. Corrin B. Bronchiolitis obliterans organizing pneumonia. *Chest* 1992;102:7S.
78. Epler GR. Bronchiolitis obliterans organizing pneumonia: definition and clinical features. *Chest* 1992;102:2S–6S.
79. Patel U, Jenkins PF. Bronchiolitis obliterans organizing pneumonia. *Respir Med* 1989;83:241–244.
80. Tan WC, Chan RKT, Sinniah R. Idiopathic bronchiolitis obliterans with organizing pneumonia in Singapore: first case report. *Singapore Med J* 1990;31:493–496.
81. Alegre-Martin J, de Sevilla TF, Garcia F, et al. Three cases of idiopathic bronchiolitis obliter-

ans with organizing pneumonia. *Eur Respir J* 1991;4:902–904.
82. Neagos GR, Lynch JP. Making sense of bronchiolitis obliterans and related disorders. *J Respir Dis* 1991;12(9):789–814.
83. Swinburn C. Bronchiolitis obliterans organizing pneumonia. *Br J Hosp Med* 1992;48(8):492–495.
84. Flowers JR, Clunie G, Burke M, Constant O. Bronchiolitis obliterans organizing pneumonia: the clinical and radiological features of seven cases and a review of the literature. *Clin Radiol* 1992;45:371–377.
85. Cordier JF, Loire R, Peyrol S. Bronchiolitis obliterans organizing pneumonia (BOOP). *Rev Mal Respir* 1991;8:139–152.
86. Myers JL, Veal CF, Shin MS, Katzenstein AA. Respiratory bronchiolitis causing interstitial lung disease. *Am Rev Respir Dis* 1967;135:880–884.
87. Hardy KA, Schidlow DV, Zaeri N. Obliterative bronchiolitis in children. *Chest* 1988;93:460–466.

SECTION 2

Bronchiolar Diseases: The Airway Disorders

Diseases of the Bronchioles, edited by
Gary R. Epler. Raven Press, Ltd.,
New York © 1994.

8

Disease of the Small Airways in Smokers: Smokers' Bronchiolitis

Richard A. Finkelstein* and Manuel G. Cosio†

**Fellow of the Canadian Lung Association, †Professor of Medicine and Director, Respiratory Division, Royal Victoria Hospital and McGill University, Montreal, Quebec, Canada.*

By far the most common cause of bronchiolitis today is self-induced by cigarette smoking. Cigarettes cause airflow limitation, most of it irreversible, in about 15% of smokers, and bronchiolitis is, in large part, responsible for the decrease in flow. This abnormality is a slowly progressive inflammatory process encompassing changes in the epithelial surface and wall of the bronchioles. These changes, by narrowing and obliterating the lumen and by actively constricting the airway, contribute significantly to the airflow limitation characteristic of smokers. Because flows are the result of a driving pressure, elastic recoil and an opposing resistance, and airway patency, it is best to refer to the changes in flows seen in smokers as airflow limitation, rather than airflow obstruction, since both loss of elastic recoil and increase in airway resistance play an important role in the observed decrease in flow. The pathological abnormalities that could account for the airflow limitation are emphysema, producing loss of recoil, and abnormalities in both large bronchi and bronchioles. Cellular inflammatory infiltrates and submucosal secretory gland enlargement in the large airways are not believed to contribute directly to the airflow limitation found in smokers. These pathological abnormalities are associated with the mucous hypersecretion found in the chronic bronchitis of smokers.

In this review will emphasize the role of the small airways in the airflow limitation in smokers and their relation to parenchymal destruction, emphysema. The small airways comprise both the membranous bronchioles (less than 2 mm in diameter) and the respiratory bronchioles. Inflammatory changes in these airways are termed *bronchiolitis* and *respiratory bronchiolitis*, respectively.

PATHOPHYSIOLOGY OF THE SMALL AIRWAYS

Macklem (1) used the novel technique of the retrograde catheter to demonstrate that, contrary to previous beliefs, the airways less than 2 mm in diameter (small airways) contributed to no more than one-quarter of the total airway resistance in dog lungs. Hogg and associates (2), applying the same technique to human lungs, found that in excised normal lungs only 25% of the total airway resistance was contributed by airways less than 2 to 3 mm in diameter. However, in smokers with mild emphysema a fourfold increase in peripheral airway resistance was found, while total airway resistance remained unchanged. More severe degrees of emphysema resulted in a marked increase in total airway resistance due almost entirely to the increase in the peripheral airway component. This work established the then new, and still prevailing, concept that peripheral airways are the major site of increased resistance and disease in smoke-induced obstructive lung disease, and that significant increases in the resistance of these airways can be present without changes in the total airway resistance of the lung. Hence the term "the silent zone of the lung" coined by Mead (3) to describe the small airways.

Niewoehner and associates (4) were the first to demonstrate that definite pathological abnormalities could already be present in the peripheral airways of young smokers. Membranous bronchioles had denuded epithelium and increased mural inflammatory cells. The most prominent finding was what they called *respiratory bronchiolitis*. This lesion was characterized by clusters of pigmented macrophages in the bronchiolar lumina frequently associated with edema, fibrosis, and epithelial hyperplasia in adjacent bronchiolar and alveolar walls. Such abnormalities were not found in the airways of nonsmokers of the same age. This study demonstrated a definite association between cigarette smoking and pathological changes in the peripheral airways, and it was hypothesized that these lesions may be responsible for subtle physiological abnormalities observed in young smokers and may be the precursor of more severe anatomical lesions.

The observation that the early structural changes and site of airflow limitation in smokers found in the small airways created an enthusiasm for tests of small airway function that could become abnormal before flow limitation by decrease in FEV_1 was obvious, and this could identify the smoker most likely to progress to chronic airflow limitation. This was based, in turn, on the hypothesis that structural changes in the small airways preceded the development of chronic obstructive pulmonary disease. If small airway disease preceded the development of emphysema and chronic obstructive pulmonary disease, it was not unreasonable to hope that tests of small airway function could be used to identify the susceptible smoker who would develop clinically significant chronic obstructive pulmonary disease. In order to test this important hypothesis it was necessary first to demonstrate that the tests of small airway function indeed reflected pathological abnormalities in the small airways before population studies were performed.

CORRELATION BETWEEN MORPHOLOGY AND FUNCTION OF THE SMALL AIRWAYS

By studying smokers who had tests of pulmonary function, including those reflecting the small airways, before undergoing resection for lung tumors, investigators (5) at McGill developed a pathological score to describe the microscopic changes in the small airways of smokers to study the correlations between the morphology and the function. Specifically, they scored luminal occlusion, goblet-cell metaplasia, squamous-cell metaplasia, mucosal ulcers, muscle hypertrophy, inflammatory cell infiltrate, fibrosis, and pigment deposition of the airway wall in airways smaller than 2 mm in diameter. The terms *small airways* and *membranous bronchioles* are used interchangeably in this chapter. This study showed that these patients had abnormalities in the small airways similar to but much more extensive than those described by Niewoehner and colleagues (4). These differences were most likely due to the fact that the patients studied at McGill were older, had smoked more, and had some degree of chronic obstructive pulmonary disease. The first abnormalities that could be seen in the older smokers were changes in the epithelium with squamous metaplasia and a chronic inflammatory infiltrate, and slight increase in the connective tissue in the walls of the small airways (Fig. 1). As the pathologic and functional abnormalities progressed, the cellular inflammatory infiltrate changed little, but there was a progressive increase in the connective-tissue pigment and muscle in the airway wall. Significant goblet-cell metaplasia could be seen in the most severely affected airways (Fig. 2).

When physiological measurements reflecting small airway abnormalities, such as nitrogen washout test,volume of isoflow, $\Delta Vmax_{50}$, and other function tests, such as the percentage of forced vital capacity in one second (FEV_1/FVC), mid flow rate, and residual volume with the pathological score were compared, all measurements showed a progressive deterioration as the score of the morphological abnormalities increased, but only the group with the most severe small airway score demonstrated a substantial amount of emphysema. The striking correlation between the progression of physiological impairment and the degree of small airway disease suggested that inflammatory changes of the small airways made an important contribution to the functional deterioration seen in chronic obstructive pulmonary disease even in the presence of emphysema. Furthermore, in subjects with normal FEV_1/FVC ratio, two tests of small airway function, the slope of phase III of the nitrogen washout and the volume of isoflow of the air–helium flow volume loops, were able to detect mild abnormalities of the small airways when spirometric tests were normal (Fig. 3) (5).

Other investigators later confirmed these findings using lungs obtained at either surgery or autopsy. Berend and others (6) showed that the tests of small airway function correlated best with the total pathological score of the small airways and, in particular, with the inflammatory score. They (7) also found that the closing volume and mid expiratory flow correlated significantly with a measure of airway lumenal size. Performing maximal expiratory flow volume curves in excised human lungs, Berend and associates (8), in another study, showed that flow at the trachea correlated significantly with the total pathological score of the small airways as well as the inflammation, fibrosis, and emphysema scores. Petty and colleagues (9) performed lung function tests on lungs obtained at autopsy. The lungs were divided into two groups on the basis of a normal or abnormal closing capacity, and the study demonstrated higher total pathological, inflammation, and fibrosis scores in the lungs with higher closing capacity. Wright and associates (10) also examined the morphologic basis of small airway obstruction in chronic obstructive pulmonary disease and attempted to determine the usefulness of tests of lung function in identifying early airway disease. In particular, they divided their group of 96 patients into those with a normal FEV_1 and those with an FEV_1 below 80% predicted. When the FEV_1 was normal, an increasing number of abnormal tests of small airway function such as VisoV, closing volume as a percentage of vital capacity, and slope of phase III of the single breath nitrogen washout were associated with increasingly severe fibrosis scores in membranous bronchioles and with worsening intralumenal and mural inflammatory scores of respiratory bronchioles (respiratory bronchiolitis).

These studies demonstrated that smokers develop abnormalities of the small airways early in life, that these abnormalities are reflected in vivo by tests of small airway disease, and that the pathological abnormalities increase as lung function deteriorates further. The scenario was then set to investigate whether abnormalities in the tests of small airways early in the lives of smokers could predict those who would eventually develop chronic obstructive pulmonary disease. Buist and colleagues (11) reported a 9- to 11-year follow-up of two groups of smokers in whom spirometry and the single-breath nitrogen test were used throughout to determine the usefulness of the single-breath nitrogen test in identifying the

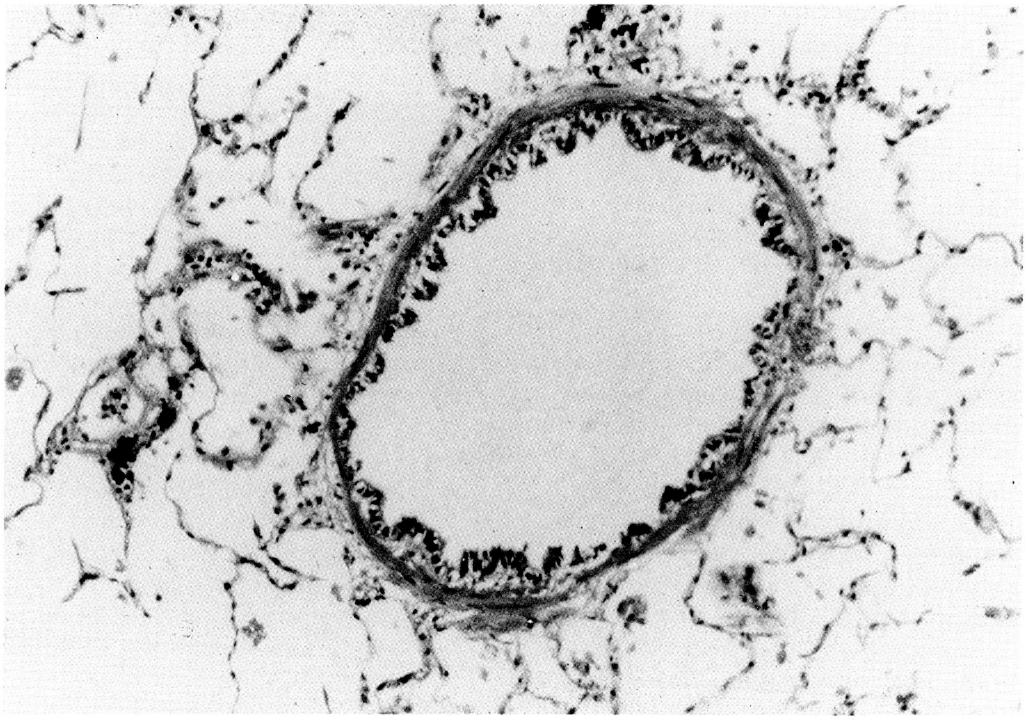

A

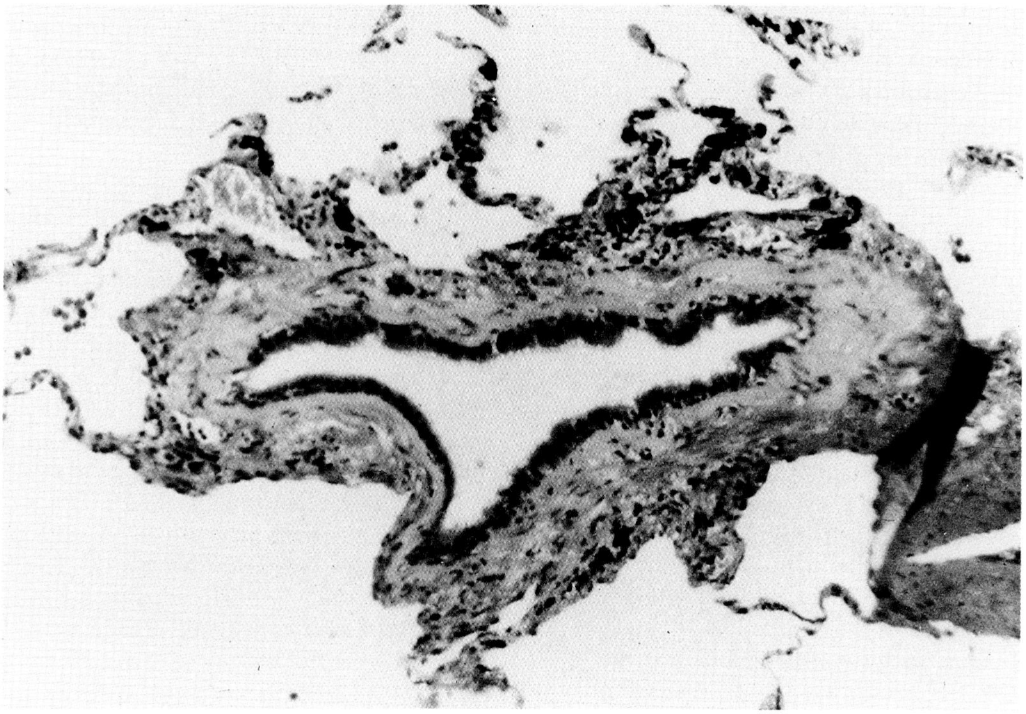

B

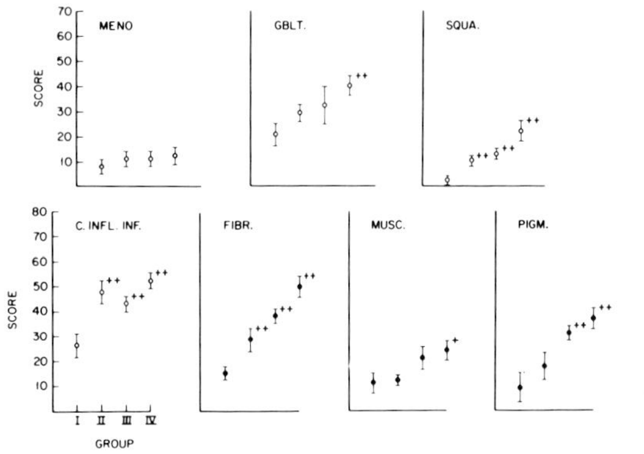

FIG. 2. Progression of the bronchiolar pathological abnormalities in four groups of smokers of increasing functional abnormalities.

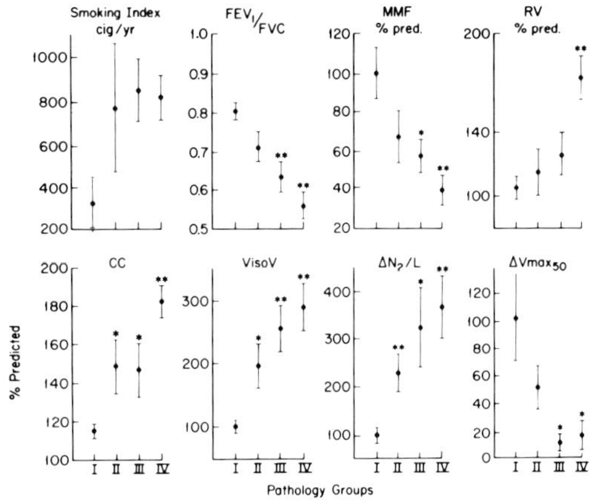

FIG. 3. Comparison of increasing small airways disease (groups 1 to IV) to smoking index (cigarettes per day times years smoked), ratio of forced expiratory volume in one second to forced vital capacity (FEV_1/FVC), and measured values as a percentage of predicted values for the maximum midexpiratory flow rate (*MMF*), residual volume (*RV*), closing capacity (*CC*), volume at isoflow comparing helium and oxygen to air on the maximum expiratory flow-volume maneuver (*VisoV*), the slope of phase III of the single breath nitrogen washout ($\Delta N_2/L$), and the increase in flow observed at 50% vital capacity comparing helium and oxygen with air on the maximum expiratory flow-volume curve ($\Delta Vmax_{50}$). Pulmonary function deteriorated progressively as the abnormality in the small airways increased. Subjects with minimal pathologic change (*group II*) could be separated from those with the most normal airways (*group I*) by the closing capacity. VisoV and ΔN_2L (ɫ, mean ± SE; *, $P < 0.05$; **, $P < 0.01$). From ref. 5. Reprinted by permission of *The New England Journal of Medicine* (298; 1277–1281, 1978).

smoker who experiences a rapid decline in FEV_1 and is therefore likely to be at risk of developing chronic airflow limitation. Of the smokers who developed an abnormal FEV_1 during the follow-up, 87% had an abnormal single-breath nitrogen test and subsequent increased rate of decline of FEV_1. It was therefore useful in identifying the smoker at risk of developing chronic airflow limitation; however, its usefulness was diminished by the high proportion of smokers who had mild functional abnormalities but did not progress to develop chronic airflow limitation.

In summary, cigarette smoke seems to elicit an inflammatory reaction in the membranous and respiratory bronchioles early in life, and this abnormality can be detected by tests of small airway function such as slope of phase III of the nitrogen washout. However, this early pathological and physiological abnormality does not progress in all smokers. Thus, physiological abnormal-

FIG. 1. **A,** Normal membranous bronchiole. Ciliated epithelium with no goblet cells, thin wall with a full layer of smooth muscle, and numerous attached alveoli are characteristic. **B,** Membranous bronchiole in a smoker with airflow limitation. The lumen is narrowed and deformed. The wall is thick with abundant fibrosis and muscle. Inflammatory cells and pigment deposition are apparent. There is a decrease in the alveolar attachments, and the ones present are severely inflamed.

ities in the small airways do not predict the 15 to 20% of smokers who progress to chronic airflow limitation. Further physiological deterioration is accompanied by such progressive pathological abnormalities as goblet-cell metaplasia, fibrosis, muscle hypertrophy, narrowing of the airways, and emphysema. A complex interaction between airflow limitation and changes in airway structure and in the lung parenchyma has emerged.

PROGRESSION OF SMALL AIRWAY ABNORMALITIES IN CHRONIC OBSTRUCTIVE PULMONARY DISEASE

The striking correlation between the progression of physiological impairment and the degree of small airway disease suggests that inflammation of the small airways makes an important contribution to the functional deterioration seen in chronic obstructive pulmonary disease, even in the presence of emphysema. Many studies have since addressed the pathological changes of the small airways in smokers and their relationship to the flow limitation found in chronic obstructive pulmonary disease. Of special interest are studies comparing the airway changes in smokers with various degrees of emphysema and chronic obstructive pulmonary disease with nonsmokers, since they give a perspective not only of the effects of smoking and emphysema but also of the effect of aging in the airways.

In one such study Cosio (12) compared abnormalities in the small airways in smokers and nonsmokers who died accidentally. Pulmonary function status was not known; however, the degree of macroscopic emphysema and microscopic emphysema, assessed by the mean linear intercept, was no different in smokers and nonsmokers, suggesting that in most cases the effects of cigarettes were mild. Nonetheless, abnormalities in the membranous and respiratory bronchioles of smokers were quite apparent, showing increased goblet cells, cellular inflammatory infiltrates, and muscle and respiratory bronchiolitis when compared with nonsmokers. The overall mean diameter of airways less than 2 mm was similar in both groups, but smokers had a significantly greater proportion of bronchioles smaller than 400 μm than nonsmokers, and this proportion was closely related to the total score of airway abnormalities. Several other studies (9,13,14) have indicated that a better relationship with airflow limitation is with the proportion of very narrowed airways of 0.2 and 0.35 mm in diameter. Of special interest, this marked narrowing may also be associated with hypoxemia and right ventricular hypertrophy (13,15–17).

Wright and co-workers (18) studied lungs of nonsmokers, smokers, and ex-smokers and reported no significant differences in individual values for total pathological scores for membranous bronchioles between current and former smokers. However respiratory bronchioles in former smokers did display a significant decrease in goblet-cell pigment, inflammation, and intralumenal macrophages in comparison with smokers. Wright and associates (19) also found that the wall thickness of membranous and respiratory bronchioles for each bronchiolar diameter was increased in almost all size ranges in smokers when compared with lifetime nonsmokers, indicating that smoking is associated with an increase in airway wall thickness independent of airway size and regardless of the presence or absence of emphysema. However, for the same level of function, the degree of airway abnormalities could be quite variable, suggesting that other abnormalities, probably elastic recoil losses, would influence the degree of flow limitation.

Hale and co-workers (20) added to the population of smokers and nonsmokers in the Cosio study (12) another group of 18 patients dying with known and measured chronic obstructive pulmonary disease. This study is of interest since it clearly shows the progression of the small airway pathological changes from nonsmoking older individuals to smokers with mild disease and finally to smokers dying with chronic obstructive pulmonary disease. The cellular inflammatory infiltrate, fibrosis, and muscle in the airway wall progressed significantly in a stepwise fashion in the three groups; and as expected from our initial study the number of airways less than 400 μm increased accordingly. The mean diameter of the small airways tended to decrease, but the range of diameters was so large that no statistical differences could be found even between patients with the most severe chronic obstructive pulmonary disease and nonsmokers. A similar wide range was found in all the airway inflammatory abnormalities measured in the two groups of smokers, indicating that not every smoker reacts in the same fashion to cigarette smoke and suggesting that some smokers are more prone than others to develop small airway abnormalities (Fig. 4). Not surprisingly, smokers dying of chronic obstructive pulmonary disease had more emphysema in their lungs than nonsmokers and patients with mild chronic obstructive pulmonary disease. The degree of emphysema assessed macroscopically correlated with all abnormalities found in the small airways. With this large degree of intercorrelation, it is not surprising that in severe chronic obstructive pulmonary disease, the degree of emphysema might override correlations between morphology of the small airways and function. Nonetheless, Hale and colleagues (20) found that the degree of airflow limitation correlated not only with emphysema but also with the average airway diameter and the proportion of airways smaller than 400 μm, a function of the total pathological score of the small airways.

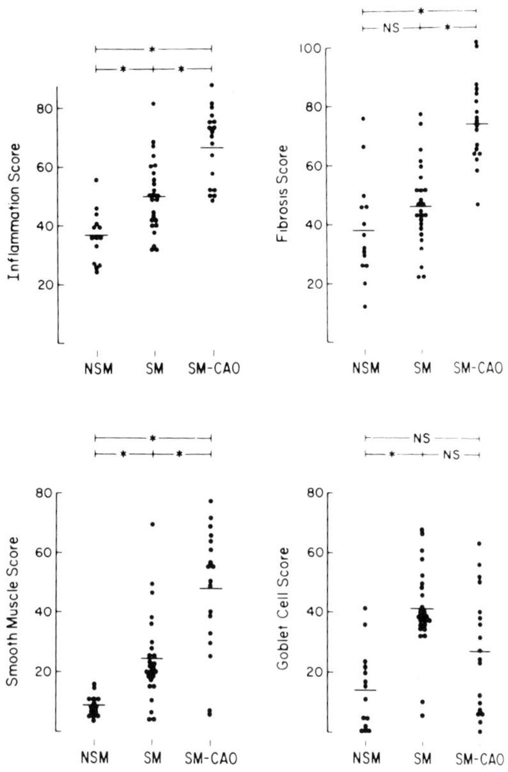

FIG. 4. Comparison of scores for peripheral airways disease among nonsmokers (*NSM*), smokers (*SM*), and smokers with chronic airflow obstruction (*SM-CAO*). From ref. 20, with permission.

Similar results were obtained by Nagai and co-workers (21) in patients dying with chronic obstructive pulmonary disease. In their study, flow rates antemortem correlated with the degree of macroscopic emphysema as well as with the proportion of airways smaller than 400 μm in diameter and the degree of deformity of bronchioles. Their interpretation of these findings was that decreases in flow were secondary to emphysema causing loss of elastic recoil and with airway obstruction caused by an excess number of very small bronchioles and deformity of bronchiolar lumina. It was also clear from this study that for the same degree of airflow limitation, smokers with lesser amounts of emphysema had more diseased small airways, suggesting that the combined effect of loss of recoil secondary to emphysema and increase in airways resistance secondary to small airway abnormalities produces the airflow limitation in chronic obstructive pulmonary disease.

The relationship between small airway diameters, a function of the proportion of the very small airways (less than 400 μm in diameter) in the lung and lung disease in smokers is of interest. Smokers in these studies had a significant excess of airways less than 400 μm in diameter when compared with nonsmokers, and this proportion correlated with the severity of pathological abnormalities in these airways. This correlation suggests that inflammatory and fibrotic reactions in the airways result in subtle degrees of airway narrowing that are best detected as an excess in airways less than 400 μm in diameter. However, this explanation may not fully account for the relationship between disease and the caliber of the small airways. The mean bronchiole diameter and the percentage of airways less than 400 μm in diameter are highly variable even in nonsmokers (12), and in one study (22) the average bronchial diameter in young adults was found to vary over a twofold range. These data might suggest that small-airway caliber may be constitutionally determined or secondary to diseases in childhood or both, and airway narrowing, as measured at total lung capacity, may not be entirely due to disease. An alternative explanation is that persons with smaller airways, because of constitution or diseases in childhood, might be more susceptible to developing disease in these airways when exposed to cigarette smoke or other irritants.

Among smokers, the severity of small airway disease correlates with the extent of centrilobular emphysema. There is also a definite tendency for small airways in the upper lung to be more diseased than those in the lower lung, a topographic distribution that corresponds to centrilobular emphysema (12). It is also known that disease in the small airways temporally precedes centrilobular emphysema (5) and that emphysema lesions first appear in the respiratory bronchiole, where the inflammatory reaction, particularly macrophage accumulation, is most intense (4,5,23). We believe these various observations are complementary and support the hypothesis that small airway disease is causally related to the development of centrilobular emphysema. Leopold and Gough (24) also showed that the small airways were usually inflamed in lungs with centrilobular emphysema but, in contrast, seldom in patients with predominant panlobular emphysema. Similar observations were reported by Anderson and Foraker (25), who believed centrilobular emphysema and panlobular emphysema were two different diseases.

THE RELATIONSHIP OF SMALL AIRWAY ABNORMALITIES AND EMPHYSEMA IN SMOKERS

Physiological evidence suggesting that smokers could develop two different types of emphysema was provided by Eidelman and co-workers (26). They found that smokers with chronic obstructive pulmonary disease had different patterns of functional abnormalities. Some exhibited pressure–volume curves that are typical of emphysema and that resemble those seen in alpha-antiprotease deficiency with high compliance and low elastic recoil pressure at high lung volumes. About one-half of their subjects had low or normal compliance and, despite similar elastic recoil, had lower FEV_1 and pressure–volume curves not typical of emphysema.

On the basis of these findings, Kim and co-workers (27) reasoned that such dissimilar functional behavior ought to correspond to different parenchymal morphological abnormalities: panlobular emphysema for the smokers with mechanical characteristics similar to alpha-antiprotease deficiency, and centrilobular emphysema for the others. They tested this hypothesis in 34 patients undergoing lung resection who had pulmonary function tests performed before surgery. Emphysema was assessed microscopically, characterized as centrilobular or panlobular using available definitions, and quantitated using the mean linear intercept. Both types of emphysema could be found in this population of smokers; 18

patients had pure or predominant centrilobular emphysema and 16 had panlobular emphysema. Mechanical properties were found to be different in both types of emphysema. Patients with panlobular emphysema had a high compliance and a higher constant of elasticity (K) than patients with centrilobular emphysema. As the emphysema worsened, compliance, K, and the elastic recoil at 90% of total lung capacity worsened in panlobular emphysema but did not change in centrilobular emphysema. Furthermore, losses of elasticity correlated significantly with the extent of emphysema in lungs with panlobular emphysema but not in those with centrilobular emphysema. These findings suggest that mechanical properties are different in the two types of emphysema, and these differences become more marked with the progression of the air space enlargement, suggesting that the two types of lung destruction are different from the start.

Another important difference between the two types of emphysema is the extent of airway abnormalities. Lungs with centrilobular emphysema had higher total pathological scores of the small airways than lungs with panlobular emphysema. This difference was mainly ascribable to increased muscle and fibrosis in the airway wall. Probably, as a result of the more severe pathological involvement, lungs with centrilobular emphysema had more airways smaller than 400 μm in diameter than those with panlobular emphysema. Not surprisingly, the pathophysiology of flow limitation in smokers, a function of airway resistance and elastic recoil pressures, differs between the two types of emphysema. Flow was shown to decrease as airway abnormalities increased in centrilobular emphysema, but no relationship between flow and airway disease could be found in panlobular emphysema. In contrast, flow decreases significantly as elasticity decreases in panlobular emphysema but not in centrilobular emphysema (Fig. 5). Some patients with centrilobular emphysema exhibited decreased flow with normal or even increased elastic recoil pressures, whereas those with panlobular emphysema had flow limitation always accompanied by loss of recoil. These findings clarify the pathogenesis of airflow limitation in smokers, indicating that in centrilobular emphysema loss of flow is primarily a function of airway abnormalities with elastic recoil loss playing an additive role. By contrast, in patients with panlobular emphysema, the flow limitation seems to be mainly a function of reduced elastic recoil; added airway abnormalities could worsen flows even further in these cases.

This study is of interest not only because it clarifies the mechanisms of airflow limitation and the role of the bronchioles in chronic obstructive pulmonary disease but also because it confirms the possibility of smokers developing two diseases with different pathogenetic mechanisms. The diffuse destruction seen in panlobular emphysema might result from a blood-borne mechanism. On the other hand, the uneven pattern of lung destruction seen in centrilobular emphysema is associated with more severe abnormalities in the small airways, suggesting that centrilobular destruction is related to airborne factors and intimately related to the airway inflammatory process. In favor of this hypothesis are the findings of Saetta and colleagues (28). These authors investigated the relationship between the inflammation of the small airways and the extent of parenchymal destruction using the destructive index (DI) (29) in smokers' lungs with centrilobular and panlobular emphysema. In lungs with centrilobular emphysema a close correlation between the inflammation of the airways and the parenchymal destruction was evident. This correlation was not present in lungs with panlobular emphysema, even though the range of inflammation of the airways in the two lungs was similar (Fig. 6). Thus it is likely that the inflammatory reaction seen in and around small airways and respiratory bronchioles spreads centrifugally to the paren-

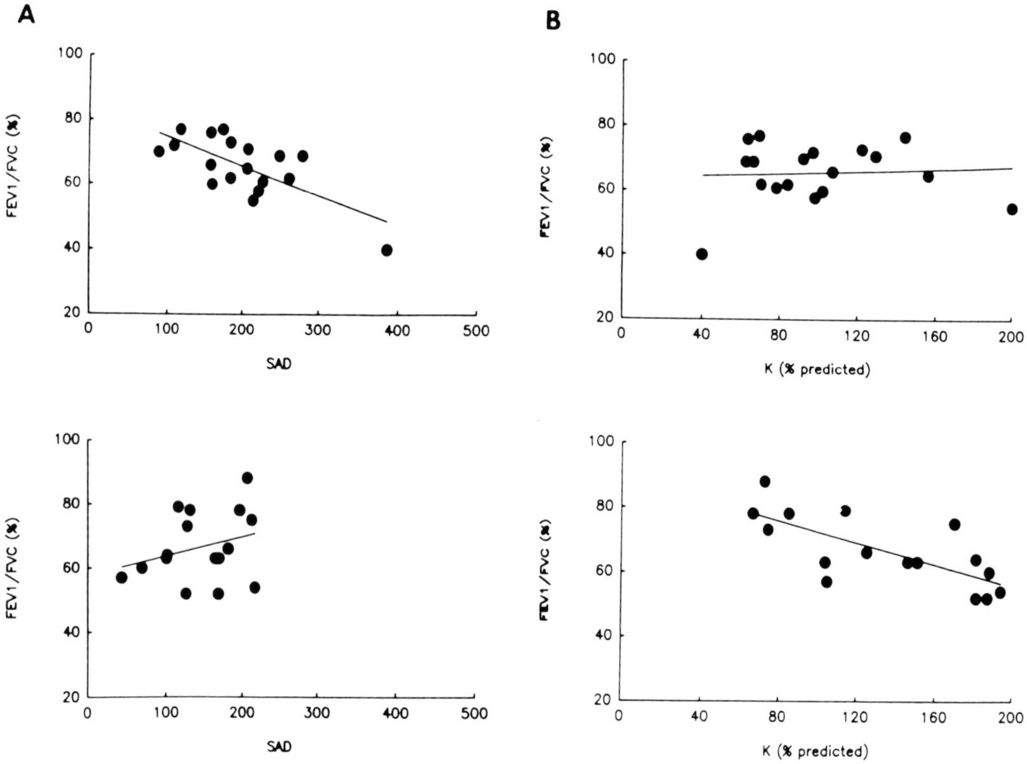

FIG. 5. **A,** Relationship between the degree of airway abnormalities (*SAD*) and the FEV_1/FVC percent in centrilobular emphysema (CLE) (*upper panel*) ($r = -0.69$, $P < 0.01$) and panlobular emphysema (PLE) (*lower panel*) ($r = 0.29$, $p > 0.05$). **B,** Relationship between the exponential constant *K* as an index of the elasticity of the lung and flow expressed as FEV_1/FVC in centrilobular emphysema (*upper panel*) ($r = 0.08$, $p > 0.05$) and panlobular emphysema (*lower panel*) ($r = -0.72$, $p < 0.01$). From ref. 27, with permission.

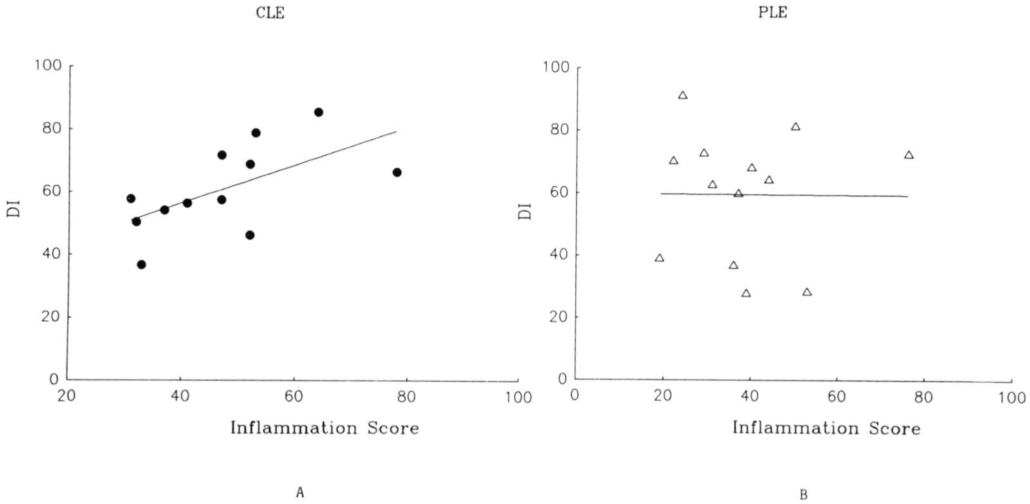

FIG. 6. Correlation between the inflammation score in the small airways and destructive index in **A,** CLE and **B,** PLE. A significant correlation is present in CLE ($r = 0.617$, $p < 0.025$) but not in PLE ($r = -0.009$, p NS).

chyma surrounding these airways and eventually destroys the alveolar walls attached to the airways and the respiratory bronchioles and alveolar ducts. The preservation of alveolar structure and size with concomitant destruction of alveolar ducts and respiratory bronchioles in centrilobular emphysema is in favor of this possibility.

These studies set a new basis for the investigation of lung disease in smokers. If the intimal pathogenetic mechanisms in the two types of emphysema in smokers are different, as the evidence suggests, the study of cigarette-induced lung disease as a single entity will delay even further the understanding of chronic obstructive pulmonary disease.

MECHANISMS OF AIRWAY INFLAMMATION AND AIRWAY CONSTRICTION

Airway dimensions are narrower in smokers than in nonsmokers. However, these differences seem to be minimal and are evident only by calculating the proportion of airways smaller than 400 μm and, by themselves, do not account for the large increases in airway resistance found in lungs of smokers. The conducting system of the lung, the airways, are not merely passive tubes, as we consider them with just morphometry, but structures able to change in size during the respiratory cycle and also to react to stimuli. It would then seem reasonable to assume that the in vitro measurements of airway diameter are an underestimate of airway dimensions in vivo. The main reasons accounting for this discrepancy are that (a) airway diameters in vitro are measured at total lung capacity, whereas expiratory flows depend on the behavior of the airways during a full lung deflation from total lung capacity to residual volume; and (b) active constriction of the airways in vivo will not necessarily be evident in fixed human lungs. Hence, the in vitro measurements cannot detect these events.

There is ample evidence demonstrating that the airways of smokers react to nonspecific stimuli by constricting with increased resistance and decreased FEV_1. Many authors (30–36) believe that smokers might have hyperreactive airways and that this hyperreactivity might contribute to the natural history of chronic obstructive pulmonary disease. However, others (37,38) believe the contrary, that the hyperresponsiveness found in smokers is a consequence of the already decreased airway dimensions and lower FEV_1. Regardless of whether hyperresponsiveness is primary or secondary to airway geometry, there is sufficient evidence indicating that airways of smokers constrict when exposed to no specific stimuli, and that the airways of smokers constrict more than those of ex-smokers and nonsmokers. The degree of hyperresponsiveness in smokers is lower than in patients with asthma, probably because the abnormal conditions of the airway smooth muscle and atopy, which are the basis for the hyperresponsiveness in asthmatics, are not present in most smokers with chronic obstructive pulmonary disease. However, the abnormalities found in the airways of smokers could contribute to the constriction of a normal airway muscle. Hence, regardless of the presence or lack of muscle hyperresponsiveness, muscle constriction in smokers is most likely an important component of airflow limitation in chronic obstructive pulmonary disease.

A number of pathological changes could be responsible for active muscle constriction and airway narrowing in chronic obstructive pulmonary disease. These include (a) airway epithelial damage resulting in increased epithelial permeability and impairment of other epithelial functions, (b) chronic airway inflammation, (c) fibrotic changes in the airway wall, (d) increased smooth muscle with altered smooth-muscle sensitivity and contractility, and (e) loss of alveolar attachments. The role of the epithelium and inflammation may be the key to the pathogenesis of airway narrowing.

Most of the knowledge in this area is derived from animal work and has been linked with the pathogenesis, inflammation, and airway constriction of asthma. However, in many respects this can also apply to chronic obstructive pulmonary disease.

Roles of the Epithelium in Airway Inflammation and Narrowing

Effects of Altered Permeability

The protective barrier formed by the airway epithelium is altered by cigarette smoke. Denuded epithelium, mucosal ulcers, and goblet and squamous metaplasia are consistently found in airways of smokers. Numerous studies (39–41) have shown that cigarette smoke causes airway epithelium to become more permeable to electron-dense tracers with damage to junctional complexes being demonstrated in smoke-exposed guinea pigs. The effects of cigarette smoke on alveolar epithelium permeability, studied in humans by Jones and colleagues (42), showed similar results. These authors speculated that the mechanism for cell damage may be mediated by carbon monoxide binding to cytochrome P450, and it is known that carbon monoxide poisoning leads to endothelial damage and increased capillary permeability (42, 43). Other possible mechanisms include the action of nicotine, catecholamines, nitrous oxide, nitrogen dioxides, and other constituents of cigarette smoke on the alveolar epithelium (42). The altered epithelium permeability leaves underlying afferent nerve endings and irritant receptors exposed to bronchoconstrictor and other proinflammatory substances. Thus, the dysfunction of the epithelial cells could contribute to bronchoconstriction and airway inflammation. Finally, altered integrity of the epithelial barrier permits access of plasma exudate to the airway lumen and also has mechanical and inflammatory effects on the small airway.

Effects of Luminal Fluid

Once across the epithelial barrier, plasma exudate and its associated macromolecules immediately fill the interstices between epithelium projections (44). Liquid-filled interstices could amplify the degree of lumenal compromise in at least two ways. First, lumenal cross-sectional area is reduced as the interstices fill with fluid (45). Second, plasma proteins could alter the surface tension of the airway lining fluid, which can further compromise the airway lumen. Macklem and colleagues (46) have reasoned that if the interstices fill with liquid, the surface tension of the airway-lining liquid increases and the radius of curvature of the interfaces joining the tips of epithelial projections increases. When the curvatures of the interfaces joining projections match the curvature of the airway lumen, a point of instability is reached and airways could close. This has been suggested as a physical mechanism that could contribute to airway hyperresponsiveness. Plasma proteins have been shown to inhibit lung-surfactant function by significantly increasing surface tension (47). Phospholipid cell mediators such as lyso-platelet activating factor (lyso-PAF), which is structurally similar to the primary surface-active component of pulmonary surfactant, likely alter surfactant function once incorporated into the air–liquid interface (45). The same mechanisms are likely to apply to airway surface tension.

Inflammatory Effects of Epithelial Disruption

Airway epithelial cells have the potential to initiate and become actively involved in the development of airway inflammation. Human tracheal epithelium metabolizes arachidonic acid predominantly via the 15-lipoxygenase pathway (48). One product of this pathway, 8S,15S-dihydroxyeicosatetraenoic acid (diHETE), is a potent signal that recruits neutrophils to the airways

(49). Furthermore, 15-hydroxyeicosatetraenoic acid (HETE) production stimulates the release of leukotriene C_4(LTC_4) from mast cells (50). The 15-lipoxygenase pathway in the human airway epithelium has the capacity to interact with neutrophils, mast cells, and macrophages by stimulating release of lipoxin A, a trihydroxy acid, from these cells (51). Lipoxin A has a variety of biological actions, including the ability to cause neutrophils to degranulate and to generate superoxide radicals (52).

Another system implicated in airway inflammatory responses, which could be triggered by the loss or alteration on the epithelial surface, is the sensory nerves. Nonadrenergic, noncholinergic sensory nerve fibers present in the airway epithelium, smooth muscle, and blood vessels release tachykinins including substance P, neurokinin A, and neurokinin B. Stimulation of these nerves causes a constellation of responses known as neurogenic inflammation. Substance P stimulates airway mucous secretion, increases airway microvascular permeability and exudation of plasma into the airway lumen (53–56), and causes contraction of smooth muscle in vitro (57). Neurokinin A, which is found in the same airway nerves and is coded by the same gene as substance P, is far more potent than substance P in contracting airway smooth muscle (58,59). Tachykinins also have important interactions with mast cells (60,61) and other inflammatory and immune cells. Specifically, tachykinins cause chemotaxis and adhesion of neutrophils in the airway circulation (62,63), activate monocytes to release inflammatory cytokines such as interleukin-6, and cause degranulation of eosinophils, which can further damage airway epithelium (64,65).

The inflammatory effects of the tachykinins are, in part, controlled by neutral endopeptidases, an enzyme that binds to the surface of the specific cells that are the site of action to tachykinins and cleaves and inactivates them. Neutral endopeptidase activity is found specifically in epithelium, glands, nerves, and smooth muscle (66). The abolition of neutral endopeptidase activity by stripping of the epithelium or by inhibition of this enzyme by specific inhibitors is known to increase smooth-muscle responses to bronchoconstrictor substances (67). If airway epithelium is shed or altered, any effects of tachykinins may be more pronounced, not only on airway smooth muscle but also on inflammatory effects of tachykinins in the mucosa and submucosa. Furthermore, damage to airway epithelium exposes afferent nerve endings, which may be stimulated by inflammatory mediators, some of which are exuded into the airway lumen from vessels. Inflammatory peptides found in exuded plasma, such as bradykinin, have been shown also to stimulate release of tachykinins (56).

Bronchodilator Effect

Respiratory epithelium seems to modulate directly the responsiveness of bronchial smooth muscle by the release of inhibitory factors for smooth-muscle contraction. In fact, the respiratory epithelium has a high density of beta-adrenoreceptors, higher than that in bronchial smooth muscle (68). The increased smooth-muscle relaxation in response to isoprotorenol in bronchial rings with intact epithelium compared with preparations denuded of epithelium highlights the importance of the beta-adrenoreceptors in the epithelial smooth muscle interaction (68,69). Furthermore, removal of the epithelium in canine bronchial rings increases the contractile responses evoked by acetylcholine, histamine, and 5-hydroxytryptamine (70). Thus, the absence of epithelial cells potentiates the reactivity of the underlying smooth muscle. These mechanisms seem to be modulated by inhibitory factors released by the epithelial cells. These factors have been identified (71), although their exact nature is unknown. Of interest is that airway mucus may inactivate these factors (72).

In summary, the integrity of the epithelial surface seems to be necessary for the normal function and regulation of the airways. Loss of the epithelium and/or possible replacement of normal epithelial ciliated cells by goblet or squamous cells might be one of the initial events in the development of an inflammatory reaction and airway narrowing in smokers. Albeit small, the chronicity of the stimulation could perpetuate the process and enhance the progress of the pathological changes in smokers.

Airway Inflammation

There is ample evidence that inflammatory cells and their mediators are key elements in the development of disease in general and of disease of the airways in particular. A myriad of cell components and mediators have been described with the potential of maintaining inflammation, recruiting other inflammatory or effector cells, and producing bronchoconstriction.

The earliest, and constant pathological abnormality in the airway of smokers is the cellular inflammatory infiltrate throughout the wall. The stimuli for this abnormality are not precisely known. However, we have reviewed in the previous section how injury to the epithelium, the first structure encountered by cigarette smoke, could promote and perpetuate an inflammatory reaction in the airway. Most of the studies of small airways in smokers have analyzed the inflammation of the airways in a quantitative fashion. Qualitative morphometric studies are much fewer. This is an area badly in need of studying, since a better understanding of the inflammatory process of smokers is the clue for the unveiling of the pathogenesis of this disease.

Inflammation, per se, may be responsible for mild airflow limitation (5,9,72); and it has been suggested that inflammation may lead to functional bronchiolar constriction by releasing mediators of inflammation that may act directly on bronchiolar smooth muscle (73). The chronicity of inflammation would, in turn, produce other changes, such as fibrosis of the airway, and could increase the smooth muscle either directly as a result of inflammation or indirectly as a result of chronically increased muscle tone. These changes, by increasing the thickness of the airway wall, will promote airway narrowing and airflow limitation. Finally, inflammation of the airway could play an important role in the destruction of the alveolar walls attached to the airway (respiratory bronchioles), and this decrease in alveolar attachments would contribute further to air-flow limitation by deforming and narrowing the airway lumen.

Neutrophil Inflammation

Bosken and colleagues (74) studied airway inflammation in smokers with chronic airflow obstruction and demonstrated no difference between smokers with no obstruction and smokers with obstruction for numbers of immunohistochemically stained neutrophils in the airways. However, the number of submucosal neutrophils correlated significantly to the amount of cigarettes smoked. In animal studies, exposure to cigarette smoke and other irritants promotes neutrophils to appear promptly in the airways. Baile and associates (75) reported that acid inhalation in dogs caused abnormalities in small airway function which were associated with an accumulation of neutrophils in noncartilaginous airways. Hulbert and colleagues (76) also showed that when the airway mucosa of guinea pigs is injured by the inhalation of cigarette smoke, edema forms within 30 minutes, and the number of neutrophils in the airway epithelium increased fivefold from control values 6 hours after injury. The earliest measured functional changes occurred in the exudative phase and before the accumulation of neutrophils in the airway (76). However, late changes in hyperresponsiveness occurred only in the presence of neutrophils (77).

The mechanism by which cigarette smoke causes neutrophil accumulation remains speculative, but several possibilities can be postulated. Components of cigarette smoke, such as nicotine, have been found to be chemotactic for human neutrophils, although they do not affect degranulation or superoxide production (78). Cigarette smoke also causes alveolar macrophages, abundantly found in the respiratory bronchioles of smokers, to release chemotactic factors that recruit neutrophils (79). Absorbed constituents of smoke could alter endothelial cells, or neutrophils directly, or the adherence of neutrophils to endothelium. Adhesion of neutrophils to vascular endothelial cells is critical for recruitment of these cells from the circulation to inflammatory tissue sites. This adhesion requires specific interactions between surface glycoproteins, including the B2 class of integrins (CD11/CD18), on neutrophils with eneothelial cell surface proteins (80). These endothelial proteins can be induced by pro-inflammatory cytokines, and include ICAM-1 (intercellular adhesion molecule-1), ICAM-2 (intercellular adhesion molecule-2), and ELAM-1 (endothelial-leucocyte adhesion molecule-1) (81–84). Expression of ICAM-1 can be induced on airway *epithelial* cells by inflammatory components. Treatment of primary tracheal epithelial cell cultures with interleukin-1 or tumor necrosis factor-alpha causes a three- to fourfold increase in cell surface ICAM-1 expression and support of neutrophil adhesion. Blocking ICAM-1 on the epithelial surface decreases neutrophil adherence by 50% (80). This suggests a role for epithelium derived ICAM-1 dependent neutrophil-epithelial cell adhesion in the pathophysiology of inflammatory airway diseases. Cox and associates (85) showed that bronchial epithelial cells markedly increase the survival of human neutrophils in vitro via the release of G-CSF (granulocyte colony stimulating factor) and GM-CSF (granulocyte-macrophage colony stimulating factor), and that their survival is unaffected by glucocorticoids. Thus, epithelial cells could modulate the cellularity of the inflammatory response in the acute phase of the smoker injury while the epithelial cell layer is still intact.

Lymphocytes

Smokers have higher total blood lymphocyte counts of the $CD3^+$, $CD4^+$, and $CD8^+$ types than nonsmokers (86). Excessive smokers have also been shown to have increased percentages of $CD3^+$ and $CD8^+$ and decreased percentages of $CD4^+$ with consequent decreases of their $CD4^+/CD8^+$ ratio. These results suggest that these smokers might have an alteration in immunoregulatory T lymphocytes (87). Natural killer cell activity is also reduced in smokers blood (88,89). These changes are reflected in the bronchoalveolar lavage (BAL) fluid. The percentage of $CD4^+$ cells is decreased in the lavage of smokers, as compared with that of nonsmokers, while $CD8^+$ percentages are increased and consequently $CD4^+/CD8^+$ ratios are decreased. There is also a significantly positive correlation between the percentage of $CD8^+$ cells in BAL fluid and the amount of cigarette smoking (90). In this study no changes in the lymphocyte subsets in the peripheral blood were seen, suggesting that alterations in immunoregulatory T lymphocyte subsets induced by smoking can be found in the lungs before systemic changes are apparent.

In the large airways of smokers with chronic bronchitis, increased numbers of $CD3^+$, $CD4^+$, and $CD8^+$ lymphocytes have been found. The $CD8^+$ lymphocytes predominated over $CD4^+$ lymphocytes, reflecting the described changes in BAL fluid and peripheral blood (91,92).

One study has examined the presence of lymphocytes in the small airways of smokers. Bosken (74) measured B lymphocytes, $CD4^+$, and $CD8^+$ in the airways of smokers with and without airflow obstruction. The B lymphocytes and CD^+ were most numerous in the adventitia, and there were more

$CD8^+$ cells in the epithelium than in the inner wall or the adventitia. The B lymphocytes in the entire wall and the adventitia accounted for about 15% of the total inflammatory cells and were the only cell type statistically increased in numbers in the airways of smokers with obstruction when compared with those without airflow obstruction. Bosken hypothesized that B lymphocytes may play a role in the deposition of connective tissue in the airways of smokers with obstruction to air flow.

The preponderance of B lymphocytes in the airways of smokers with obstructive lung disease is interesting in light of the previously noted association between cigarette smoking, increased serum levels of IgE, and airway obstruction. Chan and colleagues (93) have described seven patients with HLA-DR7 antigen in whom cigarette smoking induced immunoglobulin heavy chain gene rearrangements within the B lymphocytes and a B cell polyclonal lymphocytosis. In one patient, abnormal increase in lymphocytes and morphology reverted to normal after smoking cessation. The investigators hypothesized that smoking may select out abnormal clones of B lymphocytes.

Much remains to be learned about the inflammation of the small airways in smokers. Available results are of interest and point toward a possible alteration in the lymphocyte regulation in smokers that might be initiated locally in the lung and eventually detected in the blood, at least in excessive smokers. The study of lymphocyte inflammation in the small airways and its relationship to the inflammation of the parenchyma might give some clues about the mechanisms of lung destruction in smokers.

The function of the lymphocyte changes in the lungs of smokers is not known. However, it is known that lymphocytes play an important role in the inflammatory response. Lymphokines produced by activated T cells such as interferon-gamma, (IL-4), interleukin-5 (IL-5), and GM-CSF are key mediators in the cellular immune response (94,95). They are active in the control of many other cellular lines, such as eosinophils, neutrophils, mast cells, and monocytes, and are able to activate and degranulate these effector cells (95). Furthermore, $CD4^+$ and $CD8^+$ lymphocytes are key cells in the regulation of B lymphocytes and the cell-mediated and humoral immune systems. Lymphocytes may play an important role in the pathogenesis of emphysema in subjects with $alpha_1$-antiprotease deficiency (96–100). It has been shown that lymphocytes in these patients display hyperresponsiveness to mitogens that are inhibited by purified $alpha_1$-antiprotease and a role for the stimulated lymphocytes has been suggested in the development of chronic obstructive pulmonary disease, at least in smokers with $alpha_1$-antiprotease. This points toward the potential of the lymphocyte role in the pathogenesis of lung destruction in chronic obstructive pulmonary disease.

Airway Wall Contribution to Airway Narrowing

Cosio and others (5,10,101) have shown that as obstruction worsens so does the airway fibrosis; and this, along with the inflammatory infiltrate, will contribute to increasing the thickness of the airway wall and diminishing the airway lumen. Muscle in the airway wall is also increased in smokers when compared with nonsmokers (12), and this worsens as the air flow decreases further (20,102). Of interest are the findings of Kim and co-workers (27), who reported that smokers with centrilobular emphysema had significantly more muscle in the small airways than smokers with panlobular emphysema, even though the inflammatory infiltrate was quantitatively similar in both. Furthermore, for the same FEV_1, smokers with centrilobular emphysema are more reactive to methacholine than smokers with panlobular emphysema (103). Thus, muscle is increased in smokers, and able to constrict and at times hyperreact, and will passively contribute to increase airway wall thickness.

Both the walls internal and external to the smooth muscle layer are thicker in smokers with airflow limitation than in smokers without airflow limitation, and increasing thickness is associated with smaller airway diameters (104). The effect of such thickening not only decreases the airway lumen but also has an important effect on the mechanical behavior of the small airways. Moreno and co-workers (104,105) elegantly showed that, as the muscle constricts, the thickness of the wall increases and encroaches on the lumen in such a way that the thicker the airway wall internal to the muscle, the greater the narrowing resulting from a given degree of smooth-muscle shortening. Wiggs and co-workers (106) expanded the ideas of Moreno and associates and examined the effect of airway wall thickening, loss of elastic recoil, and airway smooth-muscle shortening on the increase in airway resistance using a model of the human tracheobronchial tree. This analysis showed that moderate amounts of airway wall thickening, which have little effect on baseline resistance, can profoundly affect the airway narrowing caused by smooth-muscle shortening—especially if the wall thickening is localized to peripheral airways. The decrease in FEV_1 in response to methacholine and histamine in many patients with chronic obstructive pulmonary disease could be, in large part, explained by the fibrosis and thickening of the airway wall that occurs internal to the smooth-muscle layer and that dramatically accentuates the airway narrowing induced by smooth-muscle shortening (104–106).

Fibrosis is not only confined to the internal part of the airway but also external to the smooth-muscle layer (105). The mechanical effects of fibrosis and increased airway wall thickness external to airway smooth muscle are different from those of increased thickness of the internal wall. In normal airways, the data of Gunst and associates (107) suggest that the forces of lung elastic recoil provide an elastic afterload to peripheral airway smooth muscle and impede its ability to shorten. This elastic load increases as lung volume and recoil increase. According to the interdependence theory, the pressure applied to the outer surface of intrapulmonary airways is equal to the sum of forces applied to the outer surface of the airway by the attached alveolar walls expressed as a fraction of the external surface area of the airway. As the airway wall thickens, the attached alveolar walls become shorter, the forces on the airway wall decrease, the outer airway surface area increases, and hence the pressure applied to the airway decreases. Macklem (108) has postulated that thickening external to the smooth muscle can influence the relationship between smooth-muscle contraction and airway narrowing by uncoupling the lung's elastic recoil forces from the airway smooth muscle, allowing it to shorten excessively.

In favor of these theories are the studies by Ding and colleagues (109) and later Bellofiore and associates (110) in elastase-induced emphysema in rats. Their results showed the importance of elastic recoil in smooth-muscle shortening and that emphysema in these animals decreases elastic recoil and probably alveolar attachments to the airways and thus profoundly influences the degree of airway narrowing that occurs in response to pharmacologic agonists.

Alveolar Attachments

From the previous discussion it is apparent that loss of the alveolar support around the airways, if it were to occur in smokers, ought to have an important effect on the patency of the small airways and consequently on the lung function. Anderson and Foraker (111) were the first to link pulmonary parenchymal disease and small airway disease in smokers. They described the inflammatory reaction in distal airways and spaces and remarked how it spread to involve surrounding alveoli. They postulated that inflammation of the small airways extends to the parenchyma, leading to weakening of the alveolar walls with destruction and loss of alveolar attachments to bronchiolar walls, which leads to a reduction in the caliber of the airways because of loss of radial traction forces. Saetta and colleagues (112) tested this hypothesis and indeed demonstrated a strong association between loss of alveolar attachments and bronchiolar narrowing in surgically obtained lungs that had mild chronic airflow obstruction (Fig. 7). As postulated by Anderson and Foraker (111), the inflammation of the small airway walls correlated closely with the number of abnormal alveolar attachments (112). Functionally, the loss of alveolar attachments was found to correlate significantly with loss of elastic recoil, increase in the closing volume, and decrease in FEV_1 (112,113). Nagai and coworkers (114) examined lungs obtained at autopsy from patients with moderate to severe chronic airflow obstruction and emphysema, and found that the loss of normal alveolar attachments was closely related to emphysema. The deformity index, used to describe the irregularity in shape and deformity of peripheral airways, was related to the loss of alveolar attachments and to the decreases in flow in these patients. Thus it seems apparent that emphysematous changes around the airways will significantly interact with airway patency in the production of airflow limitation.

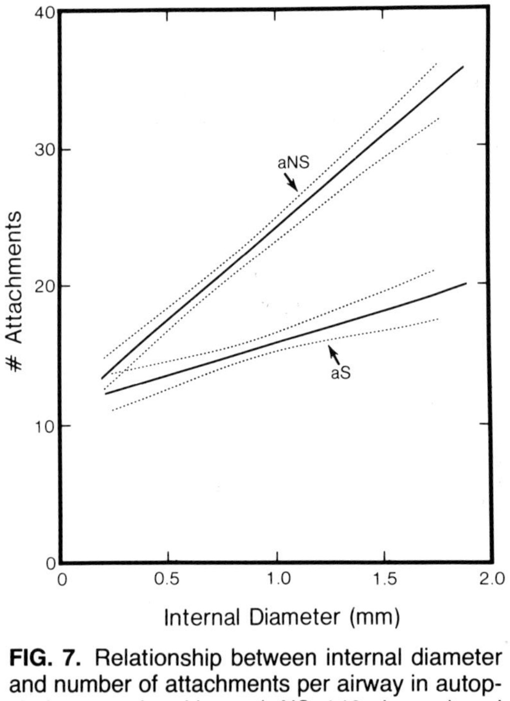

FIG. 7. Relationship between internal diameter and number of attachments per airway in autopsied nonsmokers' lungs (*aNS,* 140 airways) and autopsied smokers' lungs. (*aS,* 102 airways). The *continuous lines* represent the regression lines; the *dashed lines* are the 90% confidence limits of the regression lines. The correlation coefficients are 0.72 ($p < 0.001$ for the autopsied nonsmokers' lungs and 0.36 ($p < 0.001$) for the autopsied smokers' lungs. From ref. 112, with permission.

CONCLUSION

The role of the small airways in chronic obstructive pulmonary disease and its relationship to airflow limitation is complex and goes far beyond static measurements of pathological score and lumenal sizes. Nonetheless, it is reassuring for morphometrists that passive morphometric evaluations of airways at their maximal possible dimensions of total lung capacity relate significantly to diverse measurements of flow, such as resistance, FEV_1, FEV_1/FVC, and maximum mid expiratory flow (MMEF). However, increasing evidence suggests that active events constantly triggered by cigarette smoking can accentuate narrowing and promote a chronic inflammatory process resulting in thicker, inflamed, deformed, and narrow airways with emphysematous changes around them. Possibly alteration of the epithelium is the initial event after the first few cigarette puffs. We have described how the epithelium can initiate and maintain the inflammatory process in the airway wall and at the same time constrict the otherwise normal airway muscle. The neutrophil is probably first recruited; however, it seems that eventually alteration of the T cell subsets ensues, first in the lung and eventually in the blood. Fibrosis of the wall then develops, with increases in wall thickness that accentuate the airway narrowing produced by muscle constriction. The inflammatory process seems to migrate centrifugally toward the parenchyma, destroying it; this accentuates airway narrowing even further. It is probably that these mechanisms play an important role in centrilobular emphysema and that the uncontrolled inflammatory process in the membranous and respiratory bronchioles is eventually responsible for the centrilobular destruction of the lung. We postulate that the pathogenesis in panlobular emphysema is different, and although the functional result is the same—flow limitation—the mechanism for flow limitation is primarily due to losses of recoil. If we are finally to understand the pathogenesis of lung destruction in smokers, the separation of smokers based on their emphysema type is essential.

ACKNOWLEDGMENT

We thank Ann Wright for her expert and useful editorial assistance with this manuscript.

REFERENCES

1. Macklem PT, Mead J. Resistance of central and peripheral airways measured by a retrograde catheter. *J Appl Physiol* 1968;22:395–401.
2. Hogg JC, Macklem PT, Thurlbeck WM. Site and nature of airway obstruction in chronic obstructive lung disease. *N Engl J Med* 1968; 278:1355–1360.
3. Mead J. The lung's "quiet zone." *N Engl J Med* 1970;282:1318–1319.
4. Niewoehner DE, Kleinerman J, Rice DB. Pathologic changes in the peripheral airways of young cigarette smokers. *N Engl J Med* 1974; 291:755–758.
5. Cosio M, Ghezzo H, Hogg JC, et al. The relations between structural changes in small airways and pulmonary function tests. *N Engl J Med* 1978;298:1277–1281.
6. Berend N, Wright JL, Thurlbeck WM, Marlin GE, Woolcock AJ. Small airways disease: reproducibility of measurements and correlation with lung function. *Chest* 1981;79:263–268.
7. Berend N, Woolcock AJ, Marlin GE. Correlation between the function and structure of the lung in smokers. *Am Rev Respir Dis* 1979; 119:695–705.
8. Berend N, Skoog C, Thurlbeck WM. Single-breath nitrogen test in excised human lungs. *J Appl Physiol* 1981;51:1568–1573.
9. Petty TL, Silvers GW, Stanford RE, Baird MD, Mitchell RS. Small airway pathology is related to increased closing capacity and abnormal slope of phase III in excised human lungs. *Am Rev Respir Dis* 1980;121:449–456.
10. Wright JL, Lawson LM, Paré PD, Kennedy S, Wiggs B, Hogg JC. The detection of small airways disease. *Am Rev Respir Dis* 1984;129: 989–994.
11. Buist AS, Vollmer WM, Johnson LR, McCamant LE. Does the single-breath N_2 test identify the smoker who will develop chronic airflow limitation? *Am Rev Respir Dis* 1988; 137:293–301.
12. Cosio MG, Hale KA, Niewoehner DE. Morphologic and morphometric effects of prolonged cigarette smoking on the small airways. *Am Rev Respir Dis* 1980;122:265–271.
13. Bignon J, Khoury F, Even P, Andre J, Brouet G. Morphometric study in chronic obstructive bronchopulmonary disease: pathologic, clinical, and physiologic correlations. *Am Rev Respir Dis* 1969;99:669–695.
14. Matsuba K, Thurlbeck WM. The number and dimensions of small airways in emphysematous lungs. *Am J Pathol* 1972;67:265–276.
15. Bignon J, Andre-Bougeran J, Brouet G. Parenchymal, bronchiolar and bronchial measurements in centrilobular emphysema: relation to weight of right ventricle. *Thorax* 1970;25:556–567.
16. Jamal K, Fleetham JA, Thurlbeck WM. Cor pulmonale: correlations with central airway lesions, peripheral airway lesions, emphysema and control of breathing. *Am Rev Respir Dis* 1990;141:1172–1177.
17. Nagai A, West WW, Thurlbeck WM. The National Institutes of Health Intermittent Positive-Pressure Breathing trial: pathology studies. II: Correlation between morphologic findings, clinical findings, and evidence of expiratory air-flow obstruction. *Am Rev Respir Dis* 1985;132:946–953.
18. Wright JL, Lawson LM, Pare PD, Wiggs BJ, Kennedy S, Hogg JC. Morphology of peripheral airways in current smokers and ex-smokers. *Am Rev Respir Dis* 1983;127:474–477.
19. Wright JL, Hobson J, Wiggs BR, Pare PD. Hogg JC. Effect of cigarette smoking on structure of the small airways. *Lung* 1987;165:91–100.
20. Hale KA, Ewing SL, Gosnell BA, Niewoehner

DB. Lung disease in long-term cigarette smokers with and without chronic air-flow obstruction. *Am Rev Respir Dis* 1984;130:718–721.
21. Nagai A, West WW, Paul JL, Thurlbeck WM. The National Institutes of Health Intermittent Positive Pressure Breathing trial: pathology studies. I: Interrelationship between morphologic lesions. *Am Rev Respir Dis* 1985;132:937–945.
22. Niewoehner DE, Knoke JD, Kleinerman J. Peripheral airways as a determinant of ventilatory function in the human lung. *J Clin Invest* 1977:60:131–151.
23. McLaughlin RF, Tueller EF. Anatomic and histologic changes of early emphysema. *Chest* 1971;59:592–599.
24. Leopold JC, Gough J. The centrilobular form of hypertrophic emphysema and its relation to chronic bronchitis. *Thorax* 1957;12:219–225.
25. Anderson AE, Foraker AG, Centrilobular emphysema and panlobular emphysema: two different diseases. *Thorax* 1973;27:547–550.
26. Eidelman DH, Ghezzo H, Kim WD, Hyatt RE, Cosio MG. Pressure–volume curves in smokers: comparison with alpha-1-antitrypsin deficiency. *Am Rev Respir Dis* 1989;139:1452–1458.
27. Kim WD, Eidelman DH, Izquierdo JL, Ghezzo H, Saetta MP, Cosio MG. Centrilobular and panlobular emphysema in smokers: two distinct morphologic and functional entities. *Am Rev Respir Dis* 1991;144:1385–1390.
28. Saetta M, Izquierdo JL, Kim WD, Cosio MG. Centrilobular and panacinar emphysema in smokers: two different diseases. *Am Rev Respir Dis* 1990;141:A713.
29. Saetta M, Shiner RJ, Angus GE, et al. Destructive index (DI): a measurement of lung parenchymal destruction in smokers. *Am Rev Respir Dis* 1985;131:764–769.
30. Ramsdale EH, Morris MM, Roberts RS, Hargreave FE. Bronchial responsiveness to methacholine in chronic bronchitis: relationship to airflow obstruction and cold air responsiveness. *Thorax* 1984;39:912–918.
31. Yan K, Salome CM, Woolcock AJ. Prevalence and nature of bronchial hyperresponsiveness in subjects with chronic obstructive pulmonary disease. *Am Rev Respir Dis* 1985;132:25–29.
32. Arnup ME, Mendella LA, Anthonisen NR. Effects of cold air hyperpnea in patients with chronic obstructive lung disease. *Am Rev Respir Dis* 1983;128:236–239.
33. Benson MK. Bronchial responsiveness to inhaled histamine and isoprenaline in patients with airway obstruction. *Thorax* 1978;33:211–213.
34. Woolcock AJ, Peat JK, Salome CM, et al. Prevalence of bronchial hyperresponsiveness and asthma in a rural adult population. *Thorax* 1987;42:361–368.
35. Welty C, Weiss ST, Tager IB, et al. The relationship of airways responsiveness to cold air, cigarette smoking and atopy to respiratory symptoms and pulmonary function in adults. *Am Rev Respir Dis* 1984;130:198–203.
36. Sparrow D, O'Connor G, Colton T, Barry CL, Weiss ST. The relationship of nonspecific bronchial responsiveness to the occurrence of respiratory symptoms and decreased levels of pulmonary function: the normative aging study. *Am Rev Respir Dis* 1987;135:1255–1260.
37. Van der Lende R, Visser BF, Wever-Hess J, de Vries K, Orce NGM. Distribution of histamine threshold values in a random population. *Rev Inst Hyg Mines* 1973;28:186–190.
38. Rijcken B, Schouten JP, Weiss ST, Speizer FE, Van der Lende R. The relationship between airway responsiveness to histamine and pulmonary function level in a random population sample. *Am Rev Respir Dis* 1988;137:826–832.
39. Simani IAS, Inove S, Hogg JC. Penetration of the respiratory epithelium of guinea pigs following exposure to cigarette smoke. *Lab Invest* 1974;31:75–87.
40. Boucher RC, Johnston J, Inove S, Hulbert W, Hogg JC. The effect of cigarette smoke on the permeability of guinea pig airways. *Lab Invest* 1980;43:94–100.
41. Walker DC, Mackenzie A, Hulbert WC, Hogg JC. Cigarette smoke exposure and tight junctions of the epithelial cells of guinea pig trachea. *Am Rev Respir Dis* 1982;125[Suppl]:264.
42. Jones JG, Lawler P, Crawley JCW, Minty BD, Hulands G, Veall N. Increased alveolar epithelial permeability in cigarette smokers. *Lancet* 1980;1:66–68.
43. Astrup P, Kjeldsen K, Wanstrup J. Effects of carbon monoxide exposure on arterial walls. *Ann NY Acad Sci* 1970;174:294–300.
44. Yager D, Shore S, Drazen JM. Airway luminal liquid: sources and role as an amplifier of bronchoconstriction. *Am Rev Respir Dis* 1991;143:S52–S54.
45. Yager D, Butler JP, Bastacky J, Israel E, Smith G, Draxen JM. Amplification of airway constriction due to liquid-filling of airway interstices. *J Appl Physiol* 1989;66:2873–2884.
46. Macklem PT, Proctor DF, Hogg JC. The stability of peripheral airways. *Respir Physiol* 1970;8:191–203.
47. Phang PT, Keough MW. Inhibition of pulmonary surfactant by plasma from normal adults and from patients having cardiopulmonary bypass. *J Thorac Cardiovasc Surg* 1986;91:248–251.
48. Hunter JA, Finkbeiner WE, Nadel JA, Goetzl EJ, Holtzman MJ. Predominant generation of 15-lipoxygenase metabolites of arachidonic acid by epithelial cells from human trachea. *Proc Natl Acad Sci USA* 1985;82:4633–4637.
49. Kirsch CM, Sigal E, Djokic TD, Graf PD, Nadel JA. An in vivo chemotaxis assay in the dog trachea: evidence for chemotactic activity of 8,15-diHETE. *J Appl Physiol* 1988;64:1792–1795.
50. Goetzl EJ, Phillips MJ, Gold WM. Stimulus specificity of the generation of leukotrienes by

dog mastocytoma cells. *J Exp Med* 1983; 158:731–737.
51. Serhan CN, Nicolaou KC, Webber SE, et al. Lipoxin A: sterochemistry and biosynthesis. *J Biol Chem* 1986;261:16340–16345.
52. Dahlen S-E, Raud J, Serhan CN, Bjork J, Samuelsson B. Biological activities of lipoxin A include lung strip contraction and dilation of arterioles in vivo. *Acta Physiol Scand* 1987; 130:643–647.
53. Lundberg JM, Saria A, Brodin E, Rosell S, Folkers R. A substance P antagonist inhibits vagally induced increase in vascular permeability and bronchial smooth muscle contraction in the guinea pig. *Proc Natl Acad Sci USA* 1983;80:1120–1124.
54. Coles SJ, Neill KH, Reid LM. Potent stimulation of glycoprotein secretion in canine trachea by substance P. *J Appl Physiol* 1984;57:1323–1327.
55. Rogers DF, Awvdkij B, Barnes PJ. Effects of tachykinins on mucous secretion in human bronchi in vitro. *Eur J Pharmacol* 1989;174: 283–286.
56. McCormack DG, Salonen RO, Barnes PJ. Effect of sensory neuropeptides on canine bronchial and pulmonary vessels in vitro. *Life Sci* 1989;45:2405–2412.
57. Carstairs JR, Barnes PJ. Autoradiographic mapping of substance P receptors in the lung. *Eur J Pharmacol* 1986;127:295–296.
58. Martling C-R, Theordorsson-Norheim E, Lundberg JM. Occurrence and effects of multiple tachykinins: substance P, neurokinin A, neuropeptide K in human lower airways. *Life Sci* 1987;40:1633–1643.
59. Joos G, Pauwels R, van der Straeten M. Effect of inhaled substance P and neurokinin A on the airways of normal and asthmatic subjects. *Thorax* 1987;42:779–783.
60. Joos GF, Pauwels RA, van der Straeten ME. Mechanism of tachykinin-induced bronchoconstriction in the rat. *Am Rev Respir Dis* 1988; 137:1038–1044.
61. Joos GF, Pauwels RA, van der Straeten ME. The effect of nedocromil sodium on the bronchoconstrictor effect of neurokinin A in subjects with asthma. *J Allergy Clin Immunol* 1989;83:663–668.
62. McDonald DM. Respiratory tract infections increase susceptibility to neurogenic inflammation in the rat trachea. *Am Rev Respir Dis* 1988;137:1432–1440.
63. Marasco WA, Showell HJ, Beeker EL. Substance P binds to formylpeptide chemotaxis receptor on the rabbit neutrophil. *Biochem Biophys Res Commun* 1981;99:1065–1072.
64. Kroegel C, Giembycz MA, Barnes PJ. Characterization of eosinophil cell activation by peptides: differential effects of substance P, melittin and FMET-Leu-Phe. *J Immunol* 1990; 145:2581–2587.
65. Lotz M, Vaughan JH, Carson DM. Effect of neuropeptides on production of inflammatory cytokines by human monocytes. *Science* 1988; 241:1218–1221.
66. Johnson AR, Ashton J, Schultz WW, Erdos EG. Neutral metalloendopeptidases in human lung tissue and cultured cells. *Am Rev Respir Dis* 1985;132:564–568.
67. Frossard N, Rhoden KJ, Barnes PJ. Influence of epithelium on guinea pig airway responses to tachykinins: role of endopeptidase and cyclooxygenase. *J Pharmacol Exp Ther* 1989;248: 292–298.
68. Xue Q-F, Maurer R, Engel G. Selective distribution of beta- and alpha$_1$-adrenoreceptors in rat lung visualized by autoradiography. *Arch Int Pharmacodyn Ther* 1983;266:308–314.
69. Holroyde MC. The influence of epithelium on the responsiveness of guinea-pig isolated trachea. *Br J Pharmacol* 1986;87:501–507.
70. Flavahan NA, Aarhus LL, Rimele TJ, Vanhoutte PM. Respiratory epithelium inhibits bronchial smooth muscle tone. *J Appl Physiol* 1985;58:834–838.
71. Flavahan NA, Vanhoutte PM. The respiratory epithelium releases a smooth muscle relaxing factor. *Chest* 1985;87[Suppl]:189S–190S.
72. Vanhoutte PM. Airway epithelium and bronchial reactivity. *Can J Physiol Pharmacol* 1987; 65:448–450.
73. Berend N. Lobar distribution of bronchiolar inflammation in emphysema. *Am Rev Respir Dis* 1981;124:218–220.
74. Bosken CH, Hards J, Gatter K, Hogg JC. Characterization of the inflammatory reaction in the peripheral airways of cigarette smokers using immunocytochemistry. *Am Rev Respir Dis* 1992; 145:911–917.
75. Baile EM, Wright JL, Paré PD, Hogg JC. The effect of acute small airway inflammation on pulmonary function in dogs. *Am Rev Respir Dis* 1982;126:298–301.
76. Hulbert WM, McLean T, Hogg JC. The effect of acute airway inflammation on bronchial reactivity in guinea pigs. *Am Rev Respir Dis* 1985;132:7–11.
77. Murphy KR, Wilson MC, Irvin CG, et al. The requirement for polymorphonuclear leucocytes in the late asthmatic response and heightened airways reactivity in an animal model. *Am Rev Respir Dis* 1986;134:62–68.
78. Totti N; McCusker KT, Campbell EJ, Griffin GL, Senior RM. Nicotine is chemotactic for neutrophils and enhances neutrophil responsiveness to chemotactic peptides. *Science* 1984; 223:169–171.
79. Hunninghake GW, Crystal RG. Cigarette smoking and lung destruction: accumulation of neutrophils in the lungs of cigarette smokers. *Am Rev Respir Dis* 1983;128:833–838.
80. Tosi MF, Stark JM, Smith CW, Hamedani A, Gruenert DC, Infeld MD. Induction of ICAM-1 expression on human airway epithelial cells by inflammatory cytokines: effects on neutrophil–epithelial cell adhesion. *Am J Respir Cell Mol Biol* 1992;7:214–221.

81. Smith CW, Marlin SD, Rothlein R, Toman C, Anderson DC. Cooperative interaction of LFA-1 and Mac-1 with intercellular adhesion molecule-1 in facilitating adherence and transendothelial migration of human neutrophils in vitro. *J Clin Invest* 1989;83:2008–2017.
82. Smith CW. Molecular determinants of neutrophil adhesion. *Am J Respir Cell Mol Biol* 1990;2:487–489.
83. Lo SK, Van Seventer GA, Levin SM, Wright SD. Two leukocyte receptors (CD11a/CD18 and CD11b/CD18) mediate transient adhesion to endothelium by binding to different ligands. *J Immunol* 1989;143:3325–3329.
84. Benlacqua MP, Stengelin S, Gimbrone MA, Seed B. Endothelial leukocyte adhesion molecule 1: an inducible receptor for neutrophils related to complement regulatory proteins and lectins. *Science* 1989;243:1160–1165.
85. Cox G, Gauldie J, Jordana M. Bronchial epithelial cell-derived cytokines (G-CSF and GM-CSF) promote the survival of peripheral blood neutrophils in vitro. *Am J Respir Cell Mol Biol* 1992;7:507–513.
86. Ginns C, Goldenheim PD, Miller LG, et al. T-lymphocyte subsets in smoking and lung cancer: analysis by monoclonal antibodies and flow cytometry. *Am Rev Respir Dis* 1982; 126:265–269.
87. Miller LG, Goldstein G, Murphy M, Ginns LC. Reversible alterations in immunoregulatory T cells in smoking. *Chest* 1982;82:526–529.
88. Tollerund PJ, Clark JW, Brown LM, et al. Association of cigarette smoking with decreased numbers of circulating natural killer cells. *Am Rev Respir Dis* 1989;139:194–198.
89. Takeuchi M, Nagai S, Izumi T. Effect of smoking on natural killer cell activity in the lung. *Chest* 1988;94:688–693.
90. Costabel U, Bross KJ, Reuter C, Rühle K-H, Matthys H. Alterations in immunoregulatory T-cell subsets in cigarette smokers: a phenotypic analysis of bronchoalveolar and blood lymphocytes. *Chest* 1986;90:39–44.
91. Fournier M, Legargy F, LeRoy Ladurie F, Lenormand E, Pariente R. Intraepithelial T-lymphocyte subsets in the airways of normal subjects and of patients with chronic bronchitis. *Am Rev Respir Dis* 1989;140:737–742.
92. Saetta M, Di Stefano A, Maestrelli P, et al. Activated T-lymphocytes and macrophages in bronchial mucosa of subjects with chronic bronchitis. *Am Rev Respir Dis* 1993;147:301–306.
93. Chan MA, Benedict SH, Carstairs KC, Francombe WH, Gelfand EW. Expansion of B lymphocytes with an unusual immunoglobulin rearrangement associated with atypical lymphocytosis and cigarette smoking. *Am J Respir Cell Mol Biol* 1990;2:549–552.
94. Leung DYM, Geha RS. Regulation of the human IgE antibody response. *Int Rev Immunol* 1987;2:75–91.
95. Kay AB. "Helper" ($CD4^+$) T cells and eosinophils in allergy and asthma. *Am Rev Respir Dis* 1992;145:S22–S26.
96. Breit SN, Robinson JP, Luckhurst E, et al. Immunoregulation by $alpha_1$ antitrypsin. *J Clin Lab Immunol* 1982;7:127–121.
97. Breit SN, Luckhurst E, Penny R. The effect of $alpha_1$ antitrypsin on the proliferative response of human peripheral blood lymphocytes. *J Immunol* 1983;130:681–688.
98. Ades EW, Hinson A, Chapuis-Cellier C, Arnaud P. Modulation of the immune response by plasma protease inhibitors. I: $Alpha_2$-macroglobulin and $alpha_1$-antitrypsin inhibit natural killing and antibody-dependent cell mediated cytotoxicity. *Scand J Immunol* 1982;15:109–113.
99. Redelman D, Hudig D. The mechanism of cell-mediated cytotoxicity. I: Killing by murine T lymphocytes requires cell surface thiols and activated proteases. *J Immunol* 1980;124:870–878.
100. Hudig D, Haverty T, Fulcher C, et al. Inhibition of human natural cytotoxicity by macromolecular antiproteases. *J Immunol* 1981;126: 1569–1574.
101. Wright JL, Wiggs BJ, Hogg JC. Airway disease in upper and lower lobes in lungs of patients with and without emphysema. *Thorax* 1984;39: 282–285.
102. Petty TL, Silvers GW, Stanford RE, Baird MD, Mitchell RS. Small airway pathology is related to increased closing capacity and abnormal slope of phase III in excised human lungs. *Am Rev Respir Dis* 1980;121:449–456.
103. Cosio MG, Ghezzo H, Hogg J, Pare P. Airway reactivity in smokers and its relation with emphysema type. *Am Rev Respir Dis* 1992;145: A379.
104. Bosken CH, Wiggs BR, Paré PD, Hogg JC. Small airway dimensions in smokers with obstruction to airflow. *Am Rev Respir Dis* 1990; 142:563–570.
105. Moreno RH, Hogg JC, Paré PD. Mechanics of airway narrowing. *Am Rev Respir Dis* 1986; 133:1171–1180.
106. Wiggs BR, Bosken C, Paré PD, James A, Hogg JC. A model of airway narrowing in asthma and in chronic obstructive pulmonary disease. *Am Rev Respir Dis* 1992;145:1251–1258.
107. Gunst SJ, Warner DO, Wilson TA, Hyatt RE. Parenchymal interdependence and airway response to methacholine in excised dog lobes. *J Appl Physiol* 1988;65:2490–2497.
108. Macklem PT. Factors determining bronchial smooth muscle shortening. *Am Rev Respir Dis* 1991;143:S47–S48.
109. Ding DJ, Martin JG, Macklem PT. Effects of lung volume on maximal methacholine-induced bronchial constriction in normal humans. *J Appl Physiol* 1987;62:1324–1330.
110. Bellofiore S, Eidelman DH, Macklem PT, Martin JG. Effects of elastase-induced emphysema on airway response to methacholine in rats. *J Appl Physiol* 1990;66:606–612.

111. Anderson AE, Foraker AG. Relative dimensions of bronchioles and parenchymal spaces in lungs from normal subjects and emphysematous patients. *Am J Med* 1962;32:218–226.
112. Saetta M, Ghezzo H, Kim WD, et al. Loss of alveolar attachments in smokers: a morphometric correlate of lung function impairment. *Am Rev Respir Dis* 1985;132:894–900.
113. Petty TL, Silvers GW, Stanford RE. Radial traction and small airways disease in excised human lungs. *Am Rev Respir Dis* 1986;133:132–135.
114. Nagai A, Yamawaki I, Takizawa T, Thurlbeck WM. Alveolar attachments in emphysema of human lungs. *Am Rev Respir Dis* 1991;144:888–891.

Diseases of the Bronchioles, edited by
Gary R. Epler. Raven Press, Ltd.,
New York © 1994.

9

Mineral Dust Induced Bronchiolitis

Andrew Churg

Department of Pathology, University Hospital, University of British Columbia, Vancouver, B.C., Canada.

The notion that mineral dusts can produce abnormalities of the small airways is contrary to the typical idea of a pneumoconiosis held by most pathologists and respirologists; namely, that pneumoconioses are interstitial lesions that produce diffuse interstitial or nodular fibrosis. Traditionally also, when functional abnormalities have been associated with pneumoconioses, these have been of restrictive type.

It has become apparent in recent years that in fact mineral dust exposure can produce airflow obstruction, and it has also become apparent that a variety of mineral dusts can produce markedly abnormal membranous and respiratory bronchioles. In this chapter we discuss the concept of the fibrotic small airway changes caused by occupational exposure to inorganic dusts, a lesion we have referred to as *mineral dust induced small airways disease* (MDAD), consider what is known of the pathogenesis of these lesions, and attempt to correlate the morphologic changes with airflow abnormalities.

MORPHOLOGY OF MINERAL DUST INDUCED SMALL AIRWAYS DISEASE

MDAD consists of irregular fibrotic thickening of the walls of the membranous and respiratory bronchioles, sometimes with extension into the alveolar duct. When these lesions are viewed in cross section, the thickening of the wall and narrowing of the airway lumen is evident; longitudinal cuts show that the process distorts the airway as well (Figs. 1 and 2) (1–4).

In most but by no means all instances, the mural fibrosing process is accompanied by a large amount of pigment. This may consist of free particles of the inhaled dust, particles that have been phagocytized by macrophages, or particles that have become ferruginated; that is, they have acquired an iron protein coat. Asbestos bodies are the best known example of such ferruginous bodies, but in fact ferruginated particles of iron are probably even more frequent. If the inhaled dust is not readily visible with the light microscope, then the airway wall changes may not show extensive pigmentation, but even in this circumstance, analytical electron microscopy confirms that very large amounts of dust are present, and in fact the local degree of airway wall fibrosis appears to be proportional to the local dust burden (5).

MDAD has been described, or at least illustrated (and sometimes ignored), in workers exposed to a wide variety of inorganic dust, including iron oxide, aluminum oxide, asbestos, talc, mica, coal, silica, and slate. In experimental animals similar lesions have been seen after exposure to potassium octatitanate, brucite, fly ash, silica, and asbestos (Table 1) (6–15). Because the airway

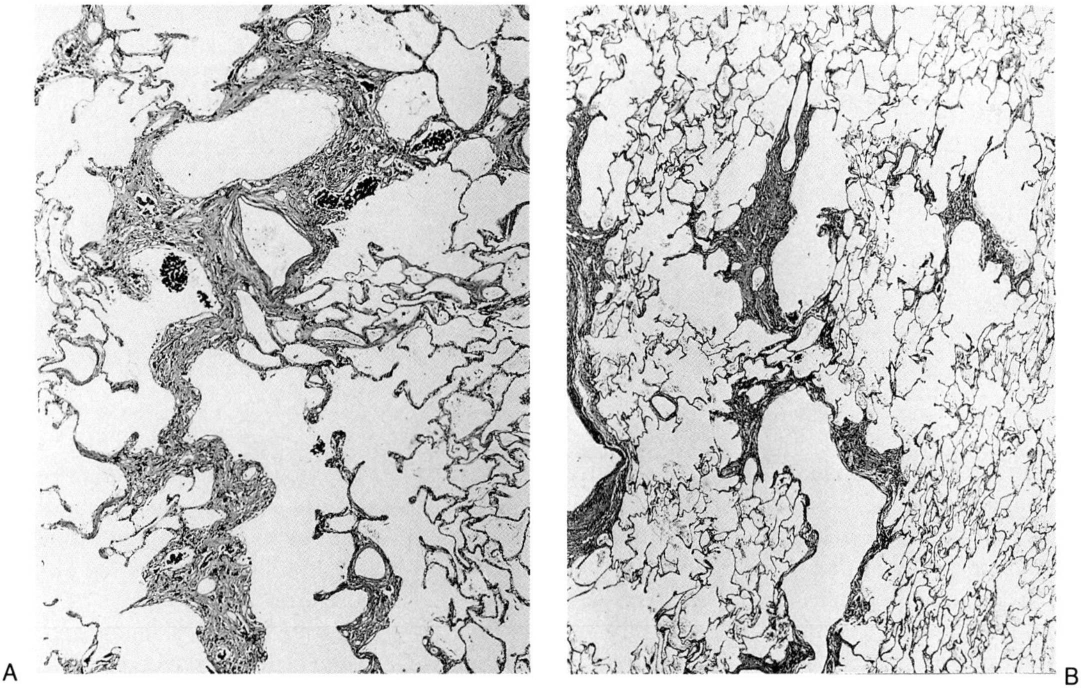

FIG. 1. Micrographs of sections from the lung of an asbestos exposed worker. **A,** A membranous bronchiole can be seen cut in cross section (*top of field*) and a respiratory bronchiole cut in longitudinal section (*bottom of field*). Note the typical mural fibrosis and distortion of the airway that we have labeled MDAD. (Hematoxylin and eosin, × 40.) **B,** Another area of the same lung demonstrates both a respiratory bronchiole with fibrotic changes in the wall (*bottom of field*) and two lesions (*top of field*) in which barely recognizable fibrotic airways are surrounded by focal emphysema. These lesions are identical to those seen in hematite miners (Fig. 2) and in simple coal workers' pneumoconiosis. (Hematoxylin and eosin, ×20.) Reproduced from ref. 15, by permission.

response is stereotypic, regardless of the dust, we have proposed that the generic term *mineral dust induced airways disease* be used for these lesions (15).

The existence of lesions of this type and their significance have been disputed issues. In part this problem arises from the fact that, at least in regard to membranous bronchioles, cigarette smoke produces changes that are morphologically similar; that is, they consist of mural fibrosis and pigmentation. By simple light microscopic observation, cigarette smoke induced lesions are generally not separable from dust induced lesions. However, if one takes series of dust exposed workers and compares them to smoking matched non-dust exposed control subjects using a morphologic grading scheme to determine the amount of fibrosis in the airway wall, then it becomes apparent that mineral dusts not only cause fibrosis of the membranous bronchioles but also that the lesions are often more severe than (and perhaps are a result of a synergistic interaction with) those caused by cigarette smoke (Table 2).

While the lesions in the membranous bronchioles are not readily distinguishable from cigarette smoke induced lesions, those in the respiratory bronchioles are easily recognized. This is particularly true when there is marked fibrosis. As indicated in Table 3, in a series of lungs from smokers without dust exposure, only 4% of respira-

A

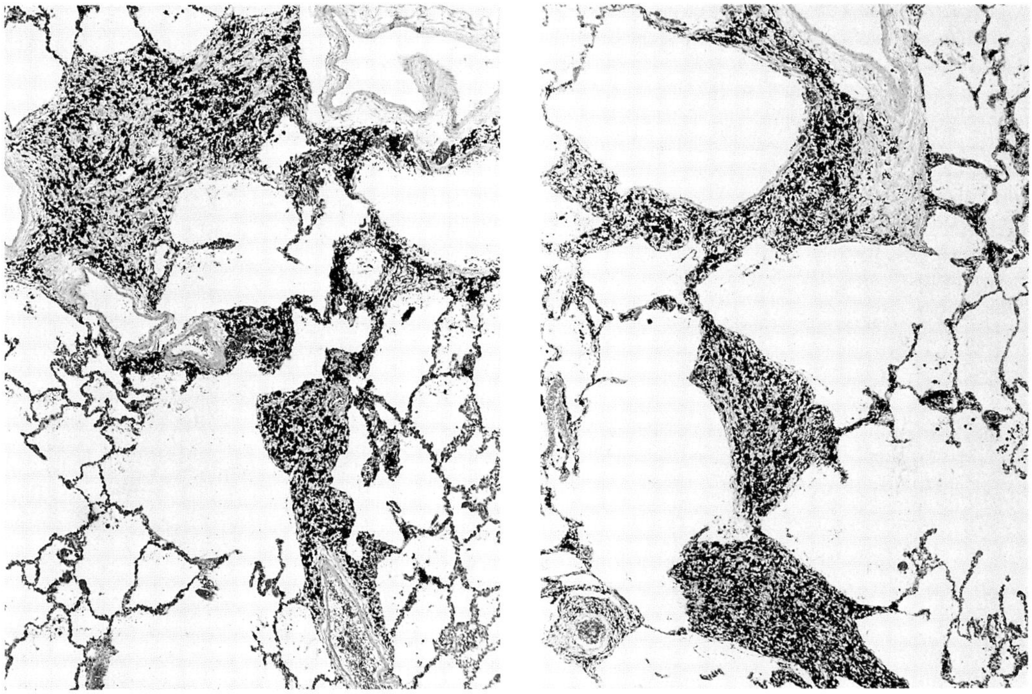

B

FIG. 2. Micrographs of lesions from the lung of a long-term hematite miner (case courtesy Dr. A. Katzenstein). **A,** Cross section of one respiratory bronchiole and another respiratory bronchiole cut longitudinally. Both airways show mural fibrosis, distortion, and pigmentation. (Hematoxylin and eosin, × 20.) **B,** Membranous bronchiole in cross section and a scarred distorted airway with surrounding focal emphysema. Note the resemblance of both these views to Fig. 1, making the point that dust-induced small airway lesions show stereotypic patterns. (Hematoxylin and eosin, × 20.) Reproduced from ref. 15, by permission.

tory bronchioles showed severe fibrosis, and this change was never seen in alveolar ducts; whereas nearly 50% of respiratory bronchioles from asbestos workers who smoked and 35% of alveolar ducts from such workers demonstrated severe fibrosis. Similar changes, but with a somewhat lower frequency, were seen in the lungs of workers with other types of dust exposure (2,3,4,8). These observations indicate that in workers with sufficient dust exposure, widespread abnormalities are often found in the small airways.

The studies just described were performed to evaluate the severity and extent of small-airway lesions in persons with known dust exposure. In order to deter-

TABLE 1. *Mineral dust exposures showing morphologic evidence of mineral dust induced airways disease*

In humans
Chrysotile asbestos
Amphibole asbestos
Coal
Sheet silicates (talc, mica)
Silica
Aluminum oxide
Iron oxide
Slate dust
In experimental animals
Chrysotile asbestos
Amphibole asbestos
Potassium octatitante
Silica
Fly ash
Brucite

TABLE 2. *Mean airway grades for fibrosis in smoking-matched control or dust exposed lungs (airways fibrosis graded on a severity scale of 0 to 3)*

Exposure	AD	RB	MB
Asbestos ($n = 15$)	1.4	1.9	1.6
Other dusts ($n = 7$)[a]	1.0	1.8	1.3
Control (no dust) ($n = 22$)	0.3	0.5	0.9

From refs. 2,3.
AD, alveolar duct; RB, respiratory bronchiole; MB, membranous bronchiole.
[a]Including silica, silicates, iron oxide.

mine whether these lesions were specific for dust exposure, we (4) reviewed, in a blinded fashion, histologic sections of a series of 174 lungs removed at surgery, almost always for carcinoma, and in almost all cases from smokers. MDAD was detected in 13 of 53 lungs from workers with a history of dust exposure, but in only 1 of 121 lungs from patients without such a history; even the single apparently false-positive patient in fact had large amounts of birefringent dust visible in his lungs, suggesting that he had had some historically occult dust exposure. These findings indicate that the lesions of MDAD (particularly the respiratory bronchiole/alveolar duct changes) are highly specific for mineral dust exposure.

With sufficient dust exposure, it is likely that the extent and incidence of such airway changes are much greater than the figures just cited might suggest, but there are few data on this point. We (Churg A, unpublished data) have found in a series of more than 300 autopsy lungs from long-term chrysotile asbestos miners and millers from Quebec, a group that had been exposed to heavy concentrations of chrysotile ore dust, MDAD was visible, either by itself or with diffuse fibrosis (asbestosis) in about two-thirds of the cases. If, as I argue in the next section, many so-called dust macules are in fact examples of MDAD, then other dust-exposed groups such as coal miners also have extremely high incidences of this lesion. Green (14) reported that so-called macular coal dust pneumoconiosis was present by itself in 46% and present combined with focal emphysema in another 36% of a series of 3,400 autopsy lungs from relatively heavily exposed U.S. coal miners.

TABLE 3. *Percent of airways showing severe (grade 2 or 3) fibrosis in a series of lungs from dust exposed workers*

Exposure	AD	RB	MB
Asbestos ($n = 15$)	35%	48%	51%
Other dusts ($n = 7$)	14%	31%	37%
Control ($n = 22$)	0%	4%	16%

From refs. 2,3.
AD, alveolar duct; RB, respiratory bronchiole; MB, membranous bronchiole.

THE RELATIONSHIP BETWEEN SO-CALLED DUST MACULES AND MINERAL DUST INDUCED SMALL AIRWAYS DISEASE

Examination of photomicrographs in the pneumoconiosis literature makes it clear that MDAD is not a new lesion. However, in general, these changes have been included under the heading of "dust macules" and thought to be of little pathologic or functional significance.

In this regard one needs to remember that the dust macule was originally defined in order to distinguish lesions that appeared to produce little fibrosis from silicosis, a disease in which obvious severe nodular fibrosis was evident. A dust macule is nominally defined as a nonpalpable pigmented lesion consisting microscopically of dust, either lying free or in macrophages, around small airways and small vessels in the lung (16). In theory, dust macules show little or no fibrosis (14,16). However, it is evident that the usage of the term "macule" has either changed over time or never been very clear, since lesions currently referred to as macules may have no associated fibrosis or may be markedly fibrotic, heavily pigmented, and quite distorted respiratory bronchioles (14). Contemporary writings still tend to lump both the fibrotic and nonfibrotic lesions under the same heading (6), and the fact that the macules of coal workers' pneumoconiosis are often markedly fibrotic is not only evident but also accepted as part of the definition of the lesion (14).

An additional source of confusion about dust macules and their associations with fibrosis is that in some conditions, particularly coal workers' pneumoconiosis, the dust macules occur in conjunction with so-called focal emphysema (14), a change that makes it difficult to realize that the underlying lesion is based on a fibrotic respiratory bronchiole. However if one examines even coal workers' macular lesions before they are associated with focal emphysema, then the linear accumulation of pigmented fibrous tissue extending down the respiratory bronchiole is evident (see, for example Figures 4.12 and 4.13 in ref. 14). Although it has not been widely appreciated, exactly the same combination of fibrotic distorted airways and focal emphysema is common in hematite miners (15) (Fig. 2) and is occasionally seen in asbestos workers (Fig. 1) and slate workers (6).

What these observations suggest is that there is in fact a stereotypic response of the central region of the pulmonary lobule to mineral dust. In its earliest stage this consists of a true macule, that is, simply a collection of pigmented dust (or occasionally nonpigmented dust) with no fibrosis. With time the dust evokes a fibrotic response, which at least initially shows a linear pattern extending down the walls of the small airways and sometimes the alveolar ducts. This lesion is the one have termed MDAD. In some instances, focal emphysema is added on, either because of cigarette smoking or because certain dusts directly produce emphysema, and once this occurs, the relationship of the lesion to MDAD becomes obscure. Nonetheless, this problem does not change the conclusion, namely, that MDAD and severely fibrotic dust macules are the same disease.

PATHOGENESIS OF MINERAL DUST INDUCED SMALL AIRWAYS DISEASE

Little direct information is available about the pathogenesis of the fibrotic changes seen in MDAD, but the limited available data suggest that two factors play a role, namely, local dust accumulation and the inflammatory response to the dust.

Simple, casual light microscopic observations suggest, as noted previously, that greater amounts of visible dust are associated with greater degrees of airway wall fibrosis. Analysis of bulk lung samples from long-term chrysotile miners and millers showed that lungs with MDAD averaged about twice the asbestos content of those without MDAD in workers matched for age and smoking status (17). Such studies, of course, say nothing about the location of the dust. We have approached this question directly (5) by preparing electron microscopic sections of the walls of airways from similar chrysotile miner lungs and determining the number of dust particles per unit area of tissue. As shown in Table 4, for either membranous or respiratory bronchioles, airways graded as 2 or 3 for fibrosis have significantly greater numbers of particles per square millimeter of airway wall than airways graded 0 or 1 for fibrosis, thus

TABLE 4. *Particle concentration in airway walls by fibrosis grade in the lungs of long-term chrysotile miners and millers*

Airway type and grade	Mean particle concentration/mm^2
MB: fibrosis grades 0 or 1	4300
MB: fibrosis grades 2 or 3	15500
RB: fibrosis grades 0 or 1	10800
RB: fibrosis grades 2 or 3	26300

From ref. 5.

MB, membranous bronchiole; RB, respiratory bronchiole.

indicating that the grade of fibrosis does correlate with the local dust burden.

However, not all workers with heavy dust exposure develop fibrotic airway lesions, and some workers with heavy dust exposure develop not only airway lesions but also nodular or diffuse fibrosis. These observations suggest that other factors must also play a role. One explanation for this process can be seen in the studies of Begin and colleagues (9), in which sheep were given intratracheal instillations of chrysotile asbestos. They found that the animals that developed diffuse fibrosis (asbestosis) had about a fourfold greater particle retention than the animals that developed only airway fibrosis. They suggested that the determining factor was the individual ability to clear particles.

Marked variations in individual rates of particle clearance are well known from experimental studies of humans inhaling inert dusts. While the basis of these differences is unclear, it is important to note that lung structure itself may play a role. Several groups (18–20) have shown, by taking measurements from chest radiographs, a correlation between the presence of mineral dust induced diseases and lung and/or airway size as measured on the radiograph. Mathematical models of particle retention suggest that airway size is the major determinant of particle deposition (21). Thus the development of airway lesions, or more severe fibrotic lesions of varying types, may have a genetic/anatomic basis.

Whatever the reason for particle retention, it is clear from the literature that most mineral dusts evoke a greater or lesser inflammatory response (21–27). The exact nature of the response depends on particle type, method of administration, and location within air space or interstitium (23,26). However, the important point is such inflammatory responses lead to the production of a variety of fibrogenic factors, both in the air spaces, and, if particles cross the bronchiolar and alveolar epithelium, in the interstitium (21–28). In this sense heavy particle deposition in the airways is entirely analogous to heavy particle deposition in the more distal parenchyma; the result of both tends to be the generation of interstitial (either airway wall or alveolar wall) fibrosis.

MINERAL DUST INDUCED EMPHYSEMA

The notion that mineral dusts could induce emphysema arose from the observation that so-called focal emphysema, a lesion morphologically similar to cigarette smoke induced centrilobular emphysema, was extremely common in the lungs of coal miners. This issue was the subject of dispute for many years, but studies using workers properly matched for smoking habit have now left no doubt that coal dust does, in and of itself, produce emphysematous changes in the center of the lobules (14,29–31). These lesions appear as enlarged air spaces around distorted fibrotic respiratory bronchioles (i.e., MDAD). The major differences between smoking-induced centrilobular emphysema and focal emphysema of coal workers is that the former may be extremely severe whereas the sizes of the enlarged air spaces in the latter is usually quite small. Also, although centrilobular emphysema in smokers may or may not be associated with obviously abnormal small airways, focal emphysema induced by dust is always associated with fibrotic MDAD.

Less information is available about the relationship between emphysema and other dusts. Becklake and co-workers (32) found a correlation between the severity of emphysema in gold miners with silica exposure and the number of shifts worked in high dust levels. Hnizdo et al. (33) subclassified the emphysema seen in gold miners and concluded that cumulative dust exposure could be related to the presence of both centrilobular and panlobular emphysema, and that centrilobular emphysema also correlated with the presence of silicosis. Emphysema can also be seen in rats after intratracheal instillation of silica (34). It is noteworthy that such animals develop not only classic silicotic nodules but also typical MDAD lesions similar to those seen in humans (34).

As noted above and illustrated in Figs. 1 and 2, the same combination of MDAD and focal emphysema can be observed more or less frequently in workers exposed to asbestos, hematite ore, or slate dust (6), and may occur with other dusts as well. In coal workers this process can be found in the absence of smoking, and this is probably true of the other dusts mentioned. There are, however, no formal studies proving this point, nor any indications of the incidence of focal emphysema with these types of dust exposure.

The pathogenesis of emphysema in dust-exposed workers is unknown, but I have proposed elsewhere (15) that the pathogenesis of emphysema caused by mineral dust is probably similar to that caused by cigarette smoking. As noted above, any inhalational dust exposure is associated with an inflammatory response, and experimental studies show that such responses are often quite prolonged but may not be of great intensity (22–28). Experimental studies of rats administered quartz (35) and analysis of lavage fluid of human coal miners (36) offer evidence that these exposures are associated with prolonged release of proteolytic enzymes into the lung, presumably from the evoked inflammatory cells. It is interesting that emphysema is also seen in addicts who abuse intravenously drugs meant for oral consumption (37,38); Schmidt et al. (38) have proposed that this phenomenon reflects delivery of a large amount of inorganic particulate matter to the lung with subsequent release of proteolytic enzymes from inflammatory cells. They noted that there appeared to be destruction of elastin in the region surrounding talc granulomas in the lungs of such patients, and we reported a decrease in morphometrically detectable elastin in the lungs of rats developing emphysema after silica exposure (35). These observations suggest that one basic mechanism of dust-induced emphysema is similar to that believed to be true for cigarette smoke induced emphysema, namely, prolonged, fairly low-grade, inflammation with continuous release of proteolytic enzymes that destroy the collagen and elastin structure of the lung.

An additional factor believed to be important in the pathogenesis of cigarette smoke induced emphysema, besides the release of proteases and elastases that attack the structure of the lung, is smoke-induced oxidation and hence neutralization of natural antiproteolytic agents such as alpha$_1$-antiprotease (39). While this question has not been examined in models of dust exposure, it is becoming increasingly clear that many dusts have the ability either to function as free radicals or to catalyze the formation of active oxygen species and other free radicals (40–43). Active oxygen species in cigarette smoke are known to inactivate alpha$_1$-antiprotease through oxidation of methionine residues (39), and presumably the same would apply to free radicals generated from mineral dusts. Thus the effects of smoke and of dust in inducing emphysema may be mechanistically similar.

A further complicating factor in humans is that many dust-exposed workers also smoke cigarettes. Whether such combined exposures produce synergistic changes both in the small airways and in the development of focal emphysema is unclear, but there are a number of reasons to presume that this is so. For one thing, smoke appears to increase the retention of many types of minerals in the lung in both humans and animals (44–48). Roentgenographic studies have suggested that smoking increases the incidence and/or severity of asbestosis in smoking humans compared to nonsmoking humans (49), an effect that presumably reflects smoke-mediated increases in asbestos fiber retention. Experimentally, we have shown (50) that the combination of smoke plus asbestos exposure produces synergistic increases in airway wall fibrosis in the lungs of guinea pigs. However, Hnizdo and colleagues (33) have concluded that, although both smoke and silica dust produce emphysema, significant emphysema (functionally important) is seen only in smokers. This topic needs further exploration.

AIRFLOW OBSTRUCTION, MINERAL DUST EXPOSURE, AND PATHOLOGIC REACTIONS

The importance of MDAD and dust-induced emphysema lies not in their interest as pathologic curiosities but in their relation to airflow obstruction in dust-exposed workers. This topic has been one of great controversy, but with the introduction of longitudinal epidemiologic methods, it is now clear that occupational dust exposure is in fact commonly associated with airflow obstruction and that, as shown by multiple regression techniques, the effects of dust may, with sufficient exposure, be comparable to that of cigarette smoke (reviewed in 51–53). Furthermore, although the initial association of dust exposure and airflow obstruction was described in coal miners, exposure to many, and perhaps all, mineral dusts in sufficient quantities likely can produce obstruction (52).

What most epidemiologic studies do not address, however, is the question of what pathologic lesion is associated with airflow obstruction. This question has proved extremely difficult to answer for cigarette smokers, a group for whom the issue of airflow obstruction is unquestioned and for whom a great deal of pathologic and functional information is available. For mineral dust, much less pathologic information has been forthcoming. Nonetheless, one can hypothesize that airflow obstruction caused by mineral dust might have the same three functional/morphologic bases as has been postulated for cigarette smokers, namely, airway hyperresponsiveness, small airways disease, and emphysema (15).

The issue of airway hyperresponsiveness and its relation to airflow obstruction in cigarette smokers is extremely controversial; in particular, there are major questions of what is cause and what is effect (15). That there is a relationship between airflow obstruction and bronchial hyperresponsiveness is, however, generally accepted. The limited data available in regard to hyperresponsiveness and dust exposure suggest that the same conclusion applies. Studies of both coal and iron miners (54,55) have shown that those who have demonstrable hyperresponsiveness as measured by acetylcholine challenge have greater functional losses over time than those who do not. But what the morphologic (both structural and inflammatory) correlates of such hyperresponsiveness to dust might be are unknown.

So-called chronic bronchitis (i.e., mucous hypersecretion) has been discredited as a cause of significant airflow obstruction in cigarette smokers, although it clearly is associated with anatomic abnormalities. A similar lesion, called industrial bronchitis (56), occurs after exposure to mineral dust. Again, little information is available about the morphologic correlates of industrial bronchitis, but the presumption is that, like chronic bronchitis in cigarette smokers, industrial bronchitis has little functional effect.

To the extent that any attempt has been made to associate a morphologic abnormality with mineral dust induced airflow obstruction it has generally been assumed that the cause of obstruction is emphysema (29–33,51–53). However, the problem with this assumption is that even in the relatively few studies in which usable quantitative data on emphysema have been obtained, no information exists about the extent and degree of small airway lesions.

In fact, a variety of functional data suggest that small airway changes are present and can produce some degree of measurable effect. This is particularly true in asbestos workers, in whom a variety of tests for small airway disease as well as FEF_{25-75} are often abnormal (58–64). Again, the major problem here is a lack of anatomic information, although Begin and colleagues (58, 59) did note the presence of MDAD-type lesions in biopsies of chrysotile miners, and these same individuals were found to have decreased flows at low lung volumes. Much stronger experimental data based on animal models suggest that small airway lesions induced by asbestos can produce significant interference with flow. Begin and colleagues (13) found, in sheep given chrysotile asbestos by intratracheal instillation, evidence of increased upstream resistance in both small and large airways. Glassroth and associates (64) found increases in functional residual capacity (FRC) and residual volume (RV) along with diminished flows in hamsters similarly given chrysotile by intratracheal installation. Wright and others (65) found that, after intratracheal instillation of amosite to guinea pigs, distinct impairment of flow with abnormal flow volume curves, diminished PEF, FEF_{25-75}, FEV_1, and FEV_1/FVC (Fig. 3). However,

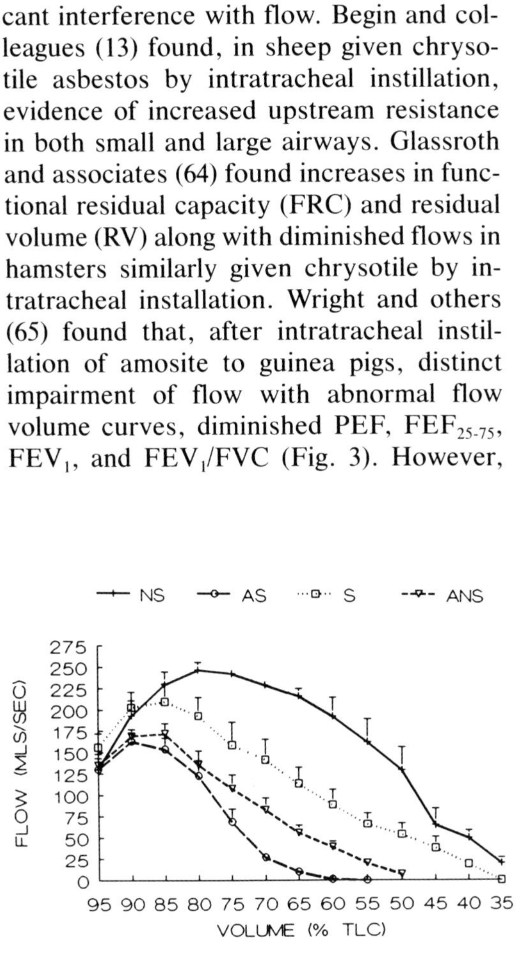

FIG. 3. Flow volume curves from a group of guinea pigs exposed to air (*NS*), cigarette smoke (*S*), amosite asbestos alone (*ANS*), or amosite asbestos and cigarette smoke (*AS*). In this animal model, both amosite and smoke produce interference with flow, and the combination of agents causes even more severe impairment. Reproduced from ref. 65, by permission.

extrapolation of these observations in rodent models to humans must be tempered by the well-known observation that intratracheal administration of asbestos to a small animal produces relatively marked airway pathology and relatively little interstitial fibrosis. Thus these experiments must serve as models of what could happen rather than what necessarily does happen.

Information also exists on the relationship of airflow abnormality and silica exposure, but here the data are confusing. Begin et al. (66) concluded that the finding of silicotic nodules on CT scans or plain chest films was associated with airflow limitation, and that the greater the profusion of nodules, the more significant the impairment. It is of particular interest that in this study, the abnormalities were seen in $Vmax_{50}$ and FEF_{25-75} but not in FEV_1/FVC, implying that small airway changes were present. The presence of emphysema was not discussed. However, Becklake and colleagues (32) and Cowie and Mabena (67) concluded that airflow obstruction in gold miners with silica exposure was related to total dust exposure and not to radiographic silicosis. Small airway lesions may be present and may be the cause of airflow obstruction in such workers. We (4) examined the correlation between morphologic abnormalities and airflow obstruction in a group of workers with many different types of occupational dust exposure. The group was initially selected because of the histologic observation of MDAD, and then was compared to age-, sex-, and smoking-matched dust-exposed workers without such lesions. As shown in Table 5, the group with mineral dust induced airway disease had considerably worse FEV_1, FEF_{25-75}, RV/TLC, and nitrogen washout, but no statistical differences in emphysema grade. These findings argue that small airway lesions may be more important than emphysema in producing airflow obstruction.

It is also important to note that in coal miners, the group of workers in whom the correlation of dust exposure and emphy-

TABLE 5. *Pulmonary function in age-, sex-, and smoking-matched dust exposed workers with or without morphologic evidence of dust-induced small airways lesions (values as % predicted ± SD, except as noted)*

Parameter	Patients with airway lesions	Patients without airway lesions
FEV_1	65 ± 11	87 ± 19[a]
FEV_1/FVC (%)	62 ± 11	66 ± 12
VC	78 ± 13	98 ± 17[a]
TLC	104 ± 15	104 ± 15
FEF_{25-75}	34 ± 16	62 ± 28[a]
RV/TLC	146 ± 19	112 ± 20[a]
FRC	124 ± 18	104 ± 25
D_{LCO}	76 ± 17	96 ± 27
N_2/L	360 ± 141	231 ± 103[a]
CC/TLC	130 ± 17	118 ± 22
Emphysema grade (absolute value)	20 ± 19	9 ± 10

From ref. 4.
[a]Significant difference between groups.

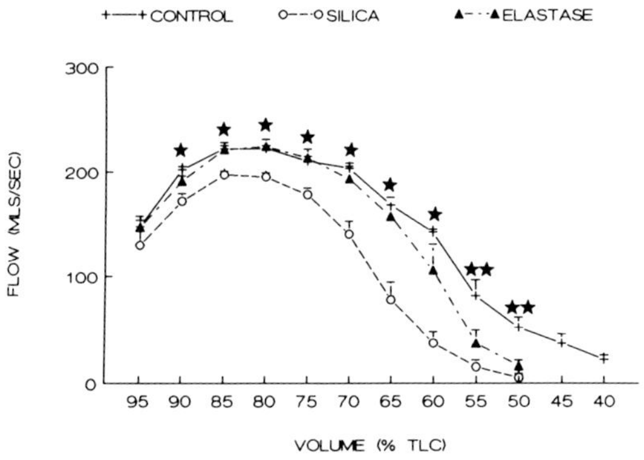

FIG. 4. Flow volume curves from rats exposed to instilled saline (control), silica, or elastase. Elastase and silica treatments produced about the same degree of emphysema, but only silica caused fibrotic small airways, which appear to be responsible for the much greater flow impairment in the silica-treated animals. Reproduced from ref. 34, by permission.

sema is best established, there is also a strong association between emphysema and the severity of simple coal workers' pneumoconiosis (i.e., dust macules or MDAD) (30–32). Since focal emphysema in coal workers is always seen in the presence of MDAD (14), it is clear that one simply cannot ascribe airflow obstruction to emphysema alone.

We have attempted to examine the question whether emphysema or small airway lesions play a greater role in airflow obstruction after dust exposure by administering either elastase or silica to rats by intratracheal instillation. Elastase administration produces emphysema but essentially no changes in the structure of the small airways, while in our model, silica instillation produces both small airway lesions and emphysema (34). In the animals administered elastase, emphysema was associated with air trapping and some flow limitation, particularly at low lung volumes, but the most significant correlations with flow abnormalities, including decreases in PEF, FEF_{25-75}, FEV_1, FEV_1/FVC, nitrogen washout, upstream resistance, and abnormal flow volume curves (Fig. 4), was the presence of markedly fibrotic small airways in the silica-treated animals (34).

Thus evidence exists that both emphysema and small airway disease can produce airflow obstruction in humans and animals exposed to dust. Which lesion is more important remains unresolved. A further confounding factor is the fact that many workers who are exposed to dust also smoke. Since, as noted, both smoke and dust produce many of the same anatomic lesions and may do so by similar mechanisms, it is not unreasonable to suppose that the two agents may produce synergistic abnormalities. Limited experimental data support this proposition. Cigarette smoke has been shown to increase the severity of elastase-induced emphysema (67) and also to increase the severity of small airway fibrosis caused by asbestos (50,65) (Table 6). In the latter study, not only were there synergistic increases in airway wall fibrosis, but there were also synergistic decrements in some parameters of flow (Fig. 3). In humans, there is much less information about synergism, and these data are hard to interpret. Begin et al. (57,58) claimed that asbestos exposure in nonsmokers produced flow abnormalities only at low lung volumes, and what they deemed significant flow limita-

TABLE 6. *Effects of smoke and asbestos on airway wall thickness in a guinea pig model*

Group	Wall thickness in mm (SD)
Saline alone	0.014 (0.01)
Smoke, no asbestos	0.017 (0.01)
Asbestos alone	0.038 (0.04)
Smoke plus asbestos	0.048 (0.04)

From ref. 50.

tion was found only in cigarette smokers. However, because their studies did not have a control group of smokers, the possibility of synergism cannot be examined; also, their studies are effectively cross-sectional, but longitudinal studies are generally required to document the presence of dust-induced flow limitation in humans (51–53).

Finally, it is worth noting an observation made by Kreiss et al. (69) concerning the effects of smoke, dust, and the combination of the two. These authors examined a group of hard-rock miners and found that nonsmokers tended to develop restrictive disease, whereas the smokers tended to develop obstructive disease; and the severity of the obstructive disease appeared to be greater than would have been expected from the amount of smoking. This observation suggests that the combination of smoke and dust may act synergistically. Again, this is an area in which further data are needed.

SUMMARY

Recent pathologic studies have documented the fact that mineral dusts can produce fibrosis of the small airways and that this lesion is morphologically recognizable and specific for dust exposure. Also, there is growing evidence that dust induces a form of centrilobular emphysema (termed "focal emphysema"), probably always in association with the fibrotic small airway changes. These reactions appear to be stereotypic and are associated with many types of dust exposure, although some dusts are implicated more frequently than others.

The development of the fibrotic lesions in the small airways appears to reflect local high dust burdens and a subsequent local inflammatory response. The pathogenesis of emphysema is less clear but may reflect destruction of alveolar walls by proteolytic enzymes released from dust-evoked inflammatory cells, accompanied by inhibition of antiproteolytic protective agents because of dust-generated active oxygen species and possibly other free radicals.

Although there is now extensive physiological support for the idea that exposure to mineral dust of many sorts is associated with airflow obstruction, the morphologic basis of this process remains unclear. Evidence exists to support bronchial hyperactivity, small airway lesions, and emphysema as anatomically important causes of airflow obstruction in dust-exposed workers, but, as is true of pure cigarette smokers, the relationship between these changes and the relative importance of each one is as yet unresolved.

ACKNOWLEDGMENTS

Supported by grants from the Medical Research Council of Canada and the National Cancer Institute of Canada.

REFERENCES

1. Churg A, Wright JL. Small airways disease and mineral dust exposure. *Pathol Ann* 1983;18:233–251.
2. Churg A, Wright JL. Small-airway lesions in patients exposed to nonasbestos mineral dusts. *Hum Pathol* 1983;14:688–693.
3. Wright JL, Churg A. Morphology of small-airway lesions in patients with asbestos exposure. *Hum Pathol* 1984;15:68–74.
4. Churg A, Wright JL, Wiggs B, Pare PD, Lazar N. Small airways disease and mineral dust exposure. *Am Rev Respir Dis* 1985;131:139–143.
5. Churg A, Wright JL: Mineral particle in airway walls in the lungs of long-term chrysotile miners. *Ann Occup Hyg* 1988;32[Suppl]:173–180.
6. Craighead JE, Emerson RJ, Stanley DE. Slate-

worker's pneumoconiosis. *Hum Pathol* 1992;23: 1098–1105.
7. Simson FW, Strachan AS. Silicosis and tuberculosis. *Publ S Afr Inst Med Res* 1935;VI:367.
8. Wright JL, Churg A. Severe diffuse small airways abnormalities in long term chrysotile asbestos miners. *Br J Indust Med* 1985;42:556–559.
9. Begin R, Masse S, Sebastien P, et al. Asbestos exposure and retention as determinants of airway disease and asbestos alveolitis. *Amer Rev Respir Dis* 1988;134:1176–1181.
10. Wehner AP, Dable GE, Milliman EM. Chronic inhalation exposure of hamsters to nickel-enriched fly ash. *Environ Res* 1981;26:195.
11. Lee KP, Barras CE, Griffith FD, Wařitz RS, Lapin CA. Comparative pulmonary responses to inhaled inorganic fibers with asbestos and fiberglass. *Environ Res* 1981;24:167.
12. Wright JL, Harrison N, Wiggs B, Churg A. Quartz but not iron oxide causes air-flow obstruction, emphysema, and small airways lesions in the rat. *Am Rev Respir Dis* 1988; 138:129–135.
13. Begin R, Masse S, Bureau MA. Morphologic features and function of the airways in early asbestosis in the sheep model. *Am Rev Respir Dis* 1982;126:870–876.
14. Green FHY. Coal workers' pneumoconiosis and pneumoconiosis due to other carbonaceous dusts. In, Churg A, Green FHY, eds. *Pathology of occupational lung disease*. New York: Igaku-Shoin; 1988:89–154.
15. Wright JL, Cagle P, Churg A, Colby TV, Myers J. State of the art: diseases of the small airways. *Am Rev Respir Dis* 1991;146:240–262.
16. Parkes WR: *Occupational lung disorders*. 2nd ed. London; Butterworth; 1982:64.
17. Churg A. Asbestos fiber content of the lungs in patients with and without asbestos airways disease. *Am Rev Respir Dis* 1983;127:470–473.
18. Becklake MR, Toyota B, Steward M, Hanson R, Janley J. Lung structure as a risk factor in adverse pulmonary responses to asbestos exposure. *Am Rev Respir Dis* 1983;128:385–388.
19. Vedal S, Enarson DA, Chan-Yeung M. Airway size and the rate of pulmonary function decline in grain handlers. *Am Rev Respir Dis* 1988; 138:1584–1588.
20. Hessel PA, Hnizdo E, Sluis-Cremer GK. Temporal patterns of silica dust exposure and lung dimensions in relation to silicosis. *Ann Occup Hyg* 1988;32[Suppl]:681–687.
21. Yu CP, Nicolaides P, Soong TT. Effect of random airway sizes on aerosol deposition. *Am Ind Hyg Assoc J* 1979;40:999–1005.
22. Rom WN, Travis WD, Brody AR. Cellular and molecular basis of the asbestos-related diseases. *Am Rev Respir Dis* 1991;143:408–422.
23. Adamson IYR, Letourneau HL, Bowden DH. Comparison of alveolar and interstitial macrophages in fibroblast stimulation after silica and long or short asbestos. *Lab Invest* 1991;64:339–344.
24. Brody AR, Hill LH, Adkins B, O'Connor RW. Chrysotile asbestos inhalation in rats: deposition pattern and reaction of alveolar epithelium and pulmonary macrophages. *Am Rev Respir Dis* 1981;123:670–679.
25. Bowden DH. Macrophages, dust, and pulmonary diseases. *Exp Lung Res* 1987;12:89–107.
26. Adamson IYR, Letourneau HL, Bowden DH. Enhanced macrophage–fibroblast interactions in the pulmonary interstitium increases fibrosis after silica injection to monocyte-depleted mice. *Am J Pathol* 1989;134:411–418.
27. Begin R, Cantin A, Masse S. Recent advances in the pathogenesis and clinical assessment of mineral dust pneumoconiosis: asbestosis, silicosis, and coal pneumoconiosis. *Eur Respir J* 1989;2: 988–1001.
28. Gore DJ, Patrick G. A quantitative study of the penetration of insoluble particles into the tissue of the conducting airways. *Ann Occup Hyg* 1982;26:149–161.
29. Leigh J, Outhred KG, McKenzie HI, Glick M, Wiles AN. Quantified pathology of emphysema, pneumoconiosis, and chronic bronchitis in coal workers. *Br J Indust Med* 1983;40:258–263.
30. Cockcroft A, Wagner JC, Ryder R, Seal RME, Lyons JP, Anderson N. Post mortem study of emphysema in coalworkers and non-coalworkers. *Lancet* 1982;2:600–603.
31. Ruckley VA, Gauld SJ, Chapman JS, et al. Emphysema and dust exposure in a group of coal workers. *Am Rev Respir Dis* 1984;129:528–532.
32. Becklake MR, Irwig L, Kielkowski D, Webster I, de Beer M, Landau S. The predictors of emphysema in South African gold miners. *Am Rev Respir Dis* 1987;135:1234–1241.
33. Hnizdo E, Sluis-Cremer K, Abramowitz J. Emphysema type in relation to silica dust exposure in South African gold miners. *Am Rev Respir Dis* 1991;143:1241–1247.
34. Churg A, Hobson J, Wright JL. A functional and morphologic comparison of silica and elastase induced airflow obstruction. *Exp Lung Res* 1989;15:813–822.
35. Brown GM, Brown DM, Slight J, Donaldson K. Persistent biological reactivity of quartz in the lung: raised protease burden compared with a nonpathogenic mineral dust and microbial particle. *Br J Indust Med* 1991;48:61–69.
36. Rom WN. Basic mechanisms leading to focal emphysema in coal worker's pneumoconiosis. *Environ Res* 1990;53:16–28.
37. Pare JP, Cote G, Fraser RS. Long-term followup of drug abusers with intravenous talcosis. *Am Rev Respir Dis* 1989;139:233–241.
38. Schmidt RA, Gleeny RW, Godwin JD, Hampson NB, Cantino ME, Reichenbach DD. Panlobular emphysema in young intravenous Ritalin abusers. *Am Rev Respir Dis* 1991;143:649–656.
39. Pryor WA. The free radical chemistry of cigarette smoke and the inactivation of alpha-1-proteinase inhibitor. In: Taylor JC, Mittman C, eds. *Pulmonary emphysema and proteolysis*. New York: Academic Press; 1987:369–392.

40. Mossman BT, Marsh JP. Evidence supporting a role for active oxygen species in asbestos induced toxicity and lung disease. *Environ Health Perspect* 1989;81:91–94.
41. Pezerat H, Zalma R, Guignard J, Jaurand MC. Production of oxygen radicals by the reduction of oxygen arising from the surface activity of mineral fibers. In: Bignon J, et al. *Biological effects of mineral fibers in the nonoccupational environment*. Lyon: IARC; 1989:100–111.
42. Kennedy TP, Dodson R, Rao NV, et al. Dust causing pneumoconiosis generate OH and produce hemolysis by acting as Fenton catalysts. *Arch Biochem Biophys* 1989;269j:359–364.
43. Dalal NS, Jafari B, Petersen M, Green FHY, Vallyathan V. Presence of stable coal radicals in autopsied coal miner's lungs and its possible correlation to coal worker's pneumonoconiosis. *Arch Environ Health* 1991;46:366–372.
44. Gilks B, Wright JL, Churg A. Effects of cigarette smoke on tissue uptake and retention of iron oxide in the guinea pig. *Am Rev Respir Dis* 1988;137:1382–1384.
45. McFadden D, Wright JL, Wiggs B, Churg A. Smoking increases the penetration of asbestos fibers into airway walls. *Am J Pathol* 1986; 123:95–99.
46. Cohen D, Arai SF, Brain JD. Smoking impairs long-term clearance from the lung. *Science* 1979; 204:514–516.
47. McFadden D, Wright JL, Wiggs B, Churg, A. Smoking inhibits asbestos clearance. *Am Rev Respir Dis* 1986;133:372–374.
48. Mauderly JM, Chen BT, Hahn FF, et al. The effect of chronic cigarette smoke inhalation on the long-term pulmonary clearance of inhaled particles in the rat. In: Wehner AP. *Biological interactions of inhaled mineral fibers and cigarette smoke*. Columbus, OH: Battelle Press; 1989: 223–240.
49. Barnhart S, Thornquist M, Omenn GS, et al. The degree of roentgenographic parenchymal opacities attributable to smoking among asbestos exposed subjects. *Am Rev Respir Dis* 1990; 141:1102–1106.
50. Tron V, Wright JL, Harrison N, Wiggs B, Churg A. Cigarette smoke makes airway and early parenchymal asbestos-induced lung disease worse in the guinea pig. *Am Rev Respir Dis* 1987; 136:271–275.
51. Becklake MR. Chronic airflow limitation: its relationship to work in dusty occupations. *Chest* 1985;88:608–617.
52. Becklake MR. Occupational exposures: evidence for a causal association with chronic obstructive pulmonary disease. *Am Rev Respir Dis* 1989;140:S85–S91.
53. Becklake MR. Occupational pollution. *Chest* 1989;96:372S–378S.
54. Minette A, Marcq M, Gepts L. Prognostic value of a positive acetylcholine test regarding VC and FEV_1 in coal miners with a history of bronchitis. *Bull Eur Physiopathol Respir* 1978;14:167–175.
55. Pham QT, Mur JM, Chau N, Gabiano M, Henquel JC, Tecelescu D. Prognostic value of acetylcholine test: a prospective study. *Br J Indust Med* 1984;41:267–271.
56. Morgan WKC. Industrial bronchitis. *Br J Indust Med* 1978;35:285–291.
57. Begin R, Cantin A, Berthiaume Y, Boileau R, Peloquin S, Masse S. Airway function in lifetime-nonsmoking older asbestos workers. *Am J Med* 1983;75:631–638.
58. Begin R, Boileau R, Peloquin S. Asbestos exposure, cigarette smoking, and airflow limitation in long-term Canadian chrysotile miners and millers. *Am J Indust Med* 1987;11:55–66.
59. Jodoin G, Gibbs GW, Macklem Pt, McDonald JC, Becklake MR. Early effects of asbestos exposure on lung function. *Am Rev Respir Dis* 1971;104:525–535.
60. Peress L, Hoag H, White F, Becklake MR. The relationship between closing volume, smoking and asbestos dust exposure. *Clin Res* 1975; 111:647A
61. Harless KW, Watanabe S, Renzetti AD. The acute effects of chrysotile asbestos exposure on lung function. *Environ Res* 1978;16:360–372.
62. Rodriquez-Roisin R, Merchant JA, Cochrane GE, et al. Maximal expiratory flow volume curves in workers exposed to asbestos. *Respiration* 1980;39:158–165.
63. Secker-Walker RH, Ho JE. Regional lung function in asbestos workers. *Respiration* 1982;43:8–22.
64. Glassroth JL, Bernardo J, Lucey EC, Center DM, Ying-Legg Y, Snider GL. Interstitial pulmonary fibrosis induced in hamsters by intratracheally administered chrysotile asbestos. *Am Rev Respir Dis* 1984;130:242–248.
65. Wright JL, Tron V, Wiggs B, Churg A. Cigarette smoke potentiates asbestos-induced airflow abnormalities. *Exp Lung Res* 1988;14:537–548.
66. Begin R, Ostiguy G, Cantin A, Bergeron D. Lung function in silica-exposed workers. *Chest* 1988;94:539–545.
67. Cowie RL, Mabena SK. Silicosis, airflow limitation, and chronic bronchitis in South African gold miners. *Am Rev Respir Dis* 1991;143:80–84.
68. Hoidal JR, Niewoehner DE. Cigarette smoke inhalation potentiates elastase-induced emphysema in hamsters. *Am Rev Respir Dis* 1983; 127:478–481.
69. Kreiss K, Greenberg LM, Kogut SJH, Lezotte DC, Irvin CG, Cherniack RM. Hard-rock mining exposures affect smokers and nonsmokers differently. *Am Rev Respir Dis* 1989;139:1487–1493.

Diseases of the Bronchioles, edited by
Gary R. Epler. Raven Press, Ltd.,
New York © 1994.

10

Diffuse Panbronchiolitis

Masatoshi Iwata,* Atsuhiko Sato,† and Thomas V. Colby‡

**Chief, Department of Respiratory Medicine, Haibara General Hospital, 2887-1 Hosoe, Haibara-cho, Haibara-gun, Shizuoka 421-04, Japan.*
†Associate Professor, Second Division, Department of Internal Medicine, Hamamatsu University School of Medicine, 3600 Handa-cho, Hamamatsu-shi, Shizuoka 431-31, Japan.
‡Department of Surgical Pathology, Mayo Clinic, 200 First Street, Rochester, MN.

Yamanaka and associates (1) first described diffuse panbronchiolitis in 1969 in Japan as a result of pathologic study of autopsy cases. Homma and colleagues (2) reported 82 cases after a nationwide survey in 1983. Although diffuse panbronchiolitis showed some similarities, Homma and co-workers concluded that it was distinct from asthma, bronchiectasis, chronic bronchitis, and emphysema. Diffuse panbronchiolitis had been recognized but had been diagnosed as other diseases since the 1950s and had proven to be a difficult condition to manage (3–9).

Diffuse panbronchiolitis is a clinicopathologic entity characterized by a number of clinical, radiographic, functional, and morphologic findings. Clinical features are chronic cough, sputum, and dyspnea. In the advanced stage, patients typically produce large amounts of purulent sputum and have chronic *Pseudomonas aeruginosa* infections of the lower respiratory tract. Once *P. aeruginosa* is present, it is rarely eradicated from their lungs, despite the use of various antibiotics. The cause of death in most patients is respiratory failure or *P. aeruginosa* pneumonia. This clinical course is similar to that of cystic fibrosis. It has recently been shown (10–12) that low-dose, long-term administration of erythromycin is effective for diffuse panbronchiolitis, although the detailed mechanisms are not understood.

Diffuse panbronchiolitis is largely restricted to Japan, but recently several case reports from North America and Europe have appeared (13–16). Homma and colleagues suggested that there might be an overlap between cases diagnosed as diffuse panbronchiolitis in Japan and those diagnosed as bronchiectasis or bronchiolitis obliterans elsewhere, although most evidence suggests that diffuse panbronchiolitis is a separate disease almost entirely restricted to the Japanese. Few pulmonologists or pathologists outside of Japan are familiar with this entity and they need to be familiar with this disease and its clinical and pathologic features, because of the major efflux of Japanese into the world.

It has recently been reported (13) that a number of other diseases, including ulcerative colitis, Churg-Strauss syndrome (17), Sjögren syndrome (18,19), adult T-cell leukemia (20), and non-Hodgkin's lymphomas (21,22), may have pulmonary changes similar to diffuse panbronchiolitis.

In this chapter, we review the clinical, radiographic, physiologic, management, and pathologic aspects of diffuse panbronchiolitis with special emphasis on differential diagnosis.

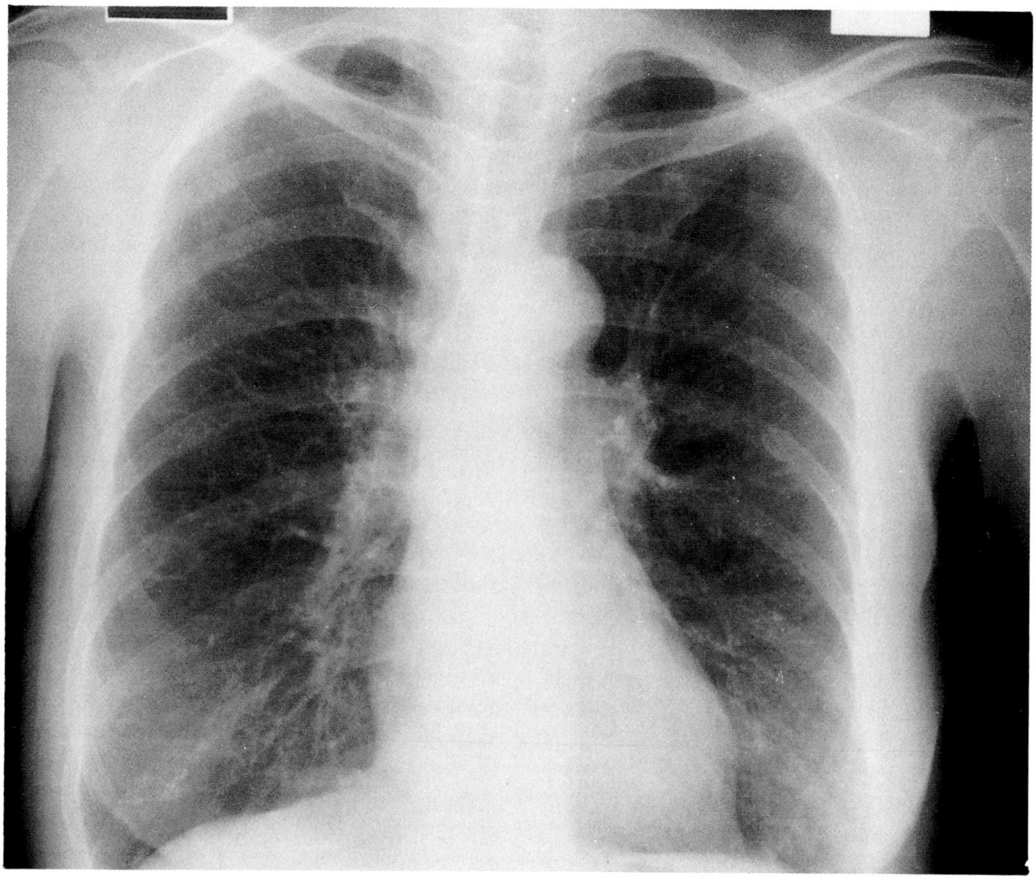

FIG. 1. Chest radiograph of a 59-year-old patient shows small nodular shadows in bilateral lower lungs and a mild degree of hyperinflation of the lung.

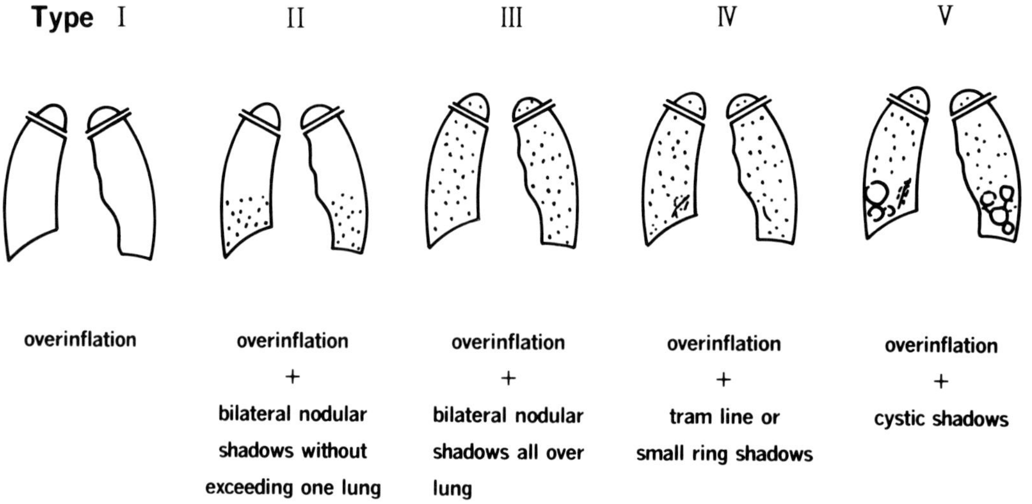

FIG. 2. Radiographic classification of diffuse panbronchiolitis.

CLINICAL SYMPTOMS

Diffuse panbronchiolitis affects males slightly more than females, but there is no significant difference of frequency between sexes (23). The patients are distributed from the first decade to the seventh decade, but middle-aged individuals are most affected. They have no evidence of toxic gas inhalation or preceding pulmonary infection (2,23). One-third of the patients have a history of smoking. The initial symptoms are chronic cough, mucous expectoration, wheezing, and exertional dyspnea. Exertional dyspnea appears relatively early, compared with other chronic obstructive lung diseases. Hemoptysis is uncommon. Cases with wheezing may initially be interpreted as asthma. With progression, large amounts of purulent expectoration (100 to 200 ml/day) and fever develop, and the patients complain of severe dyspnea (including orthopnea). Over 80% of the patients have chronic paranasal sinusitis, and 20% have a family history of paranasal sinusitis (2,23).

PHYSICAL FINDINGS

Auscultation of the chest is important in making an early diagnosis (23,24). Course crackles and rhonchi are audible over both lower lung areas. Clubbed fingers are some-

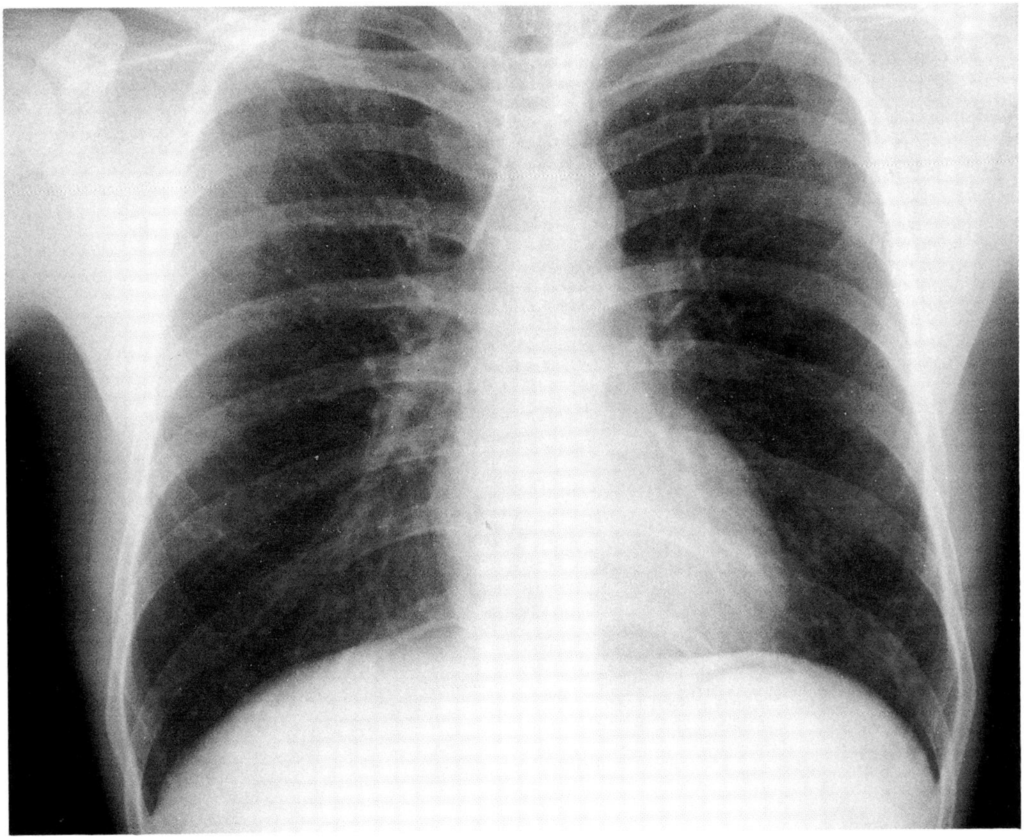

FIG. 3. Chest radiograph of a 27-year-old patient shows bilateral small nodular shadows in the costphrenic angles.

times observed at the first medical examination. In advanced stages, hypertrophy of the sternocleidomastoid muscles is often seen. The chest becomes barrel-shaped because of hyperinflation of the lung. When cor pulmonale develops, cyanosis and edema of the lower extremities appear.

RADIOGRAPHIC FINDINGS

The radiographic features of diffuse panbronchiolitis are diffusely disseminated, fine nodular shadows mainly located in the lower lung fields and hyperinflation of the lung (Fig. 1) (2,23). The nodules are 2 to 3 mm in size and have vague borders. The fine nodular shadows correlate with the inflammatory lesions of the respiratory bronchioles. Hyperinflation, reflective of increased total lung capacity, results from air trapping secondary to obstruction. The hyperinflation is due to an increase in the size of the air spaces distal to the terminal bronchiole without destructive changes in the alveolar walls; this fits with the pathology of diffuse panbronchiolitis.

Nakata and Tanimoto (25) have classified the radiographic findings into five groups according to the progression of the disease (Fig. 2). Type I shows overinflation without nodular shadows, types II and III show

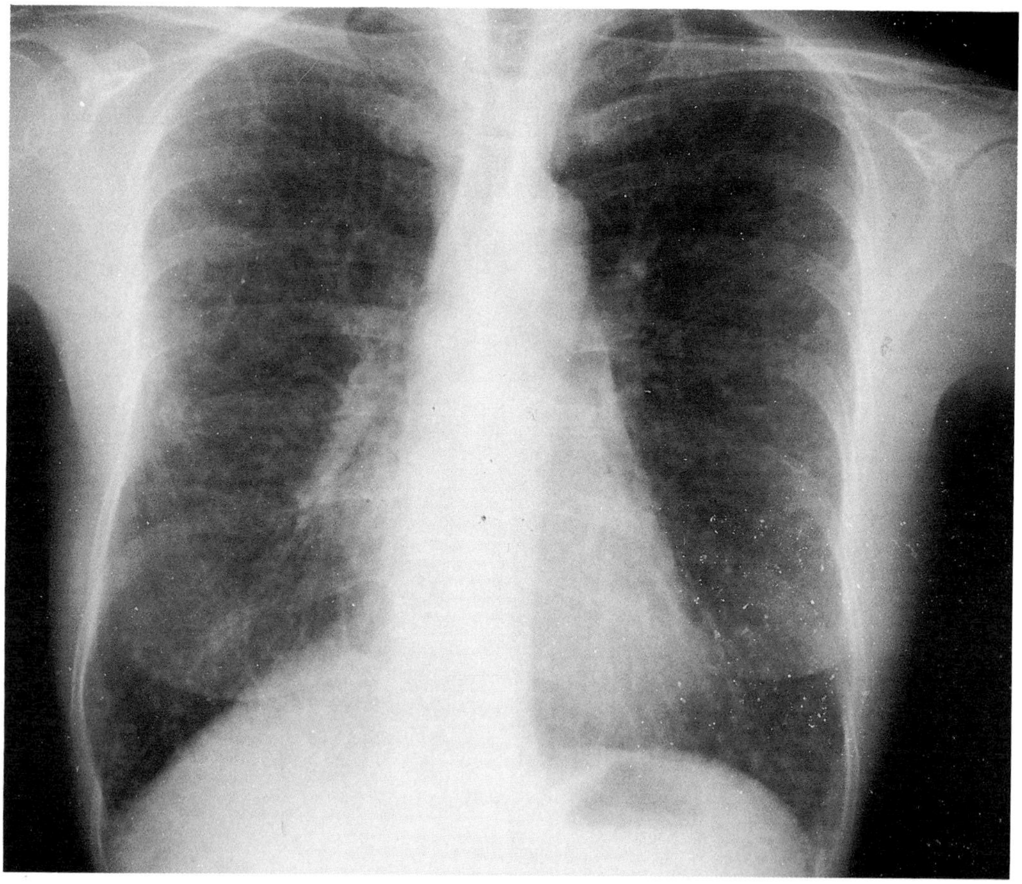

FIG. 4. Chest radiograph of a 55-year-old patient shows fine nodular shadows disseminated throughout both lungs and hyperinflation of the lung.

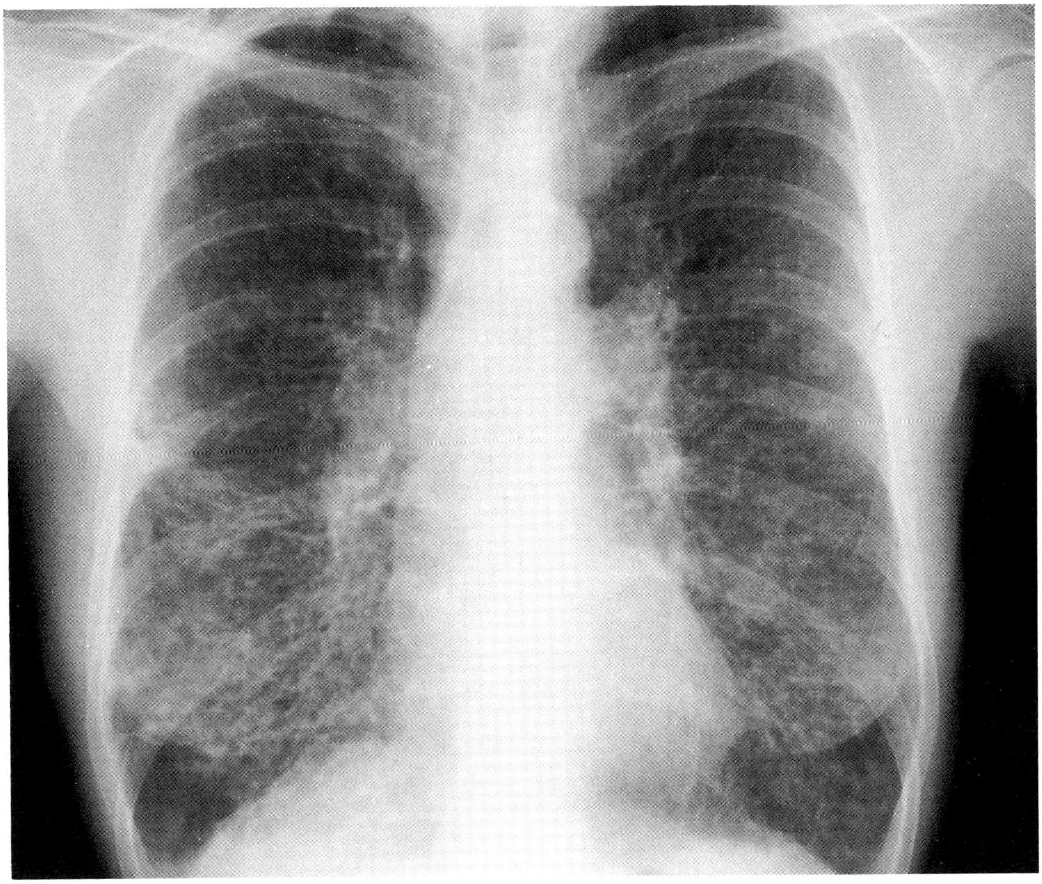

FIG. 5. Tram-line or small ring-shaped shadows are seen in both lower lungs in addition to small nodular shadows in this 52-year-old patient.

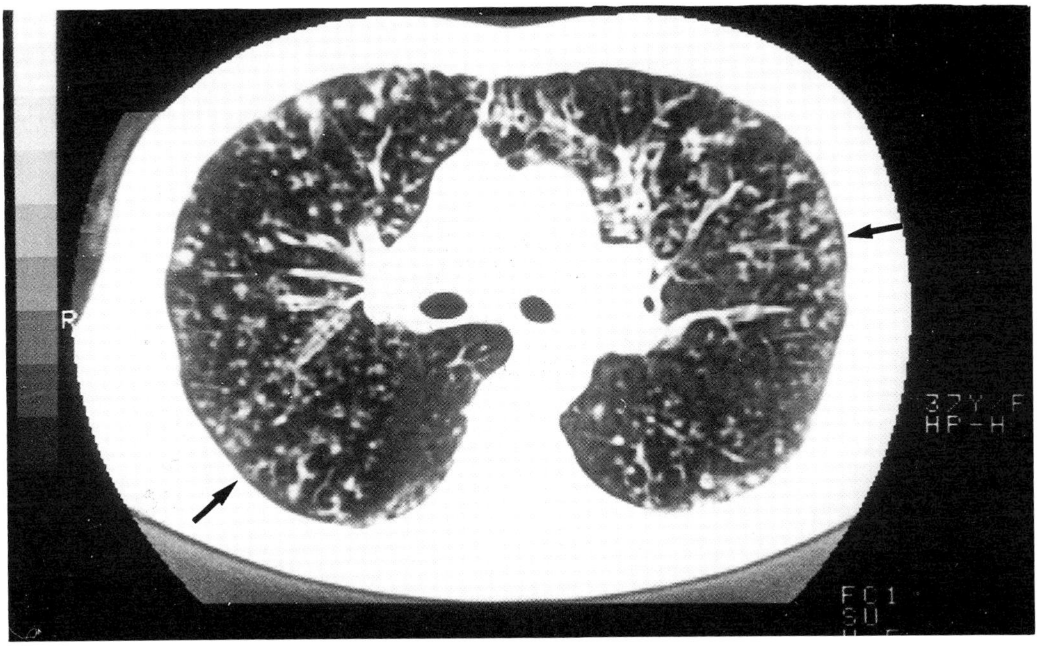

FIG. 6. CT scan of the patient of Fig. 5 shows small nodular shadows distributed away from the pleura. These are continuous from bronchovascular bundles (*arrows*). Dilatation of peripheral airways is seen.

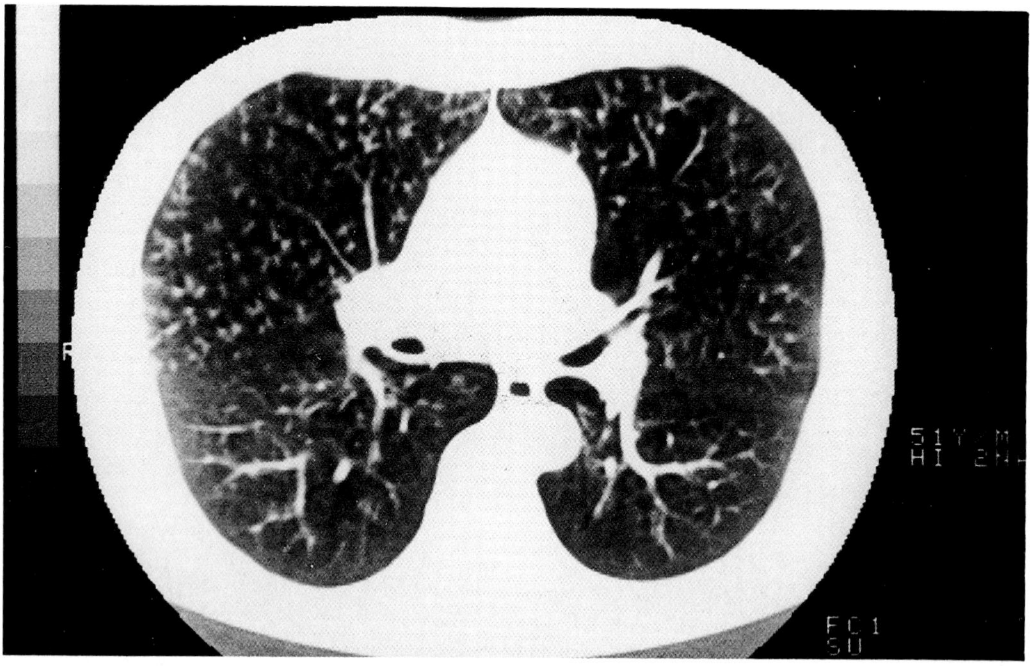

FIG. 7. Small nodular shadows are seen, but dilatation of bronchioles is not clear.

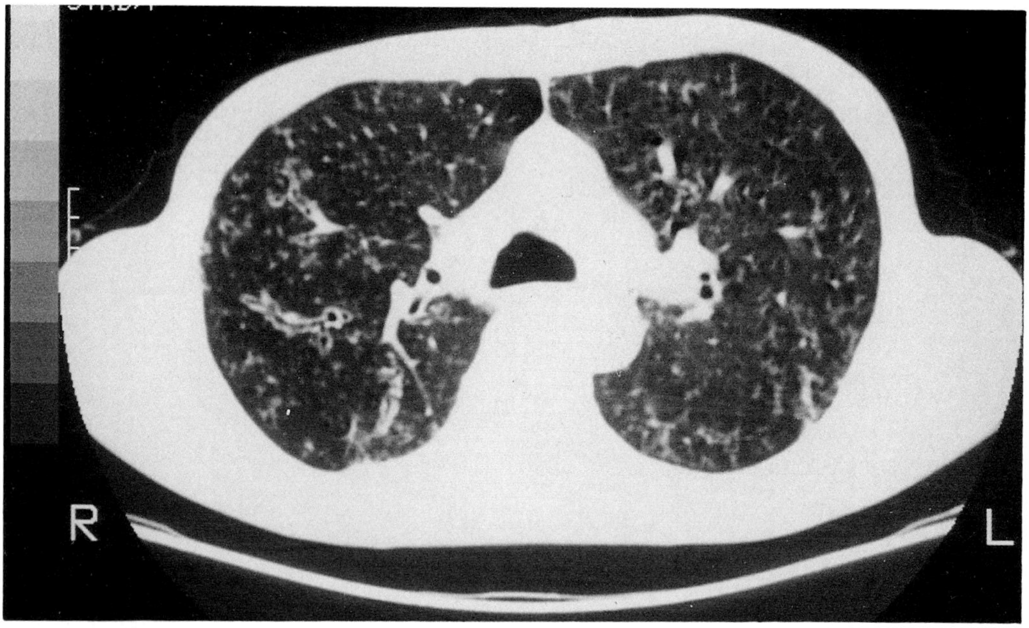

FIG. 8. CT scan shows ductal dilatation of airways with a few small nodules.

overinflation with bilateral nodular shadows whose combined area does not exceed one side of the lung in type II (Figs. 1 and 3) but occupies the entire lung in type III (Fig. 4). Type IV (Fig. 5) reveals small ring-shaped or tram-line shaped shadows associated with type III. Type V shows large ring-shaped or cystic shadows in addition to the changes of type IV.

High-resolution computed tomography (CT) is useful in the diagnosis of diffuse panbronchiolitis and evaluating its progression. The characteristic features of the disease on high-resolution CT (Fig. 6) are as follows (26–30): (a) diffuse, small nodular shadows located in the centrilobular regions, (b) dilatation of bronchioles and small bronchi, and (c) thickening of bronchiolar and bronchial walls. The small nodular shadows are distributed 2 to 3 mm away from the pleura and pulmonary vein, are continuous from bronchovascular bundles, and are located in the center of areas enclosed by pulmonary vein shadows (i.e., center of secondary lobules). Akira and colleagues (31) classified the radiographic

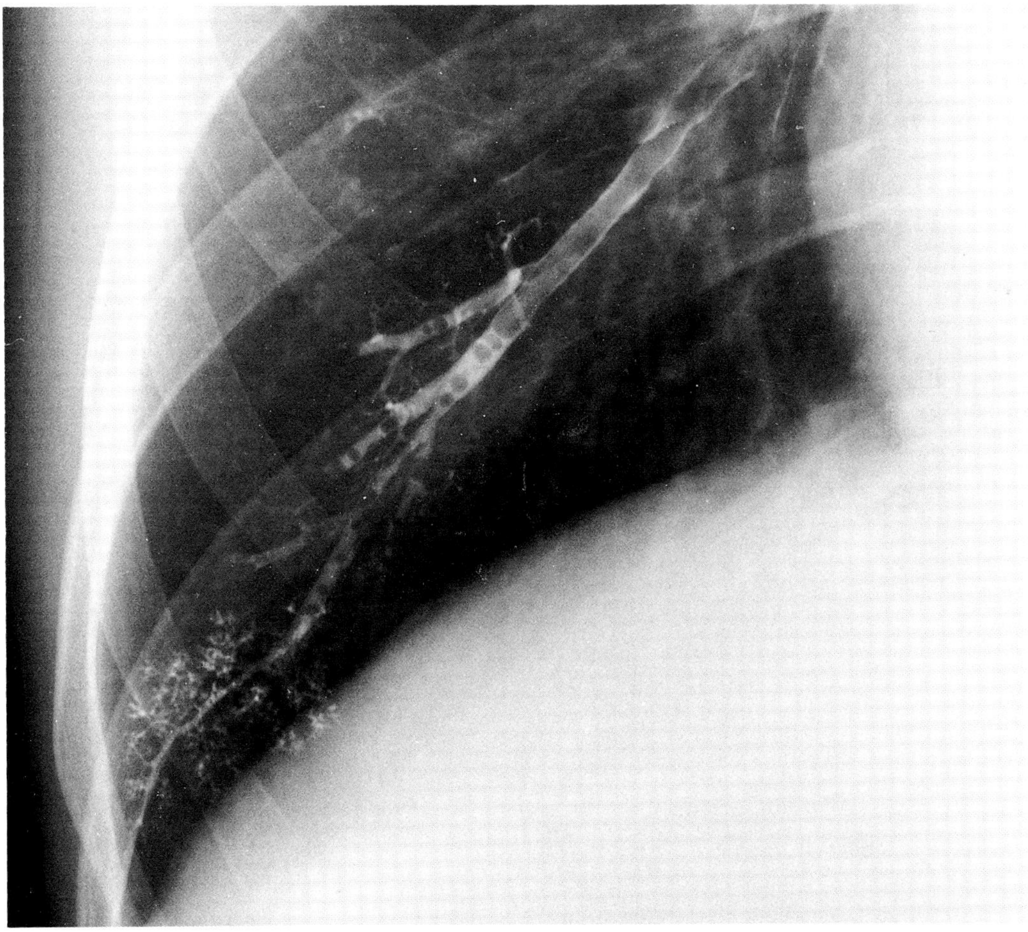

FIG. 9. Selective alveolo-bronchography in the patient of Fig. 3 shows gradual narrowing of the bronchial airways.

findings of high-resolution CT into four types as follows: type I, small nodules located around the end of bronchovascular branchings; type II, small nodules located in a centrilobular area and connected to small linear opacities branching 1 mm apart (Fig. 7); type III, nodules accompanied by ring-shaped or small ductal opacities connected to proximal bronchovascular bundles (Figs. 6 and 8); and type IV, large cystic opacities accompanied by dilated proximal bronchi. They concluded that the classification based on CT findings reflected the clinical stages and pathologic changes of the disease.

In selective alveolo-bronchography (27, 32–34), bronchioles are narrowed or obstructed, are associated with decrease of branches of proximal bronchioles in initial stages (Fig. 9), and are obstructed with accompanying dilatation of proximal bronchioles in advanced stages (Fig. 10).

PULMONARY AND CARDIAC FUNCTION

Pulmonary function tests show marked obstructive and slight restrictive impairments (2,23). The forced expiratory volume in 1 second (FEV_1) is decreased and the residual volume (RV) increased. The ratios of

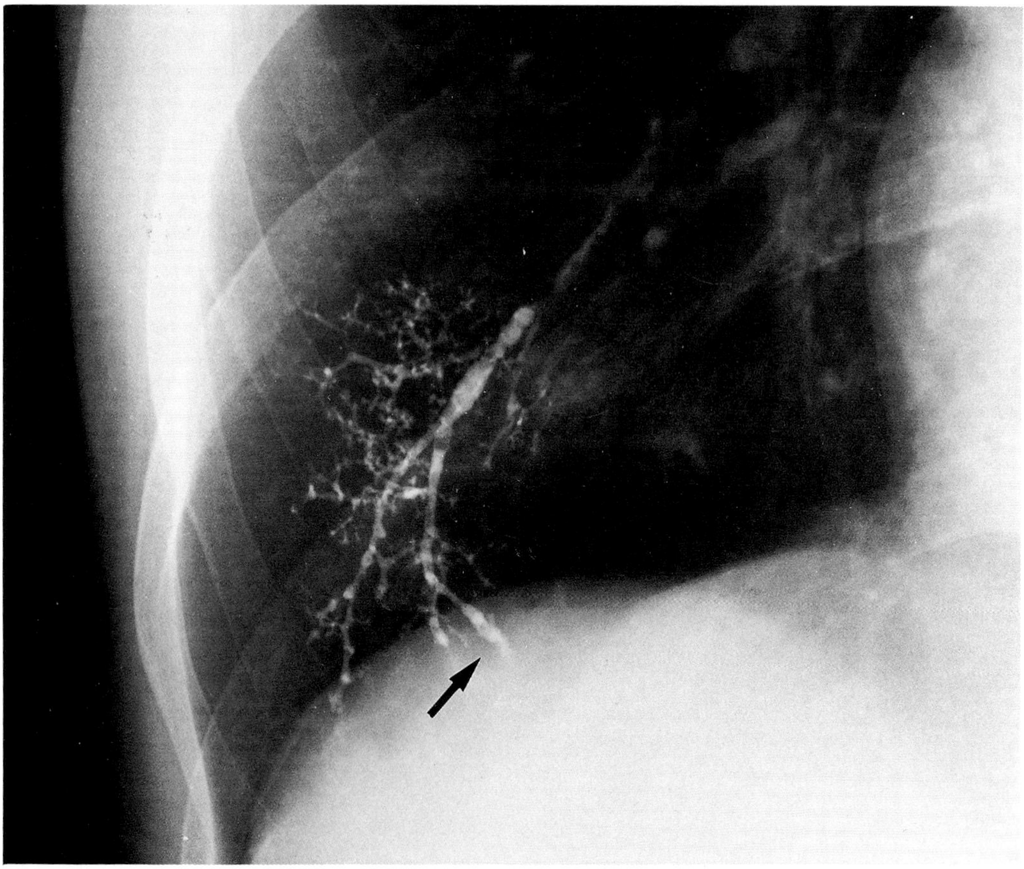

FIG. 10. Selective alveolo-bronchography in the patient of Fig. 1 shows irregular dilated bronchioles (*arrow*).

diffusing capacity with alveolar volume (DLCO/VA) and static lung compliance are often within normal limits and therefore useful in the differential diagnosis from pulmonary emphysema. Vital capacity is decreased slightly. Hypoxemia is recognized as an early abnormality in this disease, and severe hypoxemia with hypercapnea occurs. As the radiographic findings progress from type I to type V, the vital capacity (VC), FEV_1/FVC and PaO_2 decrease and the RV/TLC increase (35). In advanced stages, pulmonary arterial hypertension, right ventricular hypertrophy, and right ventricular failure appear.

CLINICAL CRITERIA FOR DIAGNOSIS AND DIFFERENTIAL DIAGNOSIS

In a nationwide survey (2) (Grant in Aid from the Ministry of Health and Welfare of Japan) of diffuse panbronchiolitis from 1978 to 1980, several clinical diagnostic criteria were agreed upon, as noted in Table 1. The characteristic findings of diffuse panbronchiolitis on histopathologic study and other clinical findings were added in 1986 (23).

Most cases of the disease show elevation of cold hemagglutinin titers (36–38). None have showed elevation of antimycoplasma antibody titer. Elevated cold agglutinin titer is not correlated with severity of the disease or any specific bacteria but is observed in initial stages. Rheumatoid factor frequently becomes positive. Serum IgA commonly increases, but other immunoglobulins including IgE do not ordinarily increase. CD4 cells (T helper/inducer) are increased, and CD8 cells (T suppressor/cytotoxic) are decreased in the peripheral blood (39,40). Consequently the CD4/CD8 ratio is elevated. Other findings include positive C-reactive protein in about 70% of patients from all stages and moderate elevation of erythrocyte sedimentation rate. The white blood cell count is about 9,000/mm^3 with 60 to 70% polymorphonuclear leukocytes. Eosinophils are not increased. HLA-Bw54 is found in 60 to 70% of the patients (41). Bronchoalveolar lavage shows higher percentages of neutrophils compared with chronic bronchitis (42).

The clinical and functional findings in diffuse panbronchiolitis have similarities to those of chronic bronchitis and emphysema, bronchiectasis, bronchiolitis obliterans, and cystic fibrosis. In chronic bronchitis and emphysema, cigarette smoking is overwhelmingly the most important factor, although other factors may play a role; the patients have no history of chronic paranasal sinusitis, and pulmonary function tests show an obstructive pattern with a decrease in diffusing capacity.

Cystic fibrosis has many similarities to this disease, including chronic pulmonary infections with *P. aeruginosa,* especially mucoid strains, which are common in patients with both cystic fibrosis and diffuse panbronchiolitis. However, cystic fibrosis is a hereditary disease with autosomal recessive transmission, and it shows abnormal sweat tests, in contrast to diffuse panbronchiolitis, which does not (43). The most common type of mutation in the cystic fibrosis gene, a 3-base deletion, is not found in this disease (44).

Bronchiectasis is ordinarily classified into three groups: cylindrical, varicose, and saccular types. Bilateral cylindrical bronchiectasis is the type that is clinically similar to diffuse panbronchiolitis. In dyskinetic cilia syndrome, roentgenographic abnormalities in the chest are present and include bronchial wall thickening, hyperinflation, and bronchiectasis (45). Clinically, the patients have chronic sinusitis and chronic and recurrent infections of the airways. Impaired mucociliary clearance is a characteristic feature of this disease (46). It has been reported that some cases of dyskinetic cilia syndrome fulfill the clinical criteria of diffuse panbronchiolitis (47). In this disease, aerosol inhalation cinescintigraphy has revealed marked impairment of the mucociliary transport function in the lower airway (48), and electron microscopic examination showed ciliary abnormalities including

TABLE 1. *Clinical diagnostic criteria of diffuse panbronchiolitis*

Symptoms	Physical examination	Chest roentgenogram	Pulmonary function[a]	Other
Chronic cough	Crackles	Diffusely disseminated fine nodular opacities, mainly in the lower lungs, with hyperinflation of the lungs	FVC $<$ 80% of the predicted volume	Past or present history of chronic paranasal sinusitis
Sputum	Rhonchi		FEV_1/FVC $<$ 70%	Immunologic findings: increase of cold hemagglutinin titer, increase of IgA, increase of CD4/CD8 ratio
Dyspnea on exertion			RV $>$ 150% of the predicted value	Proof of HLA-Bw54 antigen
			$PaO_2 < 80$ mm Hg	

FVC, forced vital capacity; FEV_1, forced expired volume in one second; RV, residual volume.
[a]Three out of four must be present.

TABLE 2. *Clinical presentations of patients with diffuse panbronchiolitis*

Case no.	Age/ Sex	Symptoms	Physical examination	Chest x-ray	Pulmonary function (% predicted)	Other
1	32 M	Cough, sputum (100–150 ml), chest pain	Rhonchi, crackles, wheeze	Bilateral reticular interstitial opacities	FVC 1.6 (39%), FEV_1 1.27 (79%), RV/TLC 34%, PO_2 67, PCO_2 55 (under 31 O_2)	Black, *H. influenzae* from sputum
2	23 M	Cough, sputum	Crackles	Bilateral diffuse bronchiectasis	VC 2.88 (58%), FEV_1 1.63 (57%), RV/TLC 28%, PO_2 66, PCO_2 40	Chinese, *H. influenzae* from sputum, HLA: A2, A24,B56, Bw73,Cw3, Cw7, DRw15(2)
3	46 M	Cough, sputum, dyspnea	Rhonchi, crackles	Bilateral micronodular opacities with hyperinflation	Mixed pattern, hypoxemia	Japanese, *P. aeruginosa* from sputum, chronic sinusitis
4	57 F	Cough, sputum		Bilateral diffuse floccular infiltrates		Caucasian, chronic sinusitis
5	51 F	Cough, dyspnea, fever		Bilateral infiltrates		Caucasian
6	53 M	Cough, green sputum		Bilateral micronodular opacities		Caucasian
7	59 M			Bilateral interstitial infiltrates		Japanese

Cases 1–3 are definite diffuse panbronchiolitis cases both clinically and pathologically.
Cases 4–7 are possible diffuse panbronchiolitis cases that showed all findings of the pathologic criteria but lack several clinical findings.

TABLE 3. *Clinical features of diffuse panbronchiolitis and various airway diseases*

	Diffuse panbronchiolitis	Bronchiectasis	Chronic bronchitis and emphysema	Constrictive bronchiolitis	Cystic fibrosis
Age	> 20	All ages	> 40	> 40	All ages (young)
Sex	M = F	M = F	M > F	M < F	M = F
Symptoms	Cough, sputum, dyspnea	Cough, sputum, hemoptysis	Dyspnea, cough, sputum	Cough, sputum, dyspnea	Cough, sputum, hemoptysis, dyspnea
Respiratory dysfunction	Mixed (obst > rest) DLCO →, RV ↑	Mixed	Obstructive, DLCO ↓, RV ↑	Obstructive	Mixed (obst > rest)
Chest x-ray	Micronodular density, overinflation (early), ectatic change (late)	Ectatic change[a]	Overinflation or increased bronchovascular markings	Overinflation	Cystic changes
Other	Chronic sinusitis (> 90%), cold hemagglutinin ↑, *Pseudomonas* infection	Chronic sinusitis (50%)	Smokers		*Pseudomonas* infection

[a]Cystic, cylindrical, or varicose type.

compound cilia and cilia beating with abnormal direction, but no cilia lacking dynein arms, unlike in dyskinetic cilia syndrome (49).

Constrictive bronchiolitis (the obstructive form of bronchiolitis obliterans) has a resemblance to diffuse panbronchiolitis symptomatically and roentgenographically (50–53). In fact, some patients with constrictive bronchiolitis fulfill the clinical criteria of diffuse panbronchiolitis (54). Two of the 7 cases of diffuse panbronchiolitis that we found among 81 cases of chronic bronchiolitis without a specific clinical diagnosis from the Charles B. Carrington Memorial Pulmonary Pathology Collection (Table 2) had been treated as bronchiectasis or bronchiolitis obliterans (54a). The clinical differential diagnosis for the disease is summarized in Table 3.

PATHOLOGIC FINDINGS

On gross examination, the lungs may be spongy and hyperinflated, and they may not deflate after biopsy or removal at autopsy. Many yellowish nodules, 2 to 3 mm in diameter or sometimes larger, are distributed in the centrilobular regions throughout both lungs (Fig. 11). Dilatation of bronchioles and bronchi are found but generally less in degree than classical bronchiectasis.

On microscopic examination, chronic inflammatory lesions are distributed in the centrilobular regions, and no pathologic changes are generally detectable in the alveoli except overinflation in the distal lobular unit (Fig. 12A) (or a secondary pneumonia). The main affected region is the respiratory bronchiole just distal to the terminal bronchiole (Fig. 12B). The walls of respiratory bronchioles are thickened by infiltration of mononuclear cells consisting of lymphocytes, plasma cells, and histiocytes (Fig. 12C). Proliferation of lymph follicle along the airways (bronchus-associated lymphoid tissue, or BALT) is frequently noted (Fig. 13). As a result, the respiratory bronchioles are narrowed or obstructed. Sato et

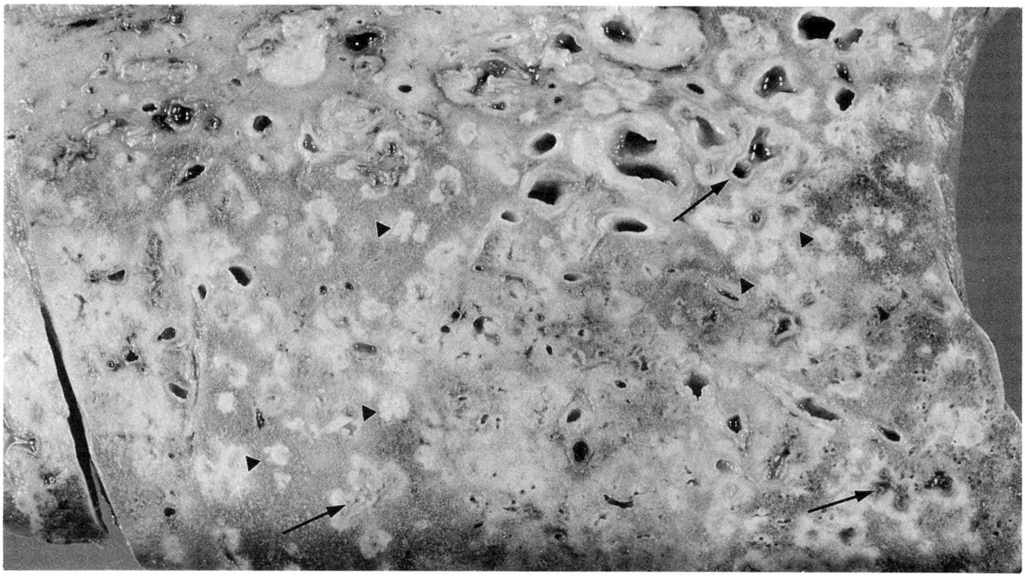

FIG. 11. Macroscopic view of a cut surface of autopsied lung. Many yellowish nodules, 2 to 3 mm in diameter (*arrowheads*) are characteristic features. Dilated bronchioles and bronchi are seen (*arrows*).

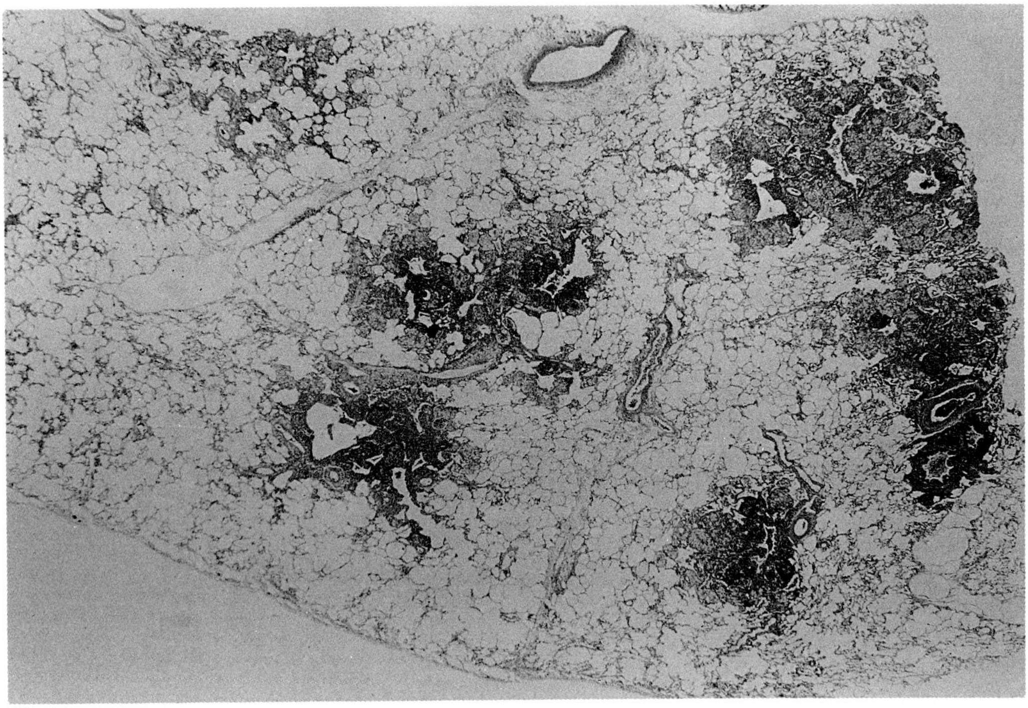

A

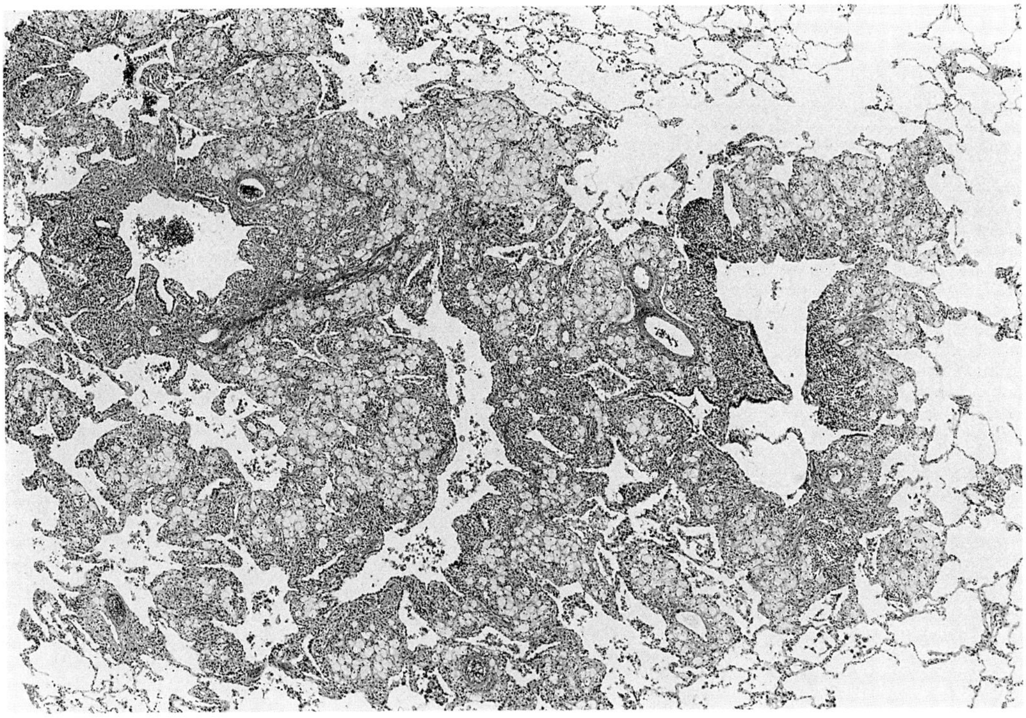

B

FIG. 12. A, Open lung biopsy specimen from the patient of Fig. 3 shows chronic inflammation in the centrilobular regions with no pathologic changes in the distal lobules. **B,** Centrilobular region (main affected region) consists of respiratory bronchiole and terminal bronchiole.

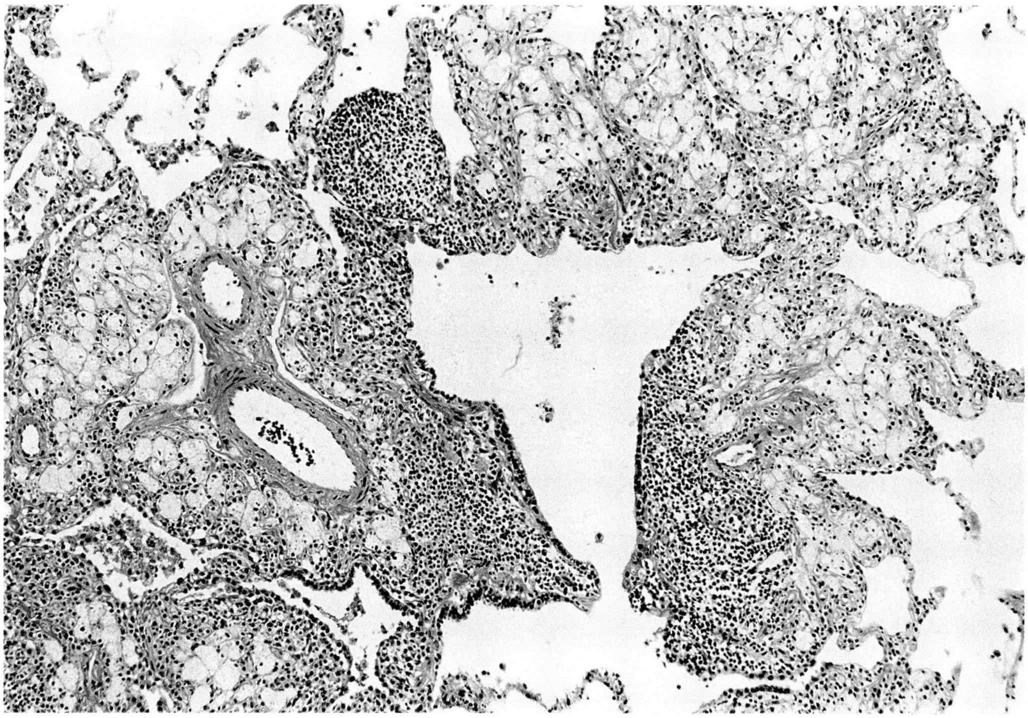

C

FIG. 12. *Continued.* **C,** High-magnification view. Accumulation of foam cells accompanied by infiltration of lymphocytes and plasma cells are seen in the walls of respiratory bronchioles. This pathologic change reveals a typical panbronchiolitis unit lesion.

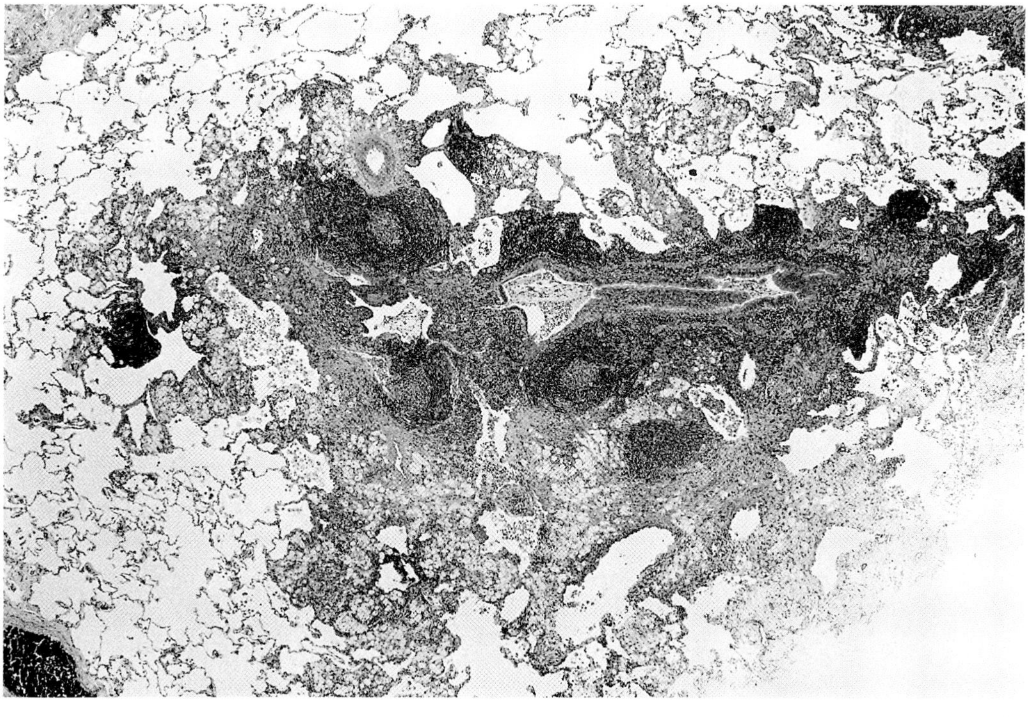

FIG. 13. Bronchus-associated lymphoid tissues are seen in the walls of respiratory bronchioles and terminal bronchioles, resulting in narrowed bronchioles.

al. (55) reported that in patients of diffuse panbronchiolitis with BALT hyperplasia the level of serum IgA was increased. Immunohistochemical study of BALT in patients with this disease showed that a number of surface IgM cells are concentrated in the center of the lymphoid tissue, associated with scattered IgG or IgA cells. The majority of T cells are confined to the parafollicular regions, with a predominance of helper T cells (Fig. 14). These results support the idea that BALT plays a vital part in the local production of immunoglobulins. Experimentally, Iwata and Sato (56) have reported that BALT regulates the local immune responses against chronic pulmonary infection due to *P. aeruginosa*.

Bronchiolar intraluminal granulation tissue, which may lead to bronchiolar stenosis, is frequently found (Fig. 15). Using a serial section and reconstruction analysis, Maeda and co-workers (57) reported the morphological changes in the region of respiratory bronchioles. These changes were classified into the three following types by the presence and size of the intraluminal granulation tissue: type 1, stenosis solely caused by the thickening of the walls of the respiratory bronchioles; type 2, stenosis caused by the localized intraluminal granulation tissue in addition to the thickened walls of the respiratory bronchioles; and type 3, stenosis caused by intraluminal granulation tissue extending to more than

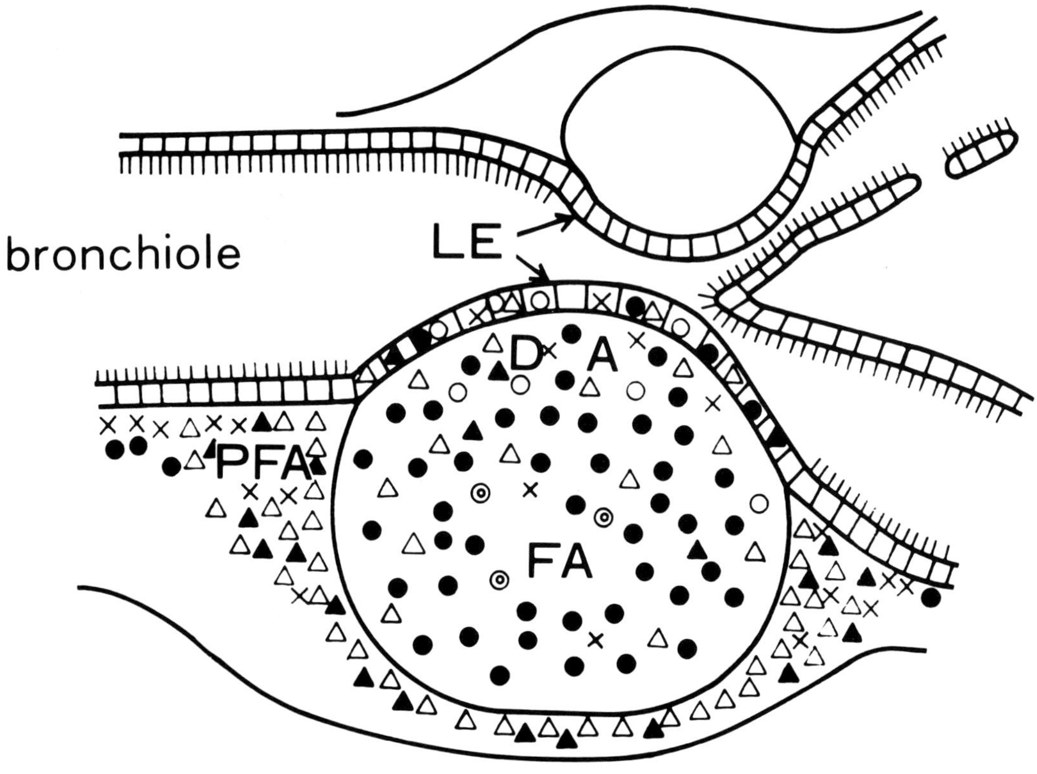

FIG. 14. Cellular distribution in hyperplastic bronchus-associated lymphoid tissue. *LE,* lymphoepithelium; *DA,* dome area; *FA,* follicular area (B cell zone); *PFA,* parafollicular area (T cell zone); *open circles,* IgG; *crosses,* IgA; *closed circles,* IgM; *closed triangles,* CD8; *open triangles,* CD4; *double circles,* CD57.

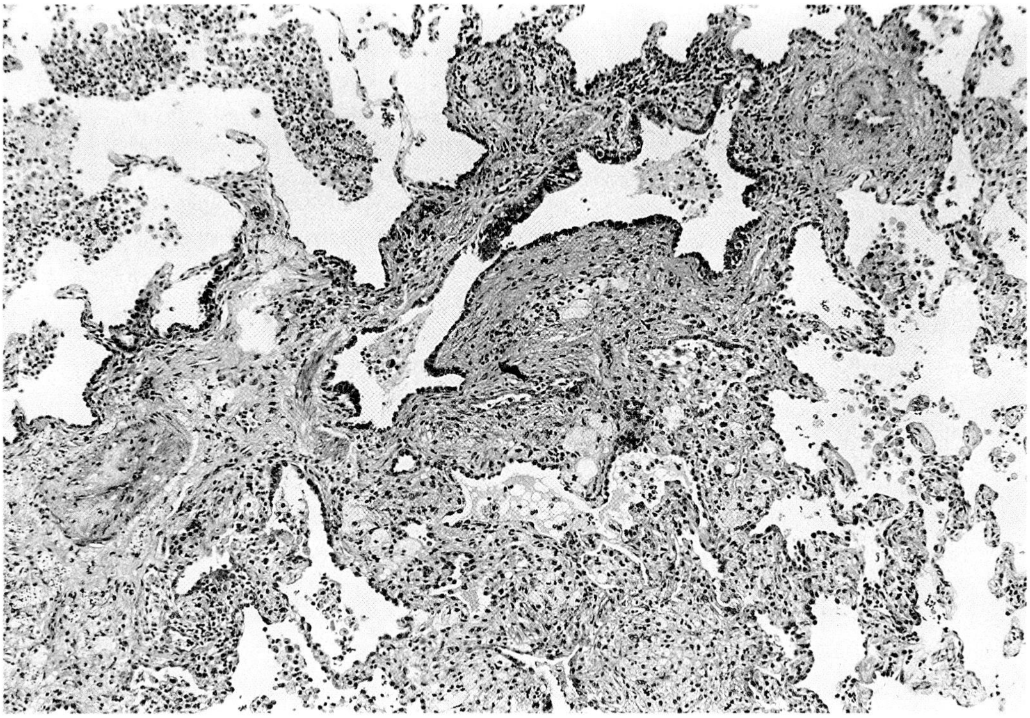

FIG. 15. Open lung biopsy specimen shows an infiltration of lymphocytes and plasma cells into the walls and peripheral tissues of terminal bronchioles and respiratory bronchioles with accumulations of foam cells and stenosis of bronchioles by intraluminal granulation tissue.

two branches of the respiratory bronchioles in addition to the type 2 findings. They concluded that the intraluminal granulation tissue in the respiratory bronchioles is an essential aspect of the disease along with the intramural bronchiolitis. The accumulation of foam cells accompanied by an infiltration of lymphocytes and plasma cells is seen in the peribronchiolar areas; these foci correspond to the yellowish nodules observed on gross examination. Typical pathologic findings and diagnostic criteria of the disease as proposed by Yamanaka and Yokoyama (58) are shown in Tables 4 and 5.

Transbronchial lung biopsy is a relatively noninvasive method of obtaining lung tissue, although it is generally accepted that the diagnosis of many diffuse lung diseases by transbronchial biopsy is not reliable (59,60). Although the tissue sampled by this

TABLE 4. *Pathologic criteria for diffuse panbronchiolitis*

1. The lesions are diffusely distributed in both lungs.
2. The lesions are composed of respiratory bronchiolitis and peribronchiolitis.
   a. The respiratory bronchioles are narrowed or obstructed as a result of proliferation of lymph-follicle and mononuclear cell infiltration and/or intraluminal granulation tissue.
   b. No pathologic changes are detectable in the alveoli except overinflation in the distal lobular unit.
   c. Accumulation of xanthoma cells (foam cells) are observed in the interstitial tissue of respiratory bronchioles, alveolar ducts, and septal walls as well as in the alveolar spaces.
3. Chronic inflammatory changes extend to proximal bronchioles and small bronchi.
   a. Cell infiltration (chronic bronchitis–bronchiolitis)
   b. Secondary bronchiectasis

TABLE 5. *Pathological grading system*

Grade	Criteria
Grade I (others) or II (questionable)	Specific findings leading to other diseases or other findings except grades III, IV, V
Grade III (compatible)	2b and 3a[a]
Grade IV (probable)	2 or 1 and 2b and 3a
Grade IV (definite)	1 and 2

[a]Refer to Table 4.

method is small, helpful information can be sometimes obtained, and it has been reported that transbronchial biopsy is sometimes useful for the diagnosis of diffuse panbronchiolitis (34,61–63). For open lung biopsies performed on 14 patients, we retrospectively studied the pathological findings of 56 specimens obtained by transbronchial biopsy (64). Only 12 (21%) of the transbronchial biopsy specimens contained respiratory bronchioles. Seven cases (50%) were interpreted pathologically as probable diffuse panbronchiolitis.

Recently it has become recognized that some cases that fulfill the above-mentioned clinical diagnostic criteria of the disease are examples of bronchiectasis, chronic cellular bronchiolitis, constrictive bronchiolitis or other disease (47,54,65–67), and conversely that there are cases that do not fulfill the clinical criteria but show typical pathologic findings of the disease in open lung biopsy material (64,67). Kitaichi (15, 67,68) reported that the most distinctive feature of diffuse panbronchiolitis in distinguishing it from other inflammatory airway disorders was chronic inflammation and an accumulation of foam cells in the walls of respiratory bronchioles, adjacent alveolar ducts, and alveoli (panbronchiolitis unit lesion). Bilateral multifocal cylindrical bronchiectasis remained a major problem in the differential diagnosis of the disease.

In addition to the Kitaichi report, we have found histologically similar lesions (panbronchiolitis-like lesion) in various pulmonary diseases including constrictive bronchiolitis, follicular bronchiolitis, cystic fibrosis (Fig. 16), bronchiectasis (group 1; see below), aspiration pneumonia, extrinsic allergic alveolitis, Wegener's granulomatosis, bronchocentric granulomatosis, and malignant lymphoma (group 2; see below) from a large review of the Charles B. Carrington Memorial Pulmonary Pathology Teaching Collection for the years 1977 through 1991 (54a).

Group 1 is clinically similar to diffuse panbronchiolitis. Bronchiectasis in cystic fibrosis involves diffusely bilateral lungs and shows a saccular morphology. The mechanism of formation of a panbronchiolitis-like lesion in cystic fibrosis or bronchiectasis may be different from that of diffuse panbronchiolitis. In cystic fibrosis, obstruction from abnormal bronchial secretions promotes infection that ultimately results in bronchiectasis (69). Esterly and Oppenheimer (69,70) reported that bronchiolar stenosis or obstruction was found only in children older than 6 months, but bronchiectasis could already been seen in children from 1 to 6 months of age, as found in a study of necropsy specimens in cystic fibrosis. Most bronchioles are also affected with chronic inflammation and are narrowed or obstructed in follicular bronchiectasis and saccular bronchiectasis (71). Thus in group 1, chronic inflammation extends from the proximal bronchioles and secondarily to respiratory bronchioles. The most striking difference between diffuse panbronchiolitis and the former group is the airway region primarily affected (1,2,23,69–72). Small biopsies in those cases could be mistaken for the disease. On the other hand, inflammatory changes involved all the airways, and secondary dilatation of the bronchioles and bronchi are seen in later stages of diffuse panbronchiolitis (Fig. 17). Therefore the main affected region, whether or not the respiratory bronchiole, sometimes becomes obscured. The results suggest that the panbronchiolitis-like lesion is a nonspecific histologic finding; the diagnosis of diffuse panbronchiolitis can be

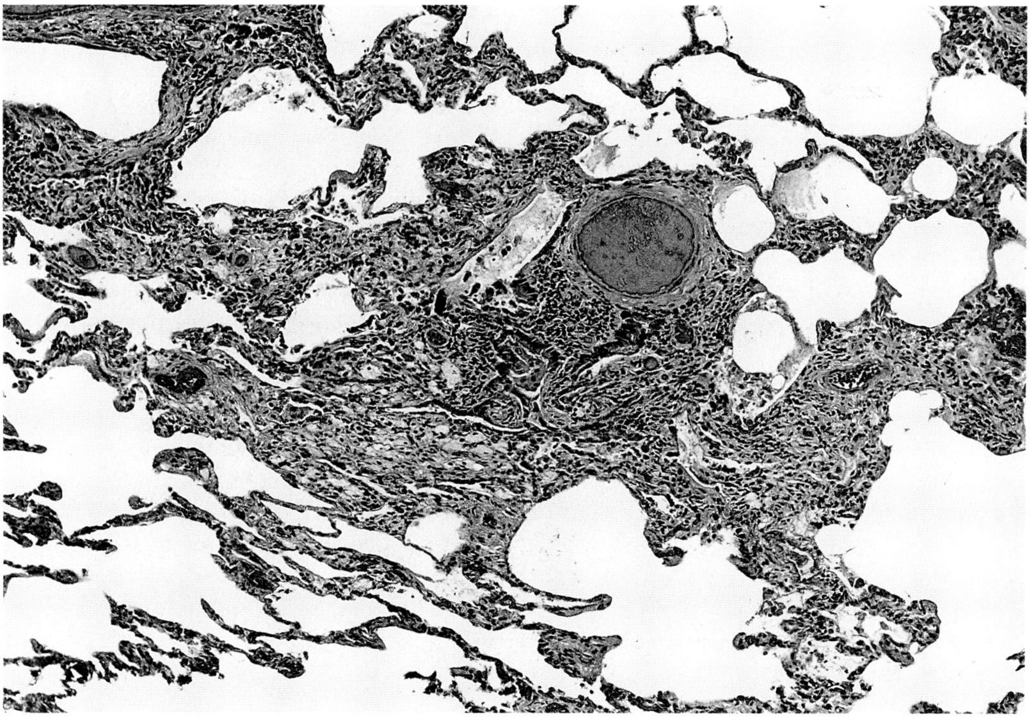

FIG. 16. Cystic fibrosis. An infiltration of lymphocytes and plasma cells can be seen in the walls of the respiratory bronchioles with accumulations of foam cells. In other sites (not shown), dense purulent mucus containing large amounts of neutrophils associated with bronchiectasis and obstructed airways were seen.

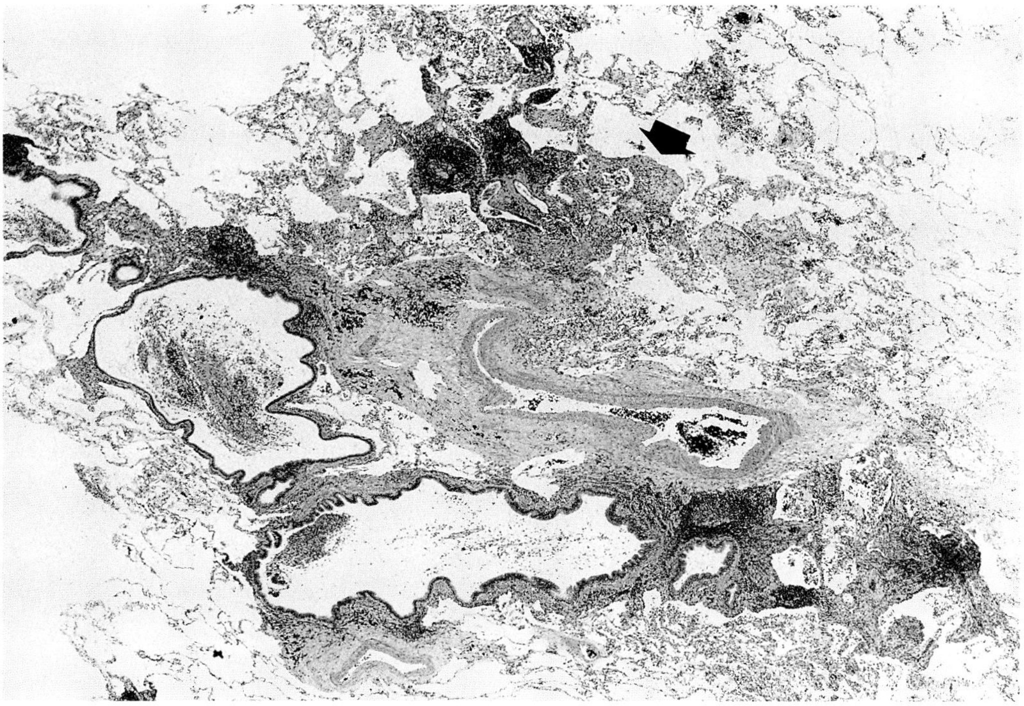

FIG. 17. Open lung biopsy specimen from the patient of Fig. 8. Dilated membranous bronchioles are accompanied by panbronchiolitis unit lesion (*arrow*).

made only in the appropriate clinical setting and when other conditions have been carefully ruled out clinically and pathologically.

Group 2 consists of miscellaneous conditions in which pathologic specific features other than a panbronchiolitis-like lesion are dominant. Cases of extrinsic allergic alveolitis show a poorly developed panbronchiolitis-like lesion, which has been noted in some cases of pigeon breeder's disease (73–75). Only a few foam cells were found within the interstitium, but numerous foam cells were seen in alveolar spaces, and marked interstitial infiltrates consisting of lymphocytes, plasma cells, and histiocytes with nonnecrotizing tiny granuloma were observed. In the cases of Wegener's granulomatosis, the inflammatory cells were infiltrated in the walls of respiratory and terminal bronchioles associated with intraluminal suppurative exudates. Foam cells were also found within the adjacent bronchiolar walls and alveolar septa (Fig. 18). The bronchi or membranous bronchioles showed acute and chronic inflammation associated with a necrotizing granulomatous process that destroyed airway walls, which were obstructed by plugs of mucus, fibrin, neutrophils, and granulomatous tissue. Necrotizing granulomatous vasculitis was observed, but it was relatively inconspicuous. This clinical finding was quite consistent with Wegener's granulomatosis. Recently it has been reported that the necrotizing process of Wegener's granulomatosis may be centered primarily on the airways (bronchocentric Wegener's granulomatosis) (76, 77).

Kitaichi (67) proposed the following pathologic diagnostic criteria for diffuse panbron-

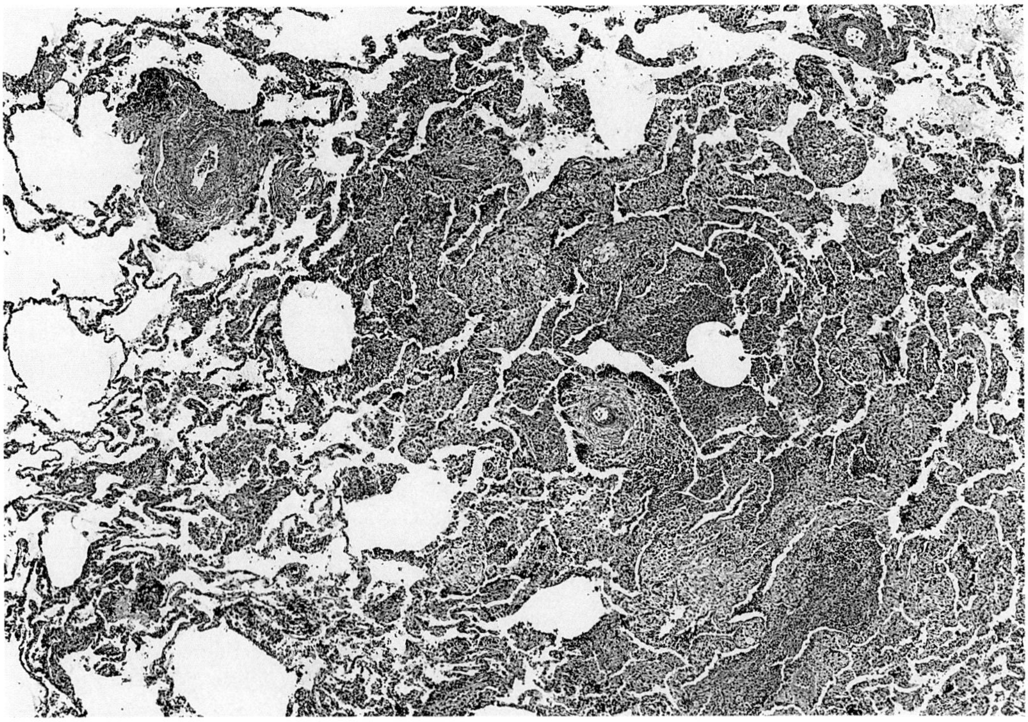

FIG. 18. Wegener's granulomatosis. The respiratory bronchiole and adjacent alveolar septa are thickened by infiltration of mononuclear cells and foam cells associated with intraluminal suppurative exudates.

chiolitis: (a) chronic airway inflammation of the lungs, involving them both diffusely and bilaterally, (b) the predominant site of the chronic inflammation in the walls of membranous and respiratory bronchioles and in the centrilobular regions, and (c) an interstitial accumulation of foam cells and lymphoid cells in the walls of respiratory bronchioles and adjacent alveolar ducts and alveoli.

There has been a report on the histologic findings of the disease after treatment (78). Scar tissue with mild infiltration of mononuclear cells and slight accumulation of foam cells was observed in the region of respiratory bronchioles, presumably a healing lesion of the disease.

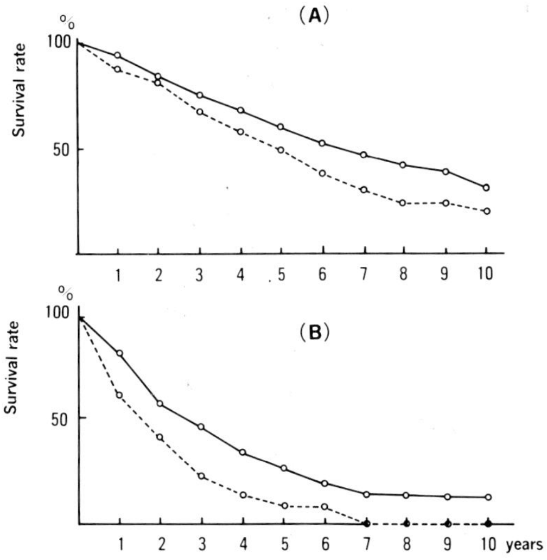

FIG. 19. The survival rates after **A,** first medical examination and **B,** *Pseudomonas aeruginosa* infection for diffuse panbronchiolitis patients. *Solid line,* clinical diagnostic group (A: $n = 318$, B: $n = 165$); *dashed line,* pathologic diagnostic group (A: $n = 80$, B: $n = 46$).

CLINICAL COURSE

Cough and sputum are usually noted first. Sputum is initially mucinous and small in amount. When secondary infections with *Haemophilus influenzae* or *Streptococcus pneumoniae* develop, purulent sputum increases and dyspnea occurs. In advanced stages, chronic intractable pulmonary infection with *P. aeruginosa* develops, and it becomes increasingly difficult to control the hypoxemia and hypercapnea; patients die of respiratory failure or consequences of respiratory infections.

In a nationwide survey in 1982 (79), the mean age at the first appearance of cough and sputum was 39.5 ± 15.0 years and that of the first medical examination was 49.8 ± 13.2 years. The 5-year survival rate after the first examination was 62.1% and at 10 years was 33.2%. After patients developed *Pseudomonas* infections, the mean survival time was 2.9 years (Fig. 19). In 1988 (80), the second nationwide survey found no difference in prognosis.

Recently Kudoh and colleagues (10) have reported that low-dose, long-term administration of erythromycin is effective for the disease. The next survey will be able to estimate if erythromycin offers long-term beneficial effects.

MANAGEMENT

Until erythromycin therapy was established, various kinds of therapy had been tried according to the therapeutic guidelines set up by the nationwide project team (23). It was suggested that patients be treated with corticosteroids in the initial stages and with antibiotics after pulmonary infections developed in advanced stages. Corticosteroids improved the symptoms by reducing sputum volume temporarily, but long-term administration of corticosteroids caused pulmonary infections. Therefore, the main therapy for the disease has been antibiotic treatment for chronic pulmonary infections. Various antibiotic regimens, including penicillin, cephalosporin, and aminoglicoside have been tried. In addition, a variety of bronchodilators including xanthine derivatives and beta-adrenergic stimulants have been frequently used. However, they appeared to result in intractable *Pseudomonas aeruginosa* superinfection.

The prognosis is poor, with rapid progression once *Pseudomonas* infection develops, despite the use of many antibiotics.

Kudoh et al. (10) first reported the usefulness of erythromycin for diffuse panbronchiolitis in 1984. They treated 18 patients with low-dose erythromycin (600 mg/day) for more than 6 months (average 19.8 months). Among the 18 patients, 16 had *H. influenzae* infection and 2 had *P. aeruginosa*. Clinical symptoms and laboratory data were improved in all cases. Dyspnea on exertion, PaO_2 level, and cold hemagglutinin titer were significantly improved 3 months after therapy. Body weight, pulmonary function data, and chest x-ray findings also improved. The therapeutic efficacy persisted during administration, and in 9 patients in whom the therapy was completed there was no difference in clinical or laboratory findings for about a year. Ultimately, 4 patients experienced relapse; 2 recovered with readministration of erythromycin. Other studies have shown similar results (81–83).

It has also been reported (84,85) that long-term administration of ofloxacin (a quinolone antibacterial agent) is effective in the disease, particularly in reducing acute exacerbations.

The long-term therapeutic effects of erythromycin and quinolone antibacterial agents on the disease have been studied retrospectively in a nationwide survey (11). Patients had been treated with either erythromycin or quinolone antibacterial agents for more than 3 months. Those treated with erythromycin showed significant improvement in dyspnea on exertion, amount of sputum, chest x-ray findings, hypoxemia, erythrocyte sedimentation rate, and cold hemagglutinin titer, compared with patients treated with quinolone antibacterial agents. Among the patients treated with erythromycin, those patients with the initial high cold hemagglutinin titer showed better improvement, but there were no differences for time of the onset of the disease, the initiation of treatment, and the initial severity of the disease.

A prospective study of the therapeutic effect of erythromycin (600 mg/day) was recently carried out in 73 patients with the disease in a double-blind placebo controlled fashion in members of institutes supported by the Ministry of Health and Welfare (12). Comparing erythromycin and placebo, respectively, 21.2% and 5.1% were "markedly improved," 57.6% and 15.4% "moderately improved," and 6.1% and 38.5% had done "poorly" 6 months after therapy. These results show that erythromycin is effective for the disease.

At present, interest is centered on the mechanism of the efficacy of erythromycin. At the prescribed dosage, erythromycin cannot be expected to act as an antibacterial agent. Among the major bacteria cultured in the disease, including *H. influenza, S. pneumoniae, Klebsiella pneumoniae,* and *P. aeruginosa,* erythromycin is probably effective for only *S. pneumoniae*. In fact, it is known that the bacteria in sputum are unchanged in the erythromycin-responsive cases (10,83). There is no relation of efficacy with absorption because the serum and sputum levels of erythromycin are higher in nonresponsive cases than in responsive cases (83). However, it may be that the intracellular antibacterial activity of erythromycin should be considered, because it has been reported that the intracellular concentration of erythromycin may be more than tenfold higher than the extracellular concentration in alveolar macrophages and polymorphonuclear leukocytes (86,87).

Chemotactic activity of neutrophils and oxygen radical production from neutrophils may be depressed by erythromycin, and thus tissue damage by proteases and oxygen radicals may also be suppressed (88–90). Other reports show that erythromycin reduces neutrophils and neutrophil-derived elastolytic-like activity in the lower respiratory tract in diffuse panbronchiolitis and follicular bronchiolitis accompanied with rheumatoid arthritis. These results suggest that erythromycin may be useful for the treatment of bronchiolitis through its direct action on host phagocytic cells (91).

Furthermore, it is thought that the improvement after erythromycin therapy could be related to a decrease of activated T cells or to inhibition of respiratory glycoconjugate secretion in the airway (92). Detailed mechanisms are not clear, and thus far, the effects of erythromycin on the pathophysiology of the disease remain to be clarified.

The 14-membered macrolides, clarithromycin and roxithromycin, are also effective, but the 16-membered macrolides are not (93). The reasons for these differences are not known.

Erythromycin is useful in the chronic sinusitis associated with the disease (94). Erythromycin is given in a daily dose of 600 mg for 6 to 12 months, but there is no information about the appropriate length of treatment. It has been reported that 200 mg once a day is also effective in some patients (83). Some patients occasionally show acute exacerbations while on erythromycin therapy. If this occurs, we treat with quinolone antibacterial agents or other intravenous antibiotics. Quinolone antibacterial agents are suitable for use in the outpatient clinic.

Treatment with erythromycin is often not effective in the advanced stages of the disease, but it is sometimes effective even for the patient with continuous *P. aeruginosa* colonization in the lung. A few patients show progression in spite of this therapy. These patients may ultimately be considered for lung transplantation.

PATHOGENESIS

Diffuse panbronchiolitis appears to be almost entirely restricted to the Japanese. It is rare in countries outside of Asia. In Japan, there have been familial cases of the disease (95,96), and the possibility that diffuse panbronchiolitis may have a genetic background and racial susceptibility has been suggested. Sugiyama and associates (41) performed HLA analysis on patients with the disease, and HLA-Bw54 is frequently found (63.2%). Among peoples of the world, the locus Bw54, or its related halotype, is limited to some mongoloid races such as Japanese, Chinese, and Korean, and to a few Ashkenazic Jews. An increase in Bw54 or Bw54-related halotype is also seen in patients with juvenile-onset or insulin-dependent diabetes mellitus (97–99), rheumatoid arthritis, and silicosis (41, 100). The frequency of HLA-Bw54 in diabetes mellitus is approximately as high as that in panbronchiolitis. It has been suggested that HLA-linked genes may control susceptibility to viral attack and/or immune responses to viral insults in diabetes mellitus (99). The detailed mechanisms of action of the HLA-linked susceptibility gene is unclear, and the relationship among these diseases remains to be clarified.

The pathogenesis of diffuse panbronchiolitis is thought to be related to immunological events because of the abnormality of immunologic parameters including cold hemagglutinin, rheumatoid factor, and CD4/CD8 ratio. It had been considered that elevated cold hemagglutinin titer might be caused by B cell activation (polyclonal stimulation) due to cell wall lipopolysaccharide associated with chronic gram-negative pulmonary infections, mainly *Hemophilus influenzae* or *Pseudomonas aeruginosa*, but was not correlated with severity of the disease and any specific bacteria. Therefore, this is probably due to a constitutional factor in the patients. In some cases there is a close relationship with human T cell lymphotropic virus type I (HTLV-I), because diffuse panbronchiolitis has preceded the development of adult T-cell leukemia (20); however, most patients with the disease do not have anti HTLV-I antibody. The pathogenesis needs further investigation.

CONCLUSION

About a quarter of a century has passed since diffuse panbronchiolitis was proposed. During that time progress has been made in diagnostic aspects and management. First, clinical and pathologic diagnostic criteria were established after a nationwide survey. Second, international communication and several reports have shown that diffuse panbronchiolitis appears to be largely restricted to the Japanese, and the reason is probably due to a genetic background. Third, the discovery that erythromycin was useful for the treatment of diffuse panbronchiolitis was important, even though it was discovered by chance and the mechanism of the efficacy of erythromycin is obscure.

As secondary bronchiectasis appears in the advanced stage, the issue of the differential diagnosis between diffuse panbronchiolitis and diffuse bronchiectasis has arisen.

REFERENCES

1. Yamanaka A, Saiki S, Tamura S, Saito K. The problems of chronic obstructive pulmonary disease: especially concerning about diffuse panbronchiolitis. *Naika* 1969;23:442–451 (in Japanese).
2. Homma H, Yamanaka A, Tanimoto S, et al. Diffuse panbronchiolitis: a disease of the transitional zone of the lung. *Chest* 1983;83:63–69.
3. Homma H, Mikami R, Yamanaka A. Pulmonary infection and acute cardiopulmonary insufficiency. *Kokyu To Junkan* 1956;4:67–75 (in Japanese).
4. Yamanaka A. Histopathology of chronic bronchitis. *Saishin Igaku* 1960;15:2035–2044 (in Japanese).
5. Kurokawa K, Yashima T, Iikawa T, Inomata K. Clinicopathology of chronic diffuse bronchiolitis. *Hai To Shin* 1961;8:200–207 (in Japanese).
6. Sawasaki H, Watabe S, Onoki S, Makita H, Naito N, Muraki A. Two cases of bronchiolitis obliterans. *Jpn J Chest Dis* 1962;21:635–647 (in Japanese).
7. Takizawa T. Diagnosis of pulmonary emphysema. *Nippon Rinsho* 1963;21:655–665 (in Japanese).
8. Okisaka S, Saiki S, Yamanaka A, Yamaguchi K, Yokoyama T, Inui M. Pathologic problems of chronic bronchitis and bronchial asthma. *Nippon Rinsho* 1966;24:851–857 (in Japanese).
9. Mikami R, Yamanaka A. Clinicopathologic study of chronic bronchitis. *Nippon Rinsho* 1967;25:2031–2053 (in Japanese).
10. Kudoh S, Uetake T, Hagiwara K, et al. Clinical effect of low-dose long-term erythromycin chemotherapy on diffuse panbronchiolitis. *Jpn J Thorac Dis* 1987;25:632–642 (in Japanese; abstract in English).
11. Yamamoto M, Kondo A, Tamura M, Izumi T, Ina Y, Noda M. Long-term therapeutic effects of erythromycin and new quinolone antibacterial agents on diffuse panbronchiolitis. *Jpn J Thorac Dis* 1990;28:1305–1313 (in Japanese; abstract in English).
12. Yamamoto M, Kudoh S, Noda M, Tamura M. Therapeutic effect of erythromycin on DPB. *Jpn J Thorac Dis* 1992;30:132 (in Japanese).
13. Desai SJ, Gephardt GN, Stoller JK. Diffuse panbronchiolitis preceding ulcerative colitis. *Chest* 1989;95:1342–1344.
14. Randhawa P, Hoagland MH, Yousem SA. Diffuse panbronchiolitis in North America: report of three cases and review of the literature. *Am J surg Pathol* 1991;15:43–47.
15. Kitaichi M, Nishimura K, Izumi T. Diffuse panbronchiolitis. In: Sharma OP, ed. *Lung disease in the tropics*. New York: Marcel Dekker; 1991:479–509.
16. Poletti V, Patelli M, Poletti G, Bertanti T, Spiga L. Diffuse panbronchiolitis observed in an Italian male. *Sarcoidosis* 1992;9:67–69.
17. Saito S, Mori M, Kawamura O, Umegai T, Kurosawa M, Kobayashi S. A case of allergic granulomatosis angitis (Churg-Strauss) associated with diffuse panbronchiolitis. *Nippon Naika Gakkai Zasshi* 1988;77:445–446 (in Japanese).
18. Okano A, Sato A, Suda T, et al. A case of diffuse panbronchiolitis complicated by malignant thymoma and Sjogren syndrome. *Jpn J Thorac Dis* 1991;29:263–268 (in Japanese; abstract in English).
19. Ubukata M, Sugiyama S, Ohno S, Sugama Y, Kitamura S. A case of Sjogren syndrome with a clinical course similar to diffuse panbronchiolitis. *Jpn J Thorac Dis* 1991;29:387–391 (in Japanese; abstract in English).
20. Ono K, Shimamoto Y, Matsuzaki M, et al. Diffuse panbronchiolitis as a pulmonary complication in patients with adult T-cell leukemia. *Am J Hematol* 1989;30:86–90.
21. Hayakawa H, Taniguchi M, Chida K, et al. A case of malignant lymphoma associated with diffuse panbronchiolitis. *Jpn J Thorac Dis* 1984;22:80 (in Japanese).
22. Mimura T, Yoshimura K, Nakamori Y, Nakata K, Tanimoto H. Non-Hodgkins' lymphoma associated with diffuse panbronchiolitis. *Jpn J Thorac Dis* 1987;19:645–651 (in Japanese; abstract in English).
23. Homma H: Diffuse panbronchiolitis. *Nippon Naika Gakkai Zasshi* 1986;75:1347–1364 (in Japanese).
24. Yamamoto M. Diagnosis of diffuse panbronchiolitis and its diagnostic criteria. *Igaku no Ayumi* 1988;147:16–19 (in Japanese).
25. Nakata K, Tanimoto H. Diffuse panbronchiolitis. *Jpn J Clin Radiol* 1981;26:1133–1142 (in Japanese).
26. Izumi T, Honda K. Computed tomography of diffuse panbronchiolitis. *Annual report on the study of diffuse disseminated lung disease* 1983;170–174 (in Japanese).
27. Honda K, Nishimura K. CT and chest X-ray of

diffuse panbronchiolitis. *Medicina* 1984;21:2624–2627 (in Japanese).
28. Nishimura K, Furue M, Kitaichi M, et al. A comparative study of computed tomography and pulmonary pathology in diffuse panbronchiolitis. *Jpn J Chest Dis* 1987;46:481–486 (in Japanese; abstract in English).
29. Nishimura K, Kitaichi M, Izumi T, Kanaoka M, Itoh H. CT pathologic correlation study of diffuse panbronchiolitis. *Jpn J Clin Radiol* 1989;34:773–782 (in Japanese; abstract in English).
30. Nishimura K, Itoh H. Radiologic findings of patients with diffuse panbronchiolitis. In: Grassi C, Rizzato G, Pozzi E, eds. *Sarcoidosis and other granulomatous disorders*. Amsterdam: Elsevier Science Publishers B.V; 1988: 747–752.
31. Akira M, Kitatani F, Yong-Sik L, et al. Diffuse panbronchiolitis: evaluation with high-resolution CT. *Radiology* 1988;168:433–438.
32. Maeno H, Chijimatsu Y, Inatomi K, Washizaki M, Homma H. The role of selective alveolobronchography in the staging of diffuse panbronchiolitis. *J Jpn Soc Bronchol* 1983;5:53–57 (in Japanese; abstract in English).
33. Iwata T. A study of chronic airway diseases: a discussion focused mainly upon bronchographic findings of diffuse panbronchiolitis. *Bull Chest Dis Inst Kyoto Univ* 1984;17:73–85 (in Japanese; abstract in English).
34. Chijimatsu Y, Uchida K, Maeno H, et al. Transbronchial lung biopsy in diagnosis of diffuse panbronchiolitis: comparison with roentgenological findings obtained by selective alveolo-bronchography. *Jpn J Chest Dis* 1985; 44:460–465 (in Japanese; abstract in English).
35. Homma Y. Respiratory function of diffuse panbronchiolitis. *Annual report on the study of diffuse disseminated lung disease* 1983;14–22 (in Japanese).
36. Kino T. Laboratory findings of diffuse panbronchiolitis. *Annual report on the study of diffuse disseminated lung disease* 1983;22–32 (in Japanese).
37. Hirata T, Nishikawa S, Izumi T. An immunological study on diffuse panbronchiolitis. *Jpn J Chest Dis* 1979;38:90–95 (in Japanese).
38. Takizawa H, Tadokoro K, Miyoshi Y, et al. Serological characterization of cold aggulutinin in patients with diffuse panbronchiolitis. *Jpn J Thorac Dis* 1986;24:257–263 (in Japanese; abstract in English).
39. Yoshimura K, Uchida Y, Nakatani T, et al. Immunological studies on diffuse panbronchiolitis: analysis of T lymphocyte subsets by monoclonal antibodies. *Jpn J Thorac Dis* 1984;22: 992–999 (in Japanese; abstract in English).
40. Sugiyama Y, Kudoh S, Urabe A, Kitamura S, Takaku. Analysis of peripheral lymphocyte subsets in patients with diffuse panbronchiolitis. *Jpn J Thorac Dis* 1984;22:1116–1121 (in Japanese; abstract in English).
41. Sugiyama Y, Kudoh S, Maeda H, Suzaki H, Takaku F. Analysis of HLA antigens in patients with diffuse panbronchiolitis. *Am Rev Respir Dis* 1990;141:1459–1462.
42. Ichikawa Y, Koga H, Tanaka M, Nakamura M, Tokunaga N, Kaji M. Neutrophilia in bronchoalveolar lavage fluid of diffuse panbronchiolitis. *Chest* 1990;98:917–923.
43. Koshobu T, Hirai H, Hikita T, Kawasaki Y, Burioka N, Sasaki T. Sweat chloride concentration and pancreatic function diagnostant in patients with diffuse panbronchiolitis. *Jpn J Thorac Dis* 1988;26:97–101 (in Japanese; abstract in English).
44. Akai S, Okayama H, Shimura S, Tanno Y, Sasaki H, Takishima T. δF508 mutation of cystic fibrosis gene is not found in chronic bronchitis with severe obstruction in Japan. *Am Rev Respir Dis* 1992;146:781–783.
45. Nadel HR, Stringer DA, Levison H, Turner JAP, Sturgess JM. The immotile cilia syndrome: radiological manifestations. *Radiology* 1985;154:651–655.
46. Mossberg B, Camner P. Impaired mucociliary transport as a pathogenetic factor in obstructive pulmonary diseases. *Chest* 1980;77:265–266.
47. Amitani R, Tomioka H, Kurosawa T, Ishida T, Kuze F. Clinical and ultrastructural study on primary ciliary dyskinesia. *Jpn J Thorac Dis* 1990;28:300–307 (in Japanese; abstract in English).
48. Ryujin Y, Ito S, Kasuga H, et al. Mucociliary clearance in diffuse panbronchiolitis, pulmonary emphysema and chronic bronchitis estimated by aerosol inhalation cine-scintigraphy. *Jpn J Thorac Dis* 1984;22:479–485 (in Japanese; abstract in English).
49. Nagai A. Ultrastructural characteristics of bronchial cilia in patients with respiratory infectious disease. *Jpn J Thorac Dis* 1983;21:564–573 (in Japanese; abstract in English).
50. Gosink B, Friedman PJ, Liebow AA. Bronchiolitis obliterans: roentgenologic–pathologic correlation. *AJR* 1973;117:816–832.
51. Tukiainen P, Poppius H, Taskinen E. Slowly progressive bronchiolitis obliterans: a case report with detailed pulmonary function studies. *Eur J Respir Dis* 1980;61:77–83.
52. Turton CW, Williams G, Green M. Cryptogenic obliterative bronchiolitis in adults. *Thorax* 1981; 36:805–810.
53. Yamanaka A, Maeda M, Yamamoto R. Chronic bronchiolitis obliterans. *Jpn J Chest Dis* 1986; 45:539–554 (in Japanese).
54. Nagai H, Nagayama N, Shishido H, et al. Three autopsy cases of chronic airway diseases indifferential clinically from diffuse panbronchiolitis. *Respir Res* 1990;9:447–455 (in Japanese; abstract in English).
54a. Iwata M, Colby TV, Kitaichi M. Diffuse Panbronchiolitis (DPB): diagnosis and distinction from various pulmonary diseases with centrilobular interstitial form cell accumulations. *Hum Pathol* (in communication).
55. Sato A, Chida K, Iwata M, Hayakawa H. Study of bronchus-associated lymphoid tissue in pa-

tients with diffuse panbronchiolitis. *Am Rev Respir Dis* 1992;146:473–478.
56. Iwata M, Sato A. Morphological and immunohistochemical studies of the lung and bronchus-associated lymphoid tissue in a rat model of chronic pulmonary infection with Pseudomonas aeruginosa. *Infect Immun* 1991;59:1514–1520.
57. Maeda M, Saiki S, Yamanaka A. Serial section analysis of the lesions in diffuse panbronchiolitis. *Acta Pathol Jpn* 1987;37:693–704.
58. Yamanaka A, Yokoyama T. Morphologic diagnostic criteria of diffuse panbronchiolitis. *Annual report on the study of diffuse disseminated lung disease* 1983;42–48 (in Japanese).
59. Dalqueen P, Oberholzen M. Lung biopsy: method, value, complications, timing and indications. *Pathol Res Pract* 1979;164:95–103.
60. Wall CP, Gaensler EA, Carrington CB, Haynes JA. Comparison of transbronchial and open biopsies in chronic infiltrative lung diseases. *Am Rev Respir Dis* 1981;123:280–285.
61. Yamanaka A, Yokoyama T, Maeda M, Saiki S, Hebisawa A, Ryuda S. Evaluation of transbronchial lung biopsy specimens on diffuse panbronchiolitis. *Annual report on the study of diffuse disseminated lung disease* 1981;95–98.
62. Nakata K, Tachibana A, Suzuki K, et al. Diffuse panbronchiolitis: diagnosis by transbronchial lung biopsy. *Rinsho Kagaku* 1981;17:177–183 (in Japanese).
63. Matsuoka R, Yamanaka K, Kobayashi H, et al. Transbronchial lung biopsy for diagnosis of diffuse panbronchiolitis. *J Jpn Soc Bronchol* 1987; 8:684–689 (in Japanese; abstract in English).
64. Sato A, Iwata M, Chida K, Okano A, Yasuda K, Shichi I. Significance of open lung biopsy on diffuse panbronchiolitis. *Annual report on the study of diffuse disseminated lung disease* 1988;142–144 (in Japanese).
65. Izumi T. Diffuse panbronchiolitis. *Chest* 1991; 100:596–597.
66. Senju R. A clinico-pathological study of 14 open lung biopsy cases of clinically suspected diffuse panbronchiolitis. *Jpn J Thorac Dis* 1992;30:1056–1062 (in Japanese; abstract in English).
67. Kitaichi M. Comparative pathology of inflammatory airways disease: a report made after the 1987 Milan congress. *Sarcoidosis* 1992; 9:625–628.
68. Kitaichi M. Pathology of diffuse panbronchiolitis from the view point of differential diagnosis. In: Grassi C, Rizzato G, Pozzi E, ed. *Sarcoidosis and other granulomatous disorders.* Amsterdam: Elsevier Science Publishers BV; 1988:741–746.
69. Esterly JR, Oppenheimer EH. Observations in cystic fibrosis of the pancreas. III: Pulmonary lesions. *Johns Hopkins Med J* 1968;122:94–101.
70. Esterly JR, Oppenheimer EH. Cystic fibrosis of the pancreas: structural changes in peripheral airways. *Thorax* 1968;23:670–675.
71. Whitwell F. A study of the pathology and pathogenesis of bronchiectasis. *Thorax* 1952;7: 213–239.
72. Bedrossian CW, Greenberg SD, Singer DB, Hansen JJ, Rosenberg HS. The lung in cystic fibrosis: a quantitative study including prevalence of pathologic findings among different age groups. *Hum Pathol* 1976;7:195–204.
73. Nash ES, Vogelpoel L, Becker WB. Pigeon breeder's lung: a case report. *S Afr Med J* 1967;41:191–193.
74. Eyckmans L, Gyslen A, Lauwerijns J, Cosemans J, Wildiers J, Willems J. Pigeon breeder's lung: report of three cases. *Dis Chest* 1968; 53:358–364.
75. Hensley GT, Garancis JC, Cherayil GD, Fink JN. Lung biopsies of pigeon breeder's disease. *Arch Pathol* 1969;87:572–579.
76. Amin R. Endobronchial involvement in Wegener's granulomatosis. *Postgrad Med J* 1983;59: 452–454.
77. Yousem SA. Bronchocentric injury in Wegener's granulomatosis: a report of five cases. *Hum Pathol* 1991;22:535–540.
78. Mimoto T, Uchida K, Sakuraba S, et al. A case of diffuse panbronchiolitis, performed an open lung biopsy after improvement with 6 years medication. *Jpn J Thorac Dis* 1991;29:893–899, (in Japanese; abstract in English).
79. Inatomi K. Prognosis of diffuse panbronchiolitis. *Annual report on the study of diffuse disseminated lung disease* 1983;38–41 (in Japanese).
80. Izumi T. A nation-wide survey of diffuse panbronchiolitis in Japan and the high incidence of diffuse panbronchiolitis seen in Japanese respiratory clinics. In: Grassi C, Rizzato G, Pozzi E, ed. *Sarcoidosis and other granulomatous disorders.* Amsterdam: Elsevier Science Publishers BV; 1988:753–757.
81. Chijimatsu Y, Tamura N, Maeno H, Inatomi K. A study of erythromycin therapy for the patients of diffuse panbronchiolitis. *Jpn J Chest Dis* 1986;45:299–305 (in Japanese; abstract in English).
82. Sawaki M, Mikami R, Mikasa K, Kunimatsu M, Itoh S, Narita N. The long term chemotherapy with erythromycin in chronic lower respiratory tract infections. *J Jpn Assoc Infect Dis* 1986;60:37–50 (in Japanese; abstract in English).
83. Nagai H, Shishido H, Yoneda R, Yamaguchi E, Tamura A, Kurashima A. Long-term low-dose administration of erythromycin to patients with diffuse panbronchiolitis. *Respiration* 1991;58: 145–149.
84. Nakamori Y, Yoshimura K, Nakatani T, Chonabayashi N, Nakata K, Tanimoto H. Against long-term therapy of ofloxacin for the respiratory infections in diffuse panbronchiolitis. *Chemotherapy* 1985;33:570–576 (in Japanese; abstract in English).
85. Sato A, Shichi I, Iwata M, Suda T, Okano A, Chida K. Long-term effects of ofloxacin on clinical course in patients with diffuse panbronchiolitis. *Chemotherapy (International Journal of Experimental and Clinical Chemotherapy)* 1991;37[Suppl 1]:55–59.

86. Johnson JD, Hand WL, Francis JB, Thompson NK, Corwin RW. Antibiotic uptake by alveolar macrophage. *J Lab Clin Med* 1980;95:429–439.
87. Prokesch RC, Hand WL. Antibiotic entry into human polymorphonuclear leukocytes. *Antimicrob Agents Chemother* 1982;21:373–380.
88. Nelson S, Summer WR, Terry PB, Warr GR, Jakab GJ. Erythromycin-induced suppression of pulmonary antibacterial defenses: a potential mechanism of superinfection in the lung. *Am Rev Respir Dis* 1987;136:1207–1212.
89. Fraschini F, Scaglione F, Ferrara F, Marelli O, Braga PC, Theodori F. Evaluation of immunostimulating activity of erythromycin in man. *Chemotherapy* 1986;32:286–291.
90. Hirata T, Matsunobe S, Matsui Y, Kado M, Mikiya K, Oshima S. Effect of erythromycin on the generation of neutrophil chemiluminescence in vitro. *Jpn J Thorac Dis* 1990;28:1066–1071 (in Japanese; abstract in English).
91. Ichikawa Y, Ninomiya H, Koga H, et al. Erythromycin reduces neutrophils and neutrophil-derived elasolytic activity in the lower respiratory tract of bronchiolitis patients. *Am Rev Respir Dis* 1992;146:196–203.
92. Goswami SK, Kivity S, Marom Z. Erythromycin inhibits respiratory glycoconjugate secretion from human airways in vitro. *Am Rev Respir Dis* 1990;141:72–78.
93. Takeda H, Miura H, Kawahira M, Kobayashi H, Kotomo S, Nakaike S. Efficacy of macrolides except erythromycin on diffuse panbronchiolitis. *Ther Res* 1990;11:970–972 (in Japanese).
94. Sugaki H, Sugita K, Kudoh S, et al. Efficacy of erythromycin in chronic sinusitis associated with diffuse panbronchiolitis. *Ther Res* 1990;11:961–963 (in Japanese).
95. Suzuki M, Usui K, Tamura N, et al. Familial cases of diffuse panbronchiolitis. *Jpn J Thorac Dis* 1982;19:645–651 (in Japanese; abstract in English).
96. Danbara T, Matsuoka R, Nukiwa T, Natori H, Arai T, Kira S. Familial occurrence of diffuse panbronchiolitis accompanied with elevation of cold agglutinin titer in a father and his two daughters. *Jpn J Thorac Dis* 1982;20:597–603 (in Japanese; abstract in English).
97. Wakisaka A, Aizawa M, Matsuura N, et al. HLA and juvenile diabetes mellitus in the Japanese. *Lancet* 1976_{∞}:970.
98. Kawa A, Nakazawa M, Sakaguchi S, et al. HLA system in Japanese patients with diabetes mellitus. *Diabetes* 1977;26:591–595.
99. Mann JI, Pyorala K, Teuscher A, eds. *Diabetes in epidemiological perspective*. London: Churchhill Livingstone; 1983:110–120.
100. Honda K, Hirayama K, Kikuchi I, Nagato H, Tamai H, Sasazaki T. HLA and silicosis in Japan. *N Engl J Med* 1988;319:1610.

Diseases of the Bronchioles, edited by Gary R. Epler. Raven Press, Ltd., New York © 1994.

11

Idiopathic Bronchiolitis Obliterans

Pentti Tukiainen* and Eero Taskinen†

**Associate Director, Department of Pulmonary Medicine, Helsinki University Central Hospital, Haartmaninkatu 4, 00290 Helsinki, Finland.*
†Associate Director of Pathology and Cytology, Transplantation Laboratory, University of Helsinki, Haartmaninkatu 3, 00290 Helsinki, Finland.

DEFINITION OF TERMS

Idiopathic bronchiolitis obliterans occurs in a heterogeneous group of patients who have evidence of obliteration of small airways either clinically or histologically without identifiable associated condition or cause (1–4). This disease is extremely rare; in 42,038 consecutive autopsies covering a 42-year period LaDue (5) found only one patient. A considerable amount of confusion has surrounded the term *bronchiolitis obliterans* because it has been used to describe clinical syndromes (6) as well as histologic lesions (7) and because of the connections to the term *bronchiolitis obliterans organizing pneumonia* (1–4). This term has been used widely since 1985, following the report of Epler and others (8). Since that time increasing numbers of patients with idiopathic bronchiolitis obliterans organizing pneumonia (BOOP) have been reported, but very few with idiopathic bronchiolitis obliterans (1–4,9). Bronchiolitis obliterans was, however, mentioned as a histologic finding in many earlier reports. The organizing pneumonia component was generally not quoted, even though, in retrospect, photomicrographs or pathologic descriptions are consistent with BOOP. An additional problem is that clinical evidence of small airway obstruction may be associated with a variety of pathologic abnormalities; histologic identification of bronchiolitis obliterans is not always associated with functional airway obstruction (6).

In this review the proliferative type of bronchiolitis obliterans is histologically defined as polypoid obliterative proliferation confined solely in the lumen of bronchioles and composed of granulation tissue and fibrosis without the organizing pneumonic component. Constrictive bronchiolitis encompasses a variety of histologic changes ranging from bronchiolar inflammation and scarring to progressive concentric fibrosis and occasionally complete occlusion of small airways (1).

IDIOPATHIC BRONCHIOLITIS OBLITERANS AS A DISEASE ENTITY

The term *bronchiolitis obliterans* is based on the 1910 report of Lange (10) who described bronchiolitis obliterans in two patients. The first died of an acute illness in 8 days, and the other died after 6 months of a progressive disease. Autopsy of both patients revealed microscopically polypoid granulation tissue in small airways. The term *bronchiolitis obliterans* was applied even though, in retrospect, the histologic description is more similar to BOOP than to bronchiolitis obliterans.

In the large series of Gosink and others

(7) the term *bronchiolitis obliterans* was used for two distinct histologic lesions: (a) the classic intraluminal polyps, and (b) a spectrum of bronchiolar constriction, narrowing, and submucosal fibrosis or complete obliteration by fibrous tissue, which they called constrictive bronchiolitis. In some patients interstitial infiltration appeared to be the predominant lesion, much more widely distributed than in bronchiolitis obliterans, or even in BOOP. One patient with interstitial pneumonia had small granulomas attributable to exposure to pigeons. Several other patients had occasional small granulomas; one had numerous sarcoid granulomas causing bronchiolar obstruction. The report included patients with BOOP and also other entities, such as hypersensitivity pneumonitis, in addition to patients with bronchiolitis obliterans. The disease of 21 of their 52 patients was reported to be idiopathic. Which of their patients had idiopathic bronchiolitis obliterans without organizing pneumonia is difficult to reconstruct.

Bronchiolitis obliterans has been found to occur after inhalation of irritant fumes, as a consequence of infections (1–5), associated with rheumatoid arthritis with or without penicillamine therapy (11,12), and as a complication of bone marrow transplantation (13), heart–lung transplantation (14), and single lung transplantation (15). The exclusion of these conditions is an essential criterion for the diagnosis of idiopathic bronchiolitis obliterans, but sometimes causes difficulties.

In the series of Geddes and colleagues (11) five of the six patients had rheumatoid arthritis, and the one without had positive rheumatoid factor. The patient described by Jacobs and others (16) was similar, having circulating antinuclear antibodies and positive rheumatoid factors without clinical rheumatoid disease. The patient described by us (17) originally as having idiopathic bronchiolitis obliterans, developed seropositive rheumatoid arthritis 3 years later. Subclinical ŕheumatoid arthritis must be taken into account.

In some reports patients have had a flu-like illness prior to the detection of bronchiolitis obliterans. The association of a past viral infection and present bronchiolitis obliterans may be difficult to prove, as in connection with BOOP (18,19). Because of the high incidence of bronchiolitis obliterans reported after adenovirus infection in children, a study (19) was designed to test the hypothesis of viral-induced bronchiolitis obliterans in adults. Of 20 lung biopsy specimens with BOOP, 4 showed the presence of adenovirus by in situ hybridization technique. In our experience of about 25,000 patients during a 10-year period, there have been many patients with bronchiolitis obliterans (clinical or histological) associated with other disease conditions, such as toxic fume inhalation, connective-tissue diseases, preceding viral infections, and bone marrow transplantation. There have also been several patients with idiopathic BOOP pneumonia during the same period, but only 1 patient was suspected to have idiopathic bronchiolitis obliterans. This 43-year-old nonsmoking woman initially had a flu-like illness resembling a viral infection. Within 2 months she developed a productive cough and progressive dyspnea. The chest radiograph showed hyperinflation but no opacities. Extensive laboratory examinations including viral antibodies did not show significant abnormalities. Pulmonary function studies showed slight restrictive and severe obstructive ventilatory impairment. The airway obstruction was not reversed by inhalation of 200 mg of salbutamol. The diffusing capacity was well preserved, and when related to alveolar volume, it was even high (Fig. 1). During 4 months of prednisolone therapy, slight worsening of pulmonary function was observed. A new trial of 5 months of prednisolone therapy was initiated 2 years after the diagnosis. Thereafter, pulmonary function parameters stabilized (Fig. 1).

The term *small airways disease* originally referred to disorders affecting airways smaller than 2 mm in diameter in cigarette smokers (20). The term has been applied to

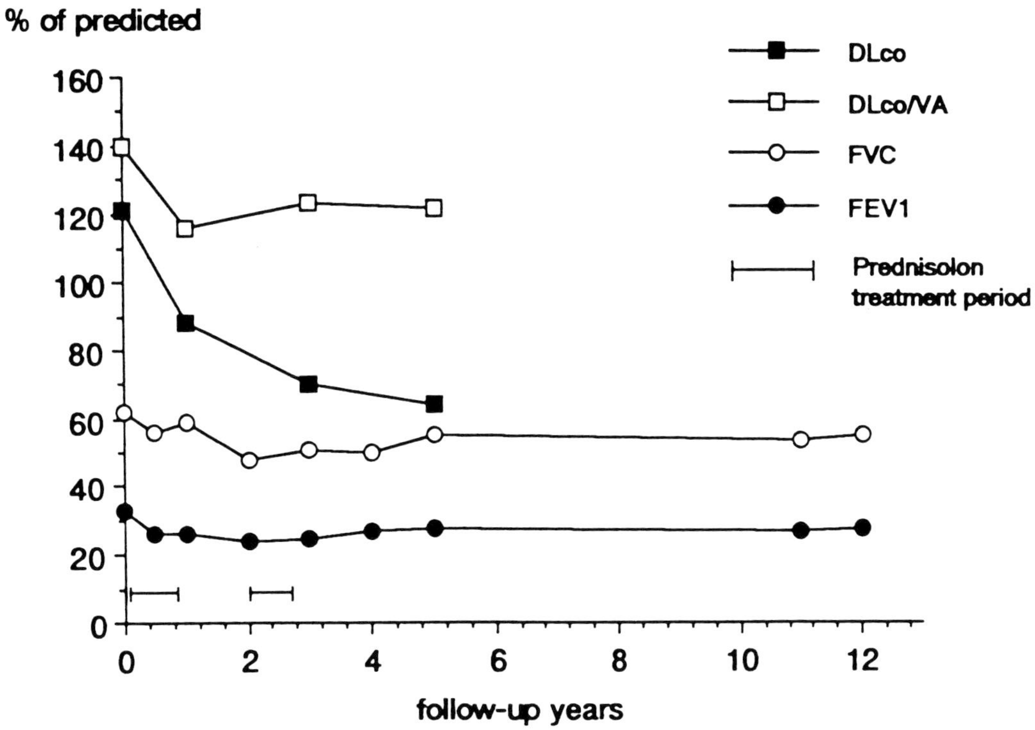

FIG. 1. Changes in forced vital capacity (*FVC*), forced expiratory volume in one second (FEV_1), diffusing capacity for carbon monoxide (*DLco*), and diffusing capacity related to alveolar volume (*DLco/VA*) during follow-up period of 12 years in a patient with idiopathic bronchiolitis obliterans.

a number of different lesions. A number of the patients described by Macklem and others (21), Guerry-Force and others (22), and Kindt and others (23) as patients with small airway disease showed histological features of bronchiolitis obliterans.

Turton and others (6) analyzed 2,094 patients with airflow obstruction. They excluded all patients who were current or ex-smokers, had a history of chronic bronchitis, asthma, or emphysema, or any other specific pulmonary disease (Table 1). This rigorous process of exclusion left a group of 10 patients with idiopathic airway obstruction, which they called cryptogenic obliterative bronchiolitis. Five patients had associated rheumatoid arthritis; in 2 there was a preceding chest infection, and the disease in 3 was idiopathic. Because histologic specimens were not available, it is difficult to confirm the histologic correlation of these clinical findings.

Sweatman and others (9) studied 15 patients with bronchiolitis obliterans (adult obliterative bronchiolitis) with chest computed tomography (CT) using the diagnostic criteria of Turton and others. Eight pa-

TABLE 1. *Criteria for the diagnosis of bronchiolitis obliterans*

Obligatory criteria
FEV_1 < 60% of predicted values at presentation
Exclusion criteria
Diurnal peak expiratory flow rate (PEFR) variability > 50 L/min
Increase in PEFR of > 50 L/min or ≥ 20% after oral corticosteroid therapy
Rise in FEV_1 or FVC of ≥ 15% after inhaled $beta_2$-agonist therapy
History of episodic wheezing
Personal/family history of atopy
Chronic bronchitis (Medical Research Council criteria)
Emphysema
Known causes of chronic airflow obstruction

From ref. 6.

tients had co-existing rheumatoid arthritis, and in 7 the disease was idiopathic. Chest CT was considered to be abnormal in 13 of 15 patients (87%), showing widespread areas of increasing attenuation of a patchy nature and variable proportion. Of interest, the chest CT findings they described resembled those found in connection with BOOP (25). Unfortunately, no tissue documentation of the underlying morphologic lesion was available in this study.

CLINICAL FEATURES OF IDIOPATHIC BRONCHIOLITIS OBLITERANS

On the basis of present knowledge, idiopathic bronchiolitis obliterans appears to be a very uncommon disease (Table 2). It seems that a great number of the patients reported before 1985 as patients with idiopathic bronchiolitis obliterans in reality had BOOP. Nevertheless, we believe that there are patients with idiopathic obliteration of small airways, which histologically show polypoid obstruction of bronchioles or constrictive bronchiolitis without organizing pneumonia (1,2,4) and/or clinically show airway obstruction of unknown cause (5,8). Middle-aged women are most commonly affected. They develop breathlessness and cough, and episodes of bronchitis may occur.

The chest radiograph is often normal but may reveal subtle peripheral vascular attenuation confined to the middle or lower zones and/or hyperinflation; in a minority of patients, diffuse opacities are seen. Bronchography may be helpful in providing supportive evidence for the diagnosis, revealing generalized, abrupt bronchial termination and incomplete distal filling (24). CT shows widespread areas of increased attenuation of a patchy nature and variable proportion, even in patients with normal chest radiographs (8). Pulmonary function studies show obstruction or, less commonly, evidence of mixed restrictive and obstructive pattern. Diffusing capacity is normal or even increased (Fig. 1).

The disease is usually chronic and slowly progressive, but some patients show a rapid progression. Corticosteroid therapy is probably the treatment of choice (23). The steroid responsive disorder usually corresponds to the proliferative lesion; and the irreversible, end-stage airflow obstruction corresponds to the constrictive lesion. Issues to be answered include whether the constrictive lesion develops after the proliferative lesion, whether it can develop directly, or whether corticosteroid therapy will prevent the constrictive lesion. The goal of therapy in these conditions is to stabilize the process. Transitory improvement can occur in some patients with an active inflammatory bronchiolitis. For patients with a progressive disease, lung transplantation can be utilized (27).

This patient group differs from those with idiopathic BOOP, which is an interstitial lung disease, the obstructive component of which is seen only in smokers (8). In addition, in BOOP the response to steroid therapy is excellent in comparison to the patients with bronchiolitis obliterans; spontaneous improvement may even occur.

The inflammatory processes involving the bronchioles may initially go unnoticed because small airways are a relatively silent area of the lungs, physiologically and symptomatically. As the disease progresses and becomes clinically evident, many of the findings may mimic chronic obstructive lung disease. Therefore, the diagnosis of idiopathic bronchiolitis obliterans should be suspected only in nonsmokers in the ab-

TABLE 2. *Spectrum of bronchiolitis obliterans*

Clinical setting	Association with organizing pneumonia
Fume exposure	rare
Postinfectious	+/−
Connective-tissue disease	+/−
Organ transplantation	+/−
Idiopathic	common

From ref. 26.

sence of evidence of asthma, chronic bronchitis, or emphysema (Table 1).

CONCLUSION

Idiopathic bronchiolitis obliterans is rare. Studies of additional patients are required to clarify the relationship of idiopathic bronchiolitis obliterans to various overlapping clinicopathologic entities causing obliteration of small airways.

ACKNOWLEDGMENTS

We thank the Paulo Foundation for their financial support.

REFERENCES

1. Colby TV, Myers JL. Clinical and histologic spectrum of bronchiolitis obliterans, including bronchiolitis obliterans organizing pneumonia. *Semin Respir Med* 1992;13:119–133.
2. Epler GR. Bronchiolitis obliterans organizing pneumonia: definition and clinical features. *Chest* 1992;102[Suppl];102:2–5.
3. King, TE. Bronchiolitis obliterans. *Lung* 1989; 167:69–93.
4. Wright JL, Cagle P, Churg A, Colby TV, Myers J. Diseases of the small airways. *Am Rev Respir Dis* 1992;146:240–262.
5. LaDue JS. Bronchiolitis fibrosa obliterans. *Arch Intern Med* 1941;68:663–673.
6. Turton CW, Williams G, Green M. Cryptogenic obliterative bronchiolitis in adults. *Thorax* 1981; 36:805–810.
7. Gosink BB, Friedman PJ, Liebow AA. Bronchiolitis obliterans. *AJR* 1973;117:816–831.
8. Epler GR, Colby TV, McLoud TC, Carrington CB, Gaensler EA. Bronchiolitis obliterans organizing pneumonia. *N Engl J Med* 1985;312: 152–158.
9. Sweatman MC, Millar AB, Strickland B, Turner-Warwick M. Computed tomography in adult obliterative bronchiolitis. *Clin Radiol* 1990;41: 116–119.
10. Lange W. Über eine eigenthümliche Erkrankung der kleinen Bronchien und Bronchiolen. (Bronchitis et Bronchiolitis obliterans.) *Dtsch Arch Klin Med* 1901;70:342–364.
11. Geddes DM, Corrin B, Brewerton DA, Davies RJ, Turner-Warwick M. Progressive airway obliteration in adults and its association with rheumatoid disease. *Q J Med* 1977;46:427–444.
12. Epler GR, Snider GL, Gaensler EA, Cathcart ES, FitzGerald MX, Carrington CB. Bronchiolitis and bronchitis in connective tissue disease. *JAMA* 1979;242:528–532.
13. Roca J, Granena A, Rodriquez-Roisin R, Alvarez P, Agusti-Vidal A, Rozman C. Fatal airway disease in an adult with chronic graft-versus-host disease. *Thorax* 1982;37:77–78.
14. Burke CM, Theodore J, Dawkins KD, Yosem SA, Blank N, Billingham ME. Post-transplant obliterative bronchiolitis and other late lung sequelae in human heart–lung transplantation. *Chest* 1984;86:824–829.
15. McGregor CGA, Dark JH, Hilton CJ. Early results of single lung transplantation in patient with end-stage pulmonary fibrosis. *J Thorac Cardiovasc Surg* 1989;98:350–354.
16. Jacobs P, Bonnyns M, Depierreux M, Ducateau J, Ergysels R. Rapidly fatal bronchiolitis obliterans with circulating antinuclear and rheumatoid factors. *Eur J Respir Dis* 1984;65:384–388.
17. Tukiainen P, Poppius H, Taskinen E. Slowly progressive bronchiolitis obliterans: a case report with detailed pulmonary function studies. *Eur J Respir Dis* 1980;61:77–83.
18. Marinopoulos GC, Huddle KRL, Waiwright H. Obliterative bronchiolitis: virus induced? *Chest* 1991;99:243–245.
19. Kuwano K, Hayashi S, MacKenzie A, Hogg JC. Detection of adenovirus DNA in paraffin-embedded lung tissues from patients with bronchiolitis obliterans and organizing pneumonia (BOOP) using in situ hybridization. *Am Rev Respir Dis* 1990;141:A319.
20. Hogg JC, Macklem PT, Thurlbeck WM. Site and nature of airway obstruction in chronic obstructive lung disease. *N Engl J Med* 1968;278:1355–1360.
21. Macklem PT, Thurlbeck WM, Fraser RG. Chronic obstructive disease of small airways. *Ann Intern Med* 1971;46:427–444.
22. Guerry-Force ML, Müller NL, Wright JL, Wiggs B, Coppin C, Pare PD. A comparison of bronchiolitis obliterans with organizing pneumonia, usual interstitial pneumonia, and small airways disease. *Am Rev Respir Dis* 1987;135: 705–712.
23. Kindt GC, Wiland JE, Davis WB, Gadek JE, Dorinsky PM. Bronchiolitis in adults: a reversible cause of airway obstruction associated with airway neutrophils and neutrophil products. *Am Rev Respir Dis* 1989;140:483–492.
24. Breatnach E, Kerr I. The radiology of cryptogenic obliterative bronchiolitis. *Clin Radiol* 1982; 33:657–661.
25. Müller NL, Guerry-Force ML, Staples CA, et al. Differential diagnosis of bronchiolitis obliterans with organizing pneumonia and usual interstitial pneumonia: clinical, functional, and radiographic findings. *Thorac Radiol* 1987;162: 151–156.
26. Epler GR, Colby TV. The spectrum of bronchiolitis obliterans. *Chest* 1983;83:161–162.
27. Cooper JD, Patterson GA, Grossman R, Maurer J, Toronto Lung Transplant Group. Double-lung transplant for advanced chronic obstructive lung disease. *Am Rev Respir Dis* 1989;139:303–307.

Diseases of the Bronchioles, edited by
Gary R. Epler. Raven Press, Ltd.,
New York © 1994.

12

Fume-Related Bronchiolitis Obliterans

William W. Douglas* and Thomas V. Colby†

**Department of Internal Medicine, Division of Thoracic Diseases, Mayo Clinic, Rochester, MN.*
†Department of Surgical Pathology, Mayo Clinic, Rochester, MN.

Inhalation of toxic gases or fumes is an uncommon cause of bronchiolitis obliterans. In the two largest series (1,2) of 109 cases of histologically confirmed bronchiolitis obliterans, only 7 were due to toxic gas inhalation injury. The nitrogen oxides are the most common cause, and the resulting clinical syndrome is relatively well defined. Only a few examples of bronchiolitis obliterans associated with other agents have been reported (Table 1). The study of bronchiolitis obliterans after exposure to toxic gases or fumes is made difficult by the sporadic nature of most incidents and the nonspecific nature of most diagnostic tests in separating bronchiolar injury from that affecting proximal bronchi or alveolar parenchyma. A firm diagnosis is therefore difficult to establish by any method other than open-lung biopsy or autopsy.

Broadly speaking, two syndromes due to bronchiolar pathology may be seen after toxic gas inhalation. Pathologically, one shows classical bronchiolitis obliterans with intraluminal polyps and the other, constrictive bronchiolitis (3). They are very different in clinical presentation, course, response to therapy, microscopic pathology, and prognosis.

The syndrome associated with classical bronchiolitis obliterans with intraluminal polyps presents with cough, fever, and dyspnea developing 10 to 14 days after exposure to nitrogen dioxide or phosgene; chest radiographs show a diffuse miliary-nodular pattern simulating miliary tuberculosis. The histologic picture is that of an inflammatory process involving nearly all bronchioles and some of the adjacent peribronchiolar alveoli, with intraluminal granulation tissue polyps within the bronchioles. Biopsies are performed frequently to exclude infection prior to initiation of corticosteroid therapy. The process usually improves with corticosteroid therapy but may leave mild functional impairment.

The syndrome associated with constrictive bronchiolitis may be suspected when the patient has persistent, severe respiratory injury, usually with a 1-second forced expire volume (FEV_1) of 60% or less of the predicted normal value that begins within 6 weeks of exposure to an irritant gas and has no response to bronchodilator or corticosteroid therapy. In suspected cases, emphysema, asthma, cystic fibrosis, or alpha$_1$-antitrypsin deficiency should be excluded (4,5). The chest radiograph must show no obvious diffuse interstitial disease or emphysema. Indeed, most radiographs are normal or show hyperinflation or bronchiectasis. Although bronchiectasis is considered an exclusion criterion for idiopathic bronchiolitis obliterans (5), bronchiectasis and constrictive bronchiolitis may coexist. Most cases have occurred after exposure to sulfur dioxide, ammonia, or fire smoke. Biopsies are rarely done for clinical reasons

TABLE 1. *Causes of bronchiolitis obliterans*

Agents causing classical bronchiolitis obliterans
Nitrogen oxides
Phosgene
Free-base cocaine (? phosgene)
Fire smoke
Agents causing constrictive bronchiolitis obliterans
Sulfur dioxide
Ammonia
Fire smoke
Agents causing histiologic focal bronchiolitis obliterans, without clinical bronchiolitis obliterans
Chlorine
Sulfur mustard

alone because the finding of constrictive bronchiolitis does not alter therapy in most patients, but the diagnosis can be established with certainty only by histologic examination. The few cases that have been biopsied have shown prominent and widespread chronic inflammation and/or fibrosis involving bronchioles, producing concentric luminal narrowing or obliteration (3).

Airflow obstruction from bronchiolar injury (bronchiolitis obliterans) due to inhalation of toxic gas occurs in three clinical settings: first, when a reactive gas of relatively low water solubility (such as the oxides of nitrogen or phosgene) is inhaled, usually with minimal symptoms; second, when a very corrosive and soluble gas such as ammonia is inhaled deeply; and third, when irritants in fire smoke are adsorbed onto soot or carbon particles and are carried deeply into the lung.

The distribution and extent of lung injury after the inhalation of a toxic gas or fume (usually defined as a fine particulate) are determined by the concentration of the agent, the duration of exposure, the route and pattern of breathing, the solubility and biologic reactivity of the agent, and the biological susceptibility, which varies among species as well as individuals (6).

Different agents cause different types of bronchiolar injury. Nitrogen oxides cause classical bronchiolitis obliterans with intraluminal polyps, whereas sulfur dioxide causes constrictive bronchiolitis obliterans. Also, Hales and colleagues (7) studied the effects of acrolein and hydrochloric acid that were adsorbed onto carbon particles and inhaled by dogs. Acrolein resulted in peribronchiolar edema, whereas hydrochloric acid produced coagulation necrosis of the epithelium of proximal airways without edema. Furthermore, acid and alkali burns also cause different patterns of injury to other tubular structures. Hydrochloric acid leads to coagulation necrosis of epithelium, which limits deeper injury; permanent scarring requires unusually protracted exposure (8). By contrast, even brief exposures to concentrated alkalis, such as lye or ammonia, quickly result in liquifaction necrosis that extends into deeper tissues; extensive scarring with stricture formation is a common outcome (9).

Airway epithelial injury and repair after acute oxidant exposure in experimental animals have been reviewed by Man and Hulbert (6). Brief exposures to ozone, nitrogen oxides, or sulfur dioxide causes focal damage to epithelial cells, which may then be shed. Ciliated cells are most easily destroyed. Denuded areas that are focal are sealed within a few hours due to proliferation of surviving nonciliated epithelial cells. When the entire epithelium is lost, exposing the basal lamina, the rate of repair is much slower and depends on the area to be covered and the rate of cell ingrowth.

An exudative reaction also is usually present after acute bronchiolar injury; the exudate contains fibrin fragments and fibronectin, which are chemotactic for inflammatory, epithelial, and endothelial cells (10,11). In experimental models, within 4 to 6 hours a dramatic influx of neutrophils is apparent. Activated neutrophils produce oxygen radicals, which are bacteriocidal but also damage healthy surviving cells, and proteases that fragment fibronectin and activate complement, thus attracting monocytes and lymphocytes. These cells in turn release growth factors and cytokines that recruit and activate fibroblasts (10,11).

Organization of the inflammatory exudate has been studied in alveoli during the proliferation phase of diffuse alveolar damage (adult respiratory distress syndrome) and in alveolar ducts of patients with bronchiolitis obliterans organizing pneumonia (BOOP) (12–14). The exudate is invaded by fibroblasts and myofibroblasts. In BOOP, these form intraluminal granulation tissue polyps. At the base of these polyps, focal disruption of basal lamina is apparent, through which the fibroblasts enter the exudate (12,14). The factors that permit resolution of the granulation tissue reaction seen in some conditions but not in others are not yet defined, but they may relate to disorganization of the basal lamina. Though not proven, this variability may relate in part to the extent of destruction of the basal lamina.

The spectrum of injury associated with the inhalation of toxic gases and fumes is wide, and a complete discussion of the subject is beyond the scope of this chapter. The interested reader is referred to several excellent reviews (15–26). This chapter focuses on histologically confirmed bronchiolar lesions and fixed airflow obstruction following exposures to high concentrations of toxic gases. The effects of chronic low-dose exposure to oxidant and irritant gases on pulmonary function, hyperreactive airways disease, and chronic bronchitis or emphysema are not considered.

OXIDES OF NITROGEN

"Nitrous fume" consists of a mixture of several nitrogen oxides. Those causing lung injury are nitrogen dioxide and nitrogen tetroxide, which are in equilibrium and together form a reddish brown gas that is heavier than air and has a low aqueous solubility relative to other irritants (27). Because of this, nitrogen oxides are not removed efficiently in the nose and upper airway, give little warning, and may be breathed deeply into the lung for prolonged periods. The threshold limit value (TLV) for nitrogen oxides is 5 parts per million (ppm). Individuals exposed to 50 to 100 ppm may experience only mild irritation of the nose and throat during exposure but may later develop pulmonary edema (28). Although nitrous oxides hydrolyze slowly on moist surfaces to form nitric and nitrous acids, their major impact on biological systems is as oxidants, with the production of free radicals that damage lipid constituents of cell membranes (6).

The histopathology of bronchiolitis obliterans due to nitrogen oxides, first described by Fraenkel (29) in 1902, was later elaborated by Wagner (30) and McAdams (31). The radiographic features were characterized by Nichols (32) in his description of the survivors of the Cleveland Clinic fire of 1929. Lowry and Schuman (33) in 1956 reported four patients with bronchiolitis obliterans after exposure to silo gas; the first two were treated with antibiotics alone and died; the second two, who had similar clinical and radiographic features, were treated with corticosteroids, rapidly improved, and survived. Since that report, corticosteroids have been used both to treat and to prevent bronchiolitis after exposure; lung biopsies have been done only rarely; serious exposures probably have occurred less often; and bronchiolitis obliterans has become a rare disease.

Exposure to nitrogen oxides may occur in industrial settings when nitric acid is heated (31,34), used to clean brass or etch zinc (29), poured into zinc-lined galvanized buckets (35,36), or spilled onto wood floors or sawdust (27). Other exposures have been associated with nitration or organic materials (37,38), the manufacture of acids, the use of contaminated nitrous oxide during anesthesia (39), the detonation of explosives in confined spaces (40–45), the decomposition of superphosphate fertilizer

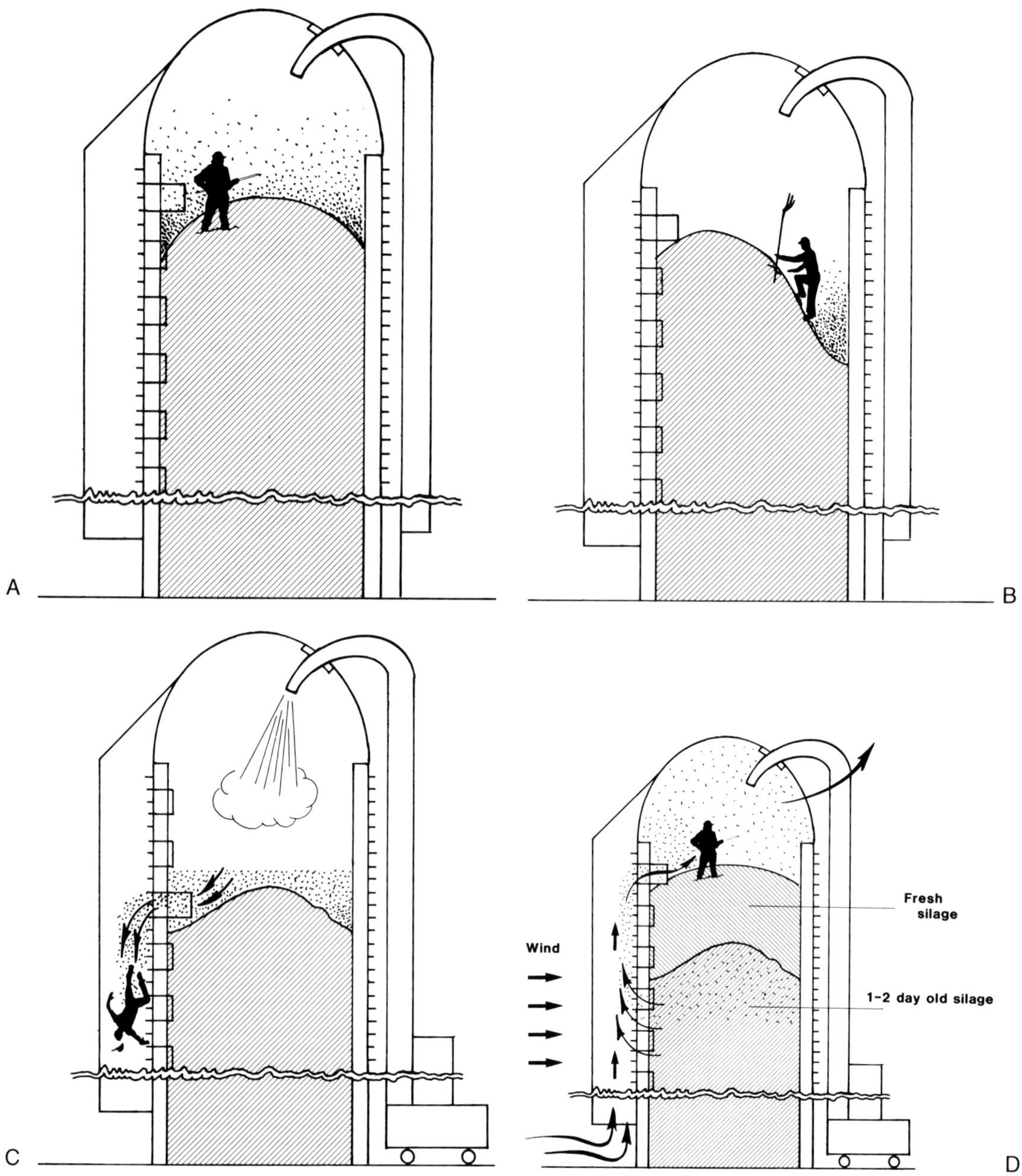

FIG. 1. Typical exposures to nitrogen oxides in agricultural silos that may result in silo-fillers' disease. **A,** Exposure usually occurs when the farmer enters the silo 1 to 4 days after the silo was filled, to level the silage then lower and connect the unloader, or to spread a plastic sheet over the silage. **B,** silo gas is heavier than air and accumulates in low places within the silo. Descent into these areas may be fatal. **C,** Opening the door just above the silage may result in concentrated exposure, causing rapid loss of consciousness and a fall down the silo chute. **D,** Entry immediately after filling is completed may not be safe, as silo gas from 1- to 2-day-old silage may leak out the silo doors and be drawn up into the working space by a chimney-like updraft.

(37), and the use of liquid fuels for rockets (46,47). Fires consuming nitrocellulose film (32,48) or shoe polish (49), and acetylene (22,50–54) or electric-arc welding in confined spaces (55) also may generate nitrogen oxides in toxic concentrations.

In many agricultural areas, silo-fillers' disease is now the most common cause of lung injury from nitrogen oxides (33,56–71). Since most physicians are unfamiliar with silos, diagrams illustrating the common exposures are given (Fig. 1). In all but one patient (63), exposures have occurred when the silo contained silage 1 to 4 days old (70,71).

The inhalation of nitrogen oxides leads to a well-defined clinical disorder characterized by biphasic lung injury. The initial phase, pulmonary edema, occurs a few hours after injury. The late phase, organizing bronchiolitis, develops 2 to 3 weeks later.

Early Phase: Immediate Symptoms, Symptom-Free Interval, Pulmonary Edema

During exposure, symptoms depend on the concentration and duration of exposure and probably also on the concentration of nitric oxide in the mixture of gases. When the concentration of nitrogen dioxide and nitrogen tetroxide is high and nitric oxide is present, loss of consciousness may be rapid, often with fatal results (27,42,56, 70,71). Most of those exposed to moderate concentrations complain of cough and lightheadedness, often with dyspnea, chest tightness, or a choking sensation. A few develop an acute asthma-like reaction accompanied by wheezing (68,70,71).

In most patients, the immediate symptoms resolve promptly after exposure ceases, but after a symptom-free interval of about 10 hours (range 30 minutes to 42 hours), pulmonary edema may develop. Symptoms

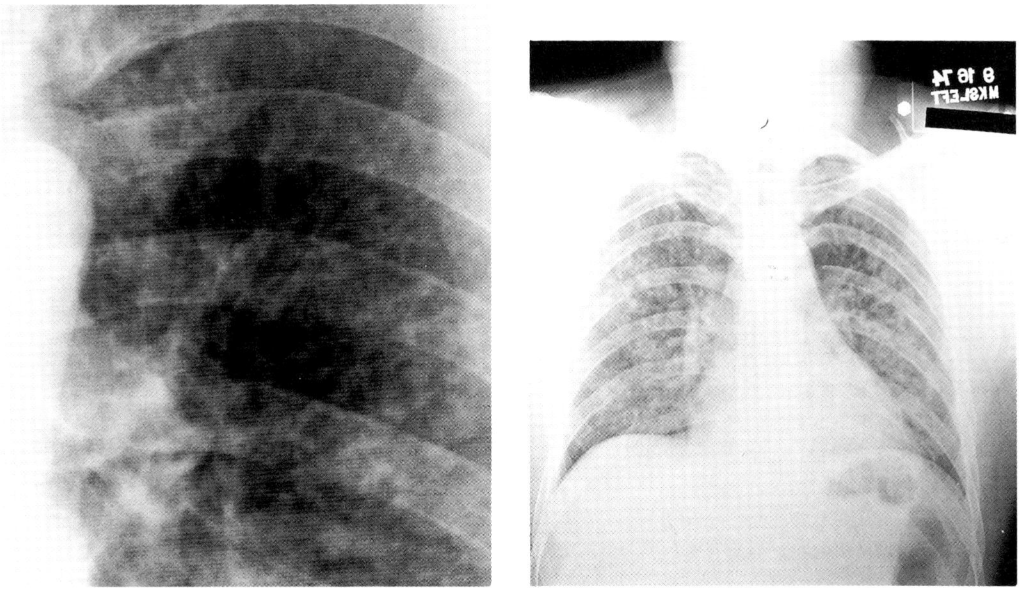

A B

FIG. 2. A and **B,** Two typical examples of the early phase of silo-fillers' disease. Chest radiographic appearance, showing multiple nodular infiltrates with indistinct borders. Both films were taken 1 day after exposure. The infiltrates cleared over the next 4 days, and subsequent pulmonary functions were entirely normal in each patient. Both were treated with corticosteroids for prophylaxis against later bronchiolitis obliterans.

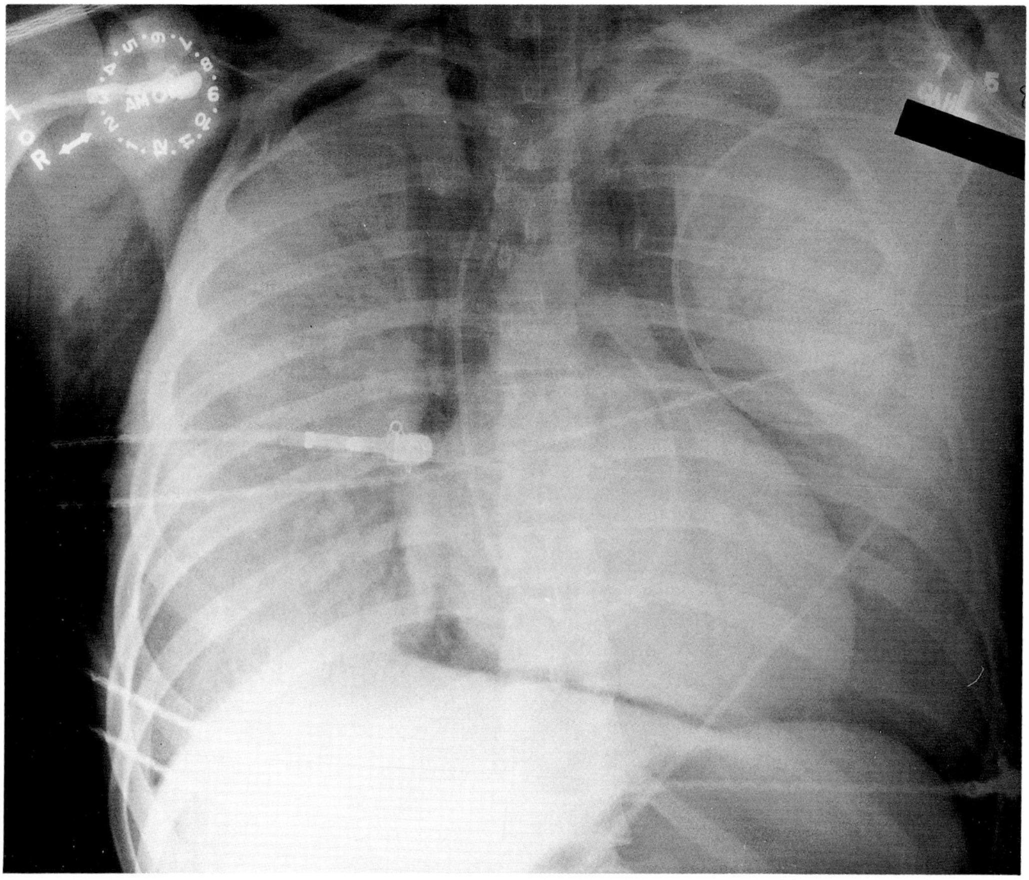

FIG. 3. Confluent pulmonary edema and pneumomediastinum in a 19-year-old farmer who later died after taking "one deep breath" of silo gas in an exposure similar to that depicted in Fig. 1C. He was rescued within 1 minute after falling to the base of the silo. Details of his course, treatment, and autopsy findings have been described elsewhere (70).

FIG. 4. Radiographic sequence of biphasic lung injury after exposure to nitrogen oxides. The patient was a 55-year-old chemist who mixed the wrong ingredients when making an experimental brine in a pickle factory. **A,** Nineteen hours after exposure, pulmonary edema is present, with multiple "woolly" nodules that have indistinct margins. The patient was wakened from sleep with dyspnea, fever, and diaphoresis. **B,** Three days after exposure, the infiltrates have resolved. The patient continued to have mild exertional dyspnea. Thirty days after exposure, he developed progressive dyspnea, wheezing, chest pain, and diaphoresis. **C,** Thirty-six days after exposure, classical bronchiolitis obliterans is apparent with discrete, tiny miliary nodules. He was hospitalized for 2 weeks and treated with antibiotics and oxygen. He slowly improved but remained dyspneic walking at a normal pace and was referred for consultation. **D,** Sixty-six days after exposure, the miliary infiltrates have resolved. Pulmonary function tests 66 days after exposure gave the following results with predicted normals in parentheses: TLC 6.41 (6.60), VC 3.56 (4.90), RV 2.87 (1.70), FEF_{25-75} 0.9 ($>$2.0) MVV 98 (119), D_LCO_{ss} 17 (30). Corticosteroids were administered for 1 month, and the patient did not significantly improve. Pulmonary function tests 31 months after exposure gave the following results: TLC 6.81, VC 3.82, RV 3.00, FEF_{25-75} 1.7, MVV 109, D_LCO_{ss} 21. (TLC, total lung capacity, liters; VC, vital capacity, liters; RV, residual volume, liters; FEF_{25-75}, forced expiratory flow between 25 and 75% of vital capacity, L/second; MVV, maximal voluntary ventilation, L/minute; D_LCO_{ss}, diffusing capacity of the lung for carbon monoxide, steady state method, ml/minute/mm Hg.) Courtesy of Dr. N. G. G. Hepper.

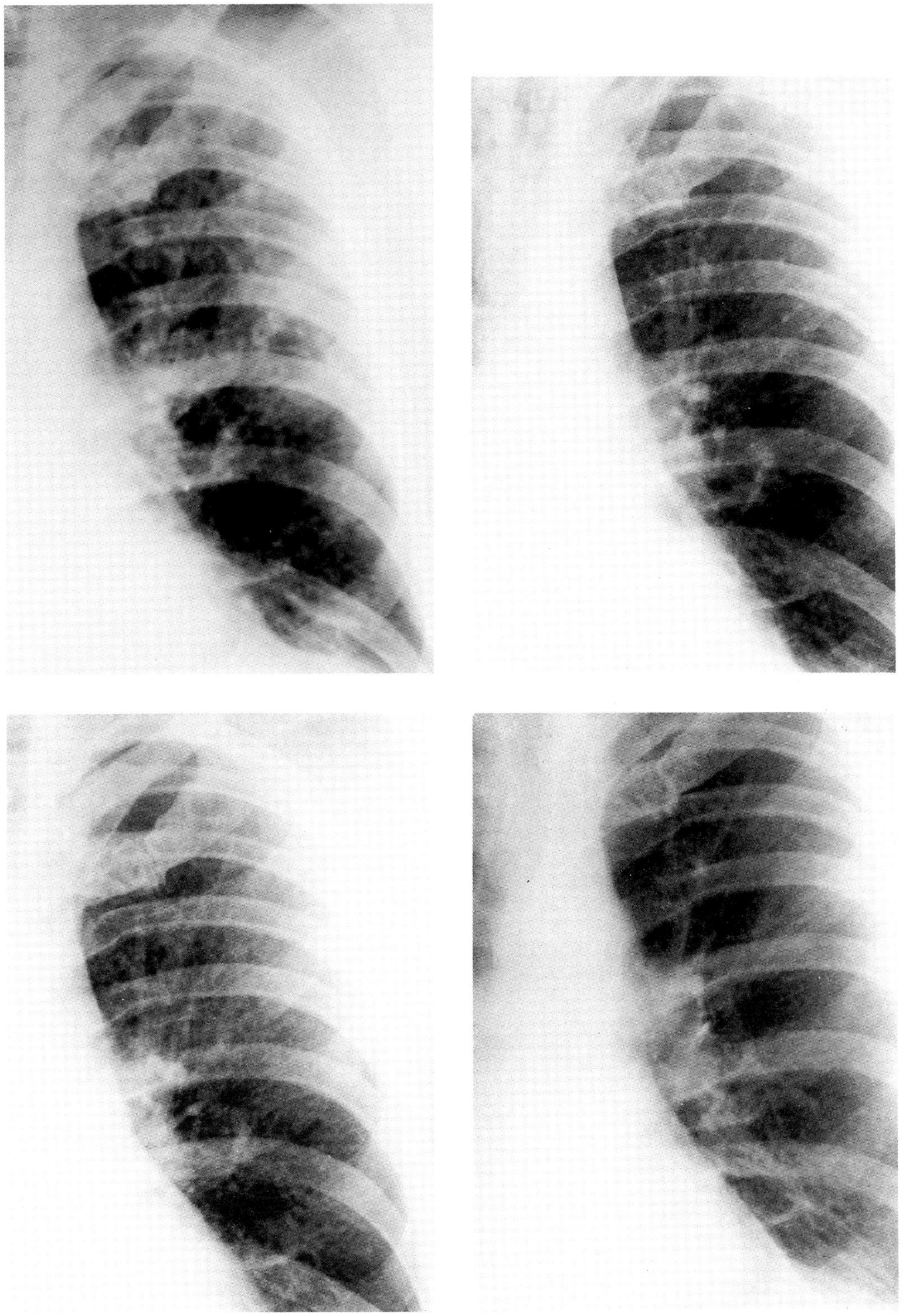
A
B
C
D

then include dyspnea, cough, and chest pain; generalized fine crackles with or without wheezes are usually present (70,71). Chest radiographs may show a miliary pattern; the nodules show indistinct borders or may become confluent and demonstrate findings typical for pulmonary edema (Figs. 2–4) (32,33,36,45,52,54).

When patients are seen after a known exposure and no evidence of lung injury has yet appeared, corticosteroids are still recommended. Although both systemic corticosteroids (70,71) and inhaled corticosteroids (72) have been employed, neither these nor antioxidant therapy, such as vitamin E or inhaled glutathione, has been studied in a controlled manner.

Mild pulmonary edema should be treated using oxygen therapy with monitoring of oxygen saturation and respiratory frequency (28). Because of concern that an oxidant-induced injury may be aggravated by hyperoxia, the minimum oxygen concentration should be used to maintain adequate arterial oxygenation. Continuous positive airway pressure may be useful. Severe pulmonary edema should be treated using standard therapy for the adult respiratory distress syndrome with endotracheal intubation and mechanical ventilation using positive end expiratory pressure.

Late Phase: Organizing Bronchiolitis

Symptoms may arise with or without preceding pulmonary edema and usually begin 2 to 3 weeks (range 8 to 45 days) following exposure. The most frequently described symptoms are dyspnea, progressing to tachypnea and orthopnea; paroxysmal cough, usually nonproductive but sometimes productive of frothy or mucoid sputum that may be blood-tinged or mucopurulent; fever, often with chills; chest pain; and wheezing or chest tightness. Physical findings include tachypnea, orthopnea, paroxysmal coughing, fever, cyanosis, tachycardia, and generalized fine crackles. Audible wheezes or decreased breath sounds also may be present (29–36,45,49,53,57,59–63,69,71,72–77).

Radiographic features are dominated by the finding of innumerable small densities consisting of irregular, rather discrete miliary nodules scattered uniformly throughout both lungs, simulating the appearance of miliary tuberculosis (Figs. 4 and 5). These nodular densities may coalesce, making a diagnosis of superimposed bronchopneumonia difficult to exclude (Fig. 6). In one autopsy-proven case involving a patient with pre-existing right lower lobe bron-

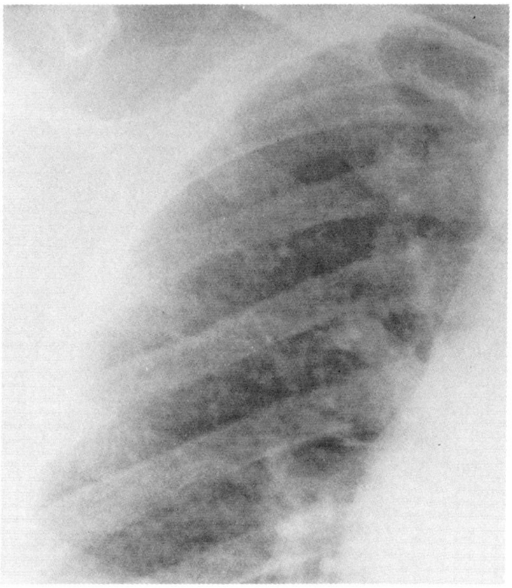

FIG. 5. Chest radiograph showing classical bronchiolitis obliterans, with miliary nodular infiltrates. Approximately 5 weeks before, this 50-year-old farmer had developed nausea, vomiting, and severe shortness of breath within 1 minute after entering a silo that had been filled the previous day. He presented with a 3-week history of anorexia and had lost 12 pounds; during the week before admission, the patient had developed a nonproductive cough, chest tightness, and night sweats. Coarse crackles were audible at the right lung base. Vital capacity was 3.67 L (predicted 4.0 L), forced expired volume in one second was 3.04 L (predicted 3.2 L). (This patient is mentioned in ref. 71.) Courtesy of Dr. John J. May, Cooperstown, NY.

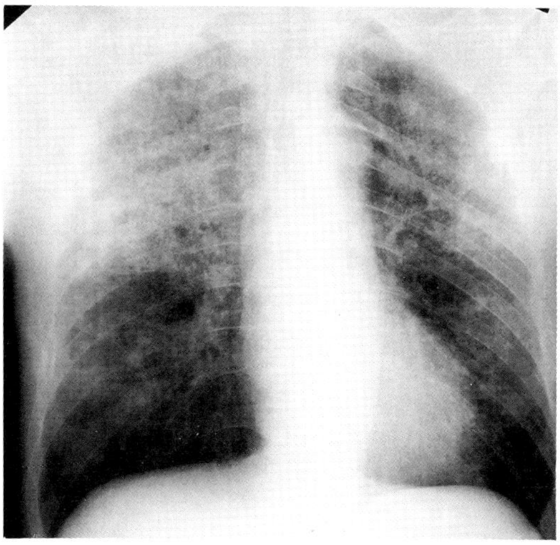

FIG. 6. Atypical bronchiolitis obliterans with confluent upper lobe infiltrates suggesting superimposed bronchopneumonia, 33 days after exposure to silo gas. Aged 59 years then and an 80-pack year smoker, the patient's mild dyspnea was somewhat worse after recovery. He developed progressively severe obstructive lung disease and died 23 years later, at age 82. His pulmonary function tests have been reported elsewhere (70).

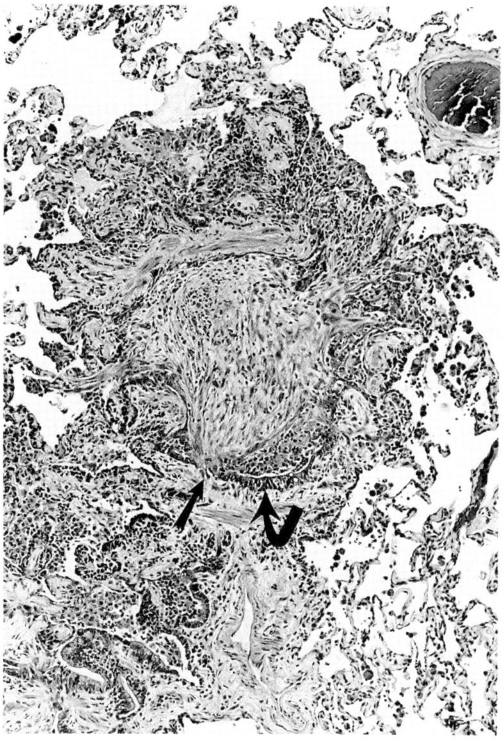

FIG. 7. Classical bronchiolitis obliterans in a 54-year-old woman who noted cough, fatigue, and dyspnea 3 weeks after being exposed to "brown fumes" in a chemical spill at a nickel-plating factory. The chest radiographs showed miliary infiltrates. Open-lung biopsy was done 3½ weeks after exposure. A membranous bronchiole is filled with a fibroblastic proliferation associated with a moderate chronic inflammatory exudate in the wall of the bronchiole. There is slight involvement of the peribronchiolar alveoli. The pattern is that of the proliferative phase of bronchiolitis obliterans with marked intraluminal fibrous tissue proliferation that can be seen to arise from the bronchiolar wall (*arrow*) adjacent to some preserved mucosa (*curved arrow*). Courtesy of Dr. T. V. Colby.

chiectasis, the miliary process spared this lobe (35), presumably because of decreased regional ventilation and delivery of nitrogen oxides to this segment.

Histologic examination demonstrates an inflammatory process centered on small bronchioles and their immediately surrounding alveoli. The characteristic lesion is intrabronchiolar granulation tissue polyps that originate from the walls of bronchioles and partially fill their lumens (Fig. 7). These bronchiolar and peribronchiolar lesions represent the nodular densities seen radiographically.

In patients not treated with corticosteroids or antibiotics, the nodular densities gradually fade and disappear over the next several months, and the symptoms (which in the series of Nichols [32] began on average 15 days after exposure) persist until approximately 50 days after exposure. In corticosteroid-treated patients, the miliary infiltrates and symptoms usually improve within a few days (33,45,53,59,60,63,75–77).

Pulmonary function tests within the first few months after exposure usually show a restrictive pattern with decreased lung volumes, decreased diffusing capacity, and arterial hypoxemia. A mixed pattern is occasionally seen, accompanied by features of obstruction (53,60,63,75,79).

During recovery these functional abnormalities improve slowly, sometimes returning to normal (53). Only a few patients have had pulmonary function tests done more than a year after bronchiolitis obliterans caused by nitrogen oxides; a few have no residua, but many have shown mild abnormalities including decreased forced expiratory flow between 25 and 75% of vital capacity and arterial hypoxemia (60), mild obstruction and decreased diffusing capacity (61), or increased residual volume and total lung capacity (59,63,76). In one patient, progressive decline in vital capacity, maximal voluntary ventilation and FEV_1 with decreased diffusing capacity and arterial hypoxemia was observed (75).

Most patients who recover from the organizing bronchiolitis obliterans after exposure to nitrogen oxides have some persistent, measurable abnormality of pulmonary function. By contrast, the majority of patients who had pulmonary edema alone have normal late pulmonary function. However, patients from either group may have residual impairment (70,71,80). Late functional impairment after exposure to the oxides of nitrogen, with or without bronchiolitis obliterans, is more common in patients over 50 years of age (44,60,70,82), when there is a history of smoking or chronic bronchitis (53,44,70,75), and after prolonged exposures (60,70). Tests more sensitive to dysfunction of small airways, including measurement of airways resistance (43) and frequency dependence of compliance (81), may be abnormal when the usual pulmonary function tests are normal. However, the documentation of arterial hypoxemia seems to be a sensitive and simpler method for the detection of mild injury. In most situations when the customary pulmonary function tests including arterial oxygen tension at rest and after exercise are normal, the patients are asymptomatic and are not impaired. Some patients reported to have persistent impairment of pulmonary function due to silo-fillers' disease may instead have had other diseases such as chronic farmers' lung disease or community-acquired pneumonia (83–85). Finally, increased airway reactivity to nonspecific irritants (reactive airways dysfunction syndrome) (86) also may develop after acute exposure to nitrogen oxides (44,62,68,70).

The selectivity of terminal bronchioles to injury related to nitrogen oxides is unknown. Speculations have included the relatively low rate of hydrolysis that allows the nitrogen oxides to be delivered deeply down to the level of alveolar ducts; beyond this level the agent is diluted by residual air (87), making the small airways more severely affected. In addition, nitrogen oxides delivered to the distal acinus may be cleared centrally into the relatively small terminal bronchioles and concentrated there by a funnel-like effect (88) enhanced by the pooling that results from the damaged bronchiolar mucociliary apparatus. The neutrophilic response that develops soon after injury probably adds proteases and oxidants. Injury also may be enhanced by oxygen therapy, positive airway pressure ventilation, and superimposed infection.

Prevention

Prevention of lung injury from nitrogen oxides centers on avoiding exposure. Education programs and improved ventilation systems have led to improved safety for chemical and electroplating workers, miners involved in underground blasting, welders, and fire fighters. Recommendations for farmers who may be exposed to silo gas have been described: avoid entering the silo within the first 2 weeks after filling; leave the chute doors open down to the level of the silage after filling; and operate the blower prior to entry (70).

Once exposure has occurred, prevention of bronchiolitis obliterans may be possible by the administration of even a short course of corticosteroids (70,71). In rabbits exposed to a mist of dilute nitric acid, the incidence and severity of bronchiolar injury with bronchiolitis obliterans was decreased dramatically by corticosteroid therapy when compared to untreated controls (89). Since the use of corticosteroids has become routine in clinical practice, the incidence of bronchiolitis obliterans seems to have decreased over the years, but no prospective study has been done in humans.

PHOSGENE

Phosgene is a heavy, toxic gas with an odor similar to that of freshly cut hay or green corn. Although phosgene hydrolyzes to hydrochloric acid, phosgene is approximately 800 times as toxic to the lung as hydrochloric acid (90); the major toxic effect on tissues is thought to be mediated by the reactive carbonyl group, which combines with amines and hydroxyl groups to produce cell injury (90). Phosgene is relatively insoluble and therefore is not efficiently removed by the upper airway and nose, causes little irritation of the upper airway, and thus gives little warning. The TLV is 0.5 ppm; the odor threshold is 1.5 ppm; cough occurs at 5 ppm; and 15 to 100 ppm may be lethal after a 20-minute exposure (90).

Used as a poison gas during World War I, phosgene was blamed for many battlefield casualties (91,92). Since then, only sporadic cases of phosgene inhalation injury have been reported, usually from manufacturing of phosgene (93) or after exposure to the combustion products of the solvents trichloroethylene or methylene dichloride (94–100). These exposures have been quite subtle, and most have followed work in confined spaces with a solvent near a flame or hot surface or welding metals that had been cleaned using these agents (100). Trichloroethylene and ethylene dichloride are widely used in homes as paint removers or paintbrush cleaners; if open containers are placed near space heaters or hot kitchen stoves, the fumes of these solvents may undergo combustion and dangerous levels of phosgene may be generated. These exposures should be considered in patients with "idiopathic" bronchiolitis obliterans. Phosgene also may have been a major toxic component of the noxious gas that caused a well-described sequence of acute lung injury following the explosion of a tank of solvents including methylene dichloride (101).

Although the acute phase of lung injury has been documented several times, the late phase of bronchiolitis obliterans is distinctly uncommon. In one patient, initial pulmonary edema resolved after 5 days; but a second episode, described as pulmonary edema with respiratory failure, occurred 10 days after exposure and required intubation with mechanical ventilation (100). Histologically confirmed classical bronchiolitis obliterans with intraluminal polyps has been documented in humans both in autopsies of World War I victims of war gas poisoning (91,92) and in victims of postwar industrial accidents (102,103). Phosgene was the probable cause of death in a patient with classical bronchiolitis obliterans found at autopsy. He attributed his illness to shoe dye: after repeated exposures, he had become progressively ill, with cough and dyspnea; the chest radiograph showed miliary infiltrates. The solvent in the shoe dye was found to contain "impure trichloroethylene" with an "irritating odor" (94).

Pulmonary function tests have been reported (92) in one group of six subjects studied 3 to 14 months after pulmonary edema due to phosgene exposure. Findings included rapid shallow breathing, decreased maximal voluntary ventilation with normal vital capacity, and either an increased alveolar to arterial oxygen tension difference or abnormal nitrogen washout curves in each patient.

The sequence of bronchiolar injury following exposure to phosgene was studied in dogs by Winternitz (104) following World War I (Figs. 8 and 9). More recent studies

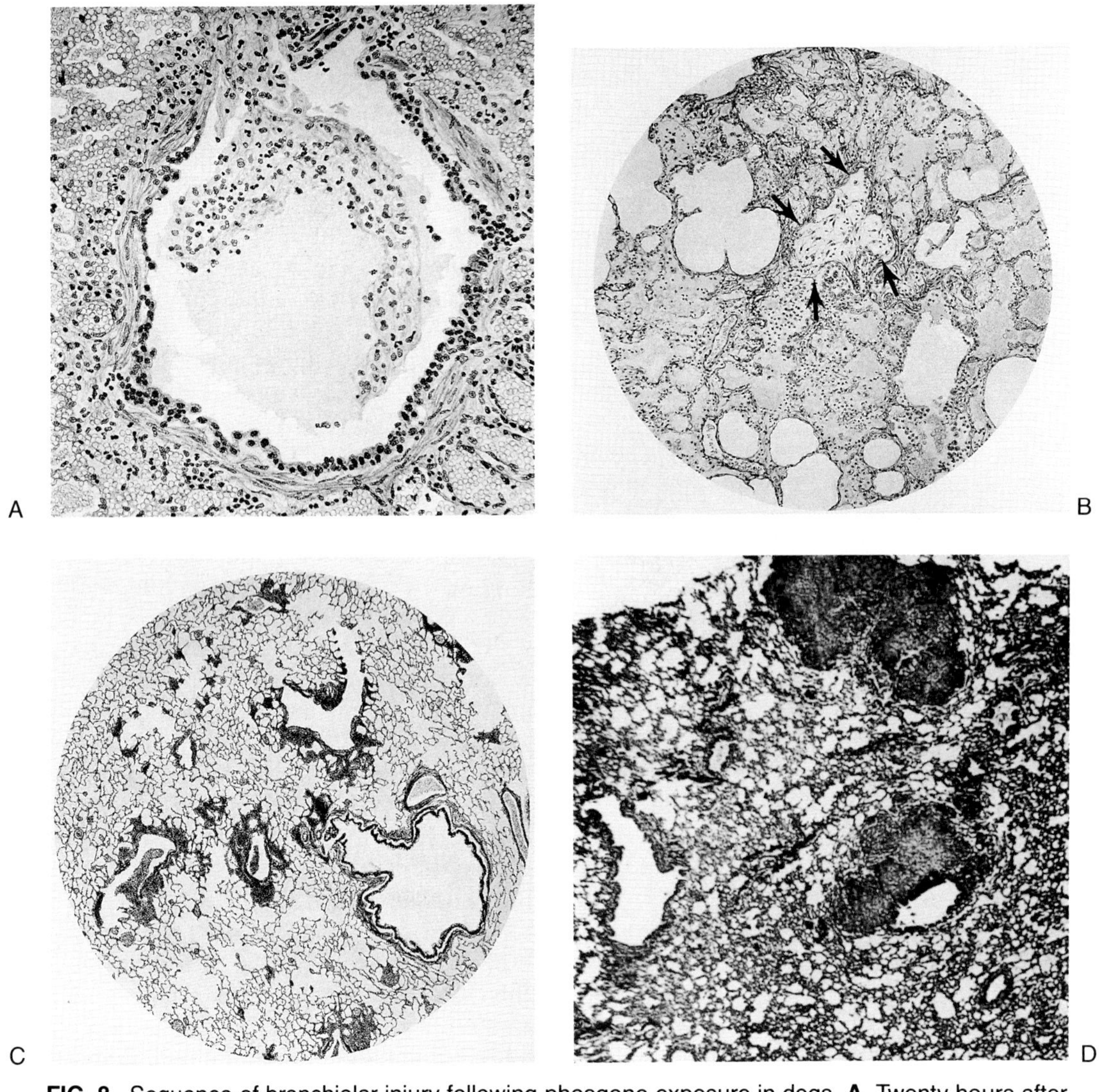

FIG. 8. Sequence of bronchiolar injury following phosgene exposure in dogs. **A,** Twenty hours after exposure. Bronchiole shows degeneration and partial desquamation of the epithelium and intraluminal exudate with neutrophilic inflammation. **B,** Four days after exposure. Beginning organization of the inflammatory exudate in a bronchiole (*arrows*). Fibrin and neutrophils are present in alveoli. **C,** Fourteen days after exposure. Later stage of organization and inflammation in and around bronchioles. **D,** Thirty-three days after exposure, showing miliary peribronchial nodules containing fibroblasts and mononuclear cells. From Winternitz MC *Collected studies on the pathology of war gas poisoning.* New Haven: Yale University Press; 1920, with permission of the publisher. Arrows have been added.

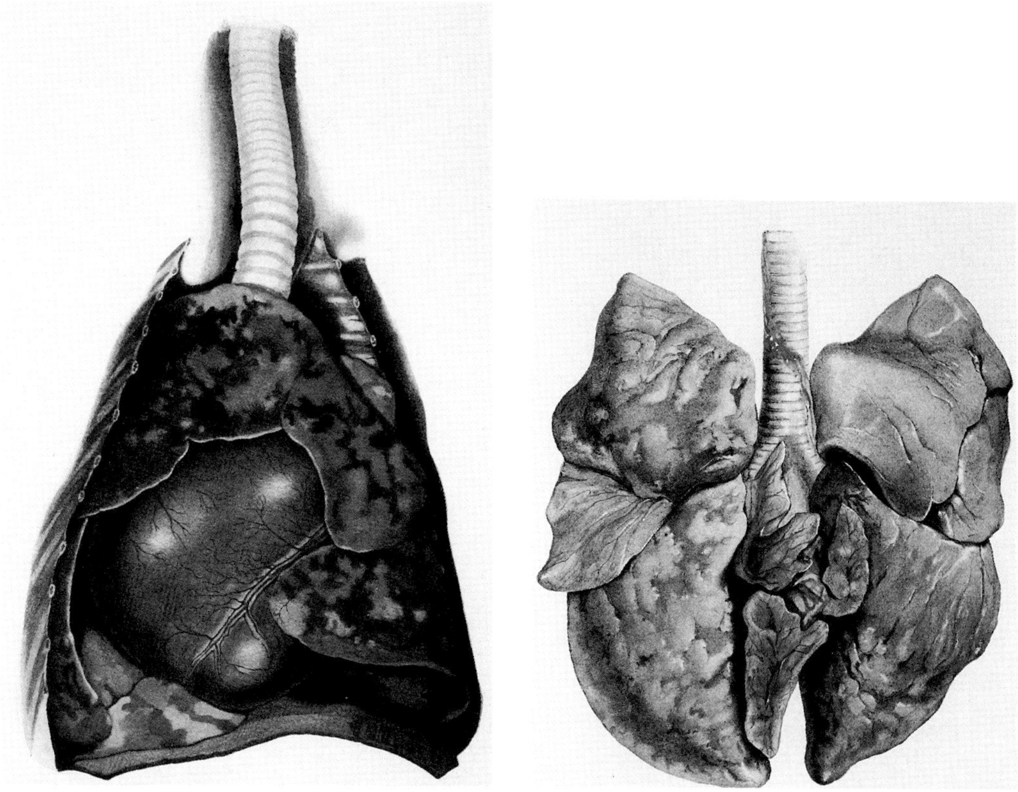

FIG. 9. Drawings of the lungs of dogs during the early and late phases of injury due to phosgene. **A,** Heart and lungs 24 hours after exposure. Light patches of acute hyperinflation alternate with dark areas of edema and atelectasis. The right ventricle is dilated. **B,** Lungs, 14 days after exposure. Marked hyperinflation is apparent with irregular patches of atelectasis. Microscopically, widespread obliterative bronchiolitis is present. From Winternitz MC *Collected studies on the pathology of war gas poisoning.* New Haven: Yale University Press; 1920, with permission of the publisher.

(105,106) have confirmed his observations.

In dogs, 30 to 40 repeated 30-minute sublethal exposures to 24 to 40 ppm phosgene result in bronchiolitis, which progresses to widespread obliterative bronchiolitis (constrictive bronchiolitis) with irreversible emphysema and hyperinflation; this protocol has been suggested as an animal model for the study of human emphysema (107). Three clinical reports suggest that repeated exposures to other toxic gases (sulfur mustard [108] and cadmium fume [109,110]) may cause a similar response in humans. Repeated exposure of rats to cadmium chloride causes repeated acute granulomatous reactions around respiratory bronchioles that may eventually produce emphysema (111).

MUSTARD GAS

Mustard gas results in delayed-onset, acute, blistering skin injury; eye damage; and desquamating tracheobronchitis with mucosal sloughing (112,113). Pulmonary edema may develop, usually on the second or third day; occasionally it is fatal. Secondary infection is common, creating another peak of deaths on the eighth and ninth days after exposure (114,115). Nevertheless, mortality is low in most series (90).

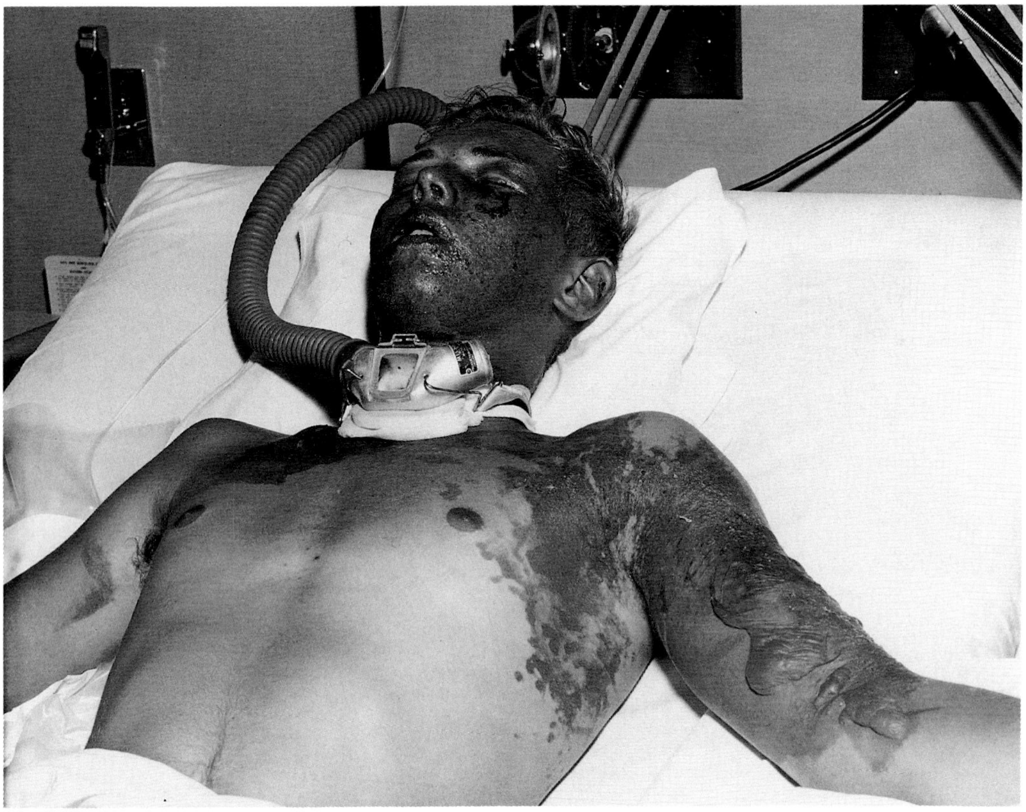

A

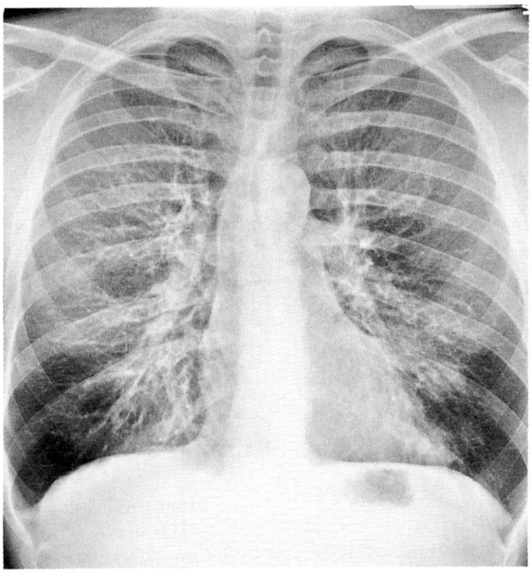

B

FIG. 10. The usual consequences of exposure to concentrated ammonia. **A,** Brief contact from a spray of anhydrous liquid ammonia results in blistering skin burns, severe eye damage, and laryngeal edema requiring endotracheal intubation or tracheostomy. This patient had no subsequent tracheobronchial or pulmonary injury. **B,** When concentrated ammonia gas is inhaled deeply, mucosal necrosis results with pseudomembranes which may slough, causing sudden major airway obstruction. Late bronchiectasis may result. Chest radiographs 8 years after recovery from respiratory failure suggest bronchiectasis.

C
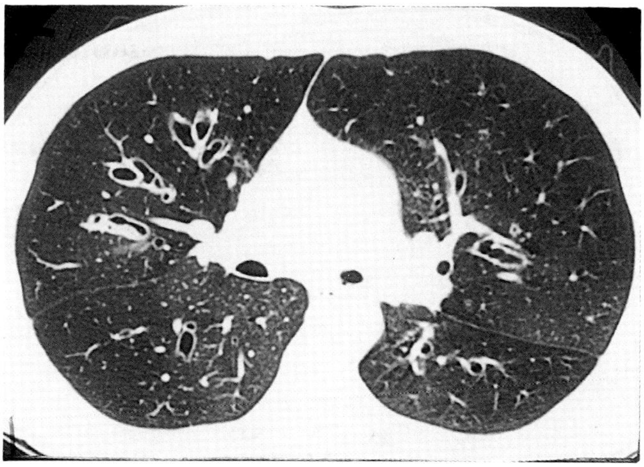

FIG. 10. *Continued.* **C,** Thin-section CT scan in the same patient, confirming bronchiectasis.

The only reports on bronchiolitis obliterans are from Winternitz's (104) study in dogs, which shows that the predominant lesion is severe tracheobronchial epithelial necrosis and pulmonary edema; histologic bronchiolitis obliterans was seen in only a few bronchioles.

SULFUR DIOXIDE

Sulfur dioxide is a heavy, colorless, irritant gas with a pungent odor, usually encountered as an air pollutant. Much more soluble than nitrogen oxides or phosgene, sulfur dioxide is readily detected, is efficiently removed in the upper airway, and causes relatively greater injury to the trachea than to the distal airways. The TLV is 5 ppm; detection threshold is 0.3 to 1.0 ppm; 20 ppm causes immediate eye irritation; and higher concentrations cause cough and a choking sensation (116). Sulfur dioxide acts as an oxidant that can generate free radicals that in turn injure lipid membranes. It hydrolyzes to form bisulfite, sulfate, and hydrogen ions; at physiologic pH bisulfite predominates and can react with many molecules, especially enzymes containing disulfide bonds (117).

Concentrated sulfur dioxide is used commercially to bleach wood pulp for paper production (118), and it may be present when sulfur or iron pyrite ore dust (119) is ignited. Lithium batteries may vent thionyl chloride into the atmosphere, resulting in toxic levels of sulfur dioxide (116).

Exposure to concentrated sulfur dioxide may cause death within a few minutes; autopsies show necrotizing laryngotracheobronchitis and pulmonary edema (120,121). Symptoms in survivors include eye, nose, and throat irritation; chest tightness; and dyspnea. Conjunctivitis, superficial corneal burns, and pharyngeal erythema may be apparent. Examination of the chest shows decreased breath sounds, crackles, and rhonchi (118,120,122). The acute phase may progress rapidly and result in death; in one report (121) autopsy at 17 days showed extensive ulcerating or desquamative neutrophilic tracheobronchitis with pseudomembranes, terminal bronchioles plugged with mucopurulent exudate, and the lamina propria replaced by fibrosis that narrowed the lumen. Treatment of the acute phase is similar to that described for nitrogen oxides. No studies of systemic or aerosolized corticosteroids, aerosolized sodium bicarbonate, or antioxidants have been reported.

In some patients, late effects may develop. About 10 days after exposure, cough and dyspnea may begin or worsen, often with purulent sputum (120,122). Crackles and wheezes or decreased breath sounds may be noted. Chest radiographs are usually normal or demonstrate only hyperinflation (118). Pulmonary function tests may be normal or show airflow obstruction with or without increased lung volumes (22, 118, 120). In most patients, dyspnea and productive cough progressed slowly and culminated in severe obstructive lung disease, unresponsive to corticosteroid therapy (22, 79–118,120,122). In some, bronchial hyperreactivity also was present (119). Chest radiographs were normal or showed hyperinflation unless bronchiectasis was superimposed. Constrictive bronchiolitis was present histologically. Bronchograms in one patient confirmed varicose bronchiectasis with lack of distal filling (22).

Corticosteroids have not been helpful once airflow obstruction is established. Bronchiectasis should be treated using antibiotics guided by cultures; if airway hyperreactivity is present, bronchodilators and perhaps corticosteroids may be useful. Prevention consists of avoiding exposure to the concentrated gas.

AMMONIA

Ammonia is a lighter-than-air, hygroscopic, colorless gas with a distinctive, irritating odor. Ammonia can be detected at 53 ppm and has excellent warning properties; it is efficiently removed from inspired air by the upper airway (123). Exposure to 400 to 450 ppm may result in death within 30 minutes, and exposure to more than 5000 ppm may induce prompt respiratory arrest (124). Ammonia quickly hydrolyzes to ammonium hydroxide, generating hydroxyl ions; lipid membranes are saponified and proteins denatured, resulting in liquifaction necrosis of tissues (123,126).

Ammonia is extensively used as a liquid agricultural fertilizer, as a refrigerant, and in chemical processes. Exposures usually result from accidental release of the pressurized liquid but also may occur with prolonged exposure to lower concentrations of the gas. Several different clinical syndromes may result from ammonia exposure, and they differ depending on the type of exposure. When the liquid is sprayed onto the victim, severe corneal injury, skin burns, laryngospasm, and laryngeal edema requiring endotracheal intubation or tracheostomy may result, with no evidence of injury below the larynx (Fig. 10A) (124,125). When an individual cannot escape exposure and is forced to breathe concentrated ammonia gas deeply, pulmonary edema and extensive necrosis of the entire airway epithelium develop, forming necrotic psuedomembranes, which may slough and obstruct airways (Fig. 10B). Autopsies of patients dying soon after prolonged exposures show necrosis and desquamation of the tracheobronchial mucosa with hemorrhagic pulmonary edema (127). When sublethal concentrations are breathed over a longer interval, usually more than 30 minutes, eye and skin injuries are mild but bronchial and bronchiolar injury may ensue, with or without pulmonary edema (126,127). Pulmonary functions show an obstructive pattern accompanied by arterial hypoxemia.

Treatment of the acute phase often requires endotracheal intubation to facilitate access to obstructing pseudomembranes and to permit the application of positive airway pressure when pulmonary edema is present (126). Although immediate copious water irrigation of the skin and eye lesions is effective in limiting the severity of these injuries (123,124), the inhalation of ultrasonic mist or lung lavage for bronchopulmonary injury has not been described. Corticosteroids have been used but have not been evaluated systematically. Antibiotics are required for infections.

Over the next 2 to 6 months after injury, pulmonary function may return to normal (124,127), or obstructive airways disease may develop (126,128). In one patient who died from a secondary infection 2 months after exposure, bronchioles showed constrictive bronchiolitis with denudation of epithelium and focal peribronchiolar fibrosis; some bronchioles were obliterated by scar tissue; no intraluminal granulation tissue polyps were seen (129).

Pulmonary function tests performed more than 6 months after exposure have demonstrated decreases in vital capacity (79), 1-second forced vital capacity (127), and maximal voluntary ventilation and diffusing capacity (79). The histologic finding of constrictive bronchiolitis has been reported in only two patients, one at the time of autopsy and the other at the time of open-lung biopsy (129,130). Another patient is shown in Fig. 11.

Chest radiographs may be normal or may show hyperinflation or bronchiectasis (Fig. 10B, C) (129–131). Although corticosteroid therapy has been useful in limiting the se-

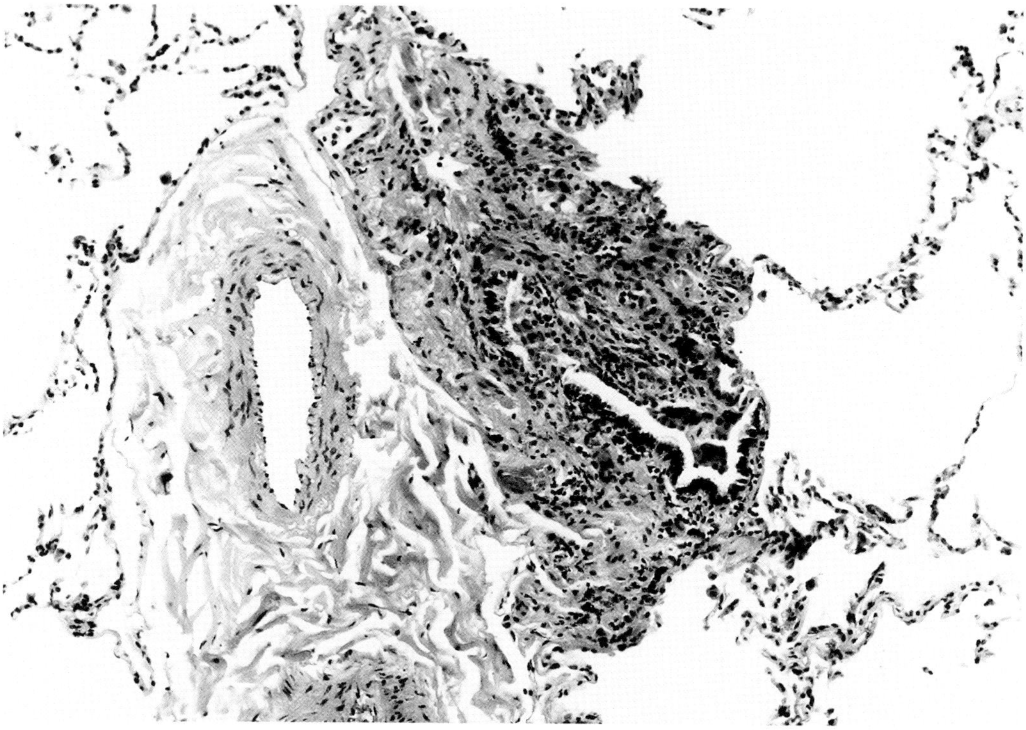

FIG. 11. Constrictive bronchiolitis due to ammonia inhalation. Pulmonary edema and bronchiolitis obliterans are more likely to occur after prolonged exposures to low concentrations of ammonia. A small bronchiole shows chronic inflammation and scarring in the walls with diminution in size of the lumen, which is partially filled with histiocytes. The pattern is that of chronic bronchiolitis consistent with constrictive bronchiolitis. The biopsy is from a patient with a history of ammonia exposure 19 years previously. An ammonia solution was poured on the floor, and he was locked in a sealed room as punishment at boot camp. He was hospitalized the next day with "pneumonia"; cough and dyspnea improved over the next several weeks but moderate exertional dyspnea persisted. He had smoked less than 1 pack year, alpha$_1$-antitrypsin values were normal, and a trial of corticosteroid therapy resulted in no improvement. Pulmonary functions were as follows, with normals in parentheses: TLC 7.92 (6.48), RV 3.32 (1.66), VC 4.59 (4.82), FEV_1 1.61 (3.93), FEF_{25-75} 0.4 (3.8), MVV 73 (163), D_LCO_{sb} 26 (32). (FEV_1, forced expired volume in one second; D_LCO_{sb}, carbon monoxide diffusing capacity of the lung, single breath method, ml/min/mm Hg). Courtesy of Drs. T. V. Colby and S. G. Peters.

verity of fibrosis and stricture formation in the esophagus after lye ingestion, similar therapy has usually been ineffective in improving late fixed airway obstruction after ammonia inhalation. The only prevention is avoidance of exposure.

METHYLISOCYANATE

Methylisocyanate caused bronchiolitis obliterans after the industrial accident in Bhopal, India, in 1984 (132). The agent is a colorless liquid that reacts with water in an exothermic reaction, forming a mixture of gases. Methylisocyanate is odorless; at 2 ppm irritation of the eyes, nose, and throat begins; exposure to 21 ppm is unbearable (132).

Bhopal survivors suffered severe skin and eye injuries acutely. Three months after injury most still complained of dyspnea, chest pains, and cough, which was usually productive (133,134); crackles or wheezes were often present. Chest radiographs showed hyperinflation or punctate and sometimes micronodular infiltrates, suggesting bronchiolar lesions (133,134). Pulmonary functions usually revealed a restrictive pattern, often with decreased flow at smaller lung volumes (133,134). Three open lung biopsies done 6 to 8 months after exposure were reported (132) to show interstitial fibrosis and an exudative reaction in terminal bronchioles with "bronchiolitis obliterans." However, five other biopsies revealed only pulmonary fibrosis (133).

FREE-BASE COCAINE

Classical bronchiolitis obliterans with intraluminal polyps has been described in one patient after intensive smoking of free-base cocaine (136). Dyspnea and fever were present, with crackles and decreased breath sounds. Chest radiographs demonstrated a miliary nodular pattern. Respiratory failure ensued; open-lung biopsy revealed classical bronchiolitis obliterans. Corticosteroid therapy resulted in dramatic improvement. Eighteen months later the patient had normal exercise tolerance and only mild airflow obstruction; the chest radiograph was normal. A similar case has been mentioned, but no further details were available (136); and it is not clear whether these cases are due to cocaine or to the combustion product (such as phosgene) of a solvent (such as trichloroethylene) used during refining.

CHLORINE AND OTHER IRRITANT GASES

Dozens of highly reactive compounds may result in acute pulmonary edema and bronchopulmonary injury with acute bronchiolitis, yet they have never been reported to result in clinical bronchiolitis obliterans with airflow obstruction. Chlorine is the most commonly encountered and best studied; other agents include hydrogen sulfide, phosphine, arsine, nickel carbonyl, ozone, hydrofluoric acid, hydrochloric acid, and acetaldehyde (16,137):

Chlorine is a heavier-than-air, greenish-yellow gas with a characteristic sharp, acrid odor that can be detected at 0.1 ppm, thus giving good warning properties. The TLV is 0.5 ppm; 1.0 ppm can result in mucosal irritation; 40 to 60 ppm is dangerous for short periods; and even brief exposure to 1,000 ppm is almost always lethal. At physiological pH on moist surfaces, chlorine is converted to hypochlorous acid, which diffuses into cells to react with the amino groups of cytoplasmic proteins, forming N-chloro derivatives (90).

Exposure to chlorine occurs after transportation accidents or leaks in paper mills, chlorine plants, and water purification or sewage treatment facilities. Chlorine also is produced when household hypochlorite bleach is mixed with weak acids such as sodium bisulfate or phosphoric acid (138,139). A related highly reactive compound, chloramine, is formed when hypochlorite bleach and ammonia are mixed (139,140).

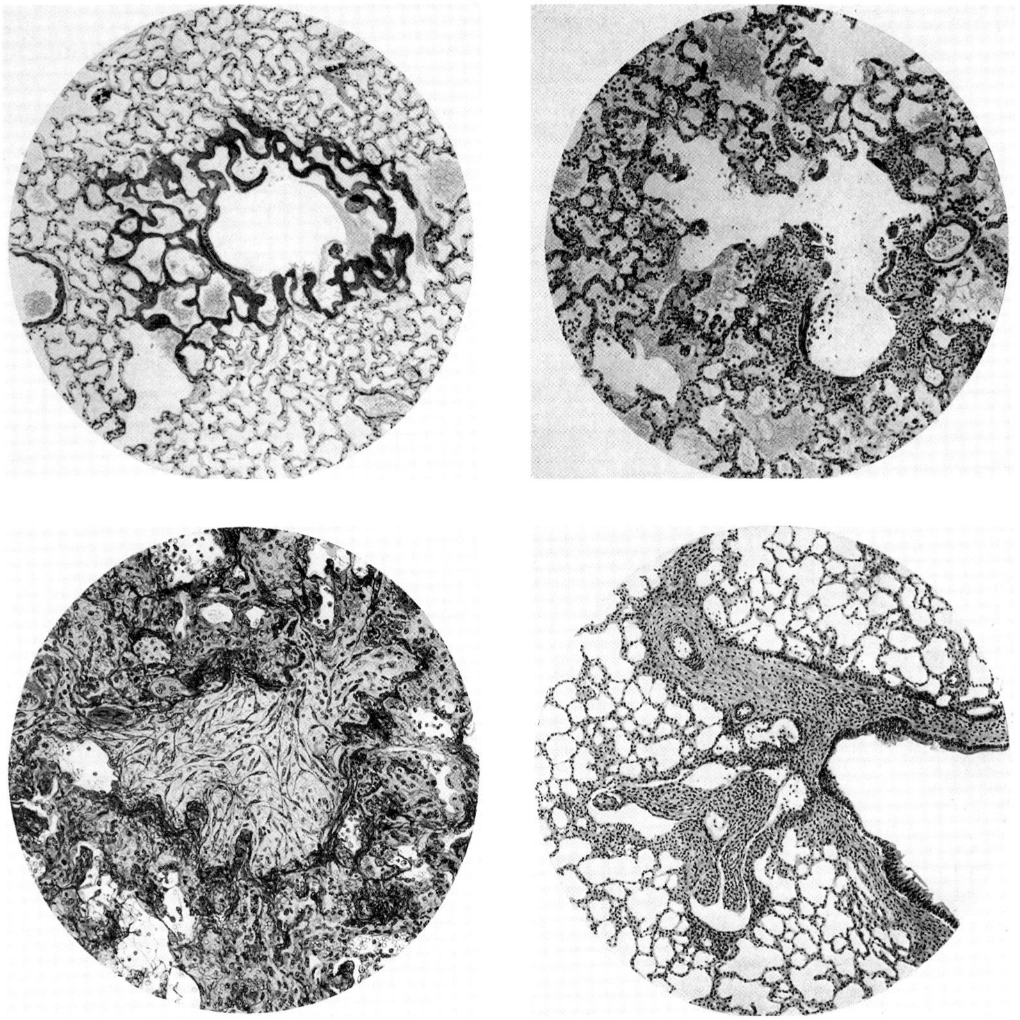

A B

C D

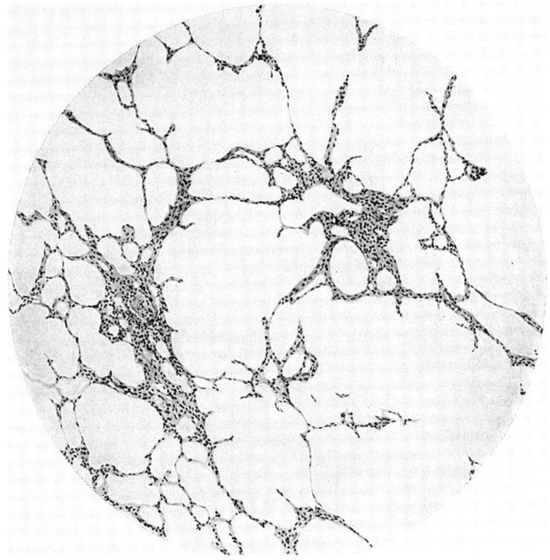

E

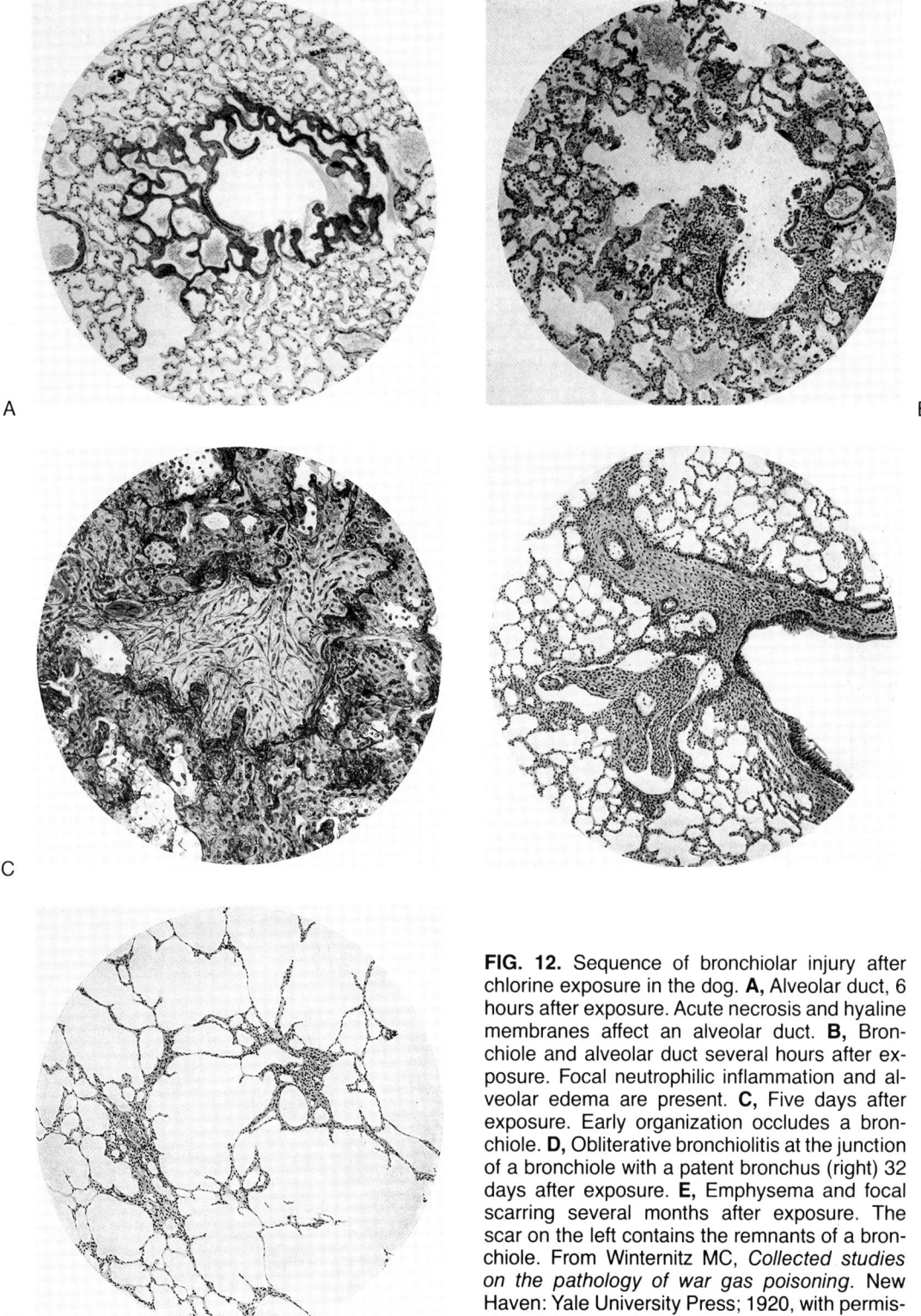

FIG. 12. Sequence of bronchiolar injury after chlorine exposure in the dog. **A,** Alveolar duct, 6 hours after exposure. Acute necrosis and hyaline membranes affect an alveolar duct. **B,** Bronchiole and alveolar duct several hours after exposure. Focal neutrophilic inflammation and alveolar edema are present. **C,** Five days after exposure. Early organization occludes a bronchiole. **D,** Obliterative bronchiolitis at the junction of a bronchiole with a patent bronchus (right) 32 days after exposure. **E,** Emphysema and focal scarring several months after exposure. The scar on the left contains the remnants of a bronchiole. From Winternitz MC, *Collected studies on the pathology of war gas poisoning.* New Haven: Yale University Press; 1920, with permission of the publisher.

Acute exposures to chlorine may cause immediate irritative effects on exposed mucous membranes; these have been reported to be relieved promptly by inhalation of a 3.75% sodium bicarbonate solution (141). Delayed-onset pulmonary edema may ensue several hours to days after exposure; the symptoms, findings, radiographic features, and treatment are identical to those described for nitrogen oxides and phosgene.

Winternitz's (104) study showed that dogs exposed to chlorine develop bronchiolar lesions (Fig. 12). In contrast to the injuries seen with phosgene, injury to the trachea and bronchi predominates, and the bronchiolar injury is more focal. Nevertheless, some bronchioles develop residual peribronchial fibrosis, and others are obliterated (Fig. 12D), forming fibrous scars (Fig. 12E). All references to bronchiolitis obliterans caused by chlorine refer only to this study.

Pulmonary function after chlorine-induced lung injury suggests an initial obstructive pattern with increased residual volume and arterial hypoxemia, which resolves quickly in those with only cough but more slowly in those who also have dyspnea (142). After the initial development of pulmonary edema, recovery proceeds slowly and may not be complete for 1 or 2 years (143–147), during which time the residual volume slowly decreases to normal, and even to subnormal values, suggesting stiffening of bronchioles by peribronchiolar fibrosis or parenchymal scarring (143). In most cases, the pulmonary function returns entirely to normal, suggesting that although some bronchioles may have been lost, the cumulative damage remains below the threshold required to cause symptoms or to be detectable by standard tests of pulmonary function (142–149). A few exceptions have been described, with expiratory flow obstruction (143,147), decreased maximal voluntary ventilation (144), and increased alveolar to arterial oxygen tension difference (144, 148).

BROMINE

Compared to chlorine, bromine is a more soluble halogen and causes a more severe and deeper injury to mucosal surfaces. In experimental animals, bronchiolar spasm, delayed-onset pneumonitis, and peribronchiolar abscesses are found (150). One patient was reported (151) to have developed delayed-onset bilateral pneumonitis after exposure, followed by relapsing migratory pulmonary infiltrates similar to those seen in idiopathic BOOP; no biopsy was done, but bronchiolitis obliterans was suggested as the most likely cause.

FIRE SMOKE

Smoke inhalation and the respiratory complications of burns have been reviewed in several reports (152–157). To summarize, bronchiolar and acinar injury are due to the toxic components in smoke, including irritant gases and particulates with adsorbed toxins. Thermal injury is limited to the upper airway to subglottic level unless steam is inhaled. The asphyxiants carbon monoxide and cyanide cause most of the immediate deaths but do not cause direct bronchiolar injury. Irritants that have been suspected to be the cause of bronchiolar injury include acrolein, ammonia, nitrogen oxides, sulfur dioxide, chlorine, isocyanates, hydrochloric acid, hydrofluoric acid, and bromine.

Acrolein is an extremely irritating, unsaturated aldehyde, which in dogs causes bronchiolar mucosal injury with desquamation, together with edema that originates more from the bronchial circulation than from the pulmonary circulation (7). Acrolein is present in fires that consume wood, petroleum products, paper, or cotton, and was the only toxic agent other than carbon monoxide found in toxic concentration in one series of fires (158). Hydrochloric acid also is commonly present in fire smoke (159), but even when adsorbed onto smoke particles and inhaled by dogs, produces coagulation necrosis of the epithelium of proximal airways, leaving bronchioles relatively uninjured (7).

In some fires, other irritants may include the following agents: phosgene from halogenated hydrocarbons or polyvinyl chloride; ammonia from wool, silk, nylon, polyurethane, or melamine resins; nitrogen oxides from nitrocellulose, fertilizer, shoe polish, and some plastics; sulfur dioxide from rubber products, including tires; chlorine from halogenated hydrocarbons and polyurethane foams; isocyanates from polyurethane and some paints or packaging materials; hydrofluoric acid from Teflons; and bromine from fire-retardant materials used in foams and fabrics (160,161).

Smoke is composed primarily of carbon particles of 0.1 to 0.5 μm (161) that deposit on the walls of small bronchioles in victims of smoke inhalation (161,162). Smoke particles not only carry adsorbed irritants but also transport short-lived oxidant radicals (161), and in aircraft fires also carry fine metallic particles derived from the skin of the aircraft (162).

Respiratory injury after smoke inhalation usually follows a sequence of immediate symptoms due to asphyxiants or thermal injury to the upper airway, followed 2 to 5 days later by delayed-onset pulmonary edema, and thereafter by infection (154–157).

Histologically proven bronchiolar lesions after exposure to fire smoke have been reported only twice. One patient had progressive cough, dyspnea, and fever after exposure to smoke from a burning automobile. The chest radiograph showed miliary infiltrates; open-lung biopsy at 10 days showed classical bronchiolitis obliterans with intraluminal polyps. Corticosteroid therapy was given for 6 months, and gradual improvement was noted. At 21 months, only mild airflow obstruction and arterial hypoxemia were found, and symptoms were only those of bronchial hyperreactivity to irritants (163). The second patient became dyspneic 2 months after exposure to smoke while fighting a fire in a plastics factory. Dyspnea progressed relentlessly despite therapy with corticosteroids, azothioprine, and bronchodilators; he died 31 months after exposure with a nocardial brain abscess. Open-lung biopsy at 5 months showed several obliterated bronchioles (constrictive bronchiolitis); autopsy disclosed mild chronic bronchiolitis and emphysema (164). A similar case is shown in Fig. 13.

Bronchiectasis is occasionally seen after smoke inhalation (165–167); and in one pa-

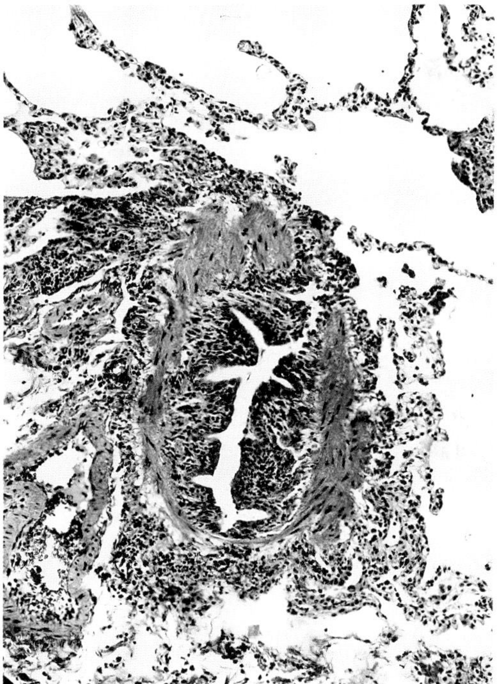

FIG. 13. Constrictive bronchiolitis following exposure to fire smoke. The patient inhaled smoke at the MGM Grand fire in Las Vegas and subsequently suffered severe respiratory disease with chronic obstruction. A membranous bronchiole shows luminal narrowing due to submucosal fibrosis and chronic inflammation and smooth-muscle hypertrophy. There is slight involvement of the peribronchiolar alveoli. The pattern is that of constrictive bronchiolitis. Courtesy of Dr. T. V. Colby.

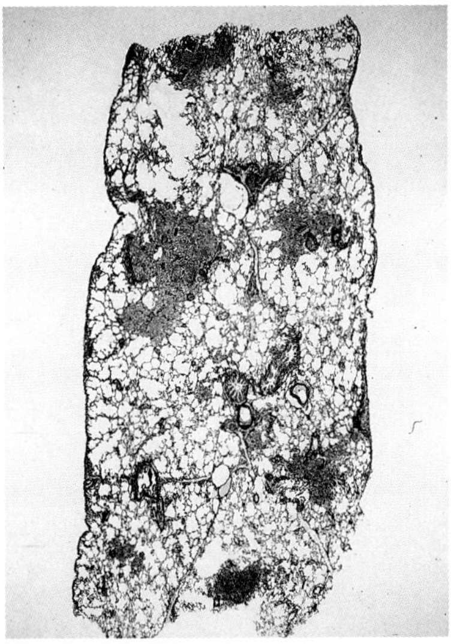

FIG. 14. 52-year-old male truck driver exposed to smoke in a house fire 22 days before open-lung biopsy. He had developed an increase in the severity of his usual cough, and his chest radiograph showed a diffuse interstitial nodular pattern. He had smoked 60 pack years prior to exposure. Preoperative pulmonary function tests were normal except for a diffusing capacity 61% predicted normal and arterial oxygen tension of 60 mm Hg. His cough improved on corticosteroid therapy. The open-lung biopsy shows nodular inflammation centered on bronchioles. From the collection of Dr. C. B. Carrington; courtesy of Dr. T. V. Colby.

tient (167), the bronchogram demonstrated absence of filling of peripheral airways by contrast material, which was ascribed to bronchiolitis obliterans (constrictive bronchiolitis). The patient progressively deteriorated and died; no autopsy was performed.

The recovery of most survivors of smoke inhalation is uneventful (168–170); some complain of dyspnea, cough, and hoarseness (170) (Fig. 14). Bronchial hyperreactivity may be present (171). In one series (172) of 54 fire fighters, smoking seemed more predictive for evidence of small airways dysfunction than did fire fighting and exposure to smoke, but one patient had severe obstructive impairment that was still present 2 ½ years after an unusually severe exposure.

Corticosteroid therapy has not improved survival during the acute phase of smoke inhalation (173) and was ineffective in the one reported patient with constrictive bronchiolitis, but it was effective in the patient with classical bronchiolitis obliterans with intraluminal polyps (163). A controlled trial evaluating the effect on late pulmonary function has not been described. Antibiotics usually are required, guided by cultures. Bronchodilators and aerosolized corticosteroid therapy may be useful when bronchial hyperreactivity is present.

ACKNOWLEDGMENTS

The authors thank Drs. A. H. Limper and P. D. Scanlon for reviewing the manuscript and offering helpful suggestions, Mr. Robert Benassi for drawing the silo diagrams, Dr. John J. May for permission to include his patient in the figures, and Mrs. Deanna Lichty for typing the manuscript.

REFERENCES

1. Gosink BB, Friedman PJ, Liebow AA. Bronchiolitis obliterans: roentenologic-pathologic correlation. *Am J Roentgenol Radium Ther Nucl Med* 1973;117:816–832.
2. Epler GR, Colby TV, McLoud TC, Carrington CB, Gaensler EA. Bronchiolitis obliterans organizing pneumonia. *N Engl J Med* 1985;312: 152–158.
3. Wright JL, Cagle P, Churg A, Colby TV, Myers J. Diseases of the small airways. *Am Rev Respir Dis* 1992;146:240–262.
4. Penington AH. War gases and chronic lung disease. *Med J Aust* 1954;1:510–516.
5. Kindt GC, Weiland JE, Davis WB, Gadek JE, Dorinsky PM. Bronchiolitis in adults. *Am Rev Respir Dis* 1989;140:483–492.
6. Man SFP, Hulbert WC. Airway repair and adaptation to inhalation injury. In: Loke J, ed. *Pathophysiology and treatment of inhalation injuries*. New York: Marcel Dekker; 1988: 1–47.
7. Hales CA, Barkin PW, Jung W, et al. Synthetic smoke with acrolein but not HC1 produces pulmonary edema. *J Appl Physiol* 1988;64:1121–1133.
8. Ingram PR, Keswani RK, Muller WH. A correlative histopathologic study of experimental surgical reflux esophagitis. *Surg Gynecol Obstet* 1960;111:403–411.
9. Johnson EE. A study of corrosive esophagitis. *Laryngoscope* 1963;73:1651–1696.
10. Roman JR, McDonald JA. Cellular processes in lung repair. *Chest* 1991;100:245–248.
11. Roman JR, Limper AH, McDonald JA. Lung extracellular matrix: physiology and pathophysiology. *Hosp Pract* 1990;125–140.
12. Kuhn C, Boldt J, King TE, Crouch EC, Vartio T, McDonald JA. An immunohistochemical study of architectural remodeling and connective tissue synthesis in pulmonary fibrosis. *Am Rev Respir Dis* 1989;140:1693–1703.
13. Myers JL, Katzenstein A-LA. Ultrastructual evidence of alveolar epithelial injury in idiopathic bronchiolitis obliterans organizing pneumonia. *Am J Pathol* 1988;132:102–109.
14. Basset F, Ferrans VJ, Soler P, Takemura T, Fukuda Y, Crystal RG. Intraluminal fibrosis in interstitial lung disorders. *Am J Pathol* 1986; 122:443–461.
15. Summer W, Haponik E. Inhalation of irritant gases. *Clin Chest Med* 1981;2:273–287.
16. Parkes WR. Non-neoplastic disorders due to metallic, chemical, and physical agents. In: *Occupational lung disorders*. 2nd ed. Boston: Butterworths; 1982:454–498.
17. Seaton A, Seaton D, Leitch AG. Occupational lung diseases. In: *Crofton and Douglas's respiratory diseases*. 4th ed. Oxford: Blackwell Scientific Publications; 1989:834–838.
18. Utell MJ. Acute and accidental inhalation injuries; diagnosis and management in the intensive care unit. In: MacDonnell KF, Fahey PJ, Segal MS, eds. *Respiratory intensive care*. Boston: Little, Brown; 1987:510–515.
19. Corwin RW, Canada AT, Irwin RS. Toxic gas, fume, and smoke inhalation. In: Rippe JM, Irwin RS, Alpert JS, Dalen JE, eds. *Intensive care medicine*. Boston: Little, Brown; 1985: 510–515.
20. Sheppard D. Noxious gases: pathogenetic mechanisms. In: Baum GL, Wolinsky E, eds. *Textbook of pulmonary diseases*. 4th ed. Boston: Little, Brown; 1989:831–846.
21. Graham DR. Noxious gases: clinical aspects. In: Baum GL, Wolinsky E, eds. *Textbook of pulmonary diseases*. 4th ed. Boston: Little, Brown; 1989:847–859.
22. Bates DV, Macklem PT, Christie RV. *Respiratory function in disease*. Philadelphia: WB Saunders; 1971:389–398.
23. Bates DV. *Respiratory function in disease*. 3rd ed. Philadelphia: WB Saunders; 1989:322–330.
24. Schwartz DA. Acute inhalational injury. *Occup Med* 1987;2:297–318.
25. Schwartz LW. Pulmonary responses to inhaled irritants and the morphological evaluation of those responses. In: Salem H, ed. *Inhalation toxicology*. New York: Marcel Dekker; 1987: 293–348.(Occupational safety and health: vol 12).
26. Overton JH, Miller FJ. Absorption of inhaled reactive gases. In: Gardner DE, Crapo JD, Massaro EJ, eds. *Toxicology of the lung*. New York: Raven Press; 1988:477–507. (*Target organ toxicology series*).
27. Von Oettingen WF. The toxicity and potential danger of nitrous fumes. *US public health bulletin*. No 272. Washington DC: US Government Printing Office; 1941:1–34.
28. Douglas WW, Hepper NGG. Silo-filler's disease. *Curr Ther Respir Dis* 1989;3:207–211.
29. Fraenkel A. Ueber bronchiolitis fibrosa obliterans, nebst bemerkungen über lungenhyperäemie und indurirende pneumonie. *Dtsch Arch Klin Med* 1902;73:484–510.
30. Wagner JH. Bronchiolitis obliterans following the inhalation of acrid fumes. *Am J Med Sci* 1917;154:511–522.
31. McAdams AJ. Bronchiolitis obliterans. *Am J Med* 1955;19:314–322.
32. Nichols BH. The clinical effects of the inhalation of nitrogen dioxide. *Am J Roentgenol* 1930;23:314–322.
33. Lowry T, Schuman LM. "Silo-filler's disease": a syndrome caused by nitrogen dioxide. *JAMA* 1956;162:153–160.
34. Beining H. Tödliche bronchopneumonie infolge vergiftung mit nitrosen gasen. *Röntgenpraxis* 1935;7:534–541.
35. Darke CS, Warrack AJN. Bronchiolitis from nitrous fumes. *Thorax* 1958;13:327–333.
36. Doub HP. Pulmonary changes from the inhalation of noxious gases. *Radiology* 1933;21:105–113.
37. Rigner KG, Swensson A. The late prognosis of nitrous fume poisoning: a follow-up study. *Acta Med Scand* 1961;170:291–299.

38. Schultz-Brauns O. Die tödlichen vergiftungen durch gasförmige stickoxyde (nitrose-gase) beim arbeiten mit saltpetersäure. *Virchows Arch* [*A*] 1930;277:174–220.
39. Clutton-Brock J. Two cases of poisoning by contamination of nitrous oxide with higher oxides of nitrogen during anesthesia. *Br J Anaesth* 1967;39:388–392.
40. Booth FJ. Cases of lung injury following exposure to blast and nitrous fumes. *Aust NZ J Surg* 1942;12:72–73.
41. Franke H, Krauland W, Ruckensteiner E. Vergiftungen durch nitrose gase aus sprengbomben. *Schweiz Med Wochenschr* 1948;78:256–260.
42. Charleroy DK. Nitrous and nitric gas casualties. *US Navy Med Bull* 1945;44:435–437.
43. Becklake MR, Goldman HI, Bosman AR, Freed CC. The long-term effects of exposure to nitrous fumes. *Am Rev Tuberc* 1957;76:398–409.
44. Müller B. Nitrogen dioxide intoxication after a mining accident. *Respiration* 1969;26:249–261.
45. Kronenberger FL. Bronchiolitis after shot-firing in a colliery. *Br J Dis Chest* 1959;53:308–313.
46. Yockey CC, Eden BM, Byrd RB. The McConnell missile accident: clinical spectrum of nitrogen dioxide exposure. *JAMA* 1980;244:1221–1223.
47. Hatton DV, Leach CS, Nicogossian AE, DiFerrante N. Collagen breakdown and nitrogen dioxide inhalation. *Arch Environ Health* 1977;32:33–36.
48. Gregory KL, Malinoski VF, Sharp CR. Cleveland Clinical fire survivorship study, 1929–1965. *Arch Environ Health* 1969;18:508–515.
49. LaFleche LR, Boivin C, Leonard C. Nitrogen dioxide: a respiratory irritant. *Can Med Assoc J* 1961;84:1438–1443.
50. Lindqvist T. Nitrous gas poisoning among welders using acetylene flame. *Acta Med Scand* 1944;118:210–243.
51. Norwood WD, Wisehart DE, Earl CA, Adley FE, Anderson DE. Nitrogen dioxide poisoning due to metal cutting with oxyacetylene torch. *J Occup Med* 1966;8:301–306.
52. Renander A. Roentgenological changes in the lungs caused by acetylene gas. *Acta Radiol* 1937;18:688–692.
53. Jones GR, Proudfoot AT, Hall JI. Pulmonary effects of acute exposure to nitrous fumes. *Thorax* 1973;28:61–65.
54. Camiel MR, Berkan HS. Inhalation pneumonia from nitric fumes. *Radiology* 1944;42:175–182.
55. Williman FL. Electric welding. II: An acute fatal pneumonia following electric welding of galvanized iron in an enclosed space. J Indust Hyg 1935;17:129–137.
56. Hayhurst ER, Scott E. Four cases of sudden death in a silo. *JAMA* 1914;63:1570–1572.
57. Delaney LT Jr, Schmidt HW, Stroebel CF. Silo-filler's disease. *Proc Mayo Clin* 1956;31:189–198.
58. Grayson RR. Silage gas poisoning: nitrogen dioxide pneumonia, a new disease in agricultural workers. *Ann Intern Med* 1956;45:393–408.
59. Ramirez-R J, Dowell AR. Silo-filler's disease: nitrogen dioxide-induced lung injury; long-term follow-up and review of the literature. *Ann Intern Med* 1971;74:569–576.
60. Horvath EP, doPico GA, Barbee RA, Dickie HA. Nitrogen dioxide-induced pulmonary disease. *J Occup Med* 1978;20:103–110.
61. Fleetham JA, Munt PW, Tunnicliffe BW. Silo-filler's disease. *Can Med Assoc J* 1978;119:482–484.
62. Cornelius EA, Betlach EH. Silo-filler's disease. *Radiology* 1960;74:232–238.
63. Moskowitz RL, Lyons HA, Cottle HR. Silo-filler's disease: clinical, physiologic, and pathologic study of a patient. *Am J Med* 1964;36:457–462.
64. McCabe WO Jr. Silo-filler's disease. *Va Med Mon* 1972;99:859–863.
65. Scott EG, Hunt WB Jr. Silo-filler's disease. *Chest* 1973;63:701–706.
66. Maurer WJ. Silo-filler's disease: a historical perspective and report of a case. *Wis Med J* 1985;84:13–16.
67. Centers for Disease Control. Silo-filler's disease in rural New York. *MMWR* 1982;31:389–391.
68. Gailitis J, Burns LE, Nally JB. Silo-fillers disease: report of a case. *N Engl J Med* 1958;258:543–544.
69. Rafii S, Godwin MC. Silo-filler's disease: relapse following latent period. *Arch Pathol* 1961;72:424–433.
70. Douglas WW, Hepper NGG, Colby TV. Silo-filler's disease. *Mayo Clin Proc* 1989;64:291–304.
71. Zwemer FL, Pratt DS, May JJ. Silo-filler's disease in New York State. *Am Rev Respir Dis* 1992;146:650–653.
72. Daunderer M. Antidottherapie bei massenvergiftungen. *Dtsch Apotheker Zeitung* 1982;122:1959–1963.
73. Edens. Über bronchiolitis obliterans. *Dtsch Arch Klin Med* 1906;85:598–617.
74. Chaumont MAJ. Le Danger des vapeurs nitreuses: a propos de 2 cas mortels. *Arch Mal Profes* 1954;15:63–64.
75. Tse RL, Bockman AA. Nitrogen dioxide toxicity: report of four cases in firemen. *JAMA* 1970;212:1341–1344.
76. Milne JEH. Nitrogen dioxide inhalation and bronchiolitis obliterans. *J Occup Med* 1969;11:538–543.
77. Woie L. Silo-filler's disease. *Tidsskr Nor Laegeforen* 1971;91:1751–1752.
78. Roche L, Nicholas A, Marin A. Pneumopathies par vapeurs nitreuses. *Rev Lyonnaise Med* 1957;6:147–158.
79. LePine C, Soucy R. Le bronchopneumopathie d'origine toxique. *Union Med Can* 1962;91:7–11.
80. Van Mechelen J, Prignot J. Intoxication collec-

tive aux vapeurs rutilantes. *Acta Tuberc Belg* 1965;1:68–79.
81. Fleming GM, Chester EH, Montenegro HD. Dysfunction of small airways following pulmonary injury to nitrogen dioxide. *Chest* 1979; 75:720–721.
82. Roche L, Marin A, Nicholas A. Les pneumopathies par vapeurs nitreuses. *Arch Mal Profes* 1957;18:20–21.
83. Leib GM, Davis WN, Brown T, McQuiggan M. Chronic pulmonary insufficiency secondary to silo-filler's disease. *Am J Med* 1958;24:471–474.
84. Schell NW. Chronic silo-filler's disease. *Conn Med J* 1958;22:546–552.
85. Morrisey WL, Gould IA, Carrington CB, Gaensler EA. Silo-fillers disease. *Respiration* 1975;32:81–92.
86. Brooks SM, Weiss MA, Bernstein IL. Reactive airways dysfunction syndrome: persistent asthma after high level irritant exposures. *Chest* 1985;88:376–384.
87. Adelheim R. Contributions to the pathological anatomy and pathogenesis of war gas poisoning. *Virchows Arch [A]* 1922;236:309–360.
88. Gross P, Rinehart WE, Hatch T. Chronic pneumonitis caused by phosgene. *Arch Environ Health* 1965;10:768–775.
89. Moran TJ, Hellstrom HR. Bronchiolitis obliterans: an experimental study of the pathogenesis and the use of cortisone in modification of the lesions. *AMA Arch Pathol* 1958;66:691–707.
90. Urbanetti JS. Battlefield chemical inhalation injury. In: Loke J, ed. *Pathophysiology and treatment of inhalation injuries*. New York: Marcel Dekker; 1988:281–348.
91. Groll H. Anatomische befunde bei vergiftungen mit phosgen (Kampfgasvergiftungen). *Virchows Arch [A]* 1921;231:480–518.
92. Galdston M, Luetscher JA Jr, Longcope WT, et al. A study of the residual effects of phosgene poisoning in human subjects. I: After acute exposure. *J Clin Invest* 1946;26:145–181.
93. Génevois M, Marin A. Pneumopathies par phosgene dans le travail exposant au trichloroéthylène. *Arch Mal Profes* 1956;307–308.
94. La Due JS. Bronchiolitis fibrosa obliterans. *Arch Int Med* 1941;68:663–673.
95. Hughes JP. Hazardous exposure to some so-called safe solvents. *JAMA* 1954;156:234–237.
96. Buie SE, Pratt DS, May JJ. Diffuse pulmonary injury following paint remover exposure. *Am J Med* 1986;81:702–704.
97. Gerritsen WB, Buschmann CH. Phosgene poisoning caused by the use of chemical paint removers containing methylene chloride in ill-ventilated rooms heated by kerosene stoves. *Br J Ind Med* 1960;17:187–189.
98. Spolyar LW, Harger RN, Keppler JF, Bumsted HE. Generation of phosgene during operation of a trichloroethylene degreaser. *AMA Arch Indust Hyg* 1951;4:156–160.
99. Snyder RW, Mishel HS, Christensen GC. Pulmonary toxicity following exposure to methylene chloride and its combustion product, phosgene. *Chest* 1992;101:860–861.
100. Sjogren B, Plato N, Alexandersson R, Eklund A, Falkenberg C. Pulmonary reactions caused by welding-induced decomposed trichloroethylene. *Chest* 1991;99:237–238.
101. Conner EH, DuBois AB, Comroe JH. Acute chemical injury of the airway and lungs: experience with six cases. *Anesthesiology* 1962; 23:538–547.
102. Wohlwill F. Ueber eine massenvergiftung durch phosgengas in Hamburg: zur pathologischen anatomie der phosgenvergiftung. *Dtsche Med Wochenschr* 1928;54:1553–1557.
103. Miller JW. Über die pathologische anatomie des spättoder nach kampf gas (Perstoff) vergiftung. *Beitr Pathol Anat Allg Pathol* 1923–1924;72:339–343.
104. Winternitz MC. *Collected studies in pathology of war gas poisoning*. New Haven: Yale University Press; 1920.
105. Durlacher SH, Bunting H. Pulmonary changes following exposure to phosgene. *Am J Pathol* 1947;23:679–693.
106. Coman DR, Bruner HD, Horn RC, et al. Studies on experimental phosgene poisoning. I: The pathologic anatomy of phosgene poisoning, with special reference to the early and late phase. *Am J Pathol* 1947;23:1037–1073.
107. Clay JR, Rossing RG. Histopathology of exposure to phosgene: an attempt to produce emphysema experimentally. *Arch Pathol* 1964; 78:544–551.
108. Roche L, Grunwald E, Rouanet J. Emphysème professionnel dû à l'ypérite. *Arch Mal Profes* 1957;18:339–342.
109. Lane RE, Campbell ACP. Fatal emphysema in two men making a copper cadmium alloy. *Br J Ind Med* 1954;11:118–122.
110. Bonnell JA. Emphysema and proteinuria in men casting copper cadmium alloys. *Br J Ind Med* 1955;12:181–195.
111. Snider GL, Hayes JA, Korthy AL, Lewis GP. Centrilobular emphysema experimentally induced by a cadmium chloride aerosol. *Am Rev Respir Dis* 1973;108:40–48.
112. Smith WJ, Dunn MA. Medical defense against blistering chemical warfare agents. *Arch Dermatol* 1991;127:1207–1213.
113. Eisenmenger W, Drasch G, von Clarmann M, Kretschmer E, Roider G. Clinical and morphological findings on mustard gas [bis (2-chloroethyl) sulfide] poisoning. *J Forensic Sci* 1991; 36:1688–1698.
114. Alexander SF. Medical report on the Bari harbor mustard casualties. *Milit Surg* 1947;101:1–17.
115. Infield G. *Disaster at Bari*. New York: Bantam Books; 1971.
116. Ducatman AM, Ducatman BS, Barnes JA. Lithium battery hazard: old-fashioned planning implications of a new technology. *J Occup Med* 1988;30:309–311.
117. Sheppard D. Mechanisms of airway responses to inhaled sulfur dioxide. In: Loke J, ed.

Pathophysiology and treatment of inhalation injuries. New York: Marcel Dekker; 1988:49–65.
118. Woodford DM, Coutu RE, Gaensler EA. Obstructive lung disease from acute sulfur dioxide exposure. *Respiration* 1979;38:238–245.
119. Härkönen H, Nordman H, Korhonen O, Winblad I. Long-term effects of exposure to sulfur dioxide: lung function four years after a pyrite dust explosion. *Am Rev Respir Dis* 1983; 128:890–893.
120. Charan NB, Myers CG, Lakshminarayan S, Spencer TM. Pulmonary injuries associated with acute sulfur dioxide inhalation. *Am Rev Respir Dis* 1979;119:555–560.
121. Galea M. Fatal sulfur dioxide inhalation. *Can Med Assoc J* 1964;91:345–347.
122. Prügger F. Ein fall von sublethaler, akuter schwefeldioxydvergiftung und deren folgeerscheinungen auf die lungenfunktion. *Pneumonologie* 1974;150:97–98.
123. Millea TP, Kucan JO, Smoot EC. Anhydrous ammonia injuries. *J Burn Care Rehabil* 1989; 10:448–53.
124. Helmers S, Top FH, Knapp LW. Ammonia injuries in agriculture. *J Iowa Med Soc* 1971; 61:271–290.
125. Close LG, Catlin FI, Cohn AM. Acute and chronic effects of ammonia burns of the respiratory tract. *Arch Otolaryngol* 1980;106:151–158.
126. Levy DM, Divertie MB, Litzow TS, Henderson JW. Ammonia burns of the face and respiratory tract. *J Am Med Assoc* 1964;190:90–98.
127. Walton M. Industrial ammonia gassing. *Br J Ind Med* 1973;30:78–86.
128. Brille MD, Hatzfeld C, Laurent MR. Emphysème pulmonaire après inhalation de vapeurs irritants (Ammoniaque en particulier). *Arch Mal Profes* 1957;18:320–326.
129. Sobonya R. Fatal anhydrous ammonia inhalation. *Hum Pathol* 1977;8:293–299.
130. Kass I, Zamel N, Dobry CA, Holzer M. Bronchiectasis following ammonia burns of the respiratory tract: a review of two cases. *Chest* 1972;62:282–285.
131. Sestier F, Bernier J, Charbonneau R. Bronchopneumopathie d'origine toxique par inhalation de vapeurs ammoniacales. *Union Med Can* 1969;98:1903–1910.
132. Mehta PS, Mehta AS, Mehta SJ, Makhijani AB. Bhopal tragedy's health effects: A review of methyl isocyanate toxicity. *JAMA* 1990; 264:2781–2787.
133. Kamat SR, Mahasur AA, Tiwari AKB, et al. Early observations on the pulmonary changes and clinical morbidity due to the isocyanate gas leak at Bhopal. *J Postgrad Med* 1985;31:63–72.
134. Naik SR, Acharya VN, Bhalerao RA, et al. Medical survey of methyl isocyanate gas affected population of Bhopal. *J Postgrad Med* 1986;32:185–191.
135. Patel RC, Dutta D, Schonfeld SA. Free-base cocaine use associated with bronchiolitis obliterans organizing pneumonia. *Ann Intern Med* 1987;107:186–187.
136. Glassroth J, Adams GD, Schnoll S. The impact of substance abuse on the respiratory system. *Chest* 1987;91:596–602.
137. Skornik WA. Inhalation toxicity of metal particles and vapors. In: Loke J, ed. *Pathophysiology and treatment of inhalation injuries*. New York: Marcel Dekker; 1988:123–186.
138. Murphy DMF, Fairman RP, Lapp NL, Morgan WKC. Severe airway disease due to inhalation of fumes from cleansing agents. *Chest* 1976; 69:372–376.
139. Chlorine gas toxicity from mixture of bleach with other cleaning products: California. *MMWR* 1991;40:619–629.
140. Gapany-Gapanavicius M, Malho M, Tirosh M. Chloramine-induced pneumonitis from mixing household cleaning agents. *Br Med J* 1982; 285:1086.
141. Vinsel PJ. Treatment of acute chlorine gas inhalation with nebulized sodium bicarbonate. *J Emerg Med* 1990;8:327–329.
142. Hasan FM, Gehshan A, Fuliehan FJD. Resolution of pulmonary dysfunction following acute chlorine exposure. *Arch Environ Health* 1983; 38:76–80.
143. Charan NB, Lakshminarayan S, Myers GC, Smith DD. Effects of accidental chlorine inhalation on pulmonary function. *West J Med* 1985;143:333–336.
144. Kaufman J, Burkons D. Clinical, roentgenologic, and physiologic effects of acute chlorine exposure. *Arch Environ Health 1971;23:29–34.*
145. Beach FXM, Jones E, Scarrow GD. Respiratory effects of chlorine gas. *Br J Ind Med* 1969;26:231–236.
146. Kowitz TA, Reba RC, Parker RT, Spicer WS. Effects of chlorine gas on respiratory function. *Arch Environ Health* 1967;14:545–558.
147. Ploysongsang Y, Beach BC, DiLisio RE. Pulmonary function changes after acute inhalation of chlorine gas. *South Med J* 1982;75:23–26.
148. Chester EH, Kaimal PJ, Payne CB, Kohn PM. Pulmonary injury following exposure to chlorine gas. *Chest* 1977;72:247–250.
149. Jones RN, Hughes JM, Glindmeyer H, Weill H. Lung function after acute exposure. *Am Rev Respir Dis* 1986;134:1190–1196.
150. Schlagbauer M, Henschler D. Toxicicät von chlor und brom bei einmaliger und wiederholter inhalation. *Int Arch Gewerbepath* 1967;23:91–98.
151. Kraut A, Lilis R. Chemical pneumonitis due to exposure to bromine compounds. *Chest* 1988; 94:208–210.
152. Crapo RO. Smoke-inhalation injuries. *JAMA* 1981;246:1694–1696.
153. Fein A, Leff A, Hopewell PC. Pathophysiology and management of the complications resulting from fire and the inhaled products of combustion. *Crit Care Med* 1980;8:94–98.
154. Loke J, Matthay RA, Smith GJW. The toxic environment and its medical implications with

special emphasis on smoke inhalation. In: Loke J, ed. *Pathophysiology and treatment of inhalation injuries*. New York: Marcel Dekker; 1988:453–504.
155. Shirani KZ, Moylan JA, Pruitt BA. Diagnosis and treatment of inhalation injury in burn patients. In: Loke J, ed. *Pathophysiology and treatment of inhalation injuries*. New York: Marcel Dekker; 1988:239–279.
156. Pruitt BA, Flemma RJ, DiVincenti FC, Foley FD, Mason AD. Pulmonary complications in burn patients: a comparative study in 697 patients. *J Thorac Cardiovasc Surg* 1970;59:7–18.
157. Herndon DN, Barrow RE, Linares HA, et al. Inhalation injury in burn patients: effects and treatment. *Burns* 1988;14:349–356.
158. Treitman RD, Burgess WA, Gold A. Air contaminants encountered by fire fighters. *Am Ind Hyg Assoc J* 1980;41:796–802.
159. Dyer RF, Esch VH. Polyvinyl chloride toxicity in firefighters. *JAMA* 1976;235:393–397.
160. Levin BC. A summary of the NBS literature reviews on the chemical nature and toxicity of the pyrolysis and combustion products from seven plastics: acrylonitrile-butadiene-styrenes (ABS), nylons, polyesters, polyethylenes, polystyrenes, poly (vinyl chlorides) and rigid polyurethane foams. *Fire and Materials* 1987;11: 143–157.
161. Einhorn IN. Physiological and toxicological aspects of smoke produced during the combustion of polymeric materials. *Environ Health Perspect* 1975;11:163–189.
162. Mitchelson BP. The electron energy-loss spectroscopic analysis of inhaled smoke particles. *J Microsc* 1992;166:381–387.
163. Arora NS, Aldrich TK. Bronchiolitis obliterans from a burning automobile. *South Med J* 1980; 73:507–510.
164. Seggev JS, Mason UG, Worthen S, Stanford RE, Fernandez E. Bronchiolitis obliterans: report of three cases with detailed physiologic studies. *Chest* 1983;83:169–174.
165. Slutzker AD, Kinn R, Said SI. Bronchiectasis and progressive respiratory failure following smoke inhalation. *Chest* 1989;95:1349–1950.
166. Donnellan WL, Poticha SM, Holinger PH. Management and complications of severe pulmonary burn. *JAMA* 1965;194:1323–1325.
167. Perez-Guerra F, Walsh RE, Sagel SS. Bronchiolitis obliterans and tracheal stenosis: late complications of inhalation burn. *JAMA* 1971; 21:1568–1570.
168. Whitener DR, Whitener LM, Robertson KJ, Baxter CR, Pierce AK. Pulmonary function measurements in patients with thermal injury and smoke inhalation. *Am Rev Respir Dis* 1980;122:731–739.
169. Morris AH, Spitzer KW. Lung function in convalescent burn patients. *Am Rev Respir Dis* 1973;108:989–993.
170. Fogarty PW, George PJM, Solomon M, Spiro SG, Armstrong RF. Long term effects of smoke inhalation in survivors of the King's Cross underground station fire. *Thorax* 1991;46:914–918.
171. Moisan TC. Prolonged asthma after smoke inhalation: a report of three cases and a review of previous reports. *J Occup Med* 1991;33:459–461.
172. Loke J, Farmer W, Matthay RA, Putman CE, Smith GJW. Acute and chronic effects of fire fighting on pulmonary function. *Chest* 1980; 77:369–373.
173. Robinson NB, Hudson LD, Riem M, et al. Steroid therapy following isolated smoke inhalation injury. *J Trauma* 1982;22:876–879.

Diseases of the Bronchioles, edited by
Gary R. Epler. Raven Press, Ltd.,
New York © 1994.

13

Postinfectious Bronchiolitis Obliterans

David B. Coultas* and Linda M. Funk†

**Associate Professor of Medicine, Pulmonary and Critical Care Division, and New Mexico Tumor Registry, Cancer Center, University of New Mexico School of Medicine, Albuquerque, NM.*
†Department of Medicine, Pulmonary and Critical Care Division, University of New Mexico School of Medicine, Albuquerque, NM.

Bronchiolitis obliterans without organizing pneumonia, also known as constrictive bronchiolitis, may be the healed lesion resulting from any lower respiratory tract infection or injury causing bronchiolar inflammation and necrosis (Fig. 1) (1,2). Although it is plausible that any infectious agent that causes bronchiolar injury could result in bronchiolitis obliterans, only a limited number of agents, primarily selected viruses and *Mycoplasma pneumoniae*, have been reported to be causes (Table 1). It is possible that diffuse lung injury resulting from infections remote from the lung may also cause bronchiolitis obliterans (2); however, the focus of this chapter is on primary infections of the lung and their association with bronchiolitis obliterans.

To provide a context for understanding postinfectious bronchiolitis obliterans, this review begins with a brief overview of lower respiratory tract infections, the necessary precursors to postinfectious bronchiolitis obliterans. The clinical syndromes of respiratory tract infection are usually divided into upper and lower respiratory tract infections; lower respiratory tract infections are categorized as bronchitis, bronchiolitis, and pneumonia (3). However, because infections may involve more than one anatomic location, making it difficult to categorize bronchiolitis rigidly as the sole precursor to the development of bronchiolitis obliterans, this review considers any lower respiratory tract infection as a potential precursor to bronchiolitis obliterans.

Worldwide, mortality and morbidity are substantial in children and adults as a result of lower respiratory tract infections (3). In developing countries, an estimated three million deaths per year are attributed to respiratory tract infections in children less than 5 years of age, with the rates from lower respiratory tract infections estimated to be 5 to 73 times higher than rates in developed countries.

Although mortality rates from lower respiratory tract infections are substantially higher in the developing countries, incidence rates are similar (3). In developed countries approximately 20% of children per year are affected by lower respiratory tract infections, and approximately 25% of all primary care visits for older children and adults are for acute respiratory illness. The 1981 National Health Interview Survey of the United States estimated that 1.5 episodes of pneumonia occur per 100 persons per year in ambulatory children and adults, totalling approximately 3.3 million cases per year (4). Over 530,000 hospitalizations for pneumonia were estimated for persons older than 15 years of age.

The agents causing lower respiratory tract infections vary primarily with age; viruses predominate during childhood, and

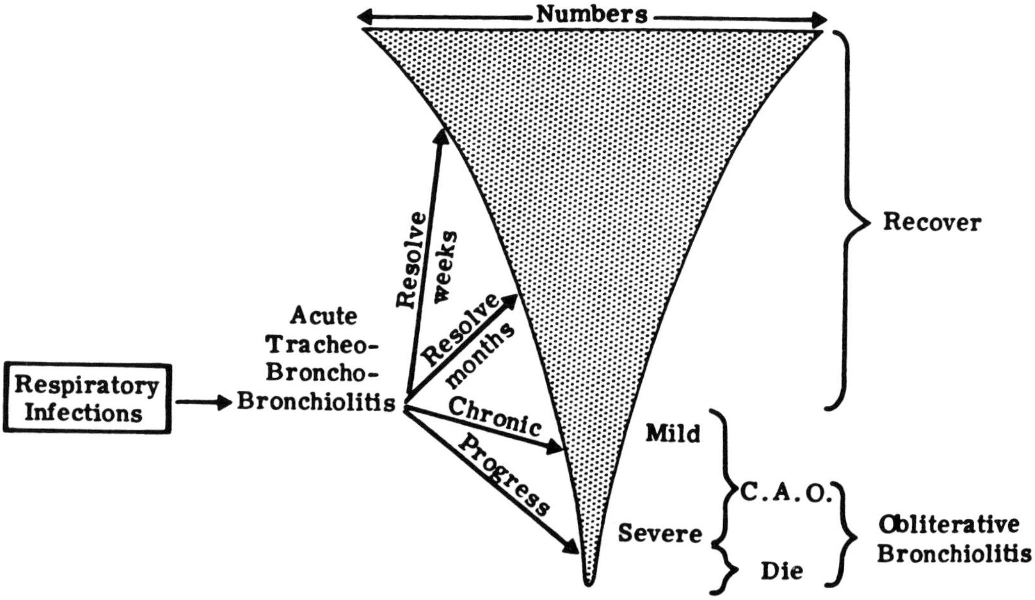

FIG. 1. Hypothesis relating the natural history of lower respiratory tract infections to the development of bronchiolitis obliterans and to chronic airways obstruction (*CAO*). From ref. 1 with permission.

bacteria occur most commonly in adolescence and adulthood (Table 2). Between May 1980 and January 1984, Taussig and co-workers (5) enrolled in a study group 1,246 newborns from a large health maintenance organization in Tucson, Arizona. These newborns were monitored for lower respiratory tract illnesses from May 1980 through October 1986. During this monitoring period 1,052 illnesses occurred in 46% of the children. Of specimens obtained to identify causative agents by culture and immunofluorescence, 62% were positive for an infectious agent by one or both methods.

TABLE 1. *Infectious agents associated with bronchiolitis obliterans*

DNA viruses
Adenovirus
Cytomegalovirus
Varicella
RNA viruses
Influenza A and B
Parainfluenza 2, 3
Respiratory syncytial virus
Mycoplasma pneumoniae

Respiratory syncytial virus and parainfluenza 1, 2, and 3 were associated with approximately 75% of the lower respiratory tract illnesses with an identified pathogen (Table 2). Bronchiolitis was the most common diagnosis (59.7%), followed by croup (23.2%), pneumonia (6.9%), bronchitis (5.1%), multiple diagnoses (3.9%), reactive airways disease (0.6%), and pertussis (0.6%) (8). Only about 1% of the children required hospitalization.

Although little information is available on agents causing lower respiratory tract infections in developing countries, measles and whooping cough may be important causes partly because of a lack of immunizations (9). Failure to immunize preschool children against measles and pertussis in the United States has also contributed to marked increases in these infections. Between 1979 and 1990, the numbers of measles cases in the United States increased by 100% and of pertussis cases by 180% (10).

In adults, information on causative agents of lower respiratory tract infections has been derived largely from patients hospital-

TABLE 2. *Distributions of infectious agents associated with lower respiratory tract infection from childhood through adulthood*

Agent	Childhood: ≤3 years[a] (%)	Childhood: Adolescence/young adulthood[b] (%)
RSV	32	—
Parainfluenza 1, 2, 3	16	4
Adenovirus	3	3
Influenza A, B	3	10
Mycoplasma pneumoniae	3	30–50
Chlamydia trachomatis	2	—
Other nonbacteria	5	—
No pathogen isolated	36	30–50
	Adulthood[c]: Outpatient	**Adulthood[c]: Inpatient**
Streptococcus pneumonia	9–36	15–47
Other bacteria	12	11–26
Mycoplasma pneumoniae	1–37	2–18
Viral	12–13	0–10
Chlamydia	1–4	1–6
Other	0–3	3–17
No pathogen isolated	45–51	29–35

[a]From ref. (5).
[b]From ref. (6).
[c]From ref. (7).

ized with pneumonia (Table 2) (7,11–13). As with children, a causative agent may not be identified in a high proportion of adults with pneumonia. Although the distribution of pathogens varies widely among case series (Table 2), bacteria account for 21 to 48% of agents in ambulatory patients and 26 to 73% in hospitalized patients. In some series, particularly outpatients, *Mycoplasma pneumoniae* may be as common as other bacteria. Viral agents comprise fewer than 15% of pneumonias in both outpatients and inpatients with pneumonia. Of all adults with pneumonia, approximately 15 to 20% may require hospitalization.

Numerous factors may contribute to the different distributions of agents associated with lower respiratory tract infections in children and adults (Table 3). Differences in exposure and immunity may largely explain differences in the epidemiologic patterns between children and adults. During childhood, exposure to viruses is common, and children often lack specific immunity to viral agents. As specific immunity to various agents is acquired, infections with bacteria and *Mycoplasma pneumoniae* begin to predominate in adolescents and adults.

Except for mortality from acute lower

TABLE 3. *Factors that may influence host response to an infectious agent*

Agent(s)	Host
Dose	Age
Virulence	Sex
Site of entry	Preexisting immunity
Multiple infections	Type and intensity of immune response
	Genetic factors
	Nutritional status
	Preexisting disease
	Personal habits: smoking, alcohol, drugs
	Other environmental exposures
	Psychological status

Adapted from ref. (6).

TABLE 4. *Selected case reports in adults with a clinical diagnosis of postinfectious bronchiolitis obliterans*

Year of report (ref.)	Number of cases	Age(s) (years)	Sex	Symptom duration	Criteria for diagnosis	Comment/outcome
1929 (17)	3	18–73	1F, 2M	4 days–2 weeks	Pathology	All patients died
1964 (18)	4	29–48	1F, 3M	4 days–4 weeks	Obstructive PFT[a] Hyperinflation on CXR[b]	All recovered
1965 (19)	1	72	F	6 days	Pathology	Died
1967 (20)	2	48, 53	M, F	2 months–1 year	Obstructive PFT	CAO[c]
1977 (21)	1	48	F	3 months	Obstructive PFT Pathology	Improved on steroids
1980 (22)	1	40	M	14 years	Obstructive PFT Pathology	No response to steroids
1981 (23)	2	27, 60	M, F	2–8 years	Obstructive PFT	CAO
1981 (24)	1	44	F	11 months	Obstructive PFT Pathology Hyperinflation on CXR	Improved on steroids
1983 (25)	1	69	F	3 months	Obstructive PFT Pathology	No improvement on steroids; died 10 months later of respiratory failure

[a]Pulmonary function test.
[b]Chest roentgenogram.
[c]Chronic air-flow obstruction.

TABLE 5. *Selected case reports in adults of specific agents causing bronchiolitis obliterans*

Year of report (ref.)	Number of cases	Age(s) (years)	Sex	Symptom duration	Criteria for diagnosis	Comment/outcome
Adenovirus-21						
1979 (26)	1	60	F	10 days	Pathology	Died
Parainfluenza-2						
1980 (27)	1	22	M	7 days	Hyperinflation on CXR[a]	Recovered with CAO[b]
Cytomegalovirus						
1981 (28)	1	71	F	10 days	Pathology	Improved on steroids
1990 (29)	1	41	M	2 weeks	Pathology	1) HIV + 2) Recovered with gancyclovir
Varicella-Zoster						
1982 (30)	1	19	M	2 weeks	Pathology	Recovered with CAO
Mycoplasma						
1986 (31)	1	37	M	3 weeks	Obstructive PFT[c] Pathology	Recovered with normal lung function after erythromycin
1986 (32)	1	48	M	Unknown	Pathology	Recovered with normal lung function after erythromycin

[a]Chest roentgenogram.
[b]Chronic air-flow obstruction.
[c]Pulmonary function tests.

respiratory tract infections, population-based data on the sequelae of these common infections are few. It may be that respiratory tract infections in childhood have long-term sequelae, including loss of lung function after severe episodes of lower respiratory tract infection, the development of asthma, the development of bronchiolitis obliterans, bronchiectasis, and an increased risk of developing chronic obstructive pulmonary disease in adulthood (14). Similar outcomes may result from lower respiratory tract infections acquired in adulthood. Many risk factors may determine the sequelae of lower respiratory tract infections, including host characteristics, the agent causing infection, and the site of infection (Table 3). However, except for identification of specific agents associated with long-term pulmonary complications, and the potential for prevention or treatment of these infections, the clinical usefulness of these other risk factors remains to be defined and is an active area of investigation. Because of the importance of specific agents as causes of bronchiolitis obliterans (Table 1), these agents are considered in greater detail in the next section.

Although the first description of bronchiolitis obliterans was attributed to Lange (15) in 1901, the two cases he described were of unknown cause. The first cases attributed to infections were described in 1904 (16), and occurred after measles and pertussis. In 1929 Blumgart and MacMahon (17) described five cases of bronchiolitis obliterans, two after a "cold," one scarlet fever, one influenza, and one asthma. Since then, sporadic cases and case series have been reported of bronchiolitis obliterans occurring after a clinical diagnosis of an infection (Table 4) or with microbiologic evidence of an infectious agent (Table 5). These reports provide the basis in this chapter for describing the agents that cause bronchiolitis obliterans and the clinical characteristics of postinfectious bronchiolitis obliterans.

SPECIFIC AGENTS

As mentioned previously, the agents that have been associated with bronchiolitis obliterans include viruses and *Mycoplasma pneumoniae* (Tables 1 and 5). The specific viral agents include the DNA viruses: adenovirus, cytomegalovirus, and varicella zoster virus; and the RNA viruses: influenza, measles, parainfluenza, and respiratory syncytial virus (RSV). This section provides a brief overview of each agent and the methods for diagnosis. (For more detailed descriptions of the viral agents see ref. 6; for a description of *Mycoplasma pneumoniae* see ref. 33.) Although the agents associated with the development of bronchiolitis obliterans have remarkable differences in their biologic characteristics, they all demonstrate a propensity to infect and injure epithelial cells of the respiratory tract. Furthermore, the injuries that result from many of these infections may be histologically indistinguishable (34). Although *Legionella pneumophila* and *Serratia marcescens* pneumonias have caused localized bronchiolitis obliterans (35,36), the clinical and pathologic descriptions in these cases are most consistent with bronchiolitis obliterans organizing pneumonia (BOOP), and are discussed in greater detail in Chapter 5.

Adenovirus

Adenoviruses are double-stranded DNA viruses; they were first isolated in 1953 and subsequently identified worldwide (37). This group of viruses currently includes 41 species that cause a wide range of diseases, primarily affecting the conjunctiva and respiratory and gastrointestinal tracts. The species associated with respiratory tract disease include 1, 2, 3, 4, 5, 6, 7, 11, 14, 16, 21, 34, and 35. Types 1, 2, 5, and 6 are usually endemic and acquired in early childhood. Most of the other types occur in epidemics or sporadically; and 3, 7, and 21 have been associated with severe lower respiratory tract infections and the development of bronchiolitis obliterans (38,39). The incidence of respiratory disease is highest in winter, spring, and early summer. Epidemics of acute respiratory disease have been extensively studied in military recruits.

Respiratory disease caused by adenoviruses is usually acute and self-limited. However, in rare cases death may result from severe bronchiolitis and/or pneumonitis (40–43). Latent infections may result from specific virus types (37,44). Although latent infections are considered asymptomatic, recent evidence suggests that they may result in chronic sequelae (44). This is discussed in greater detail in the section on treatment and prognosis.

Cytomegalovirus

Cytomegalovirus, a double-stranded DNA virus, was first isolated in 1956 and has been found worldwide (45). Although cytomegalovirus infection may cause a wide variety of diseases, including hepatitis and a mononucleosis-like illness, infections are frequently asymptomatic. The development of pneumonitis is most often associated with an immunocompromised state.

Varicella

Although the disease caused by varicella (chickenpox) has been recognized for hundreds of years, this DNA virus was not isolated until 1952 (46). Primary infection occurs most frequently in childhood; however, in tropical regions of the world, a high proportion of primary infections occur in late adolescence and adulthood.

The disease caused by varicella varies with age. In immunocompetent children the disease is usually benign, characterized by fever and development of vesicular cutaneous lesions. However, in adults, radiographic evidence of pneumonia may be apparent in as many as 16%.

Influenza

The single-stranded RNA influenza viruses are found worldwide and include types A, B, and C (47). Because of their segmented genome, influenza viruses undergo genetic reassortment in vitro, resulting in antigenic variation. Although influenza A was first isolated in 1901, it was not recognized as an influenza virus until 1955. Influenzas B and C were first isolated in 1940 and 1947, respectively.

Epidemics of disease characteristic of influenza have been described for thousands of years. Today, influenzas A and B are common causes of morbidity and mortality, causing an average of approximately 10,000 deaths per year in the United States. In contrast, influenza C usually causes uncomplicated upper respiratory tract infections.

Measles

The disease caused by the measles virus has been recognized worldwide for almost 2,000 years, but this RNA virus was not isolated until 1953 (48). Availability of the measles vaccine in 1963 resulted in marked declines of this infection in the United States, but since the early 1980s there has been an increase in its occurrence (10). The disease remains a major source of morbidity and mortality in less developed countries, particularly when associated with malnutrition.

Mucosal cells of the respiratory tract are the initial site of infection with the virus, which is spread by aerosol. Viremia results in systemic spread of the virus, which is followed by the development of oral lesions (Koplik's spots) and cutaneous rash. Although measles is usually a benign infection, severe illness and mortality can occur at the extremes of age and with malnutrition.

Parainfluenza

The RNA parainfluenza viruses were first isolated from children with croup in 1956 (49). Four parainfluenza types are associated with different clinical patterns of respiratory tract infections in children. Types 1 and 2 are most often associated with laryngotracheobronchitis (croup); type 3 is associated with bronchiolitis and pneumonia; and type 4 is of little clinical importance.

Respiratory Syncytial Virus

The RNA virus RSV is a major cause of lower respiratory tract infection that occurs commonly during infancy and early childhood (50). The isolation of RSV was first reported in 1957. Fewer than 1% of infections causing bronchiolitis or pneumonia during childhood require hospitalization.

Mycoplasma pneumoniae

Mycoplasma pneumoniae, the smallest organism capable of independent replication, is found worldwide. The organism was first recognized in 1962 as a cause of atypical pneumonia in humans (33). The occurrence of disease in infected persons appears to be highly variable, and symptoms are usually mild. Using data from studies of *Mycoplasma pneumoniae* infections conducted in the United States, Clyde (51) estimated the annual incidence of asymptomatic infections, of tracheobronchitis, and of pneumonia to be 12 per 1,000 persons, 46 per 1,000 persons, and 2 per 1,000 persons, respectively. Approximately 2% of patients with *Mycoplasma pneumoniae* pneumonia require hospitalization (52). Although the infection is endemic, epidemics may occur at 4- to 7-year intervals.

DIAGNOSTIC METHODS

The diagnosis of lower respiratory tract infections caused by the agents discussed in this chapter is frequently made from clinical and epidemiologic information. Although laboratory methods can assist the clinician in making a specific diagnoses, their clinical usefulness is limited because specific therapies are available only for selected viruses and *Mycoplasma pneumoniae.* However, as the availability of antiviral agents increases, the ability to diagnose specific viruses is likely to become more useful.

The methods for diagnosing viral and mycoplasmal infections can be categorized into two general types: (a) those for directly detecting the agent or its components, and (b) those for detecting the immune response to the agent (53). Examples of the first type include culture techniques for isolating a virus and immunofluorescence microscopy to detect antigens of a virus. Cultures to obtain a diagnosis take from several days to several weeks and require special laboratory facilities. A more rapid diagnosis may be obtained for RSV; parainfluenzas 1, 2, and 3; influenzas A and B; and adenovirus with immunofluorescence microscopy on upper and lower respiratory tract specimens.

Detection of antibodies to viruses and *Mycoplasma pneumoniae* offers an indirect method for documenting infection. Several serologic methods are available for detecting antibodies; complement fixation is the most commonly used. A fourfold increase in antibody titer comparing acute and convalescent serum is traditionally regarded as evidence of acute infection. However, the development of methods to distinguish IgM antibodies, associated with acute infection, from IgG antibodies, associated with past immunity, may be useful for a more rapid diagnosis of acute *Mycoplasma pneumoniae* infection (54).

POSTINFECTIOUS BRONCHIOLITIS OBLITERANS

Bronchiolitis obliterans is a diffuse lung disease characterized clinically by airways obstruction and pathologically by bronchiolar pathology with "partial or complete luminal obliteration accompanied by chronic bronchiolar inflammation, concentric bronchiolar luminal narrowing caused by submucosal and/or adventitial scarring, smooth muscle hypertrophy, bronchiolectasis, and stasis of mucus and macrophages within ectatic bronchiolar lumens" (2). The absence of an alveolar organizing pneumonia distinguishes bronchiolitis obliterans from BOOP. Furthermore, because bronchiolitis obliterans causes airflow obstruction it must be distinguished from airways hyperreactivity and bronchiectasis, which also cause airflow obstruction and may also result from respiratory tract infections.

Because no population-based data are available on the development of postinfectious bronchiolitis, the occurrence of this complication of lower respiratory tract infections may be qualitatively estimated only from reported case series of patients evaluated for chronic airflow obstruction and of patients who had open-lung biopsies. Turton and co-workers (23) found 10 patients with clinical and bronchographic features of bronchiolitis obliterans among 2,094 referred for evaluation of severe chronic airflow obstruction. Of these 10 patients, only 2 reported onset of symptoms after a respiratory illness. In a review of a series of approximately 2,500 open-lung biopsies from Boston-area hospitals, Epler and co-workers (55) found 57 cases of BOOP pneumonia and 10 cases of bronchiolitis obliterans without organizing pneumonia. Of these 10 cases, only 1 was attributed to an infection with *Mycoplasma pneumoniae*. Given the common occurrence of lower respiratory tract infections and the rarity of bronchiolitis obliterans in these large case series, it is apparent that clinically evident postinfectious bronchiolitis is uncommon in the general population.

Although clinically evident bronchiolitis obliterans may be uncommon, pathologic evidence may be very common, and it increases with age (56,57). McLean (56) examined approximately 20,000 histologic sections from blocks of lung tissue obtained from approximately 70 patients. The information on the characteristics of these patients was limited, but they were not selected as a group because of lower respiratory tract infection, and they "varied widely in age and in conditions leading to death." McLean presented little quantitative information on the occurrence of histologic evidence of bronchiolitis obliterans, but he reported that "relatively slight but extensive lesions were found, increasing with age" (57). McLean concluded that "these lesions represent the cumulative effect of such common episodes as childhood viral infections, colds that lingered, influenza, 'bronchitis,' and inhalation of irritating material."

Bronchiolitis Obliterans in Children

Because lower respiratory tract infections are common during childhood, and many agents that cause these infections are frequently associated with bronchiolitis, children may be particularly susceptible to development of bronchiolitis obliterans. Furthermore, the small airway diameter in children compared to that in adults may result in more clinically evident airways obstruction during the acute phase of bronchiolitis and as a complication of these infections. Although the problems of bronchiolitis and bronchiolitis obliterans in children are considered in greater detail in

Chapters 27–29, these conditions are also briefly reviewed here.

Acute bronchiolitis is the most common lower respiratory tract infection of infancy and childhood, usually resulting from a viral infection (39). Recovery from viral bronchiolitis occurs in 99% of patients in a period of days or weeks; however, in some patients the airway injury may result in airways hyperreactivity, obliterative bronchiolitis, bronchiectasis, or death (1,38). Lung specimens obtained from children dying with viral bronchiolitis have demonstrated bronchiolar necrosis and bronchiolitis obliterans (42).

Antemortem diagnosis of obliterative bronchiolitis was made by Hodges and co-workers (58) in 13 children, seen over a 4-year period, who were referred because of prolonged respiratory illnesses manifested by tachypnea and/or cough. The average age of the children when they developed acute bronchiolitis was 9 months, and symptoms persisted for an average of 5 weeks before the children were referred for evaluation. Physical findings in these children included tachypnea (respiratory rate greater than 60 per minute), hyperinflation of the chest, and widespread crackles. Only 4 children had wheezes. Pulmonary function tests demonstrated hyperinflation and varying degrees of airways obstruction. Chest roentgenograms showed hyperinflation and fine nodular opacities, with streaky densities predominantly affecting the upper lobes. Pathologic specimens were available from 3 of the children, and the histologic findings were consistent with bronchiolitis obliterans. Evidence of infection was documented in 3 patients, with positive cultures for adenovirus in 2 and rising complement fixation titer consistent with *Mycoplasma pneumoniae* infection in the third. One child with adenovirus infection died of chronic respiratory failure.

In addition to the prolonged respiratory illness described by Hodges and co-workers, progression of acute bronchiolitis to bronchiolitis obliterans in children may result in several other clinical presentations. Atelectasis, a common finding in acute bronchiolitis, may also occur in bronchiolitis obliterans and may persist for several years. Narrowing and obliteration of bronchiolar lumina combined with underdeveloped collateral channels for ventilation (pores of Kohn) both contribute to the development of atelectasis with acute bronchiolitis and bronchiolitis obliterans (38). In contrast to atelectasis, localized areas of hyperlucent lung may follow acute bronchiolitis and pneumonitis, presumably from air trapping and decreased perfusion associated with obliterative bronchiolitis (59, 60). Finally, in some patients bronchiolitis obliterans may manifest as asymptomatic airflow obstruction. Kattan and co-workers (61) examined 23 asymptomatic children approximately 10 years after resolution of acute bronchiolitis. Evidence of small airways obstruction was found in a high proportion of the children; the RV/TLC ratio was greater than 2 standard deviations above the mean in 41% of the children, and the mean flow at 60% of TLC was significantly reduced compared to the predicted value. In addition, 78% had an arterial Po_2 less than 2 standard deviations below the mean. Asthma was not a likely explanation for these findings because children with symptoms suggestive of asthma were excluded from the study group.

Several infectious agents have been associated with the development of bronchiolitis obliterans in children. These agents have included adenovirus (38,39), influenza (62), and *Mycoplasma pneumoniae* (59,60). Although respiratory syncytial virus is the most common cause of acute bronchiolitis in infancy and early childhood, and may be followed by recurrent wheezing and airflow obstruction, little information is available on the role of respiratory syncytial virus in the development of bronchiolitis obliterans (39).

Because information on bronchiolitis obliterans during childhood is derived largely from case series, it is difficult to establish definitively the risk factors for the development of this complication. However, the available literature suggests that the type of infectious agent and the racial/ethnic background of the child may predispose to bronchiolitis obliterans. Although adenovirus infections are associated with less than 5% of cases of acute bronchiolitis in the United States (38), these infections account for the majority of reported cases with chronic sequelae, including bronchiectasis and bronchiolitis obliterans, following lower respiratory tract infection. The adenoviruses, particularly serotypes 3, 7, and 21, have been associated with severe lower respiratory tract infections and the development of bronchiolitis obliterans (38,39).

Several investigations of lower respiratory tract infections in children have suggested that indigenous children of Native American and of Polynesian ancestry have more severe infections that may be complicated by bronchiolitis obliterans than nonnative children. Gold and co-workers (63) reviewed all lower respiratory tract infections due to adenovirus seen from 1963 to 1968 at the Children's Hospital of Winnipeg. They identified 69 children with this infection, of whom 67% were Native American. Of the Native American children, 52% developed chronic pulmonary disease (obliteration of small airways, bronchiectasis, and unilateral hyperlucent lung) compared to 30% of the nonnative children; and of the seven deaths from acute or chronic pulmonary disease, six were in Native American children. Lung specimens obtained from biopsy or autopsy showed necrotizing bronchiolitis in the acute phase of the disease and obliterative bronchiolitis in the chronic stage. In a subsequent study at Children's Hospital of Winnipeg from 1974 to 1978, Wenman and co-workers (41) also found a high prevalence of severe adenoviral lower respiratory tract infections in Native American children. Of 41 children identified, 78% were Native American, although Native American children accounted for only 7% of the general population of Manitoba. Furthermore, the most severe infections occurred in the native children, and all of the 5 children who died were native children.

In Auckland, New Zealand, Lang and co-workers (40) identified 25 children admitted over a 6-month period in 1965 to Princess Mary Hospital for Children with severe pneumonitis attributed to adenovirus (type 21) infection. Although native peoples accounted for only 19% of the Auckland population, 92% of the 25 children were of Polynesian ancestry. The overall outcome from the infection in these children was poor: 2 children died; 15 had residual lung abnormalities; and only 8 returned to normal. The residual lung abnormalities included chronic cough, repeated chest infections, wheezing, and dyspnea on exertion. Bronchiectasis was documented in 5 children. Pathologic specimens were subsequently obtained from 3 of the children 2 months to 3 years after the acute infections (42). Bronchiolitis obliterans was the predominate finding in all 3.

Although the results of these series suggest that race/ethnicity may predispose to severe adenovirus infections and bronchiolitis obliterans, the small number of cases and the potential for bias in the selection of cases limits definitive conclusions about these factors as risks for bronchiolitis obliterans. In addition, the role of genetic factors versus environmental factors in contributing to the possible effects of race/ethnicity in these series is unknown. Environmental tobacco smoke, an established risk factor for lower respiratory tract infections and decreased rate of lung growth in children (64), has not been systematically examined as a risk for the development of bronchiolitis obliterans following acute bronchiolitis.

Bronchiolitis Obliterans in Adults

In contrast to children, in whom postinfectious bronchiolitis obliterans has often been identified in series of patients who presented with acute bronchiolitis following adenovirus infections, adults have usually presented as isolated cases with a diversity of agents (Tables 4 and 5). The adult case reports can be categorized into two general types on the basis of the criteria used for documenting infection. The first type of report includes patients with a clinical diagnosis of a respiratory tract infection (Table 4), and the second type includes patients with microbiologic evidence of infection (Table 5).

In reports based on a clinician's diagnosis of a presumed respiratory tract infection (Table 4), the major criteria for diagnosis of bronchiolitis obliterans were an obstructive ventilatory impairment on pulmonary function tests or pathologic evidence. The subjects of these reports ranged in age from 18 to 73 years, with an equal distribution of males and females. These patients usually came to clinical attention because of persistent cough and dyspnea, but the duration of these symptoms was highly variable, ranging from 4 days to 14 years. Information on smoking and occupation, both known causes of chronic airflow obstruction, was limited.

Reports that identified a specific infectious agent associated with bronchiolitis obliterans relied primarily on pathologic findings as the criteria for diagnosis (Table 5). As in the cases based on a clinical diagnosis, the age range of these subjects was also large, ranging from 22 to 71 years. Although two-thirds of the subjects in these reports were males, this finding should be generalized cautiously because of the small number of subjects. The duration of symptoms in these patients was much shorter, ranging from days to weeks, than in the subjects with a clinical diagnosis of postinfectious bronchiolitis obliterans (Table 4). Although information on smoking and occupational exposures was provided in some reports, the numbers of cases are too small to make inferences about the interactions among these exposures.

While the histologic finding of bronchiolitis obliterans is the "gold standard" for diagnosing the disorder, several clinical findings, although not specific, should suggest the diagnosis of postinfectious bronchiolitis obliterans. The presenting symptoms are usually a persistent, nonproductive cough with varying degrees of dyspnea following a respiratory tract infection. Inspiratory crackles are a prominent finding on physical examination, with wheezing less common. Nodular opacities or a normal chest radiograph may be seen in the early phase of the illness, followed by hyperinflation in the late phase. Irreversible airflow obstruction and air trapping are hallmarks of bronchiolitis obliterans, with a normal or reduced diffusing capacity.

Risk factors that predict the development of bronchiolitis obliterans in adults have not been identified. However, characteristics of the agent and host need to be considered (Table 3). Cigarette smoking, a cause of respiratory bronchiolitis (65), may potentiate the bronchiolar injury associated with an infectious agent and may predispose to the development of bronchiolitis obliterans. The interaction of cigarette smoking and other environmental exposures with infectious agents in the development of bronchiolitis obliterans requires further investigation.

Treatment and Prognosis

The number of bronchioles injured by the infecting agent and the severity of residual bronchiolar obstruction will determine the magnitude of airways obstruction and symptomatology. Although bronchiolitis obliterans may be common pathologically (57), the development of clinically apparent chronic airflow obstruction may be less common, and some cases may resolve subacutely and return to normal function.

The information in available case reports suggests two factors that may determine the outcome of postinfectious bronchiolitis obliterans: the age at onset and the infecting agent. Hodges and co-workers (58) reported on 13 children (mean age of 9 months) with postinfectious bronchiolitis obliterans; 1 child died and the other children began to improve after 3 to 24 months. The improvement was attributed to new lung growth; however, the status of these children during later childhood and into adulthood is unknown.

Although comprehensive information on the outcome of bronchiolitis obliterans associated with specific agents is unavailable, the case reports suggest that viral infections have a worse prognosis than infections with *Mycoplasma pneumoniae* (Table 5). In the two case reports of bronchiolitis obliterans associated with *Mycoplasma pneumoniae,* treatment with erythromycin resulted in resolution of symptoms and return of normal lung function (31,32). Antiviral therapy may prove useful for specific viral infections (29).

Other therapies for postinfectious bronchiolitis obliterans have included corticosteroids and lung transplantation. The role of corticosteroid therapy in postinfectious bronchiolitis obliterans, while theoretically feasible, has not been consistently effective (Tables 4 and 5). In one patient with respiratory failure from rapidly progressive postviral bronchiolitis obliterans, lung transplantation proved life-saving (66).

The role of lower respiratory tract infections during childhood or adulthood in the development of chronic airflow obstruction, while biologically plausible, has not been definitively established (14). In fact, the development of chronic airflow obstruction following a lower respiratory tract infection may be mediated through several mechanisms, including airways hyperreactivity, bronchiolitis obliterans, and bronchiectasis (65). A recent report of latent adenoviral infection in patients with chronic obstructive pulmonary disease provides further evidence of an association between lower respiratory tract infections and development of chronic obstructive pulmonary disease (44,67). However, results from longitudinal studies from childhood to adulthood will be needed to establish the relationship between lower respiratory tract infections and the development of chronic obstructive pulmonary disease (14).

CONCLUSIONS

Although there are no population-based data on the occurrence of postinfectious bronchiolitis obliterans, the available reports suggests that bronchiolitis obliterans is a rare complication of several viral infections and *Mycoplasma pneumoniae*. Risk factors for development of this complication have not been established, but adenoviral infections and racial/genetic characteristics may be important, particularly in children. Interactions between infectious agents and cigarette smoking or other environmental exposures in the development of bronchiolitis obliterans are not known. Specific antiviral or antibiotic therapies during the acute phase of the illness may prevent permanent impairment. However, lower respiratory tract infections with development of bronchiolitis obliterans may be one of several pathways in the development of chronic obstructive pulmonary disease.

Distinguishing postinfectious bronchiolitis obliterans from other disorders characterized by chronic airflow obstruction is a clinical challenge. The presence of crackles with bronchiolitis obliterans separates it in most cases from asthma, chronic bronchitis, and emphysema, but may be less useful in separating it from cystic fibrosis and bronchiectasis. A sweat test is the cornerstone for diagnosing cystic fibrosis. Bronchiolitis obliterans and bronchiectasis, both postinfectious complications, may be particularly difficult to distinguish solely on clinical information. High-resolution CT scan may be helpful for diagnosing bronchiectasis. Ultimately, an open-lung biopsy may be necessary, if clinically indicated, for distinguishing bronchiolitis obliterans from other diffuse lung diseases.

ACKNOWLEDGMENTS

Supported in part by a FIRST Award, R29 HL40587, and a Preventive Pulmonary Academic Award, K07 HL02474, National Heart, Lung, and Blood Institute, Bethesda, Maryland. The authors thank Carolyn Lara for her assistance with preparation of the manuscript.

REFERENCES

1. Green M, Turton CW. Manifestations of diseases of the small airways. *Eur J Respir Dis* 1982; 63:36–42.
2. Wright J, Cagle P, Churg A, Colby TV, Myers J. Diseases of the small airways. *Am Rev Respir Dis* 1992;146:240–262.
3. Graham NMH. The epidemiology of acute respiratory infections in children and adults: a global perspective. *Epidemiol Rev* 1990;12:149–178.
4. Garibaldi RA. Epidemiology of community acquired respiratory tract infections in adults: incidence, etiology, impact. *Am J Med* 1985; 78:32–37.
5. Taussig LM, Wright AL, Wayne JM, Harrison HR, Ray CG, The Group Health Medical Associates. The Tucson children's respiratory study: design and implementation of a prospective study of acute and chronic respiratory illness in children. *Am J Epidemiol* 1989;129:1219–1231.
6. Evans AS, ed. *Viral infections of humans: epidemiology and control.* 3rd ed. New York: Plenum; 1989.
7. Rodnick JE, Gude JK. Diagnosis and antibiotic treatment of community-acquired pneumonia. *West J Med* 1991;154:405–409.
8. Wright AL, Taussig LM, Ray CG, Harrison HR, Holberg CJ, The Group Health Medical Associates. The Tucson children's respiratory study: lower respiratory tract illness in the first year of life. *Am J Epidemiol* 1989;129:1232–1246.
9. Chretien J, Holland W, Macklem P, Murray J, Woolcock A. Acute respiratory infections in children: a global public-health problem. *N Engl J Med* 1984;310:982–984.
10. McGinnis JM, Richmond JB, Brandt EN, Windom RE, Mason JO. Health progress in the United States. *JAMA* 1992;268:2545–2552.
11. Finch RG. Epidemiological features and chemotherapy of community-acquired respiratory tract infections. *J Antimicrob Chemother* 1990; 26:53–61.
12. Marrie TJ, Durant H, Yates L. Community acquired pneumonia requiring hospitalization: 5 year prospective study. *Rev Infect Dis* 1989; 11:586–599.
13. Carpenter JL, Huang DY. Community-acquired pulmonary infections in a public municipal hospital in the 1980s. *South Med J* 1991;84:299–306.
14. Samet JM, Tager IB, Speizer FE. The relationship between respiratory illness in childhood and chronic air-flow obstruction in adulthood. *Am Rev Respir Dis* 1983;127:508–523.
15. Lange W. Uber eine eigenthumliche Erkrangkung der kleinen Bronchien und Bronchiolen. (Bronchitis et Bronchiolitis obliterans.) *Dtsch Arch Klin Med* 1901;70:342–364.
16. LaDue JS. Bronchiolitis fibrosa obliterans. *Arch Intern Med* 1941;68:663–673.
17. Blumgart HL, MacMahon HE. Bronchiolitis fibrosa obliterans: a clinical and pathologic study. *Med Clin North Am* 1929;13:197–214.
18. Ham JC. Acute infectious obstructing bronchiolitis. *Ann Intern Med* 1964;60:47–60.
19. Harris C. Acute obstructive bronchiolitis. *JAMA* 1965;194:203–205.
20. Dines DE. Acute bronchiolitis as a cause of chronic obstructive lung disease in adults. *Lancet* 1967:281–282.
21. Dale RC, Auchincloss JH, Gilbert R, Markarian B. Bronchiolitis obliterans. *NY State J Med* 1977;77:1485–1488.
22. Tukiainen P, Poppius H, Taskinen E. Slowly progressive bronchiolitis obliterans. *Eur J Respir Dis* 1980;61:77–83.
23. Turton CW, Williams G, Green M. Cryptogenic obliterative bronchiolitis in adults. *Thorax* 1981; 36:805–810.
24. Hawley PC, Whitcomb ME. Bronchiolitis fibrosa obliterans in adults. *Arch Intern Med.* 1981;141:1324–1327.
25. Seggev JS, Mason UG, Worthen S, Stanford RE, Fernandez E. Bronchiolitis obliterans. *Chest* 1983;83:169–174.
26. Scully RE, Galdabini JJ, McNeely BU. Case records of the Massachusetts General Hospital. *N Engl J Med* 1979;300:301–309.
27. O'Reilly JF. Adult bronchiolitis and parainfluenza type 2. *Postgrad Med J* 1980;56:787–788.
28. Scully RE, Mark EJ, McNeely BU. Case records of the Massachusetts General Hospital. *N Engl J Med* 1981;305:627–635.
29. Vasudevan VP, Mascarenhas DAN, Klapper P, Lomvardias S. Cytomegalovirus necrotizing bronchiolitis with HIV infection. *Chest* 1990; 97:483–484.
30. Nikki P, Meretoja O, Valtonen V, et al. Severe bronchiolitis probably caused by varicella-zoster virus. *Crit Care Med* 1982;10:344–346.
31. Coultas DB, Samet JM, Butler C. Bronchiolitis obliterans due to mycoplasma pneumoniae. *West J Med* 1986;144:471–474.
32. Rollins S, Colby T, Clayton F. Open lung biopsy in mycoplasma pneumoniae pneumonia. *Arch Pathol Lab Med* 1986;110:34–41.

33. Willett HP. Mycoplasma. In: Joklik WK, Willett HP, Amos DB, Wilfert CM, eds. *Zinsser microbiology*. 20th ed. Norwalk, CT: Appleton & Lange; 1992:730–7.
34. Aherne W, Bird T, Court SDM, Gardner PS, McQuillin J. Pathological changes in virus infections of the lower respiratory tract in children. *J Clin Pathol* 1970;23:7–18.
35. Sato P, Madtes DK, Thorning D. Albert RK. Bronchiolitis obliterans caused by legionella pneumophila. *Chest* 1985;87:840–842.
36. Goldstein JD, Godleski JJ, Balikian JP, Herman PG. Pathologic patterns of serratia marcescens pneumonia. *Hum Pathol* 1982;13:479–484.
37. Foy HM. Adenoviruses. In: Evans AS, ed. *Viral infections of humans: epidemiology and control*. 3rd ed. New York: Plenum; 1989:77–94.
38. Wohl MEB, Chernick V. Bronchiolitis. *Am Rev Respir Dis* 1978;118:759–781.
39. Milner AD, Murray M. Acute bronchiolitis in infancy: treatment and prognosis. *Thorax* 1989; 44:1–5.
40. Lang WR, Howden CW, Laws J, Burton JF. Bronchopneumonia with serious sequelae in children with evidence of adenovirus type 21 infection. *Br Med J* 1969;1:73–79.
41. Wenman WM, Pagtakhan RD, Chernick V, Albritton W. Adenovirus bronchiolitis in Manitoba. *Chest* 1982;81:605–609.
42. Becroft DMO. Bronchiolitis obliterans, bronchiectasis, and other sequelae of adenovirus type 21 infection in young children. *J Clin Pathol* 1971;24:72–82.
43. Dudding BA, Wagner SC, Zeller JA, Gmelich JT, French GR, Top FH Jr. Fatal pneumonia associated with adenovirus type 7 in three military trainees. *N Engl J Med* 1972;286:1289–1292.
44. Hogg, JC. Latent viral infections in airway epithelium. *Chest* 1992;101:80S–802S.
45. Gold E, Nankervis GA. Cytomegalovirus. In: Evans AS, ed. *Viral infections of humans: epidemiology and control*. 3rd ed. New York: Plenum; 1989:77–94.
46. Weller TH. Varicella-herpes zoster virus. In Evans AS, ed. *Viral infection of humans: epidemiology and control*. 3rd ed. New York: Plenum; 1989:659–683.
47. Glezen WP, Couch RB. Influenza viruses. In: Evans AS, ed. *Viral infections of humans: epidemiology and control*. 3rd ed. New York: Plenum; 1989:419–449.
48. Black FL. Measles. In: Evans AS, ed. *Viral infections of humans: epidemiology and control*. 3rd ed. New York: Plenum; 1989:451–469.
49. Glezen WP, Loda FA, Denny FW. Parainfluenza viruses. In Evans AS, ed. *Viral infections of humans: epidemiology and control*. 3rd ed. New York: Plenum; 1989:493–507.
50. Chanock RM, McIntosh K, Murphy BR, Parrott RH. Respiratory syncytial virus. In: Evans AS, ed. *Viral infections of humans: epidemiology and control*. 3rd ed. New York: Plenum; 1989: 525–544.
51. Clyde WA Jr. Mycoplasma pneumoniae respiratory disease symposium: summation and significance. *Yale J Biol Med* 1983;56:523–527.
52. Foy HM, Nolan CM, Allan ID. Epidemiologic aspects of M. pneumoniae disease complications: a review. *Yale J Biol Med* 1983;56:469–473.
53. Henshaw NG. Rapid viral diagnosis. In: Joklik WK, Willett HP, Amos DB, Wilfert CM, eds. *Zinsser microbiology*. 20th ed. Norwalk, CT: Appleton & Lange; 1992:941–948.
54. Smith TF. Mycoplasma pneumoniae infections: diagnosis based on immunofluorescence titer of IgG and IgM antibodies. *Mayo Clin Proc* 1986; 61:830–831.
55. Epler GR, Colby TV, McLoud TC, Carrington CB, Gaensler EA. Bronchiolitis obliterans organizing pneumonia. *N Engl J Med* 1985;312: 152–157.
56. McLean KH. The pathology of acute bronchiolitis: a study of its evolution. I: The exudative phase. *Australas Ann Med* 1956;5:254–267.
57. McLean KH. The pathology of acute bronchiolitis: a study of its evolution. II: The repair phase. *Australas Ann Med* 1957;6:29–43.
58. Hodges IGC, Milner AD, Groggins RC, Stokes GM. Causes and management of bronchiolitis with chronic obstructive features. *Arch Dis Child* 1982;57:495–499.
59. Stokes D, Sigler A, Kouri NF, Talamo RC. Unilateral hyperlucent lung (Swyer-James syndrome) after severe mycoplasma pneumoniae infection. *Am Rev Respir Dis* 1978;117:145–152.
60. Isles AF, Masel J, O'Duffy J. Obliterative bronchiolitis due to mycoplasma pneumoniae infection in a child. *Pediatr Radiol* 1987;17:109–111.
61. Kattan M, Keens TG, Lapierre JG, Levison H, Bryan C, Reilly BJ. Pulmonary function abnormalities in symptom-free children after bronchiolitis. *Pediatrics* 1977;59:683–688.
62. Laraya-Cuasay LR, DeForest A, Huff D, Lischner H, Huang NN. Chronic pulmonary complications of early influenza virus infection in children. *Am Rev Respir Dis* 1977;116:617–625.
63. Gold R, Wilt JC, Adhikari PK, MacPherson RI. Adenoviral pneumonia and its complications in infancy and childhood. *J Can Assoc Radiol* 1969;20:218–224.
64. U S Department of Health and Human Services. *The health consequences of involuntary smoking*. Washington, DC: US Government Printing Office; 1986. DHHS Publication No. (CDC) 87-8398.
65. Wright JL. Small airways disease: its role in chronic airflow obstruction. *Semin Respir Med* 1992;13:72–84.
66. Cooper JD, Patterson GA, Grossman R, Maurer, Toronto Lung Transplant Group. Double-lung transplant for advanced chronic obstructive lung disease. *Am Rev Respir Dis* 1989;139:303–307.
67. Matsuse T, Hayashi S, Kuwano K, Keunecke H, Jefferies WA, Hogg JC. Latent adenoviral infection in the pathogenesis of chronic airways obstruction. *Am Rev Respir Dis* 1992;146:177–184.

Diseases of the Bronchioles, edited by
Gary R. Epler. Raven Press, Ltd.,
New York © 1994.

14

Rheumatoid Arthritis and Connective-Tissue Disease Related Bronchiolitis Obliterans

D.M.G. Halpin* and Duncan M. Geddes*

**Royal Brompton National Heart and Lung Hospital, Sydney Street, London, England.*

The connective-tissue diseases are a heterogeneous group of immunologically mediated chronic inflammatory disorders characterized clinically by inflammation of joints, serosal membranes, connective tissue, and blood vessels. The classical connective-tissue diseases merge into the vasculitides, and there are a number of overlap syndromes. In this chapter we review the evidence concerning the occurrence of bronchiolitis obliterans in the "classical" connective-tissue diseases: rheumatoid arthritis, systemic lupus erythematosus (SLE), ankylosing spondylitis, Sjögren's syndrome, systemic sclerosis, Behçet's disease, and mixed connective-tissue disease.

Pulmonary involvement in some of the connective-tissue diseases has been recognized for many years. Osler (1) described a case of systemic lupus erythematosus with interstitial pulmonary infiltrates in 1904, and pulmonary involvement in scleroderma was described as early as 1870 (2). However, it was not until 1948 that Ellman and Ball (3) first drew attention to the fact that rheumatoid arthritis was not simply confined to the musculoskeletal system, but was a multisystem disorder affecting the lungs as well as other organs. They described diffuse interstitial fibrosis; and subsequently pleural effusions (4), Caplan's syndrome (5), pulmonary rheumatoid nodules (6), and bronchiectasis (7,8) were described. Reports of lung function test results in patients with rheumatoid arthritis showed obstructive findings, but these were largely ignored or attributed to smoking. It was not until the pathological description of bronchiolitis obliterans in rheumatoid arthritis in 1977 that small airway involvement was recognized (9).

It is now clear that small airway narrowing in patients with connective-tissue disease may occur as a result of the distinct clinicopathological syndromes of bronchiolitis obliterans and bronchiolitis obliterans organizing pneumonia (BOOP), and that it may be detected functionally on routine lung function testing without any additional evidence of an underlying disease process. Because of similar nomenclature, bronchiolitis obliterans and BOOP are sometimes confused; however, connective-tissue associated BOOP differs both clinically and pathologically from bronchiolitis obliterans and is dealt with in Chapter 3. The relationship between small airways obstruction detected on lung function testing and the presence or nature of underlying pathological processes is still unclear.

The obstructive bronchiolitis seen in rheumatoid arthritis is the most common of the connective-tissue disease related bronchiolopathies.

RHEUMATOID ARTHRITIS

Bronchiolitis obliterans in patients with rheumatoid arthritis was first described following the observation of the development of rapidly progressive airway obstruction in five patients (9). Since then there have been numerous other case reports (10–31). The association with rheumatoid arthritis seems specific, but there has been considerable debate as to whether the bronchiolitis obliterans is a feature of the chronic inflammation caused by the rheumatoid arthritis or whether it is induced by drugs used to treat the disease.

Occurrence

It is impossible to determine the prevalence of bronchiolitis obliterans in patients with rheumatoid arthritis from the published case reports and small series. There have been no attempts to determine the prevalence of bronchiolitis obliterans in large unselected populations of patients with rheumatoid arthritis, but there have been a number of studies describing the results of lung function testing. Some of these have considered only patients with interstitial fibrosis (32–34) and therefore do not give information about the prevalence of airflow obstruction. Davidson and colleagues (35) found a 24% prevalence of decreased FEV_1/FVC ratios; and Schernthaner and associates (36) found that 21% had decreased FEV_1/FVC ratios, while 42% had increased residual volumes. However, these studies were primarily designed to assess abnormalities of gas transfer, and the numbers of patients were small. Collins and co-workers (37) studied 43 patients and reported airflow obstruction in 60%; but 92% of these had smoked, and the contribution of their rheumatoid arthritis to the development of airflow obstruction was impossible to assess. Geddes and colleagues (38) found that compared with a control group matched for age, sex, and smoking habit, the prevalence of abnormal FEV_1/FVC ratios and midexpiratory flow rates in 100 unselected patients with rheumatoid arthritis was 32%. Mountz and co-workers (39) showed abnormalities of small airway function in 12 unselected nonsmokers with rheumatoid arthritis; but other studies (40, 41) have failed to show airflow limitation except in those patients who were, or had been, smokers. Thus the true prevalence of nonsmoking-related small airways obstruction in patients with rheumatoid arthritis remains unknown. The observation of airflow obstruction in nonsmokers suggests that there is airway obliteration in these patients; however, the relationship of the lesions causing this obstruction to the pathologically well characterized lesions seen in bronchiolitis obliterans is also not known.

It has been reported that bronchiolitis obliterans is more common in patients with specific human leukocyte antigen (HLA) types. Sweatman and co-workers (42) found that HLA-B40 was significantly more common in patients with bronchiolitis obliterans and rheumatoid arthritis than in patients with bronchiolitis obliterans alone or in healthy control subjects, but they did not include a control group of patients with rheumatoid arthritis without bronchiolitis obliterans. Scott and associates (43) found no association of airflow limitation with HLA-DR4 status, although there was a significant reduction in both FEV_1 and FVC in DR4-positive patients compared with DR4 negative.

Clinical Features

The diagnosis of bronchiolitis obliterans can be made with reasonable certainty on clinical grounds. Patients present with progressive breathlessness often preceded by a cough, which is generally nonproductive. They may identify an initial "influenza-

like" episode, but more commonly the onset is insidious. On examination, patients are breathless at rest, and about two-thirds have early or midinspiratory crackles, generally more prominent at the lung bases. Half have associated midinspiratory "squeaks." These are brief and high pitched and may be temporarily abolished by repeated deep breathing. They are often best heard anteriorly over the upper chest, where the crackles are quietest. These sounds probably come from explosive opening and oscillation of the narrowed bronchioles. The mean age of the 46 patients in the literature is 52.3 ± 1.6 (range 27 to 72) years, and all but 3 of these patients were women.

The clinical course may be static or show progressive deterioration. The initial description of obstructive bronchiolitis in rheumatoid arthritis followed the observation of rapidly progressive breathlessness leading to death over a few months (9). Bégin and associates (44) reported that airway disease in nonsmoking patients with rheumatoid disease progressed more rapidly than in smokers with chronic airflow limitation, but there was considerable variation in the rate of decline among individuals.

Investigations

Of the 46 patients reported, 43 had positive rheumatoid factor titers; and other autoantibodies, especially antinuclear antibodies, may be detected. One case of bronchiolitis obliterans has been reported (45) in a woman who had both rheumatoid factor and antinuclear antibodies in her blood but no joint disease. Chest radiographs may be normal or may show overinflated hypertransradiant lungs (46). The obliteration of small airways is well shown by bronchography (Fig. 1) (46), but this has been largely replaced by inspiratory and expiratory CT scan images, which show patchy areas of transradiancy representing air trapping at the secondary pulmonary lobule and widespread bronchial wall thickening (Fig. 2) (47). Lung function tests show a reduced FEV_1/FVC ratio, which is not increased after inhalation of bronchodilator agents. The total lung capacity (TLC) and residual volume (RV) are increased, consistent with small airways obstruction; and carbon monoxide gas transfer coefficients are usually normal, reflecting normal alveolar function. Lung volumes measured by helium dilution are found to be considerably lower than those measured by body plethysmography. This has been shown to be due to poor mixing of the helium gas mixture, presumably as a result of ventilation of lung units distal to obstructed bronchi by collateral drift (9).

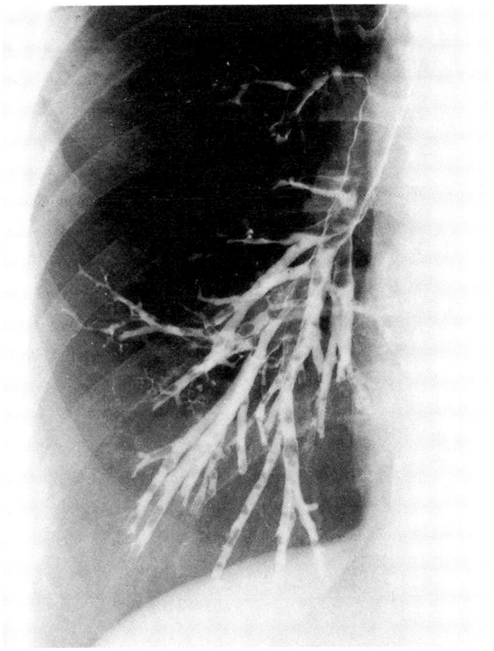

FIG. 1. Pruning of the peripheral airways in a patient with rheumatoid arthritis associated bronchiolitis obliterans shown by bronchography.

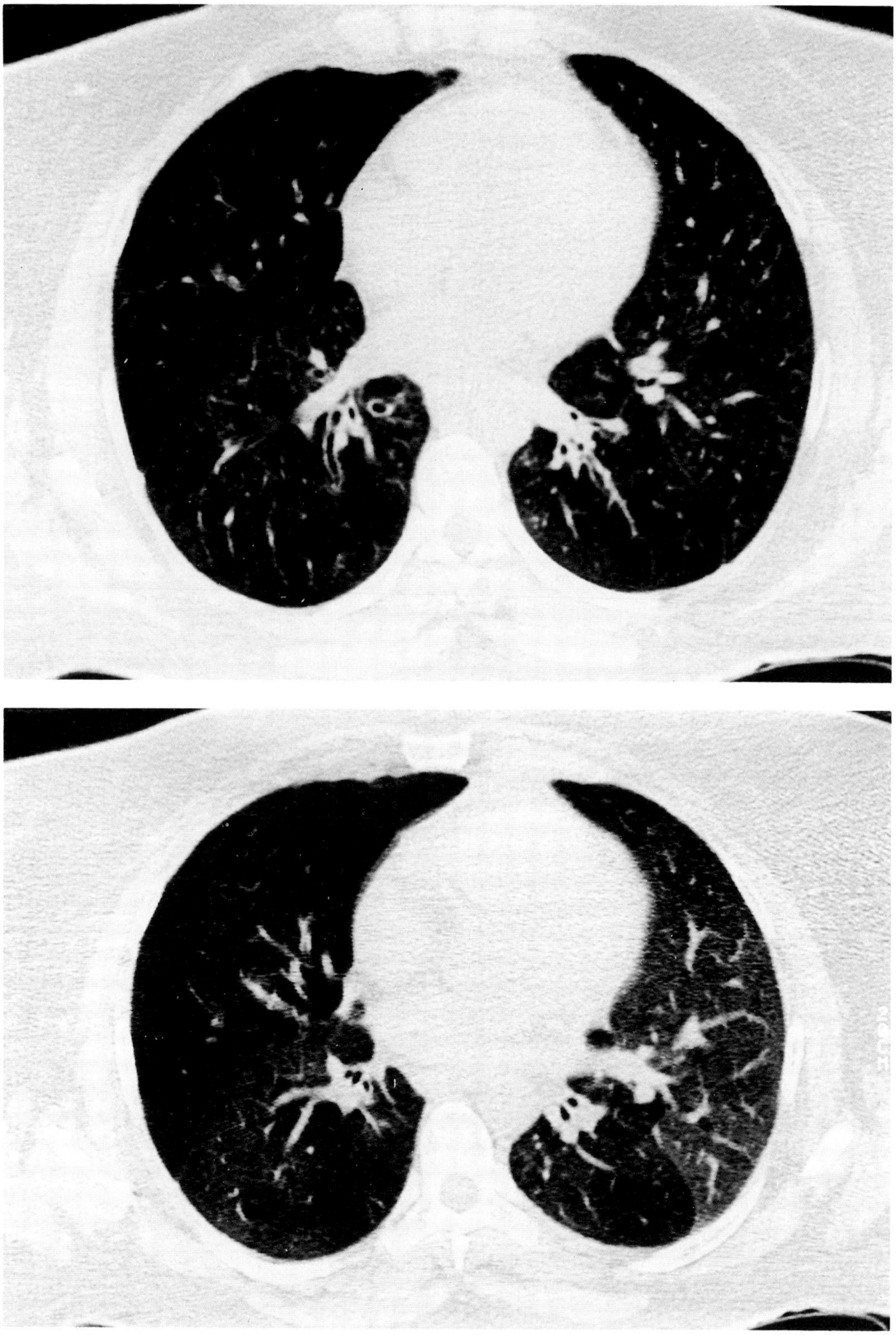

A

B

FIG. 2. CT scan of the lungs **A,** in inspiration showing areas of hypertransradiancy and bronchial wall thickening and **B,** in expiration showing the air trapping.

Pathology

The pathological appearances may easily be overlooked in both biopsy and postmortem material, as the lung tissue may look relatively normal macroscopically. The main abnormality is fibrous narrowing or obliteration of airways, with diameters in the range of 1 to 6 mm (9,48). The fibrosis occurs predominantly in bronchioles, but may extend to small bronchi. The alveolar ducts and alveoli are spared, in contrast to the situation in BOOP. The airway narrowing is due to mural scar tissue, which predominantly affects the mucosa but also spreads into the smooth muscle and peribronchiolar tissues. Mucosal thickening causes circumferential constriction or total obliteration of the airway lumen (Fig. 3). The intraluminal polyps of granulation tissue seen in other forms of bronchiolitis obliterans (49) are not usually seen. The airway obliteration is patchy but widespread. The airways may be completely destroyed, and in this situation they can be identified only as stellate scars accompanying pulmonary arteries. Serial sectioning shows that the obstruction or obliteration affects a discrete segment of the airway over a length of only a few millimeters (9). Beyond this the airway lumen is preserved and distal alveoli are aerated.

It is likely that these fibrotic appearances represent the end stage of a chronic inflammatory process, and occasionally more active chronic inflammation is also seen. There may be severe necrotizing ulceration of the bronchial mucosa, with granulation tissue densely infiltrated with lymphocytes.

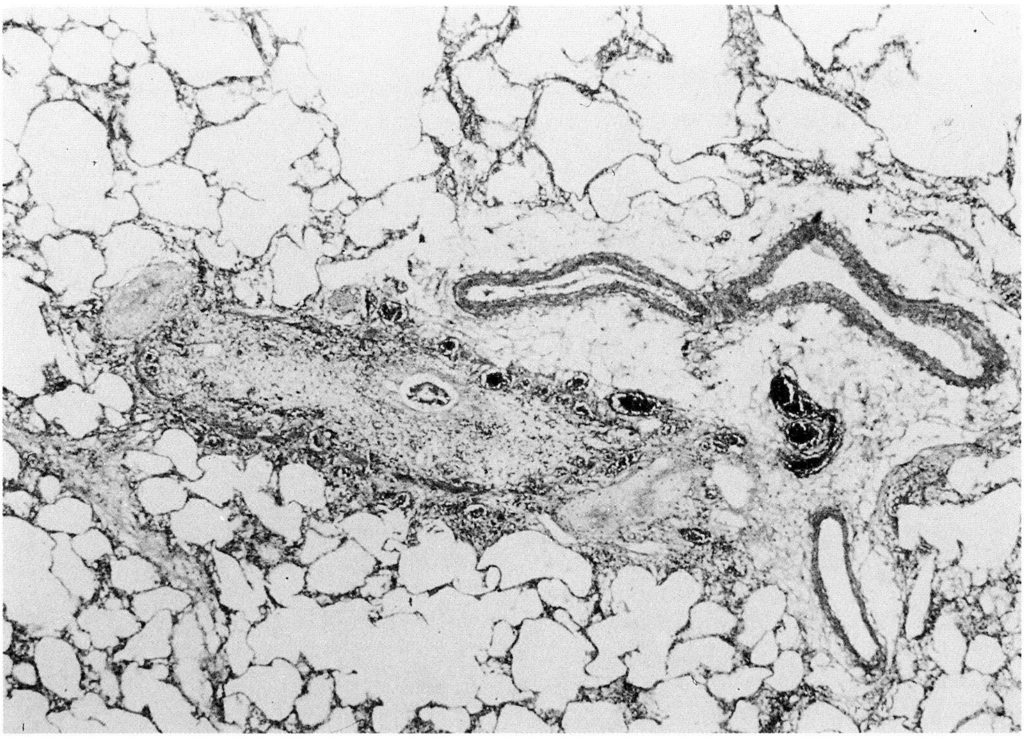

FIG. 3. Histological appearance of an obliterated bronchus in a patient with rheumatoid arthritis associated bronchiolitis obliterans showing the circumferential scar tissue and complete obliteration of the lumen. (Photomicrograph kindly provided by Professor B. Corrin, who retains the copyright.)

Pathogenesis

The pathogenesis of the chronic inflammation remains unclear, but it has been suggested that it may have an autoimmune basis, result from increased susceptibility to infections, or be related to therapy.

Early studies (9) found no serum autoantibodies directed against components of the airway, and direct immunofluorescence of the lesions was negative. Herzog and coworkers (14) described linear IgG staining of alveolar walls in patients with rheumatoid arthritis and acute bronchiolitis, suggesting direct immune-mediated lung injury; and IgG and IgM deposition in alveolar walls has been reported (17,50) in the lungs of patients with rheumatoid arthritis. Further evidence in support of an immune mediated process comes from studies (51–53) on post lung and bone marrow transplant bronchiolitis obliterans.

Pulmonary infections have been reported (54) to be more common in rheumatoid arthritis; however, whether the rheumatoid process itself or the immunosuppressive drugs used in the disease predispose to viral infections is uncertain.

One-half of the patients in the original series (9) had been treated with D-penicillamine, and one had received gold. Other reports (10–26,29,31) that followed suggested an association between the development of bronchiolitis obliterans and penicillamine treatment, but this may represent reporting bias. More recent studies (9,27,28,30) have not supported this association, and patients undoubtedly develop bronchiolitis obliterans never having been treated with penicillamine.

D-penicillamine has also been implicated in the development of other pulmonary complications, including Goodpasture's syndrome (55) and pulmonary interstitial infiltrates (56), as well as autoimmune disorders associated with autoantibody production, including a systemic lupus erythematosus–like syndrome (57,58), polymyositis (59), and myaesthenia gravis (60). The mechanisms by which penicillamine leads to the production of autoantibodies remain unclear, but it is known that penicillamine modulates both humoral and cellular immune responses (61). It may alter the balance between T-helper and T-suppressor cell function in such a way as to allow the formation of autoantibodies and immune complexes. Penicillamine may also stimulate autoimmune reactions by modifying endogenous antigens through its chelating and reducing properties. Jansen and colleagues (17) have reported increased levels of circulating immune complexes and granular IgM deposits along alveolar septae in a patient with bronchiolitis obliterans who had been treated with penicillamine. Further evidence for an immune-mediated tissue damage in patients treated with penicillamine comes from the work of Woodley and associates (62), who found that penicillamine-induced proteinuria was more common in patients who were HLA-DRw3 positive.

A retrospective survey (63) of 3,356 patients treated with D-penicillamine found two definite and two possible deaths attributable to the development of bronchiolitis obliterans. A prospective study (64) of 259 rheumatoid patients treated over 3 years found two cases of bronchiolitis obliterans. Wolfe and co-workers (22) described two definite occurrences and one probably occurrence of bronchiolitis obliterans in 133 patients treated with penicillamine over a 4-year period, compared with none in both the 89 patients treated with gold salts alone and the 380 patients not receiving gold or penicillamine.

As well as the initial patient treated with gold, 17 other patients of the 46 reported in the literature had received gold salts (13,16,17,19,20,22–24,28,29,31). Wolfe and colleagues (22) did not observe any cases of bronchiolitis obliterans in their 89 patients treated with gold, and there is no direct evidence linking chrysotherapy with the development of bronchiolitis obliterans.

Treatment

Treatment is generally unsuccessful. Corticosteroids with or without immunosuppressive agents have been tried, with occasional reports of success (26); but in our experience, although there is sometimes a slight improvement in symptoms, this is not maintained. Despite the uncertainty about the role of penicillamine or gold in the pathogenesis of bronchiolitis obliterans, it seems wise to stop treatment with these agents if bronchiolitis obliterans develops. Lung transplantation may offer the best hope for treatment in patients who are severely limited by their lung disease but who are otherwise well.

SYSTEMIC LUPUS ERYTHEMATOSUS

Pulmonary abnormalities are common in patients with systemic lupus erythematosus (65) and bronchial obliteration in a patient with systemic lupus erythematosus pneumonitis was first described by Matthay and colleagues (66) in 1974, although this was not discussed. A similar finding was described in 1977 (67) but the first conscious description of bronchiolitis obliterans in systemic lupus erythematosus was in 1980 (12), and an additional patient was described by Kinney and Angelillo in 1982 (68).

Pulmonary function studies in patients with systemic lupus erythematosus have shown an obstructive picture in less than 5% (69), and it seems that bronchiolitis obliterans, although it occurs in patients with systemic lupus erythematosus, is rare. The clinical and radiological features and the results of lung function tests are similar to those in patients with rheumatoid arthritis, and the diagnosis can usually be established by the clinical features. Pathologically, small airway obliteration is found to be due to inflammation within the walls of small bronchi and bronchioli, with buds of granulation tissue within the lumen. This proliferative appearance, which may improve with corticosteroid therapy, is similar to that found in bronchiolitis obliterans due to other causes, but differs from that seen in rheumatoid-associated bronchiolitis obliterans.

In one case (12) the patient had been treated with penicillamine; and in another (68) there was focal deposition of IgG and IgM in the alveolar walls, together with some IgA, IgE, C3, and C4, suggesting immune-mediated lung injury.

The response to treatment appears to be as disappointing as that seen in rheumatoid arthritis.

ANKYLOSING SPONDYLITIS

Unlike the other connective-tissue diseases, over 90% of those affected by ankylosing spondylitis are men, and 90 to 95% have HLA B27 (70). Chest wall restriction is an almost invariable finding, and upper lobe fibrosis occurs in some (65). Spencer (71) states, presumably on the basis of postmortem studies, that bronchiolitis obliterans commonly occurs in patients with ankylosing spondylitis; however, there are only two case reports in the literature (27,28). The clinical, radiological, and pathological features of these patients were similar to those found in patients with rheumatoid arthritis. In the one patient for whom the data were presented, the lung function studies showed a restrictive pattern compatible with chest wall restriction. There was no deterioration in this patient's lung function over 5 years, but it is impossible to generalize about prognosis on the basis of this single report.

SJÖGREN'S SYNDROME

Sjögren's syndrome generally occurs in association with other connective-tissue diseases. Approximately one-half of patients with Sjögren's syndrome have rheumatoid arthritis, but systemic lupus erythematosus and systemic sclerosis may be associated, as well as other systemic vasculitides (72). Pulmonary abnormalities are common in patients with Sjögren's syndrome, but it may be difficult to distinguish those that reflect an associated disease from those that characterize Sjögren's syndrome itself. Airflow obstruction has been reported in patients with Sjögren's syndrome. In one series (44) all the patients were nonsmokers but also had rheumatoid arthritis. In another (73) only 2 out of 13 had an associated arthritis, and the results showed an obstructive pattern predominantly due to small airways disease that was unresponsive to bronchodilators, suggesting that bronchiolitis obliterans may occur in Sjögren's syndrome. The majority of the clinicopathological data concerning bronchiolitis obliterans in Sjögren's syndrome comes from patients who also had rheumatoid arthritis or who had high titers of rheumatoid factor; however, Fortoul and colleagues (27) reported bronchiolitis obliterans in a patient without rheumatoid arthritis. The findings in these patients were similar to those found in patients with rheumatoid arthritis alone, and it is not possible to comment on whether there are specific features of bronchiolitis obliterans in Sjögren's syndrome.

SYSTEMIC SCLEROSIS

Clinical or radiological evidence of pulmonary disease is found in most patients with systemic sclerosis: interstitial fibrosis is the commonest abnormality. Airflow obstruction due to small airways disease is not a common finding in patients with systemic sclerosis (74,75). Two cases of bronchiolitis obliterans in patients with systemic sclerosis have been published (10,28). No specific features of these patients distinguish them from those with rheumatoid arthritis-associated bronchiolitis obliterans.

BEHÇET'S DISEASE

Pulmonary involvement of any sort is rare in Behçet's disease (65). There have been no reports of an association with bronchiolitis obliterans.

MIXED CONNECTIVE-TISSUE DISEASE

Patients with mixed connective-tissue disease have clinical features and pulmonary abnormalities that resemble those found in patients with systemic lupus erythematosus, systemic sclerosis, and polymyositis/dermatomyositis (65). Bronchiolitis obliterans has not been reported in association with mixed connective-tissue disease.

OTHER CONNECTIVE-TISSUE DISEASES

Bronchiolitis obliterans has been described in a 22-year-old woman with juvenile chronic arthritis (76) with features similar to those found in rheumatoid arthritis. Bronchiolitis obliterans may also occur in polymyositis/dermatomyositis (77).

REFERENCES

1. Osler W. On the visceral manifestations of the erythema group of skin diseases. *Am J Med Sci* 1904;127:1–23.
2. Day W. Case of scleroderma with the autopsy and remarks. *Am J Med Sci* 1870;59:350–359.
3. Ellman P, Ball RE. "Rheumatoid disease" with joint and pulmonary manifestations. *Br Med J* 1948;2:816–820.
4. Walker WC, Wright V. Rheumatoid pleuritis. *Ann Rheum Dis* 1967;26:467–474.
5. Caplan A, Payne RB, Withey JL. A broader concept of Caplan's syndrome. *Thorax* 1962;17:205–212.
6. Rubin EH, Gordon M, Thelma WL. Nodular pleuropulmonary rheumatoid disease. *Am J Med* 1967;42:567–581.
7. Aronoff A, Bywaters EGL, Fearnley GR. Lung lesions in rheumatoid arthritis. *Br Med J* 1955; 2:228–232.
8. Macfarlane JD, Dieppe PA, Rigden BG, Clark

TJH. Pulmonary and pleural lesions in rheumatoid disease. *Br J Dis Chest* 1978;72:288–300.
9. Geddes DM, Corrin B, Brewerton DA, Davies RJ, Turner-Warwick M. Progressive airway obliteration in adults and its association with rheumatoid disease. *Q J Med* 1977;46:427–444.
10. Epler GR, Snider GL, Gaensler EA, Catchcart ES, FitzGerald MX, Carrington CB. Bronchiolitis and bronchitis in connective tissue disease: a possible relationship to the use of penicillamine. *JAMA* 1979;242:528–532.
11. Cordier JF, Falconnet M, Moulin J, Brune J, Touraine R. Bronchiolite severe et polyarthrite rhumatoide role tres probable de la D-penicillamine dans deux observations. *Lyon Med* 1980; 244:113–114.
12. Chebat J, Seigneur F, Lechien J, Menkes CJ, Simon F, Martin JL. Obliterating bronchiolitis during D-penicillamine treatments [Letter]. *Nouv Presse Med* 1980;9:2655.
13. Murphy KC, Atkins CJ, Offer RC, Hogg JC, Stein HB. Obliterative bronchiolitis in two rheumatoid arthritis patients treated with penicillamine. *Arthritis Rheum* 1981;24:557–560.
14. Herzog CA, Miller RR, Hoidal JR. Bronchiolitis and rheumatoid arthritis. *Am Rev Respir Dis* 1981;124:636–639.
15. Turton CW, Williams G, Green M. Cryptogenic obliterative bronchiolitis in adults. *Thorax* 1981; 36:805–810.
16. Herne N, Jaubert D, Camilleri G, Prieur J. Obliterating bronchiolitis in rheumatoid arthritis: responsibility of D-penicillamine [Letter]. *Rev Rhum* 1981;48:744.
17. Jansen HM, Elema JD, Hylkema BS, et al. Progressive obliterative bronchiolitis in a patient with rheumatoid arthritis. *Eur J Respir Dis* 1982;121[Suppl]:43–52.
18. Penny WJ, Knight RK, Rees AM, Thomas AL, Smith AP. Obliterative bronchiolitis in rheumatoid arthritis. *Ann Rheum Dis* 1982;41:469–472.
19. Pieters R, Martens J, Dequeker J. Rheumatoid arthritis associated with bronchiolitis obliterans and immunoblastic sarcoma. *Clin Rheumatol* 1982;1:35–40.
20. Holness L, Tenenbaum J, Cooter NB, Grossman RF. Fatal bronchiolitis obliterans associated with chrysotherapy. *Ann Rheum Dis* 1983;42: 593–596.
21. McCann BG, Hart GJ, Stokes TC, Harrison BD. Obliterative bronchiolitis and upper-zone pulmonary consolidation in rheumatoid arthritis. *Thorax* 1983;38:73–74.
22. Wolfe F, Schurle DR, Lin JJ, et al. Upper and lower airway disease in penicillamine treated patients with rheumatoid arthritis. *J Rheumatol* 1983;10:406–410.
23. Geraads A, Brambilla E, Hohn B, Piton JL, Blanc-Jouvan F, Kamel A. Rheumatoid arthritis, obliterating bronchiolitis and D-penicillamine: apropos of a new case with ultrastructural examination and review of the literature. *Poumon Coeur* 1983;39:257–262.
24. Lahdensuo A, Mattila J, Vilppula A. Bronchiolitis in rheumatoid arthritis. *Chest* 1984;85:705–708.
25. Heyn J, Rasmussen EK. Obliterative bronchiolitis in rheumatoid arthritis. *Ugeskr Laeger* 1984; 146:4036–4037.
26. van de Laar MAFJ, Westermann CJJ, Wagenaar S, Dinant HJ. Beneficial effect of intravenous cyclophosphamide and oral prednisolone on D-penicillamine-associated bronchiolitis obliterans. *Arthritis Rheum* 1985;28:93–97.
27. Fortoul TI, Cano-Valle F, Oliva E, Barrios R. Follicular bronchiolitis in association with connective tissue diseases. *Lung* 1985;163:305–314.
28. Hakala M, Pääkkö P, Sutinen S, Huhti E, Koivisto O, Tarkka M. Association of bronchiolitis with connective tissue disorders. *Ann Rheum Dis* 1986;45:656–662.
29. Renier JC, Bontoux-Carre E, Racineux JL. Three cases of obliterating bronchiolitis during treatment of rheumatoid polyarthritis with D-penicillamine. *Rev Rhum* 1986;53:25–26.
30. Garcia Flores A, Martinez Pardo S, Soler Bel J, Garces Jarque JM. Bronchiolitis and rheumatoid arthritis: presentation of a case associated with therapy with gold salts [Letter]. *Rev Clin Esp* 1988;182:501–502.
31. Quijada C, Galleguillos F. Rheumatoid arthritis treated with penicillamine and bronchiolitis obliterans. *Rev Med Chil* 1988;116:164–168.
32. Newcomer AD, Miller RD, Hepper NG. Pulmonary dysfunction in rheumatoid arthritis and systemic lupus erythematosus. *Dis Chest* 1964; 46:562–570.
33. Patterson CD, Harville WE, Pierce JA. Rheumatoid lung disease. *Ann Intern Med* 1965;62: 685–697.
34. Walker WC, Wright V. Diffuse interstitial pulmonary fibrosis and rheumatoid arthritis. *Ann Rheum Dis* 1969;28:252–259.
35. Davidson C, Brook AGF, Bacon PA. Lung function in rheumatoid arthritis. *Ann Rheum Dis* 1974;33:293–297.
36. Schernthaner G, Scherak D, Kolarz G, Kummer F. Seropositive rheumatoid arthritis associated with decreased diffusion capacity of the lung. *Ann Rheum Dis* 1976;35:258–262.
37. Collins RL, Turner RA, Johnson AM, Whitley NO, McLean RL. Obstructive pulmonary disease in rheumatoid arthritis. *Arthritis Rheum* 1976;19:623–628.
38. Geddes DM, Webley M, Emerson PA. Airways obstruction in rheumatoid arthritis. *Ann Rheum Dis* 1979;38:222–225.
39. Mountz JD, Turner RA, Collins RL, Gallup KR, Semble EL. Rheumatoid arthritis and small airways function: effects of disease activity, smoking and α_1-antitrypsin deficiency. *Arthritis Rheum* 1984;27:728–736.
40. Sassoon CSH, McAlpine SW, Tashkin DP, Baydur A, Quismoro FP, Mongan ES. Small airways function in nonsmokers with rheumatoid arthritis. *Arthritis Rheum* 1984;27:1218–1226.
41. Hyland RH, Gordon DA, Broder I, et al. A systematic controlled study of pulmonary abnor-

malities in rheumatoid arthritis. *J Rheumatol* 1983;10:395–405.
42. Sweatman MC, Markwick JR, Charles PJ, et al. Histocompatibility antigens in adult obliterative bronchiolitis with or without rheumatoid arthritis. *Disease Markers* 1986;4:19–26.
43. Scott TE, Wise RA, Hochberg MC, Wigley FM. HLA-DR4 and pulmonary dysfunction in rheumatoid arthritis. *Am J Med* 1987;82:765–771.
44. Bégin R, Masse S, Menard H-A, Bureau M-A. Airways disease in a subset of nonsmoking rheumatoid patients. *Am J Med* 1982;72:743–750.
45. Jacobs P, Bonnyns M, Depierreux M, Duchateau J, Sergysels R. Rapidly fatal bronchiolitis obliterans with circulating antinuclear and rheumatoid factors. *Eur J Respir Dis* 1984;65:384–388.
46. Breatnach E, Kerr I. The radiology of cryptogenic obliterative bronchiolitis. *Clin Radiol* 1982; 33:657–661.
47. Padley SPG, Adler B, Hansell DM, Muller NL. Bronchiolitis obliterans: high resolution CT findings and correlation with pulmonary function tests. *Clin Radiol* 1993;47:236–249.
48. Corrin B. Volume 5: the lungs. In: *Systemic pathology*. 3rd ed. Edinburgh: Churchill Livingstone; 1990.
49. Gosnik BB, Friedman PJ, Liebow AA. Bronchiolitis obliterans: roentgenologic-pathologic correlation. *AJR* 1973;117:816–832.
50. DeHoratius RJ, Abruzzo JL, Williams RC. Immunofluorescent and immunologic studies of rheumatoid lung. *Arch Intern Med* 1992;129: 441–446.
51. King TE Jr. Bronchiolitis obliterans. *Lung* 1989; 167:69–93.
52. Griffith BP, Paradis IL, Zeevi A, et al. Immunologically mediated disease of the airways after pulmonary transplantation. *Ann Surg* 1988;208: 371–378.
53. Holland HK, Wingard JR, Beschorner WE, Saral R, Santos GW. Bronchiolitis obliterans in bone marrow transplantation and its relationship to chronic graft-versus-host disease and low serum IgG. *Blood* 1988;72:621–627.
54. Walker WC. Pulmonary infections in rheumatoid arthritis. *Q J Med* 1967;36:239–251.
55. Sternlieb I, Bennett B, Scheinberg IH. D-penicillamine induced Goodpasture's syndrome in Wilson's disease. *Ann Intern Med* 1975;82:673–676.
56. Eastmond CJ. Diffuse alveolitis as a complication of penicillamine treatment for rheumatoid arthritis. *Br Med J* 1976;1:1506.
57. Crouzet J, Camus JP, Leca AP. Lupus induit par la D-penicillamine au cours du traitment de la polyarthrite rhumatoide. *Ann Med Interne* 1974; 125:71–79.
58. Harpey JP, Caille B, Merilias P, Goust JM. Lupus-like syndrome induced by D(-)penicillamine in Wilson's disease. *Lancet* 1971;i:292.
59. Schraeder PL, Peters HA, Dahls DS. Polymyositis and penicillamine. *Arch Neurol* 1972;27: 456–457.
60. Bucknall RC, Dixon AStJ, Glick EN, Woodland J, Zutshi DW. Myasthenia gravis associated with penicillamine treatment for rheumatoid arthritis. *Br Med J* 1975;1:600–602.
61. Dawkins RL, Zilko PJ, Carrano J, Garlepp MJ, McDonald BL. Immunobiology of D-penicillamine. *J Rheumatol* 1981;8[Suppl 7]:56–61.
62. Woodley PH, Griffin J, Panayi GS, Batchelor JR, Welsh KI, Gibson TJ. HLA-DR antigens and toxic reactions to sodium aurothiomalate and D-penicillamine in patients with rheumatoid arthritis. *N Engl J Med* 1980;303:300–302.
63. Lyle WH. D-penicillamine and fatal obliterative bronchiolitis. *Br Med J* 1977;1:105.
64. Stein HB, Patterson C, Offer RC, Atkins C, Teufel A, Robinson HS. Adverse effects of D-penicillamine in rheumatoid arthritis. *Ann Intern Med* 1980;92:24–29.
65. Hunninghake GW, Fauci AS. Pulmonary involvement in the collagen vascular diseases. *Am Rev Respir Dis* 1979;119:471–503.
66. Matthay RA, Schwarz MI, Petty TL, et al. Pulmonary manifestations of systemic lupus erythematosus: review of twelve cases of acute lupus pneumonitis. *Medicine* 1974;54:397–409.
67. Pertschuk LP, Moccia LF, Rosen Y, et al. Acute pulmonary complications in systemic lupus erythematosus: immunofluorescence and light microscopic study. *Am J Clin Pathol* 1977;68:553–557.
68. Kinney WW, Angelillo VA. Bronchiolitis in systemic lupus erythematosus. *Chest* 1982;82:646–649.
69. Venizelos PC, Al-Bazzaz. Pulmonary function abnormalities in systemic lupus erythematosus responsive to glucocorticoid therapy. *Chest* 1981; 79:702–704.
70. Brewerton DA. HLA-B27 and the inheritance of susceptibility to rheumatic disease. *Arthritis Rheum* 1976;19:656–668.
71. Spencer H. *Pathology of the lung;* vol 2. 4th ed. Oxford: Pergamon; 1985:813.
72. Webb KW, McAvoy BA, Hughes GRV, Lee HP, MacSweeny RNM, Buchanan WW. Sjögren's syndrome: clinical associations and immunological phenomena. *Q J Med* 1973;42:513–548.
73. Newball HH, Brahim SA. Chronic obstructive airways disease in patients with Sjögren's syndrome. *Am Rev Respir Dis* 1977;115:295–304.
74. Bjerke RD, Tashkin DP, Clements DJ, Chopra SK, Gong H Jr, Bein M. Small airways in progressive systemic sclerosis. *Am J Med* 1979;66: 201–209.
75. Guttadauria M, Ellman H, Kaplan D, Diamond H. Pulmonary function in scleroderma. *Arthritis Rheum* 1977;20:1071–1079.
76. Porter DR, Stevenson RD, Sturrock RD. Obliterative bronchiolitis in juvenile chronic arthritis. *J Rheumatol* 1992;19:476–477.

Diseases of the Bronchioles, edited by
Gary R. Epler. Raven Press, Ltd.,
New York © 1994.

15

Drug-Related Bronchiolitis Obliterans

Gary R. Epler

Associate Clinical Professor, Boston University School of Medicine. Chairman, Department of Medicine, New England Baptist Hospital, 125 Parker Hill Avenue, Boston, MA.

Bronchiolitis obliterans is a rare lesion with limited causes and associated disorders. The first consideration of the possibility that the lesion could result from a drug-related effect was from a report in the late 1970s. Although several agents are a cause of bronchiolitis obliterans organizing pneumonia (BOOP), direct evidence of drug-related bronchiolitis obliterans continues to be difficult to confirm because the two possible agents, penicillamine and gold, are both used for rheumatoid arthritis, a disease itself that is related to bronchiolitis obliterans in the absence of any therapy. Most reports regarding these two agents and bronchiolitis obliterans were published between 1977 and 1986. This chapter reviews the perspective of these reports as they relate to drug-related bronchiolitis obliterans.

PENICILLAMINE

Bronchiolitis obliterans was not associated with an adverse drug reaction until 1977, when Geddes and colleagues (1) reported three patients with rheumatoid arthritis and obliterative bronchiolitis who had also received penicillamine. All three had chest radiographs showing distended lungs, crackles and a midinspiratory squeak on examination of the chest, and severe reduction in the forced expired volume in one second (FEV_1) of only 0.56 to 0.70 L. The first was a 45-year-old woman who had had rheumatoid arthritis for 11 years and smoked. She was admitted to the hospital because of 6 weeks of progressive dyspnea. She had been taking 55 g of penicillamine for 7 months, which was stopped at about the time of admission because of a rash that suggested drug hypersensitivity. Respiratory distress progressed, requiring mechanical ventilation. She died 5 months after hospital admission. The histology showed marked constriction of the bronchiolar lumen by fibrous tissue. The second patient was a 50-year-old woman who had had rheumatoid arthritis for 10 years. She was admitted to the hospital because of 3 months of nonproductive cough and progressive dyspnea. She had received a total dose of penicillamine of 400 g during the previous year. It was stopped during the hospitalization. Treated with corticosteroid therapy, she improved initially but then deteriorated and died. At autopsy, the bronchioles showed constrictive bronchiolitis. The lumina of some bronchioles were completely obliterated by fibrous tissue. Intraluminal polyps were not observed. The third patient was a 37-year-old woman who had had rheumatoid arthritis for 10 years. She developed severe breathlessness after an episode of bronchitis. She had been treated briefly with gold 9 years previously without adverse pulmonary effects. Penicillamine therapy had been started 1 year before the onset of dyspnea. After a course of prednisone, 30 mg daily, pulmonary function tests improved but incapacitating breathlessness persisted.

Two years later, there was a report of two patients treated with penicillamine who developed bronchiolar disease (2). The first was a 42-year-old woman who had never smoked. Her initial diagnosis was scleroderma, and she received penicillamine therapy, 500 mg daily. During the next 5 months, stiffness and thickening of the skin persisted and the penicillamine was increased to 1,250 mg daily. This therapy was discontinued 1 month later because of leukopenia; however, she had also developed dyspnea that became so severe that hospitalization was required. It was thought that the scleroderma illness more closely resembled eosinophilic fasciitis. The FEV_1 increased dramatically from a normal value of 2.33 L before penicillamine treatment to a severely decreased value of 0.52 L, and the FEV_1/FVC ratio decreased from 75 to 40%. Lung biopsy showed severe chronic bronchitis and bronchiolitis. There were many irregular foci of granulation tissue in the thickened bronchial wall but no intraluminal polyps. The intensity of the cellular infiltrate diminished progressively until none was apparent at the level of the respiratory bronchioles. The second patient was a 54-year-old woman who had developed progressive rheumatoid arthritis that did not respond to conventional therapy. Penicillamine, 750 mg daily, was started with a dramatic improvement in arthritic symptoms. Ten months later, she developed a nonproductive cough and then dyspnea; the penicillamine was stopped. The chest roentgenogram was normal. Distinctive early inspiratory crackles were heard and graphically documented. There was no mid-inspiratory squeak. The FEV_1 was 0.94 L. Lung biopsy showed that most lesions involved the conducting airways. One small bronchus included in the biopsy was narrowed to about one-half of its original diameter by scar tissue. The walls of bronchioles were infiltrated by a mixture of mononuclear cells, and some bronchioles were surrounded by lymphoid follicles consistent with follicular bronchiolitis. Some of the bronchioles were obliterated by irregular polypoid masses of maturing granulation tissue. After 3 months of prednisone, 60 mg daily, pulmonary function remained unchanged. It was noted that penicillamine blocks cross-linkage of newly synthesized collagen and elastin, which could cause impaired wound healing. Patients with connective-tissue disorders, especially rheumatoid arthritis, are prone to develop bronchiolitis obliterans, and penicillamine could interfere with or modify this process.

Two patients were reported (3) to have developed bronchiolitis obliterans in a prospective study of 259 patients with rheumatoid arthritis treated with penicillamine. Of these patients, 99% had received gold therapy before administration of penicillamine. A report (4) describing these two patients indicated that the first was a 61-year-old woman who had had rheumatoid arthritis for 3 years and had received gold, but because of continuing active rheumatologic disease, she was given penicillamine, 750 mg daily. Six months later she developed dyspnea and a nonproductive cough, and 2 months aftr that she was admitted to the hospital with acute respiratory failure. The penicillamine was discontinued, leading to some improvement in her clinical status. Chest examination noted a "clicking" sound synchronous with respiration. She progressively deteriorated and died. Autopsy showed marked bronchiolitis. The second patient was a 52-year-old woman who had had rheumatoid arthritis for 3 years. Gold therapy failed to control her arthritis; thus penicillamine at 500 mg daily was given. This agent was stopped in 4 months because of widespread urticaria. Five weeks later, dyspnea and a nonproductive cough developed with coarse inspiratory crackles. Pulmonary function studies showed severe airflow obstruction. Open lung biopsy showed marked bronchiolitis; the airway lumen was distorted by the inflammatory process, which was heaped up in a polypoid-like fashion. The authors noted that this report was written as a warning of the possible relationship between penicillamine and obliterative bronchiolitis. They recommended the cessation of penicillamine in any patient with unexplained respiratory symptoms.

A report in 1982 (5) described two patients with rheumatoid arthritis who had received penicillamine and developed obliterative bronchiolitis. The first was a 63-year-old woman who had had rheumatoid arthritis for 5 years. She was admitted to the hospital because of rapidly worsening dyspnea and a nonproductive cough. She had been treated with nonsteroidal antiinflammatory agents for 4 years, but because of active arthritis disease, penicillamine was given at a dosage not exceeding 375 mg daily. Fifteen months later she developed dyspnea. Coarse crackles and a variable wheeze were heard on examination of the chest. The FEV_1 was severely decreased to 0.6 L, only 29% of the predicted value. Transbronchial biopsy showed no parenchymal lung disease. After several weeks of therapy and a trial of azathioprine therapy, which was rapidly discontinued because of severe oral ulceration, she steadily deteriorated and died of respiratory failure 5 months after the initial symptoms. Autopsy showed bronchiolitis obliterans. Bronchioles were occluded by chronic inflammatory cells, and their walls were thickened by granulation tissue. In some bronchioles the mucosa was ulcerated with the formation of granulation tissue polyps. The alveolar ducts and alveoli were not involved. The second patient had a diagnosis of nonbiopsy confirmed bronchiolitis obliterans. She was a 56-year-old woman who was admitted to the hospital after experiencing cough and wheezing for 8 months and worsening dyspnea for 4 months. She had had rheumatoid arthritis for 11 years and Sjögren's syndrome for 3 years. More than 2 years before these symptoms appeared, she had received penicillamine 125 mg daily, and the dose was progressively increased to 375 mg daily. The rheumatoid arthritis improved, although she had recurrent episodes of penicillamine-related thrombocytopenia, and the dosage was stabilized at 50 mg daily. On admission she had dyspnea at rest. Bilateral coarse crackles and a midinspiratory squeak were heard throughout the lungs. The chest radiograph showed hyperinflation. Pulmonary function tests showed airflow obstruction with FEV_1 of 1.20 L (52% predicted) and FEV_1/FVC of 56% with no improvement after bronchodilator inhalation. The penicillamine was stopped. The pulmonary function tests showed stabilization with persistent airflow obstruction after corticosteroid and azathioprine therapy. The authors noted that although the evidence implicating penicillamine as a causal agent was conflicting because obliterative bronchiolitis had been reported in patients not receiving penicillamine, they recommended that patients receiving this agent who develop unexplained respiratory symptoms should be evaluated for obliterative bronchiolitis.

A second report (6) in 1982 from the Netherlands described a 62-year-old woman who had had seropositive rheumatoid arthritis for 4 years. She was treated with gold injections and indomethacine for 2 years and then penicillamine and indomethacine for 1 year. During the time of penicillamine therapy, she developed increasing shortness of breath and wheezing. Pulmonary function studies showed nonreversible airflow obstruction with FEV_1 of 0.78 L and FEV_1/FVC of 34%. Auscultation of the lungs revealed inspiratory wheezing, crackles, and prolonged expiration. The sedimentation rate was 12 mm/hour. The chest roentgenogram showed hyperinflation and normal lungs. The patient deteriorated rapidly and required mechanical ventilation. An open lung biopsy showed mononuclear infiltration of alveolar septa and respiratory bronchioles obliterated by young fibrous tissue. Lobular and terminal bronchioles showed submucosal edema with lymphocytic and plasma-cellular infiltration. Some bronchioles showed ulceration of the epithelium and obliteration of the lumen by inflammatory cells. The patient was treated with corticosteroid therapy and azathioprine, but this treatment had no effect on the course of the illness and the patient died. The authors of this report concluded that it was unlikely that penicillamine played a causal role because only three of the six patients described in Geddes and colleagues (1) were treated with the drug, and there was no improvement in this patient after the treatment was stopped.

A 1983 report (7) noted that up to that time, 20 patients with rheumatoid arthritis had developed obliterative bronchiolitis during penicillamine therapy and 15 patients with rheumatoid arthritis who had not received penicillamine had developed bronchiolitis obliterans. The authors also reported 3 additional patients with rheumatoid arthritis and obliterative bronchiolitis who had received penicillamine. One was a 61-year-old woman who had had rheumatoid arthritis for 6 years who developed severe, obstructive airway disease 6 months after penicillamine therapy. The FEV_1 was 0.85 L, and the chest radiograph showed hyperinflation. The disease progressed despite corticosteroid therapy. She died 7 months after the development of symptoms. Autopsy showed luminal occlusion of the bronchioles by polypoid granulation tissue.

A second report (8) in 1985 from the Netherlands discussed a 32-year-old woman who was admitted to the hospital because of progressive dyspnea and nonproductive cough. She had had rheumatoid arthritis for 2 years and had received penicillamine, 250 mg daily, for 6 months. On admission, she was dyspneic and in obvious respiratory distress. Auscultation of the chest revealed inspiratory crackles. A graphic illustration of the respiratory sounds confirmed the midinspiratory squeak as noted by Geddes and colleagues (1). The sedimentation rate was normal. The chest radiograph showed hyperinflation. Pulmonary function studies showed severe airflow obstruction with an FEV_1 of 0.90 L. The histological findings of the open lung biopsy indicated a concentric bronchiolar process consisting of reparative tissue with predominant fibroblasts and disruption of the muscularis mucosa and constriction of the bronchiolar lumen. A diagnosis of penicillamine-associated bronchiolitis obliterans was made, and prednisone was given. After initial improvement, progressive dyspnea resumed, and cyclophosphamide at 2 mg/kg daily was started. Ten days later her dyspnea improved. Twelve weeks later, she was able to return home. After 1 year of cyclophosphamide, 100 to 125 mg daily, the prednisone, 10 to 25 mg daily, the pulmonary function had stopped declining and her clinical condition had improved, although she continued to have severe airflow obstruction with an FEV_1 of less than 0.8 L.

These authors also reviewed 12 patients from the literature who had what they called penicillamine-associated bronchiolitis obliterans. All were women aged 36 to 66 years. The dose of penicillamine ranged from 375 to 1,250 mg daily for 3 to 14 months. All were treated with prednisone and 3 also with azathioprine. Among the 12, the mortality was high, approaching 50%. Five dead, two were unchanged, one worsened, and one improved. The authors noted that direct proof of an etiologic relationship between the drug and this highly aggressive form of bronchiolitis obliterans was lacking and probably difficult to obtain because of the usually fatal course of the disease, which precludes rechallenging.

A histocompatibility antigen study (9) of 16 patients with rheumatoid arthritis who also had obliterative bronchiolitis showed an increase in HLA-B40 and DR4. The DR4 antigen may suggest an association between the pathogenesis of both obliterative bronchiolitis and rheumatoid arthritis. Patients who had received penicillamine did not show an increase in antigens such as DR2/3 that are associated with other gold and penicillamine toxicity.

PENICILLAMINE AND GOLD

Of the patients reported as possibly having penicillamine-related obliterative bronchiolitis, most of them had received gold prior to the penicillamine treatment (1,3,4, 6,7,9), and occasional patients had not received gold (2,5,8). For most of these patients, the gold had been given in the distant past and was not related to pulmonary symptoms. The effects of penicillamine and gold are most likely separate events; there has been no evidence suggesting a synergistic effect of these two agents.

GOLD

Gold therapy for rheumatoid arthritis is a possible cause of bronchiolitis obliterans, but the relationship has not been firmly established. There was a report (10) of a 65-year-old woman with rheumatoid arthritis who developed increasing dyspnea after she received a total of 1.125 g of gold therapy over several months. On examination, there were diffuse wheezes and decreased breath sounds. The chest radiograph showed hyperinflation with no parenchymal infiltrates. She developed progressive respiratory failure and died. Autopsy showed extensive obliterative bronchiolitis with ulceration of the respiratory mucosa and peribronchial inflammation. The surrounding lung parenchyma was normal.

An additional report (11) indicated that irreversible airway obstruction developed in a 44-year-old woman with severe rheumatoid arthritis. She had been treated with penicillamine for 1 year, with improvement in her arthritic symptoms; but with reactivation of her disease 3 years later, gold therapy was started. She received 1.620 g of gold during a 1-year period. The patient developed dyspnea and wheezes 2 days after a gold injection, and the therapy was stopped. On physical examination, a midinspiratory squeak was heard. The sedimentation rate was 58 mm/hour. The chest radiograph was normal. Pulmonary function showed a normal FEV_1; however, the residual volume and residual volume to total lung capacity (RV/TLC) ratio were increased. Penicillamine therapy and low-dose corticosteroid therapy was reinstituted because of progressive activity of the rheumatoid arthritis. Eight months later an open lung biopsy showed that the walls of the repository bronchioles were densely infiltrated with lymphocytes and histiocytes, and collection of histiocytes were forming small granulomatous foci in the bronchial wall. There was no evidence of bronchiolar scarring, obliteration, or intraluminal polyps. IgM and IgG containing plasma cells were seen in the bronchiolar walls, which suggested direct immune-mediated lung injury, although linear deposition of IgG in alveolar walls has been reported (12) in a patient with rheumatoid arthritis and obliterative bronchiolitis who had not received penicillamine or gold therapy.

The effects of gold and penicillamine therapy in this patient were not clear. The first course of penicillamine was several years before bronchiolitis was detected. Her respiratory symptoms developed 2 days after gold injections at the beginning of the pulmonary disease, suggesting a gold-related event; yet when the resumed penicillamine therapy was stopped, the respiratory symptoms diminished and disappeared and her lung function improved. The authors suggested caution with rheumatoid patients receiving antirheumatic drugs who develop respiratory symptoms. The auscultatory findings and measurement of lung volumes may be important in detection of early bronchiolitis.

A 44-year-old woman who had had rheumatoid arthritis for 2 years developed progressive dyspnea and a persistent nonproductive cough for 10 days, 5 months after oral gold therapy had been given (13). She was part of a penicillamine-oral gold therapy trial and had been randomly selected to receive gold at 3 mg twice daily. On examination, inspiratory crackles were heard at both lung bases. The chest roentgenogram showed no new infiltrates. Pulmonary function showed severe airflow obstruction with FEV_1 of 0.84 L. Histologic findings of the open lung biopsy showed the bronchocentric nature of the infiltrate with unaffected intervening pulmonary parenchyma. Bronchioles showed destruction of the wall by mononuclear cell infiltration with mucus plugging and macrophage infiltration of the lumen. There was some improvement with corticosteroid therapy, but severe airflow obstruction persisted. The authors noted that the link between gold or penicillamine and bronchiolitis was in dispute; and that nevertheless, the problem should be approached with open-minded caution. It may be impractical to perform regular pulmonary function testing to preempt bronchiolitis, especially since the complication is rare, (one patient of 100 studied received gold and one received penicillamine); but patients should be informed of possible serious lung injury. Unexplained cough or development of dyspnea are late warning symptoms and mandate immediate withdrawal of the agent.

In summary, penicillamine and gold have been implicated in the cause of bronchiolitis obliterans, but the cause and effect have been difficult to establish with certainty because obliterative bronchiolitis occurs in patients with rheumatoid arthritis who have not had either of these agents. Whether weekly or monthly spirometric monitoring is feasible and could prevent serious effects has not been established. It remains prudent to discontinue these agents at the first sign of unexplained pulmonary symptoms.

REFERENCES

1. Geddes DM, Corrin B, Brewerton DA, et al. Progressive airway obliteration in adults and its association with rheumatoid disease. *Q J Med* 1977;46(184):427–444.
2. Epler GR, Snider GL, Gaensler EA, et al. Bronchiolitis and bronchitis in connective tissue disease: a possible relationship to the use of penicillamine. *JAMA* 1979;242:528–532.
3. Stein HB, Patterson AC, Offer RC, et al. Adverse effects of D-penicillamine in rheumatoid arthritis. *Ann Intern Med* 1980;92:24–29.
4. Murphy KC, Atkins CJ, Offer RC, et al. Obliterative bronchiolitis in two rheumatoid arthritis patients treated with penicillamine. *Arthritis Rheum* 1981;24:557–560.
5. Penny WJ, Knight RK, Rees AM, et al. Obliterative bronchiolitis in rheumatoid arthritis. *Ann Rheum Dis* 1982;41:469–472.
6. Jansen HM, Elema JD, Hylkema BS, et al. Progressive obliterative bronchiolitis in a patient with rheumatoid arthritis. *Eur J Respir Dis* 1982;63[Suppl 121]:43–52.
7. Wolfe F, Schurle DR, Lin JJ, et al. Upper and lower airway disease in penicillamine treated patients with rheumatoid arthritis. *J Rheumatol* 1983;10:406–410.
8. Van de Laar MAFJ, Westermann CJJ, Wagenaar SS, Dinant HJ. Beneficial effect of intravenous cyclophosphamide and oral prednisone on D-penicillamine associated bronchiolitis obliterans. *Arthritis Rheum* 1985;28:93–97.
9. Sweatman MC, Markwick JR, Charles PJ, et al. Histocompatibility antigens in adult obliterative bronchiolitis with or without rheumatoid arthritis. *Dis Markers* 1986;4:19–26.
10. Holness L, Tenenbaum J, Cooter NBE, Grossman RF. Fatal bronchiolitis obliterans associated with chrysotherapy. *Ann Rheum Dis* 1983; 42:593–596.
11. Lahdensuo A, Mattila J, Vilppula A. Bronchiolitis in rheumatoid arthritis. *Chest* 1984;85:705–708.
12. Herzog CA, Miller RR, Hoidal JR. Bronchiolitis and rheumatoid arthritis. *Am Rev Respir Dis* 1981;124:636–639.
13. O'Duffy JD, Luthra HS, Unni KK, Hyatt RE. Bronchiolitis in a rheumatoid arthritis patient receiving auranofin. *Arthritis Rheum* 1986;29: 556–559.

Diseases of the Bronchioles, edited by
Gary R. Epler. Raven Press, Ltd.,
New York © 1994.

16

Bone Marrow Transplantation Bronchiolitis Obliterans

Charles K. Chan

Assistant professor of medicine; Director, pulmonary fellowship program, University of Toronto. Consultant in respiratory medicine and critical care medicine, The Wellesley and Princess Margaret Hospitals, Toronto, Ontario, Canada.

Since 1968, allogeneic and autologous bone marrow transplantations have been established as a principal modality of therapy in the provision of long-term disease-free survival for patients with acute or chronic leukemia, aplastic anemia, and various immunodeficiency syndromes (1). The major limitations to further improvements in successful bone marrow transplantation are multiorgan graft-versus-host disease, recurrence of primary malignancies, and respiratory complications after organ transplantation (1).

Pulmonary complications with bone marrow transplantation affect 40 to 60% of patients after engraftment and are the major causes of morbidity and mortality (2). The spectrum of respiratory complications post-transplant include infectious and noninfectious pneumonitis, obstructive airways disease, sinopulmonary infections, chronic aspiration, and pulmonary vascular disease (Fig. 1).

Infectious pulmonary complications tend to arise in the first 100 days after engraftment, whereas noninfectious respiratory disorders such as obstructive airways disease tend to develop much later (Fig. 1). Obstructive airways disease is the most common post-transplant noninfectious respiratory complication, usually developing after day 100 and during the same time interval as that for chronic graft-versus-host disease (2,3).

Airways disease was first described in a postmortem study by Beschorner and colleagues (4) in 1978. Lymphocytic bronchitis was observed in about 10% of the autopsies on patients who died from complications on bone marrow transplantation. This large airways inflammatory process was thought to be distinct from idiopathic interstitial pneumonitis and perhaps graft-versus-host disease of the lungs. Because this was a postmortem study, the clinical significance of airways involvement in bone marrow recipients remained uncertain until the first case of fatal bronchiolitis obliterans was described in 1982 (5).

Roca and colleagues (5) reported a 22-year-old patient who received an allogeneic bone marrow transplant for aplastic anemia. The patient's post-transplant clinical course was complicated by severe graft-versus-host disease, and the patient subsequently developed progressive obstructive airways disease. The patient died despite aggressive therapies. Lung pathology showed bronchiolitis obliterans. In the ensuing years, reports (6) from various transplant centers led to the recognition of the increasing frequency and severity of bronchiolitis obliterans in recipients of allogeneic bone marrow transplantations.

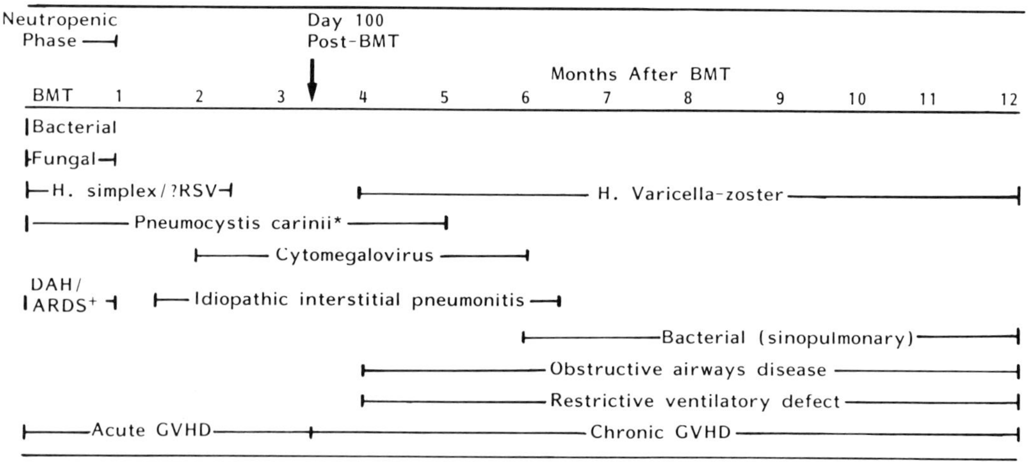

FIG. 1. The spectrum and usual time of onset of major pulmonary complications after bone marrow transplant. *DAH,* diffuse alveolar hemorrhage; *ARDS,* adult respiratory distress syndrome; *RSV,* respiratory syncytial virus; *BMT,* bone marrow transplantation; *GVHD,* graft-versus-host disease. Reprinted with permission from Chan CK, Hyland RH, Hutcheon MA. Pulmonary complications following bone marrow transplantation. *Clin Chest Med* 1990; 11(2): 323–332. Copyright W. B. Saunders.

The incidence of obstructive airways disease consistent with bronchiolitis obliterans after transplantation is estimated at 5 to 10% of allogeneic transplant recipients (3,6–8) and can be as high as 15% in patients with severe graft-versus-host disease (3,9).

It is generally believed that since graft-versus-host disease is not a problem with autologous bone marrow transplant, bronchiolitis obliterans should not be a respiratory complication after autologous transplantation; however, patients with bronchiolitis obliterans after autologous bone marrow transplant have been reported in a recent publication (10). Other unpublished cases at a number of transplant centers during recent years seem to indicate that bronchiolitis obliterans can affect autologous transplant recipients, although the frequency seems to be low.

The observations to date point toward bronchiolitis obliterans in bone marrow transplantation as a multifactorial process (2–3,6–10). Since the underlying pathophysiology is not well understood, it is not at all surprising that attempts at treatment that primarily involve aggressive immunosuppressive therapies have done poorly in reducing the morbidity and mortality associated with this complication (2–10).

This chapter reviews the pertinent clinical, radiographic, pulmonary physiological, and pathological features of bronchioli-

TABLE 1. *Profile of patients with bone marrow transplantation bronchiolitis obliterans*

Clinical
Cough and dyspnea 6 to 12 months after transplantation
Hyperinflation with or without wheezing
Sinusitis and multisystem chronic graft-versus-host disease
Methotrexate in the pretransplant conditioning regimen
? Chronic myelogenous leukemia as an underlying disease
Radiographic
Hyperinflation without parenchymal infiltrate
Presence or absence of a pneumothorax
Thickening of small airways on high-resolution computerized tomography
Physiology
Hyperinflation and gas trapping
Air-flow obstruction at mid to low lung volumes
No response to bronchodilator
Reduced diffusing capacity
Bronchoalveolar lavage
Poor returns
Absence of infectious agents
Increased lymphocytes or mixed lymphocytes–neutrophils

tis obliterans as a respiratory complication after allogeneic bone marrow transplantation. Current pathogenetic concepts, usual clinical course, and various therapeutic strategies that have been used for management are also highlighted. The typical patient profile is summarized in Table 1 and described in detail in the sections below.

CLINICAL FEATURES

Time of Occurrence

Bronchiolitis obliterans usually develops 6 to 12 months after transplantation, but has been described as early as 41 days and as late as 2 years (6).

Symptoms and Physical Findings

The predominant symptoms are a nonproductive cough and progressive dyspnea (3,6). Fever is generally not a presenting feature; however, nasal congestion due to sinusitis is a frequent comorbidity at presentation. The cough can continue for weeks to months, waxing and waning, and may even respond symptomatically to bronchodilator or topical steroids, mimicking new-onset asthma early in the clinical course. Since the majority of these patients have concurrent or antecedent graft-versus-host disease, immunosuppressive agents in the form of systemic corticosteroids are frequently administered (3,6). Corticosteroids may mask the full-blown picture of bronchiolitis obliterans; however, airflow obstruction invariably progresses and dyspnea on exertion follows.

On physical examination, wheezing or expiratory squeaky noises are frequently detected in up to one-half of the patients early in the clinical course. The absence of wheezing or squeak does not exclude bronchiolitis obliterans. However, clinical signs of hyperinflation and diminished breath sounds are the most consistent physical findings in all patients with bronchiolitis obliterans (3,6). Occasionally, basal crackles may be detected in 5 to 10% of patients (3,6).

High-Risk Clinical Profiles

Additional clinical features pointing toward bronchiolitis obliterans include a history of recurrent sinusitis and graft-versus-host disease (6,9). Recurrent sinusitis may be related to impairment of mucociliary clearance secondary to epithelial damages as a consequence of graft-versus-host disease. Mucus membrane graft-versus-host disease resulting in upper airways sicca syndrome is common in bone marrow transplant recipients with bronchiolitis obliterans.

Usually, chronic graft-versus-host disease in patients who develop bronchiolitis obliterans is severe and affects various organs, frequently involving the skin, conjunctiva, mucus membrane, gastrointestinal tract, and liver (6). Furthermore, bronchiolitis obliterans typically occurs in patients with poorly controlled chronic graft-versus-host disease despite intense immunosuppressive therapies (6). Evidence of chronic graft-versus-host disease is usually obvious clinically, but in a few patients the only significant abnormality may be persistent or worsening liver function tests.

Other established risk factors for the development of bronchiolitis obliterans include the use of methotrexate prophylaxis for graft-versus-host disease as part of the transplantation protocol (7), and the development of serum hypogammaglobulinemia (11). Methotrexate is thought to be associated with bronchiolitis obliterans through an immunological process (7). Low serum immunoglobulins may either represent a marker for chronic graft-versus-host disease or predisposes transplant recipients to yet unidentified infectious processes leading to bronchiolitis obliterans (11).

There is some indirect evidence to suggest a difference in either the incidence or severity of bronchiolitis obliterans among the various underlying disease processes resulting in bone marrow transplantation; i.e., bronchiolitis obliterans tends to be more severe in patients with chronic myelogenous leukemia than in patients who underwent transplantation for aplastic anemia (3,12–14). Whether the difference observed in these preliminary studies is due to the underlying disease process or a reflection of the pretransplant conditioning regimens remains unclear (2–3).

RADIOGRAPHIC FINDINGS

Routine Chest Radiographs

Chest radiographs in patients with bronchiolitis obliterans usually do not reveal any parenchymal infiltrate, consolidation, or air space disease. The typical findings are relatively normal with radiographic evidence of hyperinflation (2–3,6). In some patients, focal and, rarely, diffuse infiltrates may be present (2,6). Infiltrative processes or air space disease found radiographically tend to be more likely to be associated with infectious etiologies due primarily to viruses. Alternatively, such patients have evidence of interstitial pneumonitis in conjunction with bronchiolitis obliterans on lung biopsy examination (6). Recurrent pneumothoraces causing major morbidity and mortality are frequently observed in patients with advanced bronchiolitis obliterans but are rarely the presenting finding (6).

Therefore, the typical radiographic features of patients with uncomplicated bronchiolitis obliterans are very similar to those of patients with poorly controlled asthma with hyperinflation infrequently complicated by pneumothoraces. Radiographic features of simple bronchiolitis obliterans are distinctly different from those of bronchiolitis obliterans organizing pneumonia (BOOP), which typically show patchy infiltrates, both focal and diffuse patterns, and reduced or normal lung volumes instead of hyperinflation (15).

High-Resolution Computerized Tomography

There is limited published data on the utility of high-resolution computerized tomography (CT) in the diagnostic workups of patients with bronchiolitis obliterans (2). Unlike BOOP, in which there is diffuse pulmonary parenchymal involvement, high-resolution CT can help in defining air space consolidation from ground-glass opacities in a panlobular distribution (16–19). High-resolution CT has a more limited role in bronchiolitis obliterans. Patients with bronchiolitis obliterans, whose chest radiographs either are normal or show hyperinflation, usually have a relatively normal high-resolution CT examination. Careful scrutiny may reveal areas of reduced density in a lobular distribution with associated reduction of small airways caliber. These features are consistent with but not diagnostic of bronchiolitis obliterans. However, in a patient at risk of bronchiolitis obliterans and with the appropriate clinical features and physiological findings, the high-resolution CT features support the clinical diagnosis of bronchiolitis obliterans (2).

PULMONARY PHYSIOLOGICAL FEATURES

Basic Pulmonary Function Testing

Due to careful screening of candidates for bone marrow transplantation, most patients have relatively normal pulmonary function tests pretransplantation. When bronchiolitis obliterans develops and as the patient becomes more symptomatic, pulmonary function tests reveal a new onset of moderate to severe airflow obstruction (3,6).

At an earlier stage of bronchiolitis obliterans, the most common pulmonary function test abnormalities are hyperinflation with gas trapping by lung volumes measurement and reduced flow rates at mid to low lung volumes (3,6). Differing from asthma, the airflow obstruction in bronchiolitis obliterans is not reversible with bronchodilator; thus the obstruction is fixed (6). And in contrast to large airways disease, such as acute bronchitis or lymphocytic bronchitis, the site of airflow obstruction is localized to the level of the small airways in patients with bronchiolitis obliterans, as described in the assessment below (6).

Diffusing capacity, despite correction for hemoglobin, is usually reduced even though the chest radiograph is normal. Unfortunately, a reduced diffusing capacity cannot differentiate bronchiolitis obliterans from other late pulmonary complications, as shown in Fig. 1 (6). Diffusing capacity corrected for hemoglobin level is usually reduced within the first 3 to 6 months after transplantation. The diffusing capacity then gradually returns to the normal range in the majority of patients from the 6th month onwards. In most of these patients without respiratory complications, the diffusing capacity is usually within the normal range by the end of the first year after bone marrow transplantation.

Advanced Physiological Assessments

Where physiological documentation of small airways disease is desirable, helium-oxygen maximum expiratory flow studies can be applied to demonstrate obstruction at the level of the distal small airways (6). Helium-oxygen maximum expiratory flow studies demonstrate high volume of isoflow, with no significant improvement in flow rates in breathing the mixture at 50% of the vital capacity as compared to studies breathing ambient air (6,20–21).

Advanced pulmonary physiological tests, including the static lung compliance, have also been studied (6). Patients with bronchiolitis obliterans usually have normal lung compliance or elastic recoil when the complication is in the mild to moderate range (6). As the airflow obstruction and gas trapping worsen, the pressure–volume curve is shifted to the left, similar to individuals with severe emphysema (6). These physiological studies are of limited clinical value in the assessment of a transplant recipient with bronchiolitis obliterans, but they add to the understanding of the pathophysiology of this disabling complication.

Prognostic Value of Pulmonary Function Testing

The prognostic values of pretransplant pulmonary function in the prediction of patients at risk of bronchiolitis obliterans have been studied (7–8). Clark and colleagues (7) retrospectively found that a pretransplant reduction in the ratio of the forced expiratory volume in one second to the forced vital capacity (FEV_1/FVC) is associated with post-transplant airways dysfunction but not necessarily worsening airflow obstruction. Krowka and colleagues (8) prospectively assessed the prognostic significance of airway reactivity as measured by the methacholine challenge test in predicting the development of small airways disease in these patients. They found that 21% of the patients assessed responded positively to the methacholine challenge test prior to transplantation; thus reactive airways was a common phenomenon before bone marrow transplantation. However, a positive response to methacholine challenge test was not associated with the development of bronchiolitis obliterans or small airways disease. These findings offer further proof that clinical or pathologically proven bronchiolitis obliterans is distinct from asthma, and that the presence of airflow obstruction before transplant is not directly associated with the development of bronchiolitis obliterans.

BRONCHOALVEOLAR LAVAGE AND LUNG PATHOLOGY FINDINGS

Bronchoalveolar Lavage

Systematic and detailed assessments of bronchoalveolar lavage findings in patients with post-transplant bronchiolitis obliterans are not as well studied as those in patients with idiopathic BOOP (22–25). Nevertheless, lavage is frequently used in the diagnostic evaluation of transplant patients suspected of developing bronchiolitis obliterans on the basis of clinical, radiographic, and physiological investigations (2,6).

Bronchoscopy and lavage are performed primarily to exclude infectious etiologies such as cytomegalovirus, herpes simplex virus, and other opportunistic infections that may need consideration, depending on the time of occurrence, as illustrated in Fig. 1 (2). Lavage is especially important in patients suspected to have bronchiolitis obliterans whose radiographic examinations show parenchymal infiltrates because these findings are more likely to be associated with one or more infectious pathogens than those of patients with only hyperinflation (6).

Bronchoalveolar lavage should be performed cautiously in patients with advanced bronchiolitis obliterans. Because of the airways narrowing and obliteration, the return of the lavage is generally poor in patients with severe bronchiolitis obliterans. The risk of inducing barotrauma resulting in pneumothorax is increased in patients with FEV_1 below 1 L or 25% of the predicted (2).

Apart from the identification of infectious pathogens that may complicate post-transplant bronchiolitis obliterans, bronchoalveolar lavage remains an investigative tool and cannot establish the diagnosis of this complication. Preliminary data on a small number of patients with bronchiolitis obliterans without evidence of infectious agents suggest that the lavage findings are similar to those of idiopathic BOOP (22–25).

The total number of cells in the lavage returns, obtained from patients with bronchiolitis obliterans, increases after bone marrow transplantation. Cellular profile of the bronchoalveolar lavage shows either lymphocyte predominance or an increase in mixed lymphocyte–neutrophil percentage in the lavage cell population. However, the lymphocytosis tends to be in the range of 30 to 50%. A higher percentage of lymphocytes in the bronchoalveolar lavage (60 to 70%) usually suggest a concurrent or associated infectious process, including cytomegalovirus and pneumocystis carinii (2,6). The lavage profile in patients with complicated bronchiolitis obliterans, and especially those who develop BOOP, is similar to that in patients with idiopathic BOOP (26). Protein and immunoglobulin profiles of the lavage in patients with bronchiolitis obliterans are still being investigated.

Transbronchial Lung Biopsy

Transbronchial lung biopsy specimens are often too small to demonstrate pathology in the small airways because the parenchyma is less likely to be affected in bronchiolitis obliterans than in BOOP (2–3, 6,22). In patients for whom a definitive diagnosis is believed to be important, the best approach is through an open-lung biopsy (2–3,6,22,26). Since the process tends to be diffuse, more recent advances in lung biopsy through thoracoscopy may provide a less invasive alternative to thoracotomy and biopsy. However, the diagnostic yield and procedure-related complications need to be carefully assessed.

Lung Biopsy Pathology

Lung pathology findings from open-lung biopsies or autopsy specimens show a spectrum of histopathologic changes (3,5–6,11–13,27). In almost all patients, the major pathological process is in and around the bronchioles. The bronchioles are diseased by a moderate to severe peribronchiolar mononuclear inflammatory infiltrate accompanied by exocytosis into the bronchiolar epithelium. In some of the affected bronchioles, the airway lumen is completely obliterated. Usually, a moderate interstitial lymphocytic infiltrate is found immediately adjacent to the affected bronchioles. These pathological features correlate with the poor returns on the bronchoalveolar lavage and explain some of the lavage cellular features. Elsewhere, the parenchyma is typically normal.

In some cases, lung pathology includes mixed inflammatory infiltrates with a combination of neutrophils and lymphocytes in the peribronchiolar lung parenchyma (27). The bronchiolar lumen also tends to show varying degrees of narrowing, depending on the stage of the disease of bronchiolitis obliterans and sampling. Bronchiolar obstruction is caused by a combination of factors including bronchiolar wall edema; connective-tissue proliferation; smooth-muscle hyperplasia; and intraluminal plugs formed by degenerated epithelium, cellular debris, and mucus (27). These pathological features of bronchiolitis obliterans correlate with the lack of response of the airflow obstruction to bronchodilator agents and explain the difficulty in reversing the airflow obstruction and gas trapping even with aggressive immunosuppressive therapy.

PATHOGENETIC MECHANISMS

The pathogenesis of bone marrow transplantation bronchiolitis obliterans is not well understood. The most supported concept is a primary immunologic mechanism (2–3,9) similar to that found in heart–lung and lung transplant recipients (28–30) and patients with connective-tissue disease (3,31–32). This concept is supported by the strong association between bronchiolitis obliterans and chronic graft-versus-host disease in various reports (5–7,11–14,26). Thus the lungs, and especially the crucial areas around the bronchioles, may be a specific target organ of immune-mediated chronic graft-versus-host disease.

Lung epithelium can express Ia antigens that may activate donor T lymphocytes, making the bronchial mucosa a perfect target for immune-mediated injury that results in bronchiolitis obliterans (3,7,9,28). Methotrexate, which is a risk factor, is thought to induce the Ia complex in the bronchial epithelium and set the stage for bronchiolitis obliterans (2,7,9). Similarly, an autoimmune process directed against the bronchiolar epithelium secondary to prior chemotherapy and radiation treatment resulting in bronchiolitis obliterans after transplantation is the most common mechanism in autologous transplant recipients (10).

Additional immunologic abnormalities in bone marrow transplant recipients include reduced serum immunoglobulins, low salivary IgA, and decreased skin reactivity after transplantation (3,11). As a consequence of the impairment in both the humoral and cellular-mediated immunity, a secondary mechanism involving infectious processes may be important in the development of bronchiolitis obliterans (3,6,9). The secondary or infectious process is likely significantly enhanced by the intense immunosuppression used in the treatment of chronic graft-versus-host disease, which is usually present prior to the development of bronchiolitis obliterans.

Patients with bronchiolitis obliterans often have recurrent sinusitis, repeated bronchitis, and lingering cough as a preamble to the development of full-blow obliterative process (2–3,5–6,9,12–13). These may be the clinical manifestations of poor systemic immunity compounded by impairment of local secretory immunoglobulin plus sinobronchial sicca resulting in poor mucociliary transport (9). The natural consequence is airway colonization of infectious pathogens including both bacteria and viruses, ongoing irritation, and inflammation leading to bronchiolitis obliterans (9). An example of this immunologic–infection interaction after bone marrow transplant is the serial study of a patient with cytomegalovirus pneumonia 2 months post-transplant; despite recovering from the viral infection, the patient developed bronchiolitis obliterans complicated by organizing pneumonia, i.e., BOOP, 4 months later (26). Serial lavages and, eventually, open lung biopsy showed clearance of cytomegalovirus, and yet the patient developed BOOP (26). Had the infectious process not been documented at the onset, then the role it played in the development of the eventual immune-mediated BOOP could not have been appreciated.

CLINICAL COURSE AND MANAGEMENT

In the early 1980s, when bronchiolitis obliterans was first recognized in bone marrow recipients, it was almost always fatal despite attempts at treatment (5–6). In part, the initial failure at stabilizing the process may have been due to a lack of recognition of the immunological aspects. Because of this, patients were generally treated with bronchodilators and antibiotics at the onset. As the condition deteriorated, immunosuppression was tried in a desperate attempt at salvage (6). Another explanation of the bad outcomes is likely the lack of recognition of the relatively high prevalence of post-transplant bronchiolitis obliterans; thus patients were usually severely ill by the time the diagnosis was made (5–6). Alternatively, part of the failure in the control of bronchiolitis obliterans early in the 1980s may be a reflection of poor strategies in the overall prevention and treatment of graft-versus-host disease.

Since then, pulmonary surveillance protocols have become routine procedures at various transplant centers, and patients with bronchiolitis obliterans are diagnosed much earlier. Early detection and prompt immunosuppression likely contribute to a somewhat more favorable outcome. Nevertheless, reversal of the pulmonary function to normal is rare, mortality is still high, and the best-case scenario is stabilization with permanent respiratory impairment due to chronic irreversible airflow obstruction (2–3,6,9). Some long-term survivors of bronchiolitis obliterans develop bronchiectasis with frequent exacerbations due to bacterial infections. Infrequently, fungal colonization due to *Aspergillus* species can develop.

Patients who develop bronchiolitis obliterans after heart–lung and lung transplantations are reported to have a better response to immunosuppressive therapy than bone marrow recipients (3,9,33). Whether the better response reflects early detection, differences in the rejection versus graft-versus-host disease pathogenesis, or a more aggressive immunosuppression approach remains unclear.

Therapy for bone marrow transplant bronchiolitis obliterans, after the exclusion of infection, usually consists of reimplementation or increased immunosuppression. Corticosteroid therapy remains the mainstay of treatment, usually 100 mg/day for about 2 weeks. If stabilization is observed both clinically and by pulmonary function tests, then the dosage is gradually decreased every 2 weeks with the introduction of azathioprine as a double regimen immunosuppression. Other than subjective improvement, reduction in the hyperinflation and gas trapping on the follow-up pulmonary function tests is usually seen when the immunosuppression is effective. Most patients require 3 to 6 months of treatment. Exacerbations are managed in a similar fashion, but patients who stabilize usually do not relapse despite subsequent discontinuation of immunosuppression (2,6). After an apparent arrest in the progression of bronchiolitis obliterans, subsequent respiratory decompensations are more likely to be due to infectious complications of the residual chronic obstructive airways disease in these patients. Triple immunosuppressive therapy may offer better results, but experience in bone marrow transplant recipients is limited.

Cyclosporin-A seems to be relatively ineffective in the arrest of bronchiolitis obliterans once it has developed. However, cumulative data to date at our center show a strong correlation between the introduction of cyclosporin-A in the late 1980s and the reduction in the incidence of post-transplant obstructive airways disease (41). In multivariate analysis, the use of cyclosporin-A for graft-versus-host disease prophylaxis correlates strongly with the reduction in the occurrence of airflow obstruction. This association is independent of the concomitant reduction in the incidence and severity of both acute and chronic graft-versus-host disease (42).

Patients who develop bronchiolitis obliterans earlier during the post-transplant course tend to have more severe airflow obstruction and are less likely to respond to therapy (6,9). These patients also tend to have more infectious respiratory complications (6). However, earlier recognition of the development of obstructive airways disease by a regular and close clinical and pulmonary function test surveillance protocol is associated with a better chance of stabilization. In some patients in whom early and aggressive immunosuppression are instituted, significant improvement in flow rates and reduction of gas trapping can be achieved (3,6).

Another immunosuppressive agent that has been tried in patients who continue to deteriorate despite conventional immunosuppressive drugs is thalidomide. Even though thalidomide has shown some potential in animal models (34–35) and human cutaneous graft-versus-host disease (36–37), anecdotal reports and limited experience at our center using thalidomide for post-transplant bronchiolitis obliterans have been disappointing (38).

The idea of adding immunoglobulins is intriguing and is not totally unreasonable considering their use in conjunction with ganciclovir for the treatment of another immunopathological process, post-transplant cytomegalovirus pneumonitis (26,39). However, critical assessments are needed to evaluate the role of immunoglobulins as part of the immune-modulating strategy in bronchiolitis obliterans.

FUTURE DIRECTIONS

After a decade of struggle with post-transplant bronchiolitis obliterans, the outlook for the 1990s appears bright. Cyclosporin-A has made an important impact in the control of graft-versus-host disease, which may indirectly lead to a reduction in the incidence or the severity of bronchiolitis obliterans. The routine use of acyclovir in the immediate post-bone marrow transplant period not only controls herpes simplex virus disease but also reduces the occurrence of cytomegalovirus pneumonitis. Implementation of regular and close pulmonary surveillance protocols has led to the earlier detection of cytomegalovirus excretion, and early treatment using ganciclovir has prevented overt and severe cytomegalovirus disease (41). Thus, if a viral infectious process is important in the pathogenesis of, or contributes to the severity of, bronchiolitis obliterans, then suppression of viral respiratory complications in the early post-transplant period may also reduce the incidence of bronchiolitis obliterans later. Increased awareness and regular post-transplant pulmonary surveillance is resulting in the diagnosis of bronchiolitis obliterans at a much earlier stage, when it is usually more responsive to treatment. With all of the above measures, the incidence of obstructive airways disease seems to be decreasing (41) rather than increasing as we move into the second decade of the recognition of bronchiolitis obliterans as an important post-bone marrow transplant respiratory complication.

REFERENCES

1. Thomas ED. Bone marrow transplantation. In: Braunwald E, Isselbacher KJ, Petersdorf RG, Wilson JD, Martin JB, Fauci AS, eds. *Harrison's principles of internal medicine*. 11th ed. New York: McGraw-Hill; 1987:1536–1542.
2. Chan CK, Hyland RH, Hutcheon MA. Pulmonary complications following bone marrow transplantation. *Clin Chest Med* 1990;11:323–332.

3. Epler GR. Bronchiolitis obliterans and airways obstruction associated with graft-versus-host disease. *Clin Chest Med* 1988;9:551–556.
4. Beschorner WE, Saral R, Hutchins GM, Tutschka PJ, Santos GW. Lymphocytic bronchitis associated with graft-vs-host disease in recipients of bone marrow transplants. *N Engl J Med* 1978;299:1030–1036.
5. Roca J, Granena A, Rodrigues-Roisin R, Alvareg P, Agusti-Vidal A, Rozman C. Fatal airway disease in an adult with chronic graft-vs-host disease. *Thorax* 1982;37:77–78.
6. Chan CK, Hyland RH, Hutcheon MA, et al. Small airways disease in recipients of allogeneic bone marrow transplants. *Medicine* 1987;66: 327–340.
7. Clark JG, Schwartz DA, Florunoy N, Sullivan KM, Crawford SW, Thomas ED. Risk factors for airflow obstruction in recipients of bone marrow transplants. *Ann Intern Med* 1987;107:648–656.
8. Krowka MJ, Staats BA, Hoagland HC. A prospective study of airway reactivity before bone marrow transplantation. *Mayo Clin Proc* 1990; 65:5–12.
9. Sullivan KM, Shulman HM. Chronic graft-vs-host disease, obliterative bronchiolitis, and graft-vs-leukemia effect: case histories. *Transplant Proc* 1989;21[Suppl 1]:51–62.
10. Paz HL, Crilley P, Patchefsky A, Schiffman RL, Brodsky I. Bronchiolitis obliterans after autologous bone marrow transplantation. *Chest* 1992; 101:775–778.
11. Holland HK, Wingard JR, Beschorner WE, Saral R, Santos GW. Bronchiolitis obliterans in bone marrow transplantation and its relationship to chronic graft-vs-host disease and low serum IgG. *Blood* 1988;72:621–627.
12. Wyatt SE, Nunn P, Hows JM, et al. Airways obstruction associated with graft-vs-host disease after bone marrow transplantation. *Thorax* 1984; 39:887–894.
13. Link H, Reinhard LI, Blaurock M, Ostendorf P. Lung function changes after allogeneic bone marrow transplantation. *Thorax* 1986;41:508–512.
14. Chan CK, Hyland RH, Hutcheon MA, et al. Risk factors for obstructive airways disease after allogeneic bone marrow transplantation. *Am Rev Respir Dis* 1988;137[Suppl]:111.
15. Epler GR, Colby TV, McCloud TC, et al. Bronchiolitis obliterans organizing pneumonia. *N Engl J Med* 1985;312:152–158.
16. Webb WR, Stein MG, Finkbeiner WE, Im JG, Lynch D, Gamsu G. Normal and diseased isolated lungs: high resolution CT. *Radiology* 1988; 166:81–87.
17. Muller NL, Staples CA, Miller RR. Bronchiolitis obliterans organizing pneumonia: CT features in 14 patients. *AJR* 1990;154:983–987.
18. Guerry-Force ML, Muller NL, et al. A comparison of bronchiolitis obliterans with organizing pneumonia, usual interstitial pneumonia, and small airways disease. *Am Rev Respir Dis* 1987;135:705–712.
19. Nishimura K, Itoh H. High-resolution computed tomographic features of bronchiolitis obliterans organizing pneumonia. *Chest* 1992;102[Suppl]: 26S–31S.
20. Despas PJ, Leroux M, Macklem PT. Site of airway obstruction in asthma as determined by maximum expiratory flows breathing air and a helium-oxygen mixture. *J Clin Invest* 1972;51: 3025–3043.
21. Schilder DP, Roberts A, Fry DL. Effect of gas density and viscosity on the maximal expiratory flow volume relationship. *J Clin Invest* 1963; 42:1705–1713.
22. Epler GR. Bronchiolitis obliterans organizing pneumonia: definition and clinical features. *Chest* 1992;102[Suppl]:2S–6S.
23. King TE Jr, Mortenson RL. Cryptogenic organizing pneumonitis: the North American experience. *Chest* 1992;102[Suppl]:14S–20S.
24. Costabel U, Teschler H, Schoenfeld B, et al. Bronchiolitis obliterans op in Europe. *Chest* 1992;102[Suppl]:14S–20S.
25. Nagai S, Aung H, Tanaka S, et al. Bronchoalveolar lavage cell findings in patients with bronchiolitis obliterans organizing pneumonia and related diseases. *Chest* 1992;102[Suppl]:32S–37S.
26. Chien J, Chan CK, Chamberlain D, et al. Cytomegalovirus pneumonia in allogeneic bone marrow transplantation: an immunopathologic process? *Chest* 1990;98:1034–1037.
27. Urbanski SJ, Kossakowska AE, Curtis J, et al. Idiopathic small airways pathology in patients with graft-versus-host disease following allogeneic bone marrow transplantation. *Am J Surg Pathol* 1987;11(12):965–971.
28. Burke CM, Glanville AR, Theordore J, Robin ED. Lung immunogenicity, rejection and obliterative bronchiolitis. *Chest* 1984;86:824–829.
29. Burke CM, Theodore J, Dawkins KD, et al. Post-transplant obliterative bronchiolitis and other late lung sequelae in human heart–lung transplantation. *Chest* 1984;86:824–829.
30. Estenne M, Ketelbant P, Primo G, Yernault JC. Human heart–lung transplantation: physiological aspects of the denervated lung and post-transplant obliterative bronchiolitis. *Am Rev Respir Dis* 1987;135:976–978.
31. Epler GR, Snider GL, Saensler EA, et al. Bronchiolitis and bronchitis in connective tissue disease. *JAMA* 1979;242:528–532.
32. Kinney WW, Angelillo VA. Bronchiolitis in systemic lupus erythematosus. *Chest* 1982;82:646–648.
33. Glanville AR, Galdwin JC, Burke CM, et al. Obliterative bronchiolitis after heart–lung transplantation: apparent arrest by augmented immunosuppression. *Ann Intern Med* 1987;107: 300–304.
34. Field EO, Gibbs JE, Tucker DF, Hellmann K. Effect of thalidomide on the graft-versus-host reaction. *Nature* 1966;211:1308–1310.
35. Vogelsang GB, Hess AD, Gordon G, Santos GW. Treatment and prevention of acute graft-

versus-host disease with thalidomide in a rat model. *Transplantation* 1986;21:644–647f.
36. Aurat JH, Camenzind M, Helg C, Chapuis B. Thalidomide for graft-versus-host disease after bone marrow transplantation. *Lancet* 1988;i: 359.
37. Heney D, Lewis IJ, Bailey CC. Thalidomide for chronic graft-versus-host disease in children. *Lancet* 1988;ii:1317.
38. Heaton DC. Failure of thalidomide to control bronchiolitis obliterans post bone marrow transplant. *Bone Marrow Transplant* 1989;4(5):598.
39. Emanuel D, Cunningham L, Jules-Elysee K, et al. Cytomegalovirus pneumonia after bone marrow transplantation successfully treated with the combination of ganciclovir and high-dose intravenous immune globulin. *Ann Intern Med* 1988;109:777–782.
40. Goodrich JM, Motomi M, Gleaves CA, et al. Early treatment with ganciclovir to prevent allogeneic bone marrow transplantation. *N Engl J Med* 1991;325:1601–1607.
41. Payne L, Chan CK, Fyles G, et al. Cyclosporin may prevent obstructive airways disease after allogeneic bone marrow transplantation. *Chest* 1993;104:114–118.

Diseases of the Bronchioles, edited by Gary R. Epler. Raven Press, Ltd., New York © 1994.

17
Heart–Lung Transplantation

Connor M. Burke,* Samuel A. Yousem,† and Paul A. Corris‡

**Consultant Respiratory Physician, James Connolly Memorial Hospital, Blanchardstown, Dublin 15, Ireland.*
†Department of Pathology, NW 625, Montefiore University Hospital, University of Pittsburgh, School of Medicine, 3459 Fifth Avenue, Pittsburgh, PA.
‡Consultant Respiratory Physician and Associate Medical Director, Department of Cardiopulmonary Transplantation, Regional Cardiopulmonary Centre, Freeman Hospital, High Heaton, Newcastle Upon Tyne, England.

Successful heart–lung transplantation in humans was first achieved in 1981, when a 45-year-old woman with primary pulmonary hypertension underwent combined heart–lung transplantation at Stanford University Medical Center (1). This fundamental advance was achieved as a consequence of research over 40 years in a variety of animal models to optimize surgical technique and immunosuppressant regimens. Furthermore, the Stanford University unit had successfully carried out 350 cardiac transplantations before embarking on the heart–lung transplant program.

Although lung function replacement was first achieved in the context of combined heart–lung transplantation, advances in surgical technique pioneered by the Toronto group and improved, less toxic, immunosuppressant regimens, made lung transplantation without cardiac transplantation (i.e., single or bilateral lung transplantation) possible by 1985 (2). Currently three forms of lung function replacement are possible, namely, combined heart–lung, single lung, or bilateral lung transplantation.

Since the first successful human heart–lung transplant in 1981, sufficient follow-up data are now available to show that long-term survival of the transplanted lung is possible notwithstanding loss of bronchial circulation, innervation, and lymphatic drainage channels (3,4). The demonstration that essentially normal pulmonary function can be achieved and maintained indefinitely in uncomplicated heart–lung transplant recipients (4) highlights the necessity to improve the understanding and treatment of the major clinical problems in the transplanted lung, which currently limit 4-year survival to about 50% of heart–lung transplant recipients. Although infection and rejection are and will remain an ongoing concern in any allograft, the major long-term complication after human heart–lung transplantation is bronchiolitis obliterans, which is evident in up to 50% of recipients (3,6–11). This review focuses on the problem of bronchiolitis obliterans after combined heart–lung transplantation. Clinical symptoms, physical findings, radiographic findings, pulmonary functional indices, clinical course, management, and preventative measures are reviewed. Theories of pathogenesis also are considered.

HISTORICAL REVIEW OF HEART–LUNG TRANSPLANTATION

Demikhov (12) initiated cardiopulmonary transplantation using a dog model 50 years ago. He reported maximum survival of 5 days in 2 of 67 dogs who underwent heart–lung transplantation without the use of cardiopulmonary bypass or hypothermia. In 1953, Neptune and colleagues (13) used the techniques of hypothermia and circulatory arrest and reported survival limited to 6 hours in dog recipients. In 1957, Webb and Howard (14) reported survival up to 22 hours in dogs with cardiopulmonary bypass techniques. With similar techniques, Lower and Shumway (15) in 1961 achieved survival of up to 6 days in dogs. Grinnan and colleagues (16) reported one 10-day survivor in 1970. These poor results, obtained in different centers via a variety of techniques, called into question the viability of lung transplantation; and it was suggested that the denervated lung was incapable of normal respiration because of the loss of lung afferent reflexes, in particular the Hering-Breuer stretch reflex.

In 1967, Nakae (17) demonstrated that although pulmonary denervation in the dog resulted in an abnormal respiratory pattern and early death, this was not the case in primates. This fundamental observation was made after a variety of experiments of cardiopulmonary denervation in dog, cat, and monkey models. In 1972, Castaneda and colleagues (18) were the first to demonstrate prolonged survival after cardiopulmonary autotransplantation in primates. Of a total of 25 baboons, 5 survived for longer than 6 months postoperatively. In 1980, Reitz and others (19) obtained extended survival in primates after autotransplantation and allotransplantation of the heart and lungs using cyclosporin immunosuppression. The successful development of an animal model of cardiopulmonary transplantation after 40 years of research provided the springboard for clinical heart–lung transplantation (1).

In the clinical arena prior to 1981, three patients underwent heart–lung transplantation. In 1969, Cooley and colleagues (20) performed heart–lung transplantation on an infant girl who died of respiratory failure 14 hours postoperatively. Lillihei and coworkers (21) carried out cardiopulmonary transplantation in 1969 on a 43-year-old man with end-stage emphysema who died 8 days postoperatively. The third human heart–lung transplantation was performed by Barnard (22) in 1971; the patient died 23 days postoperatively of bronchial dehiscence and pneumonia. Finally in 1981, Reitz and colleagues (1) successfully achieved cardiopulmonary transplantation in a 45-year-old woman with primary pulmonary hypertension.

Thus, a period of 40 years elapsed between the original experiments of Demikhov in dogs and the clinical introduction of cardiopulmonary transplantation. The gap between the original unsuccessful animal experiments and the successful clinical introduction of heart–lung transplantation was bridged by innovative and painstaking surgical experimentation in a variety of animal models, significant advances in immunology, the introduction of cyclosporin, and the experience gained with clinical heart transplant programs.

The major long-term complication of cardiopulmonary transplantation is bronchiolitis obliterans, which develops in up to 50% of long-term survivors (3,5). Bronchiolitis obliterans is a rare condition (23), classically associated with toxic gas exposure (24), viral infection (25), or systemic connective-tissue diseases (26,27). More recently, bronchiolitis obliterans has been described in bone marrow transplant recipients (28–32). The diagnosis and treatment of post-transplant bronchiolitis obliterans is currently the major challenge facing physicians caring for heart–lung transplant recipients (33).

PULMONARY FUNCTION IN HEART–LUNG TRANSPLANT RECIPIENTS

The Natural History of the Transplanted Lung

The identification of lung complications in heart–lung transplant recipients necessarily demands an understanding of the "normal" function of lung allografts. The functional capacity of transplanted lungs, deprived of innervation, bronchial arterial supply, and lymphatic channels, was unknown at the time of the first heart–lung transplant in 1981, although grossly normal lung function and gas exchange had been documented in a small number of animal models for some years after heart–lung transplantation (18). The lung is uniquely exposed to environmental antigenic, infectious, and noxious influences; and the functional impact of denervation on bronchial reactivity, cough, and irritant receptors, mucociliary clearance, hypoxic pulmonary vasoconstriction reflexes, respiratory control mechanisms, sighing mechanisms, and other protective functions was largely unknown (36,37,38). The long-term functional capacity of airways deprived of their bronchial arterial supply was also unknown. When bronchiolitis obliterans emerged in many heart–lung transplant recipients, these considerations raised the possibility that progressive airway obstruction associated with bronchiolitis obliterans might be an inevitable consequence of lung transplantation, perhaps triggered by concurrent infection or rejection. Fortunately, recent information that documents normal long-term lung function in uncomplicated transplant recipients suggests that bronchiolitis obliterans is a complication rather than an inevitable consequence of heart–lung transplantation (3,4).

The initial evidence in support of normal long-term functional capacity of transplanted lungs was reported by the Stanford University Group (3) in 1986. A total of 10 heart–lung transplant recipients were studied in the immediate postoperative period, and comparable studies were available in 9, 8, and 6 recipients at 1, 2, and 3 years after transplantation, respectively. Functional variables studied included computerized spirometry, static lung volumes, diffusion capacity for carbon monoxide, specific airway conductance, and arterial oxygen and carbon dioxide levels. None of these variables showed any deterioration with time after transplantation; no airway obstruction was seen, and a minor postoperative restrictive ventilatory defect persisted but showed no evidence of progression. The restrictive ventilatory defect in these patients may be explained by deliberate selection of donors with smaller thoracic cavities than recipients.

More recent data are available for 21 heart–lung transplant recipients at Stanford University who survived for 3 years or more (4). Functional parameters, including serial measurements of spirometrically derived flow rates, static lung volumes, and

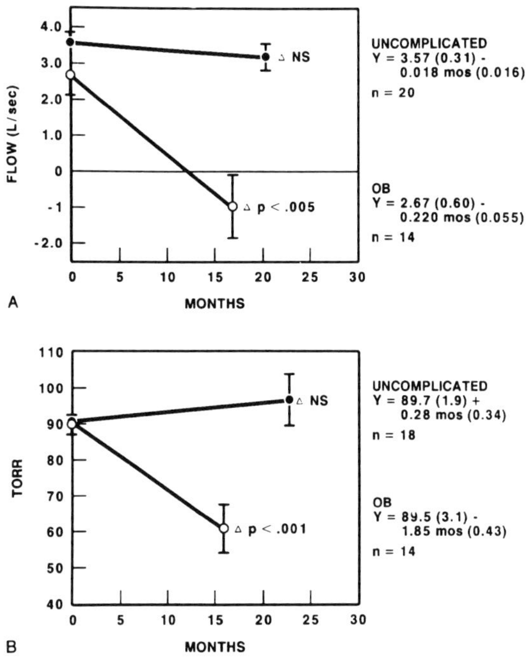

FIG. 1. Changes in **A,** FEF_{25-75} and **B,** PaO_2 over time as determined by linear regression analysis are shown for patients with bronchiolitis obliterans (*open circles*) and patients without complications (*solid circles*) after heart–lung transplantation. The figures show the means for the total number (*n*) of individual regressions obtained within the respective groups. The changes in FEF_{25-75} and PaO_2 are not significant for the group without complications, whereas the rates of decline for both parameters are quite significant in patients with obliterative bronchiolitis. From ref. 33, with permission.

arterial oxygen levels, were analyzed by linear regression to determine the rate of functional change with time after transplantation. A total of nine patients without complications were assessed for a mean period of 4.6 years (range 3.4 to 7.3 years). Pulmonary function was essentially normal at a mean of 4.6 years after transplantation. Furthermore, the slope of the linear regression showed a positive trend for all functional variables after transplantation, although only the positive changes in forced vital capacity (FVC) attained statistical significance. Serial measurements in 20 heart–lung transplant recipients without complications demonstrated no decline in FEF_{25-75} or PaO_2 over a mean 20.1 months after transplantation (33) (Fig. 1).

Similar data from the Newcastle Transplant Group in nine patients show that heart–lung transplant recipients without complications show no decline in lung function over a period of 3 years (Paul Corris; unpublished observations).

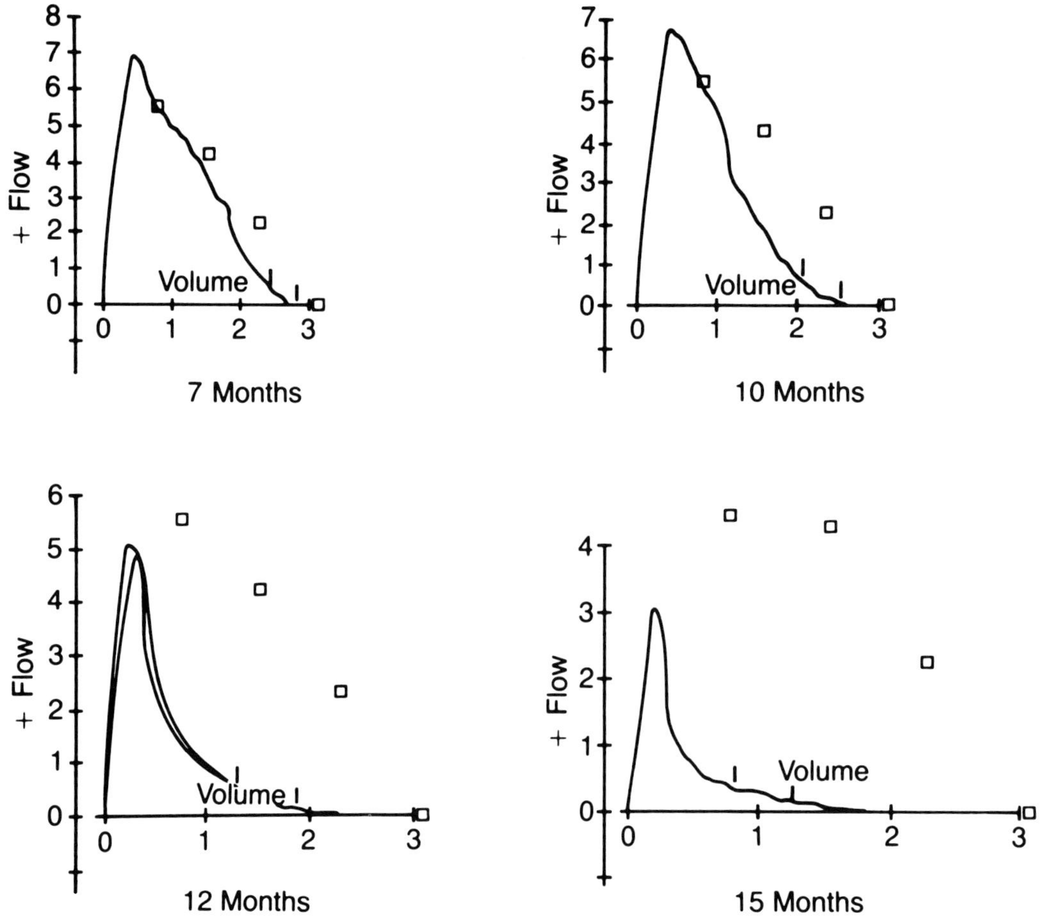

FIG. 2. Sequential changes that occur typically in the forced expiratory flow–volume curve with bronchiolitis obliterans. These values are for a 33-year-old woman at 7, 10, 12, and 15 months after heart–lung transplantation. The curve at 7 months is essentially normal. The curve at 10 months shows early "coving" of the expiratory flow limb over the middle 50% of the forced vital capacity. The progression and typical patterns of obstruction are present at 12 and 15 months. Flow is expressed in L/second; volume is expressed in L. From ref. 33, with permission.

These data support the concept that lung function remains normal over extended periods in uncomplicated heart–lung transplant recipients; i.e., the "natural history" of the transplanted lung is not one of inevitable decline but rather of sustained normal mechanical and gas-exchange capacity.

DEFINITION

Post heart–lung transplant bronchiolitis obliterans is an inflammatory disorder of small airways that causes distortion and narrowing of bronchioles (5,6,33). Progressive obliteration of the small airways results in a severe obstructive ventilatory defect. The initial physiological defect reflects the pattern associated with small airway (less than 2 mm in diameter) obstruction (Fig. 2) and is manifest by diminished FEF_{50}/FVC ratio and $FEF_{25\text{-}75}$ and "bowing" of the expiratory limb of the flow-volume loop (33). Post-transplant bronchiolitis obliterans causes rapidly progressive airway obstruction in most affected patients; the obstructive ventilatory defect does not respond to bronchodilator drugs, and spontaneous remissions have not been described.

PREVALENCE

The initial reports from Stanford University (3,35) indicated that bronchiolitis obliterans arose in 50% of long-term survivors of heart–lung transplantation. More detailed analysis of the Stanford University data (3,33,35) showed a prevalence of 68% in patients who received transplants between 1981 and 1986 and 20% in patients who received transplants between 1986 and 1989. This reduction in prevalence probably reflects augmented immunosuppression regimens and improved surveillance of recipients (33). The Pittsburgh (10) and Papworth (11) programs reported a prevalence of 54% and 10%, respectively. The Newcastle Group (39) have recently reported a prevalence of 23%.

CLINICAL SYMPTOMS AND PHYSICAL FINDINGS

Post heart–lung transplant bronchiolitis obliterans was first reported (5) in 1986 in 5 of 14 cardiopulmonary transplant recipients who survived the perioperative period. The 5 affected recipients were diagnosed 36, 26, 14, 2, and 1 month after transplantation, respectively. Since the patients were clinically reviewed on a regular basis, the widely varying intervals between transplantation and diagnosis of the lesion suggested that post-transplant bronchiolitis obliterans was not an inevitable complication of lung transplantation but rather the result of infection or rejection or both.

The clinical course of disease in these affected patients was characterized by recurrent bronchitic symptoms including cough; mucoid sputum; a propensity to infective bronchitis initially responsive to antibiotics; and clinical (5), radiologic (33), and bronchoscopic evidence of mucus plugging in small airways. Although dyspnea was not a prominent early symptom, all patients developed progressive dyspnea on exertion within weeks or months of the onset of bronchitic symptoms. A particular clinical feature related to the patients' perception of dyspnea; since all these patients suffered dyspnea at rest prior to transplantation, their expectation of exercise capacity after transplantation was limited. By the time they complained of dyspnea, lung function was invariably significantly impaired with an obstructive ventilatory defect in all cases. It is clear that overreliance on lung transplant recipients' perception of dyspnea or impaired exercise capacity resulted in significant delay in the diagnosis of post-transplant bronchiolitis. These initial reports demonstrated the critical importance of obtaining sequential pulmonary function tests and other objective indices of lung function in heart–lung recipients; overreliance on symptomatology resulted in critical delay in diagnosis of bronchiolitis obliterans at a time when treatment was most likely to influence outcome. Bronchitic symptoms, however minor, warrant further investigation in these patients. With more advanced disease, complaints of wheeze on exertion, and sometimes at rest, are common. Hemoptysis and chest pain are not prominent features in most reports (5,35).

Few abnormal signs can be detected on chest examination in the early stages of post-transplant bronchiolitis obliterans. The physical stigmata of chronic airway obstruction are manifest in well established disease, including increased anteroposterior diameter, diminished chest expansion, hyperresonant percussion note, and diminished intensity of breath sounds. The expiratory phase of the breath sounds is prolonged, and expiratory rhonchi are manifest in advanced cases. Late inspiratory high-pitched rhonchi—so-called *inspiratory squeaks*—are audible in the lower zones bilaterally. These represent a classical clinical feature and may relate to late opening of small airways secondary to accumulation of excess mucus and altered elastic properties. In advanced cases, bilateral basal crackles, which may relate to bronchiectasis or interstitial fibrosis or both, are audible throughout inspiration (5,33).

Ventilation perfusion mismatch results in hypoxia and cyanosis in well established disease, but hypercapnia and the associated clinical signs are late manifestations of terminal disease. In this regard, patients with established post-transplant bronchiolitis obliterans may be termed "blue puffers" (5,33). Although sharing the common feature of airway obstruction, post-transplant bronchiolitis obliterans differs from bronchial asthma in demonstrating minimal spontaneous variation in symptoms or indices of pulmonary function, and the obstructive ventilatory defect is at best only partially reversible on treatment with beta-agonist, anticholinergic, or theophylline bronchodilators. Augmented immunosuppression, if introduced early, may be effective in improving or arresting the decline in lung function in at least some patients (34,35).

DIAGNOSIS

Early diagnosis of bronchiolitis obliterans in heart–lung transplant recipients is vital for at least three reasons. First, current evidence suggests that pulmonary mechanical function and gas exchange shows no evidence of deterioration with time in recipients without complications (4). The potential for normal long-term pulmonary function provides a major incentive for early diagnosis and treatment of post-transplant bronchiolitis obliterans. Second, although spontaneous remissions have not been described and no response to bronchodilators is seen, bronchiolitis obliterans has been successfully treated in the acute stage of early airway obstruction by augmented immunosuppression with resolution of the obstructive ventilatory defect and restoration of normal pulmonary function and gas exchange (34). Furthermore, the addition of azathioprine to corticosteroid and cyclosporin in recipients with established bronchiolitis obliterans slows the rate of lung function loss (35) (Fig. 3). These functional data, although limited, support the concept that post-transplant bronchiolitis obliterans can be successfully treated only when identified in the acute phase before irreversible airway damage is established. Third, histopathology and immunopathological studies of post-transplant bronchiolitis obliterans demonstrate a cell-mediated immune response in the airway in the acute phase (9). However, chronic bronchiolitis obliterans is manifest by fibrous scarring and obliterated bronchioles (6). The former acute inflammatory response is at least theoretically completely reversible, whereas the latter fixed structural changes are not amenable to any therapy.

It is generally accepted that open lung biopsy is the gold standard for diagnosis of bronchiolitis obliterans (40). However, sequential open lung biopsy in transplant recipients is clearly impractical. A variety of clinical, radiological, pathological, immunological, and physiological indices have

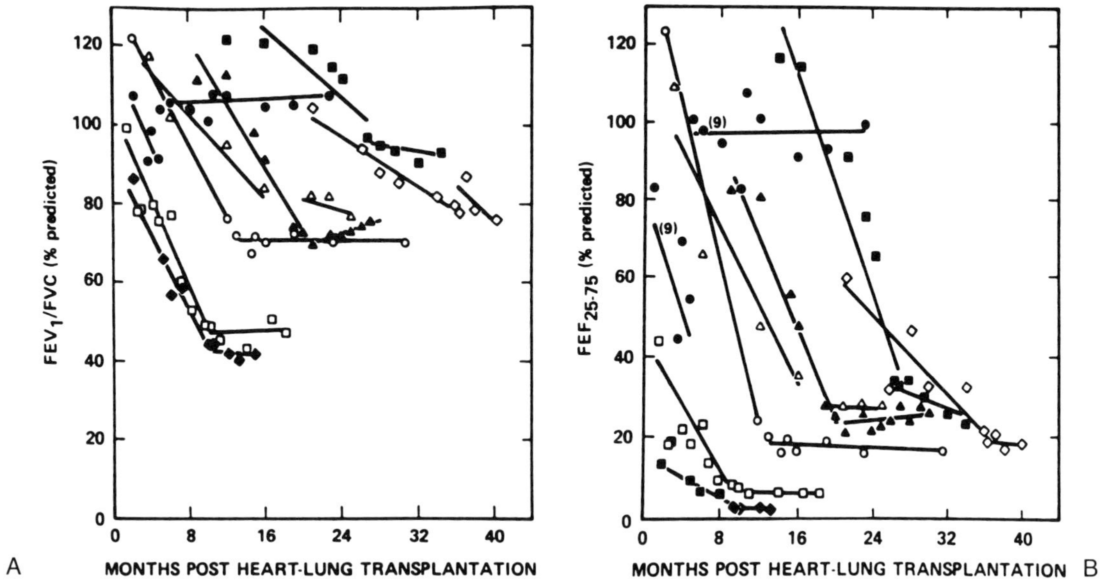

FIG. 3. Effect of the initiation of azathioprine therapy on airflow variables after heart–lung transplantation in eight patients with bronchiolitis obliterans. Each patient is represented by a different symbol. Values and regression lines are plotted for each patient for **A,** FEV_1/FVC and **B,** FEF_{25-75}. The left portion of each regression line represents values obtained while the patient was receiving only cyclosporine and prednisone; the right portion of each line represents the regression line after the addition of azathioprine to this regimen. Reproduced with permission from Glanville A, Baldwin J, Burke C, et al. Obliterative bronchiolitis after heart–lung transplantation: apparent arrest by augmented immunosuppression. *Ann Intern Med* 1987; 107:300–304.

been investigated to determine diagnostic criteria for bronchiolitis obliterans which are sufficiently noninvasive to permit regular surveillance of recipients (9,41–48). Current evidence suggests that no one test can equal the sensitivity and specificity of open lung biopsy. However, recent reports (9,41–46) suggest that a combination of studies, in particular, pulmonary function tests, bronchoalveolar lavage, and transbronchial biopsies, permit early diagnosis and treatment of post-transplant bronchiolitis obliterans without the need for open lung biopsy. Because many noninvasive approaches to the diagnosis are based on the premise that bronchiolitis obliterans represents chronic lung rejection, it is critical to review current concepts of lung allograft rejection and the association of allograft rejection with the disease.

DIAGNOSIS OF LUNG REJECTION

The first manifestation of lung rejection in nonimmunosuppressed rats is a perivascular lymphocytic infiltrate. Previous work in dogs that used identical protocols in autografted and allografted lungs to separate the effects of rejection from those of surgery documented peribronchial and alveolar lymphatic infiltration in addition to perivascular infiltrates during early rejection reactions in nonimmunosuppressed allograft recipients. When allograft recipients were treated with immunosuppressants including azathioprine, corticosteroids, and antithymocyte globulin, the rejection response was not only attenuated but also changed in that the vascular manifestations of rejection were differentially suppressed. These data suggest that the pathology of lung rejection differs in different species and also that the pattern of rejection is changed both quantitatively and qualitatively by immunosuppressant drugs. Results from animal studies or even from clinical studies in which different immunosuppressant regimens were used should be interpreted with caution for these reasons.

The early clinical experience of heart–lung transplantation together with animal studies in dogs and primates demonstrated a similar perivascular lymphocytic infiltrate in both heart and lungs during rejection episodes. It was therefore assumed that simultaneous rejection of both heart and lungs occurred, and so the diagnosis of lung rejection in heart–lung transplant recipients was made on the basis of endomyocardial biopsy findings of cardiac rejection. However, in 1985 lethal pulmonary rejection with normal cardiac histology was reported in a primate; and the first clinical documentation of isolated lung rejection was recorded in the same year when open lung biopsy showed lung rejection on the twenty-third postoperative day in a heart–lung transplant recipient with normal cardiac biopsies (49). These reports ended the practice of monitoring lung rejection by cardiac biopsy, removed one of the principal reasons for offering combined heart–lung transplantation rather than single or double lung transplantation to patients with end-stage lung disease and normal hearts, and underlined the urgency of developing sensitive and specific indices of lung rejection. In retrospect, the erroneous assumption that lung rejection was excluded by a normal endomyocardial biopsy probably contributed to the high prevalence of bronchiolitis obliterans in the early years of heart–lung transplantation.

HISTOPATHOLOGY OF LUNG REJECTION

Acute Rejection

Most authorities now believe that lung allografts are subject to both acute and chronic rejection and that airway injury occurs in both settings. Acute rejection is classically manifested by perivascular mononuclear infiltrates, which extend into alveolar septae as the intensity and grade of rejection increases (50,51) (Figs. 4 and 5). Coexistent with this vascular damage in acute rejection is airway injury. This epithelial damage is seen in both the large cartilaginous bronchi and terminal and respiratory bronchioles (52). The submucosa of the airways becomes expanded by a mixed mononuclear infiltrate of small, round, angulated, and transformed lymphocytes (Fig. 6). Macrophages, tissue histiocytes, and dendritic cells are prominent and are also increased in number directly within the epithelium (53). As the intensity of the infiltrate increases, eosinophilic infiltration is seen (42,54,55). Within the respiratory epithelium, individual cells may undergo necrosis or dyskeratosis with squamous metaplasia. In severe cases of acute rejection, the epithelium may slough, resulting in an intraluminal fibropurulent exudate rich in neutrophils, fibrin, and mucus. At this phase, the neutrophils are nonspecifically attracted by inflammatory mediators, and it may become difficult to separate alloreactive lymphocyte induced bronchitis from an

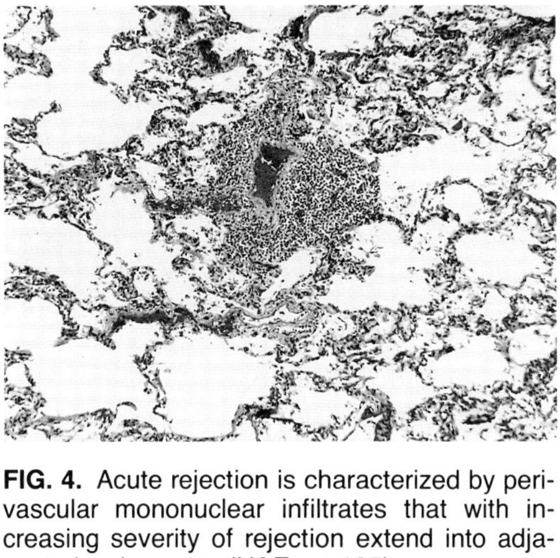

FIG. 4. Acute rejection is characterized by perivascular mononuclear infiltrates that with increasing severity of rejection extend into adjacent alveolar septa (H&E, × 125).

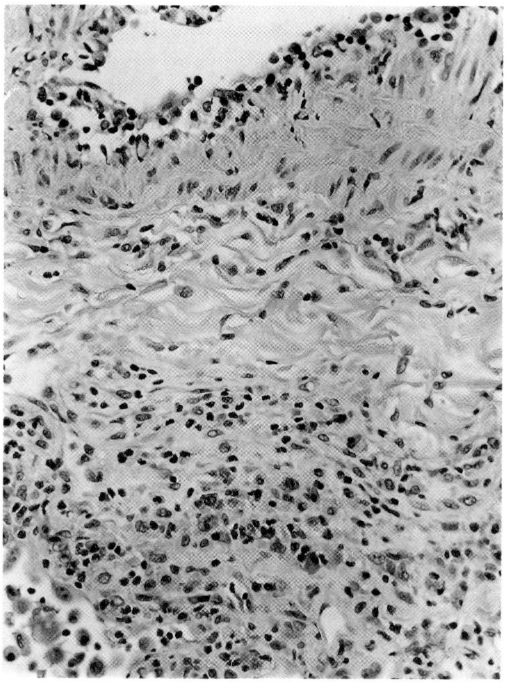

FIG. 5. Acute rejection displays perivascular lymphocytes, plasma cells, and blastic large lymphoid cells. Subendothelial infiltration by these mononuclear cells (*top*) may also be seen in higher grades of acute rejection (H&E, × 350).

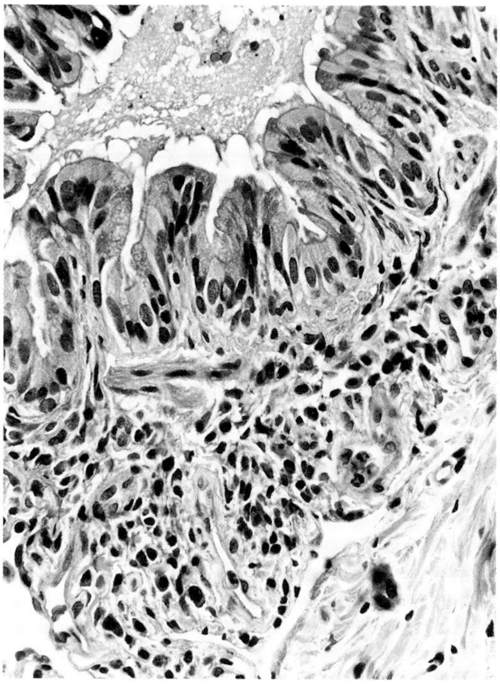

FIG. 6. Small airway inflammation without fibrosis may be seen as part of acute rejection or can be noted as isolated lymphocytic bronchiolitis (H&E, × 350).

infectious bronchitis or bronchiolitis (41,56, 57).

If epithelial necrosis occurs, granulation tissue may form within the airway. Fibroblasts, myofibroblasts, and histiocytes migrate into the exudate from the submucosa and lay down a loose acid mucopolysaccharide (hyaluronic acid) rich matrix with young collagen (58). There is a second proliferation of regenerating epithelial cells over this matrix incorporating it into the submucosa of the airway. If the alloreactive response is successfully controlled, the histiocytic component of the infiltrate elaborates tissue collagenases and hyaluronidases, which digest this matrix, and the airway heals without residual injury (59, 60). In other instances, the reaction may leave an eccentric or concentric scar or may completely obliterate the lumen by eosinophilic scar tissue (50,59,60).

If injury is severe, collagen deposits become cross-linked and form a dense eosinophilic fibrous plaque. This plaque may be submucosal or may extend in a stellate fashion into the adjacent centrilobular zones of the pulmonary lobule. Atrophy or even reactive hyperplasia of the bronchiolar smooth muscle may be noted with fragmentation or reduplication of the basal elastica.

In acute rejection, immunohistochemical studies (53,61) have demonstrated a predominant population of helper T cells with increased dendritic cells. Presumably, the CD4 population mediates the class II donor-specific reactivity (53,62,63,64,65). Increased numbers of Leu 7 positive natural killer cells within the submucosa and intraepithelial zones have been reported (66). Lavage studies have shown increased levels of platelet-derived growth factor, fibroblast growth factor, and hyaluronic acid in lavage fluid in cases of acute rejection with airway injury (which corresponds to the inflammatory reaction and reparative response induced by the alloreactive injury). In pediatric patients, animal models, and some adult recipients, the alloreactive in situ mixed lymphocyte response affects the bronchus-associated lymphoid tissue (67). This occurs in large, well circumscribed models of immunoblasts and small, round, and angulated lymphocytes at the junction of the submucosa and second interlobular septae. Large, reactive germinal cells may also be seen.

Chronic Rejection

Chronic rejection of the lung manifests as extensive scarring of the large and small airways. This may be a consequence of repeated or severe acute rejection episodes or can represent a separate chronic, insidious, and distinct immunologic reaction directed at the large and small airways (50,59,68). The histopathological form of chronic airway rejection is bronchiolitis obliterans in which the submucosa of the large and small airways is infiltrated by the dense eosinophilic scar tissue described above (Figs. 7 and 8). The collagen commonly forms compact lamellae and is associated with an infiltration of small round lymphocyte and plasma cells that phenotypically are a mixture of B cells and cytotoxic T lymphocytes (65,69). These T cells are thought to mediate class I donor antigen specific injury to the respiratory epithelium. Reports (65) have indicated increased expression of class I antigens on bronchiolar epithelium and increased expression of class II antigens on both bronchiolar epithelium and vascular endothelium in bronchiolitis obliterans. Immunohistochemical studies (67) have shown reduced amounts of bronchus-associated lymphoid tissue and IgA and IgG secreting plasma cells in the submucosa, which may predispose the patient to respiratory tract infections.

Pulmonary vascular occlusive disease, or accelerated graft atheroma in both pulmonary and cardiac vessels, appears to be correlated with the incidence and degree of bronchiolitis obliterans (6), although it is not emphasized in current reports as much as the obstructive ventilatory defect. This feature does not appear to be seen in nontransplant patients who have bronchiolitis obliterans.

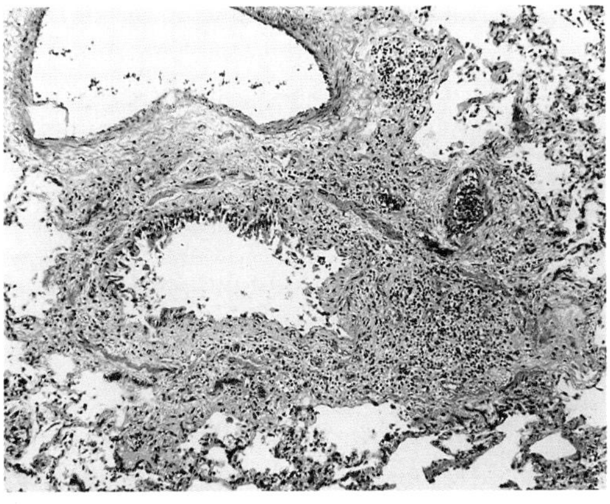

FIG. 7. Subtotal bronchiolitis obliterans is manifested by partial eccentric or concentric occlusion of the airway lumen by dense eosinophilic scar tissue, which expands the submucosa and peribronchiolar soft tissues (H&E, × 125).

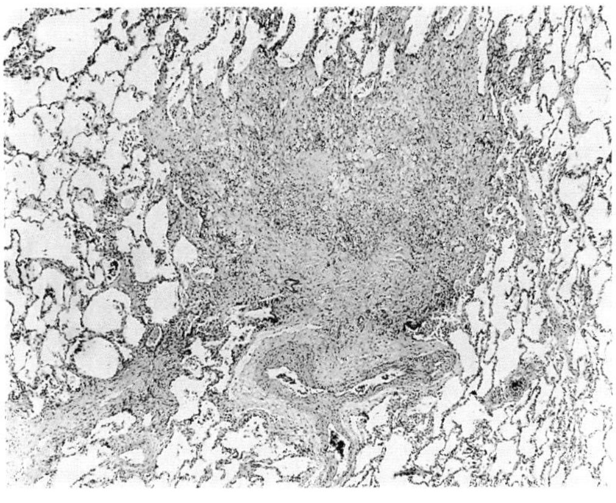

FIG. 8. Total bronchiolitis obliterans is recognized in bronchovascular bundles as rounded or stellate scars that have replaced the airway in zones adjacent to small arteries (H&E, × 50).

PATHOGENESIS

Although most investigators believe that bronchiolitis obliterans represents an immunologic event, there is still controversy about the role of infection in the pathogenesis of the obliterative airway changes (70). Most reports suggest that the primary event is alloreactive injury by activated mononuclear cells, which in its later stages is exacerbated by superimposed infectious bronchitis or bronchiolitis (33). This represents the most common form of airway fibrosis in lung transplant recipients, although rare cases of apparent primary postinfectious bronchiolitis obliterans have been described (70).

Much evidence from a variety of sources is now available linking bronchiolitis obliterans with an immunological rejection reaction. The intensity and persistence of early acute rejection episodes with associated airway injury correlate with the subsequent development of bronchiolitis obliterans (71). Histological grading of transbronchial biopsies in terms of acute rejection is of predictive value for the subsequent development of bronchiolitis obliterans (55). Specific immunological events associated with bronchiolitis obliterans include the presence of specific T cell subsets, increased numbers of dendritic cells within the respiratory epithelium and submucosa, and an increase in class II HLA antigens on the respiratory epithelium (65). A positive primed lymphocyte test also coincides with the development of bronchiolitis obliterans. Lymphocytes infiltrating the airway of allografts are positive for Leu 7, a marker for antigen-reactive cytotoxic T lymphocytes (66). The appearance of alloreactive T lymphocytes in bronchoalveolar lavage fluids precedes the emergence of clinical symptoms related to bronchiolitis obliterans, and enhanced immunosuppression results in disappearance of both alloreactivity and respiratory symptoms (72). Bronchiolitis obliterans responds to treatment with immunosuppressant drugs including corticosteroids (34) and azathioprine (35). The incidence of bronchiolitis obliterans has diminished after the introduction of augmented immunosuppressant regimens (33). Paradis (10) reports that 77% of high-risk patients develop bronchiolitis obliterans after an episode of acute rejection. Some evidence suggests that the degree of donor recipient HLA locus mismatch is directly proportional to both the incidence and severity of subsequent bronchiolitis obliterans (73). Finally, most heart–lung transplant recipients with bronchiolitis obliterans have no evidence of infection at the time of diagnosis (5,6,33).

However, lower respiratory tract infection, including respiratory syncytial virus, adenovirus, mycoplasma, and legionella, are well documented causes of bronchiolitis obliterans in native lungs in patients of all ages (23,25,39,74). Heart–lung transplant recipients are at increased risk for lower respiratory tract infection not only because of their immunosuppressant regimens but also because lung denervation may damage local defense mechanisms including cough reflex and mucociliary clearance. Furthermore, loss of bronchial circulation may impair bronchial defense mechanisms. The Pittsburgh group (10) reported that 56% of at-risk heart–lung transplant recipients developed bronchiolitis obliterans after cytomegalovirus infection and 50% after pneumocystis carinii infection. Other groups (75) have documented a link between cytomegalovirus infection and bronchiolitis obliterans.

The possibility that rejection and infection may not operate in an either/or fashion in the pathogenesis of bronchiolitis obliterans should also be considered (36). Up-regulation of antigens in the presence of infection may provide an initial immunologic stimulus to a rejection response (76). Lymphokines, including interferon gamma and interferon alpha, amplify the expression of major histocompatibility antigens (77). Cytomegalovirus activates the host immune system and induces donor-specific cytotoxicity (78,79). These and other mechanisms may up-regulate the immunogenicity of the transplanted lung in the presence of infection and in this way precipitate a recipient immune response against the airway. Although infection may be the primary cause of bronchiolitis obliterans in some patients (70), most authorities believe that lung allograft infection occurs predominantly in the setting of prior immunologic damage to the tracheobronchial tree; i.e., infection is secondary to post-transplant bronchiolitis obliterans rather than a primary cause (33,80).

CURRENT MANAGEMENT

The major challenge for clinicians caring for long-term survivors of heart–lung transplantation relates to the diagnosis and treatment of chronic rejection causing bronchiolitis obliterans on the one hand, and respiratory tract infections on the other. Clinical symptoms and signs and chest imaging techniques including CT scans fail to distinguish between rejection and infection; these tests may be normal despite significant rejection or infection. Furthermore, bronchoscopy showed rejection or infection in 15% of asymptomatic patients in one study (45). Since the treatment of rejection involves increased immunosuppression, which is dangerous in the presence of infection, the distinction between allograft infection and rejection is critical.

Babatunde and others (81) demonstrated a pivotal role for pulmonary function tests in the surveillance of heart–lung transplant recipients. They showed that FEV_1 diminished significantly in the presence of both infection and rejection. Using biopsy diagnosis as the gold standard, they found that pulmonary function tests had a sensitivity of 86% in the diagnosis of rejection in the first 3 months postoperatively and 75% subsequently, together with a sensitivity of 75% for the detection of infection. Pulmonary function tests had a specificity of 84% in the detection of infection or rejection but were unable to distinguish between them. These and similar results have led to the use of regular pulmonary function tests, in particular computerized spirometry, in the routine surveillance of heart–lung transplant recipients. Decreases in pulmonary function signal the necessity for further investigations to detect rejection or infection or both. The use of indices of small airway disease, including $FEF_{25\text{-}75}$ and FEF_{50}/FVC, may further enhance the usefulness of lung function tests in this setting (33).

Abnormal lung function tests should be followed by bronchoscopy with bronchoalveolar lavage and transbronchial biopsy using large alligator forceps to obtain at least four biopsy specimens. The sensitivity of transbronchial biopsy in the diagnosis of rejection is 84% (9). The role of bronchoscopy is emphasized by the finding of rejection or infection at bronchoscopy in 15% of asymptomatic patients (45). Sensitivity of the chest radiograph in diagnosis of obliterative bronchiolitis is poor; and more sophisticated imaging techniques such as high-resolution CT scan, although demonstrating typical changes in advanced bronchiolitis obliterans, have not been shown to be either sensitive or specific in the diagnosis to date.

TREATMENT

The treatment of bronchiolitis obliterans depends on the presence or absence of acute rejection (perivascular infiltrates) or infection. Bronchiolitis obliterans associated with acute rejection is treated with high-dose corticosteroid therapy (usually 1 g of hydrocortisone daily intravenously for 3 days). Infections are treated with appropriate antimicrobial agents. Treatment of bronchiolitis obliterans without evidence of acute rejection is more variable, but increased corticosteroid dosages are given in most cases and titrated against clinical symptoms, lung function tests, and repeat biopsies. Patients with declining lung function tests, but no evidence of bronchiolitis obliterans, rejection, or infection at bronchoscopy are usually given a trial of increased corticosteroid dosage (33). Open lung biopsy may still be necessary in a small minority of patients for precise evaluation.

The available data (33) suggest that both the prevalence and severity of bronchiolitis obliterans in heart–lung transplant recipients has diminished significantly. Three-year cumulative survival (i.e., patients at risk who did not die of bronchiolitis obliterans) has increased from 77.3% initially to 100% more recently at the Stanford University program. The prevalence of bronchiolitis obliterans has decreased from 68% initially to 20% of current long-term survivors. This improved outlook has been related to the addition of azathioprine to the immunosuppressant regimens of corticosteroids and cyclosporin and to regular-surveillance lung function tests and bronchoscopy (33).

Notwithstanding the evidence that increased immunosuppression slows the progress of established bronchiolitis obliterans, it should be stressed that with current drugs the majority of affected patients show an inexorable decline leading to retransplantation or death. This unsatisfactory situation is currently being addressed by studies of alternative immunosuppressant regimens, including nebulized corticosteroids, nebulized cyclosporin, murine monoclonal anti-T-cell antibodies, and total lymphoid irradiation (82).

FUTURE PRIORITIES

More accurate donor–recipient matching should reduce the incidence of post-transplantation bronchiolitis obliterans, but advances in this area will necessitate the capacity to preserve heart–lung donor blocks for longer periods than the few hours currently possible. Advances in immunosuppressant regimens have already had a positive impact on bronchiolitis obliterans, and further developments in this area are anticipated. The diagnostic modalities of lung rejection are becoming more sensitive and specific, and more sophisticated immunological monitoring of lung allografts to detect the onset of rejection will reduce the incidence of bronchiolitis obliterans. Further advances in rapid diagnostic techniques for allograft infection will allow earlier use of specific antimicrobial treatment and, by excluding infection, facilitate the diagnosis of rejection and bronchiolitis obliterans.

Advances in these and related areas should continue to reduce the prevalence and severity of bronchiolitis obliterans in heart–lung transplant recipients. Such a trend is already apparent. A fuller understanding of the pathogenesis of the disease not only will improve the prognosis of heart–lung transplant recipients but, it is not unreasonable to suggest, also will make a major contribution to the treatment of other more common diseases caused by airway inflammation, including bronchial asthma.

ACKNOWLEDGMENTS

We gratefully acknowledge the expert advice of Dr. James Theodore, Department of Respiratory Medicine, Stanford University School of Medicine, California, and also the secretarial services of Ms. Paula Hearne, James Connolly Memorial Hospital, Dublin 15, Ireland.

REFERENCES

1. Reitz BA, Wallwork JL, Hunt SA, et al. Heart–lung transplantation: successful therapy for patients with pulmonary vascular disease. *N Engl J Med* 1982;306:557–564.
2. Toronto Lung Transplant Group. Experience with single lung transplantation for pulmonary fibrosis. *JAMA* 1988;259:2258–2263.
3. Burke CM, Theodore J, Baldwin JC, et al.

Twenty-eight cases of human heart–lung transplantation. *Lancet* 1986;1:517–519.
4. Theodore J, Marshall S, Kramer M, Duncan S, Lewiston N, Starnes V. "The natural history" of the transplanted lung: rates of pulmonary functional change in long-term survivors of heart–lung transplantation. *Transplant Proc* 1991;23:1165–1166.
5. Burke CM, Dawkins KD, Blank M, et al. Post-transplant obliterative bronchiolitis and other late lung sequelae in human heart–lung transplantation. *CHEST* December 1984;86:824–829.
6. Yousem S, Burke C, Billingham M, et al. Pathologic pulmonary alterations in long-term human heart–lung transplantation. *Hum Pathol* 1985;16:911–923.
7. Estenne M, Ketelbant P, Primo G, et al. Human heart–lung transplantation: physiologic aspects of the denervated lung and post-transplant obliterative bronchiolitis. *Am Rev Respir Dis* 1987;135:976–978.
8. Griffith B, Hardesty R, Trento A, et al. Heart–lung transplantations: lessons learned and future directions. *Ann Thorac Surg* 1987;43:6–16.
9. Higenbottam T, Stewart S, Penketh A, et al. Trans-bronchial lung biopsies for the diagnosis of rejection in heart–lung transplant patients. *Transplant Proc* 1988;20:767–769.
10. Paradis I, Dummer S, Dauber J, et al. Risk factors for the development of chronic rejection of the human allograft. *Am Rev Respir Dis* 1989;139:529A.
11. Scott J, Higinbottam T, Clelland C, et al. The natural history of chronic lung rejection in heart–lung transplantation. *Am Rev Respir Dis* 1989;139:242A.
12. Demikhov VP. *Some essential points of the techniques of transplantation of the heart, lungs and other organs*. Moscow: Medgiz State Press for Medical Literature in Moscow; 1960:29–48.
13. Neptune WB, Cookson BA, Bailey CP, Appler, Rajkowski. Complete homologous heart transplantation. *Arch Surg* 1953;66:174–178.
14. Webb WR, Howard HS. Cardiopulmonary transplantation. *Surg Forum* 1957;8:313–317.
15. Lower RR, Shumway NE. Studies on orthotopic transplantation of the canine heart. *Surg Forum* 1960;11:18–19.
16. Grinnan GLB, Graham WH, Childs JW, Lower RR. Cardiopulmonary homotransplantation. *J Thorac Cardiovasc Surg* 1970;60:609–615.
17. Nakae S, Webb WR, Theodorides T, Gregg WL. Respiratory function following cardiopulmonary denervation in dog, cat and monkey. *Surg Gynecol Obstet* 1967;125:1285–1292.
18. Castaneda AR, Zamora R, Schmidt-Habelman P, et al. Cardiopulmonary autotransplantation in primates (baboons): late functional results. *Surgery* 1972;72:1064–1070.
19. Reitz BA, Burton NA, Jamieson SW, et al. Heart and lung transplantation: autotransplantation and allotransplantation in primates with extended survival. *J Thorac Cardiovasc Surg* 1980;80:360–371.
20. Cooley DA, Bloodwell RD, Hallman GL, Nora JJ, Harrison GM, Leachman RD. Organ transplantation for advanced cardiopulmonary disease. *Ann Thorac Surg* 1969;8:30–46.
21. Lillehei CW, Wildevuur CRH, Benfield JR. Review of 23 human lung transplantations by 20 surgeons. *Ann Thorac Surg* 1970;9:515–521.
22. Barnard CN. The present status of heterotopic cardiac transplantation. *J Thorac Cardiovasc Surg* 1981;81:433–439.
23. [Anonymous]. Obliterative bronchiolitis [Editorial]. *Lancet* 1982;1:603–604.
24. Ramirez RJ, Dowell AR. Silo-fillers disease: nitrogen dioxide induced lung injury. *Ann Intern Med* 1971;74:569–576.
25. Becroft DMO. Bronchiolitis obliterans bronchiectasis and other sequelae of adenovirus type 21 infection in young children. *J Clin Pathol* 1971;24:72–82.
26. Epler GR, Snider GL, Gansler EA, Cathcart ES, Fitzgerald MX, Carrington CB. Bronchiolitis and bronchitis in connective tissue disease. *JAMA* 1979;242:528–532.
27. Geddes DM, Corran B, Brewerton DA, Davis RJ, Turner-Warrick M. Progressive airways obliteration in adults and its association with rheumatoid disease. *Q J Med* 1977;46:427–444.
28. Ralph DD, Springmeyer SC, Sullivan KM, Hackman RC, Storb B, Thomas ED. Rapidly progressive airflow obstruction in bone marrow transplant recipients. *Am Rev Respir Dis* 1984;129:641–644.
29. Wyatt SE, Nunn P, Hows JM, et al. Airway obstruction associated with graft-versus-host disease after bone marrow transplantation. *Thorax* 1984;39:887–894.
30. Schulman HM, Sullivan KM, Weidem PL, et al. Chronic graft-versus-host syndrome in man: a longterm clinical-pathological study of 20 Seattle patients. *Am J Med* 1980;69:204–217.
31. Link H, Reinhart U, Niethammer D, Kruger GRF, Waller HD, Wilms K. Obstructive ventilation disorder as a severe complication of chronic graft-versus-host disease after bone marrow transplantation. *Exp Hematol* 1982;[Suppl]10:92–93.
32. Roca J, Granena A, Rodriguez-Roisim R, Alvarez P, Augusta-Vidal A, Rozman C. Fatal airways disease in an adult with chronic graft-versus-host disease. *Thorax* 1982;37:77–78.
33. Theodore J, Starnes Vaughan A, Lewiston NJ. Obliterative bronchiolitis. *Clin Chest Med* 1990;11:309–321.
34. Allen M, Burke C, McGregor C, et al. Steroid-responsive bronchiolitis after human heart–lung transplantation. *J Thorac Cardiovasc Surg* 1986;92:440–451.
35. Glanville A, Baldwin J, Burke CM, et al. Obliterative bronchiolitis after heart–lung transplantation: apparent arrest by augmented immunosuppression. *Ann Intern Med* 1987;107:300–304.
36. Burke CM, Glanville A, Theodore J, et al. Lung immunogenicity, rejection, and obliterative bronchiolitis. *Chest* 1987;92:547–549.
37. Glanville AR, Burke CM, Theodore J, et al. Bronchial hyperresponsiveness after human car-

diopulmonary transplantation. *Clin Science* 1987; 73:299–303.

38. Robin ED, Theodore J, Burke CM, et al. Hypoxic pulmonary vasoconstriction persists in the human transplanted lung. *Clin Sci* 1987;72:283–287.
39. Gascoigne AD, Milne DS, Wilkes J, et al. Obliterative bronchiolitis following lung transplantation. *Thorax* 1993 (*in press*).
40. Epler G, Colby T, McLoud T, et al. Bronchiolitis obliterans organizing pneumonia. *N Engl J Med* 1985;312:152–158.
41. Tazelaar HD. Perivascular inflammation in pulmonary infections: implications for the diagnosis of lung rejection. *J Heart Lung Transplant* 1991;10:437–441.
42. Hutter JA, Stewart S, Higenbottam T, et al. Histologic changes in heart–lung transplant recipients during rejection episodes and at routine biopsy. *J Heart Transplant* 1988;7:440–444.
43. Hutter JA, Stewart S, Higenbottam T, et al. *Transplant Proc* 1989;21:435–436.
44. Cagle PT, Truong LD, Holland VA, et al. Lung biopsy evaluation of acute rejection versus opportunistic infection in lung transplant patients. *Transplantation* 1989;47:713–715.
45. Starnes VA, Theodore J, Oyer PE, et al. Pulmonary infiltrates after heart–lung transplantation: evaluation by serial transbronchial biopsies. *J Thorac Cardiovasc Surg* 1989;98:945–950.
46. Starnes VA, Theodore J, Oyer PE, et al. Evaluation of heart–lung transplant recipients with prospective, serial transbronchial biopsies and pulmonary function studies. *J Thorac Cardiovasc Surg* 1989;98:689–690.
47. May RM, Cooper DKC, Du Toit ED, Reichart B. Cytoimmunologic monitoring after heart–lung transplantation. *J Heart Transplant* 1990;9: 133–135.
48. Rabinowich H, Zeevi A, Paradis IL, et al. Proliferative responses of bronchoalveolar lavage lymphocytes from heart–lung transplant patients. *Transplantation* 1990;49:115–121.
49. McGregor CGA, Baldwin JC, Jamieson SW, et al. Isolated pulmonary rejection after combined heart–lung transplantation. *J Thorac Cardiovasc Surg* 1985;90:623–630.
50. Yousem SA, Berry G, Brunt E, et al. A working formulation for the standardization of nomenclature in the diagnosis of heart and lung rejection. *J Heart Transplant* 1990;9:593–601.
51. Uyama T, Winter JB, Groen G, Wildevuur CRH, Monden Y, Prop J. Late airway changes caused by chronic rejection in rat lung allografts. *Transplantation* 1992;54:809–812.
52. Yousem SA, Paradis IL, Dauber JA, et al. Large airway inflammation in heart–lung transplant recipients. *Transplantation* 1990;49:654–656.
53. Yousem SA, Ray L, Paradis IL, Dauber JA, Griffith BP. The role of dendritic cells in bronchiolitis obliterans in heart–lung transplantation. *Ann Thorac Surg* 1990;49:424–428.
54. Yousem SA. Graft eosinophilia in lung transplantation. *Hum Pathol* 1992 (*in press*).
55. Clelland CA, Higenbottam T, Otulana B, et al. Histologic prognostic indicators for the lung allografts of heart–lung transplants. *J Heart Transplant* 1990;9:177–186.
56. Paradis IL, Duncan SR, Dauber JH, Yousem SA, Hardesty R, Griffith B. Distinguishing between infection, rejection and the adult respiratory distress syndrome after human lung transplantation. *J Heart Lung Transplant* 1992;11: 232–236.
57. Nakleh RE, Bolman RM, Hertz MI. Lung transplant pathology: a comparative study of acute rejection and CMV infection. *Lab Invest* 1991; 64:118A.
58. Yousem SA, Duncan SR, Griffith BP. Intra-airspace granulation tissue reactions in lung allograft recipients. *Am J Surg Pathol* 1992;16:877–884.
59. Tazelaar H, Yousem SA. Pathologic findings in heart–lung transplantation: an autopsy study. *Hum Pathol* 1988;19:1403–1416.
60. Yousem SA, Duncan S, Ohori P, Soumez-Alpan E. Architectural remodelling of lung allografts in acute and chronic rejection. *Arch Pathol Lab Med* 1992;116:1175–1180.
61. De Blic J, Penchmar M, Carnot F, et al. Rejection in lung transplantation: an immunohistochemical study of transbronchial biopsies. *Transplantation* 1992;54:639–644.
62. Glanville AR, Tazelaar HD, Theodore J, et al. The distribution of MHC class I and II antigens on bronchial epithelium. *Am Rev Respir Dis* 1989;139:330–334.
63. Taylor PM, Rose ML, Yacoub MH. Expression of MHC antigens in normal human lungs and transplanted lungs with obliterative bronchiolitis. *Transplantation* 1989;48:506–510.
64. Romaniuk A, Prop J, Petersen AH, Wildevuur ChRH, Nieuwenhuis P. Expression of class II major histocompatibility complex antigens by bronchial epithelium in rat lung allografts. *Transplantation* 1987;44:209–214.
65. Yousem SA, Curley JM, Dauber J, et al. HLA class II antigen expression in heart–lung allografts. *Transplantation* 1990;49:991–995.
66. Hruban R, Beschomer W, Baumgartner W, et al. Diagnosis of lung allograft rejection by bronchial intraepithelial leu-7 positive T lymphocytes. *J Thorac Cardiovasc Surg* 1988;96:939–946.
67. Hruban Rh, Beschorner WE, Baumgartner WA, et al. Depletion of bronchus associated lymphoid tissue associated with lung allograft rejection. *Am J Pathol* 1988;132:6–11.
68. Yousem SA. Lymphocytic bronchitis: bronchiolitis in lung allograft recipients. *Am J Surg Pathol* 1992 (*in press*).
69. Milne DS, Gascoigne A, Wilkes J, et al. The immunopathology of obliterative bronchiolitis following lung transplantation. *Transplantation* 1992; 54:748–750.
70. Abernathy EC, Hruban RH, Baumgartner WA, Reiz BA, Hutchins GM. The two forms of bronchiolitis obliterans in heart–lung transplant recipients. *Hum Pathol* 1991;22:1102–1110.
71. Yousem SA, Dauber JA, Keenan R, Paradis IL,

Zeevi A, Griffith B. Does histologic acute rejection in lung allografts predict the development of bronchiolitis obliterans? *Transplantation* 1992; 52:306–309.
72. Dauber J, Zeevi A. Lung transplantation: local immune function and pulmonary defense mechanism. In: Daniele R, ed. *Immunology and immunologic diseases of the lung*. Boston: Blackwell Scientific Press; 1988:625–657.
73. Harujla A, Baldwin J, Glanville A, et al. Human leukocyte antigen compatibility in heart–lung transplantation. *J Heart Transplant* 1987;6:162–166.
74. Epler G, Colby T. The spectrum of bronchiolitis obliterans. *Chest* 1983;83:161–162.
75. Burke CM, Glanville A, Macoviak M, et al. The spectrum of cytomegalovirus infection following human heart–lung transplantation. *J Heart Transplant* 1986;5:267–272.
76. Lopez C, Simmons R, Mauer S, et al. Association of renal allograft rejection with virus infections. *Am J Med* 1984;56:280–289.
77. Halloran P, Wadgymar A, Autenried P. The regulation of expression of major histocompatibility complex products. *Transplantation* 1986;41:413–420.
78. McDevitt H. The molecular basis of autoimmunity. *Clin Res* 1986;34:163–175.
79. Tourkantonis A, Lazardis A. Interaction between cytomegalovirus infection and renal transplant rejection. *Kidney Int* 1983;23:546–549.
80. Griffith BP, Paradis IL, Zeevi A, et al. Immunologically mediated disease of the airways after pulmonary transplantation. *Ann Surg* 1988;208: 371–378.
81. Babatunde A, Otulana T, Higenbottam, et al. Lung function associated with histologically diagnosed acute lung rejection and pulmonary infection in heart–lung transplant patients. *Am Rev Respir Dis* 1990;142:329–332.
82. Hunt SA, Strober S, Hoppe RT, Stintston EB. Total lymphoid irradiation for treatment of intractible cardiac allograft rejection. *J Heart Lung Transplant* 1991;10:211–216.

Diseases of the Bronchioles, edited by
Gary R. Epler. Raven Press, Ltd.,
New York © 1994.

18

Lung Transplantation Bronchiolitis Obliterans

Janet R. Maurer

Department of Medicine, Division of Respirology, The Toronto Hospital, University of Toronto, Toronto, Ontario, Canada.

It has only been a few years since the first long-term clinical survivor of a single lung transplant (1) and fewer years since a successful double lung transplantation (2). Thus, although lung transplantation has moved from the realm of experimental curiosity to that of accepted therapy in selected patients with end-stage pulmonary parenchymal or vascular lung disease, it is still in its infancy with a variety of poorly understood complications, chief among them bronchiolitis obliterans.

The St. Louis International Lung Transplant Registry (3), the most complete record of worldwide lung transplant activity, had recorded only about 1,900 total procedures through April 1993 (65% were unilateral transplants), and more than 85% were reported after 1989 (3). This means that only small numbers of patients have been observed for longer than 3 years, and available information about the impact of such complications as bronchiolitis obliterans on overall outcome must be interpreted in this light.

Bronchiolitis obliterans, reported first as a complication of heart–lung transplantation in 1984 by Burke and colleagues (4), was alarming in both its rate of occurrence in heart–lung recipients and its impact on outcome. A similar phenomenon had been reported (5) in allogeneic bone marrow transplant recipients as a presumed manifestation of graft-versus-host disease or at least occurring predominantly in patients who had other manifestations of graft-versus-host disease, but in that population it occurred in a smaller proportion of patients, usually in less severe form, and often within the first year.

INCIDENCE

In initial reports of bronchiolitis obliterans from the Stanford University group (6), of patients who received heart–lung transplants, 50% of those who survived the operative period developed this complication at a mean of 10.4 ± 8.3 months post transplant. Although the highest incidence appeared within the first year after transplant, new cases have appeared throughout the length of follow-up (at least 49 months). Investigators from Pittsburgh (7) reported a 54% rate of bronchiolitis obliterans, but a third group from Papworth Hospital, Cambridge, United Kingdom (8), reported only a 10% occurrence. The reason for this difference is not clear but might reflect earlier detection and aggressive management, as more recent reports (9) from the Stanford investigators suggest that the incidence of bronchiolitis obliterans can be lessened or delayed with careful monitoring and intervention. In contrast to the heart–lung transplant results, isolated lung recipients did not appear initially to have the same prob-

TABLE 1. *Obliterative bronchiolitis in isolated lung transplants*

Time of onset of OB:						
Months post-transplant	1–3	4–6	7–9	10–12	12–24	>24
SLT	1	3	1	0	3	2
DLT	1	2	1	2	1	3
Survival of patients with OB:						
Months post-OB diagnosis	1–3	4–6	7–9	10–12	12–24	>24
SLT	8	6	6	5	3	3
DLT	9	9	8	8	6	5

Data from the Toronto lung transplant program for single lung transplants (SLT) and double lung transplants (DLT) are shown above. Survivals are similar between the two groups at 12–24 months, though the early death rate in single lung transplants is higher. Rates of obliterative bronchiolitis in the two groups are similar.

lems with bronchiolitis obliterans (10). However, as the length of survivals and the numbers of survivors of isolated lung recipients increase, it is becoming clear that the incidence of this complication increases with length of follow-up and is probably similar to that of the heart–lung transplant population. The first reports (11) of bronchiolitis obliterans in isolated lung transplants from the Toronto group noted a 20% incidence in single lung recipients and a 14% incidence in double lung transplant recipients. In 1991 Bolman and others (12) reported a 19% incidence in a relatively small group of single lung recipients and a 22% incidence in heart–lung recipients from the same institution. San Antonio's program (13) has reported a 20% incidence in 50 single lung recipients.

The Toronto group has recently updated their series. In single lung recipients, 10 of 53 patients (19%) have developed bronchiolitis obliterans, and 10 of 81 double or bilateral sequential single lung recipients (12%) have developed bronchiolitis obliterans. This apparent discrepancy likely reflects the shorter length of time that double or bilateral sequential single lung transplants have been followed. Some patients in the single lung recipient group have been followed for more than 7 years, and 48 of 53 have had at least 2 years of follow-up. In contrast, a few patients in the bilateral group have been followed up to 6 years, but 50 of the bilateral recipients received transplants within the last 2 years.

Time of onset after transplant is similar in single and bilateral sequential transplant recipients (Table 1). Bronchiolitis obliterans is detected as early as 3 months after transplant, and one-half of our patients developed disease within the first year. However, as in recipients of heart–lung transplants, recipients of lung transplants continue to be at risk: two cases in our series occurred in the sixth year after transplant.

One group of researchers (14) has published a paper comparing the onset of and incidence of acute and chronic rejection in isolated lung transplants and heart–lung transplants. In this report (exclusively double lung recipients) there was no difference in the incidences of acute and chronic rejection in the two groups, although the number in each group in the study was small.

PATHOGENESIS

The most widely accepted theory of pathogenesis of bronchiolitis obliterans in the transplanted lung is that it is the primary manifestation of chronic rejection in this organ (Table 2). Epithelial tissues have often been the target of the immune system

TABLE 2. *Etiology of obliterative bronchiolitis*

Evidence Supporting "Chronic Rejection":
Increased bronchial/bronchiole major histocompatibility antigen expression in animal models during lung rejection
Positive primed lymphocyte testing studies on bronchoalveolar lavage derived lymphocytes in patients with acute rejection and those going on to develop obliterative bronchiolitis
Leu-7 positive T-lymphocytes found in bronchial epithelium of transplanted tissue in patients dying of obliterative bronchiolitis
High incidence of dendritic cells in bronchial and bronchiolar epithelium of patients dying of obliterative bronchiolitis

in its effort to rid the body of donor-derived tissue, e.g., the so-called *vanishing bile ducts* of liver transplant chronic rejection. The bronchial epithelium is abundant and well situated as a target. It is in nearly constant contact with a wide variety of antigenic stimuli such as viruses, other environmental organisms, aspirated material deposited on it by normal respiration, and a panoply of immune-competent cells that are constantly present to respond to these stimuli. It has been postulated by Burke and others (15) that this environment is conducive to ongoing airway inflammation, which in turn results in up-regulation of the donor airway epithelium major histocompatibility class II antigen (MHCII) expression. The graft bronchial epithelium would thus be easily recognized as foreign by recipient cells and become a prime target for activated T cells. The resultant airway injury could lead to chronic scarring and obliteration of the bronchiole lumen.

A number of animal and human studies have suggested that up-regulation of the class II antigens on the bronchiole epithelium does indeed occur in lung transplant rejection. Romaniuk and colleagues (16) identified class II antigen expression in bronchial epithelial tissue in rejecting rat lungs but not in normal lungs. The same investigators (17) later showed that the induction of the class II antigen expression occurred as rejection of the lung proceeded. A similar study (18) in dogs produced identical results. This study also evaluated the components of bronchoalveolar lavage fluid. Elevated levels of cytokines known to be involved in class II antigen expression were found, e.g., tumor necrosis factor and gamma interferon.

Progressive or persistent expression of class II antigens in human lung transplants with the subsequent development of bronchiolitis obliterans has not been clearly demonstrated. One study (19) has shown that explanted lungs in patients undergoing retransplant for severe bronchiolitis obliterans consistently show class II expression on the bronchial epithelium. In this study, however, normal donor lungs also sometimes expressed the antigens, as did lungs resected for carcinoma.

Recently Reinsmoen and co-workers (20) published a report showing that lavage derived cells from four patients undergoing acute rejection demonstrated a $CD4^+$ phenotype consistent with the class II antigen reactivity seen in primed lymphocyte testing; but the results were not different from those obtained from nonrejecting patients. However, lavage derived T cells from patients with bronchiolitis obliterans showed predominantly $CD8^+$ phenotype, consistent with class I directed reactivity observed in primed lymphocyte testing, but the cells were not cytotoxic. That $CD8^+$ T cells are a predominant subtype in lung and other solid organ rejection has been shown by others (21–23), but their role in terms of pathogenesis has never been elucidated. This may be a first step in a better understanding of their importance in the bronchiolitis obliterans lesion.

The largest body of evidence that human lung transplant supports the immunologic pathogenesis of bronchiolitis obliterans comes from the transplant program in Pittsburgh. Zeevi and colleagues (24) published a series of reports demonstrating donor-specific primed lymphocyte testing activity of cells from bronchoalveolar lavage fluid in acute rejection and in patients with bronchiolitis obliterans. Lymphocyte cultures from transbronchial biopsy tissue in patients with acute rejection or bronchiolitis obliterans show donor-specific alloreactivity as well (24–26). Of particular interest was the finding (27) that donor-specific alloreactivity noted from routine surveillance bronchoscopy material appeared to predict in 5 of 6 patients the eventual development of bronchiolitis obliterans. Conversely, 10 of 11 patients without the donor-specific alloreactivity had not developed bronchiolitis obliterans at the time the article was published. The ability to identify patients likely to develop obliterative bronchiolitis would be invaluable in tailoring their immune suppression, but the numbers in this study are small and the results need to be reproduced before it can be recommended for widespread use by transplant programs.

Finally, it has been demonstrated in renal transplants that the Leu-7 positive T lymphocytes are a specific marker of rejection. A small autopsy study (28) of heart–lung recipients dying of histologically confirmed bronchiolitis obliterans showed intraepithelial Leu-7 positive lymphocytes in the affected lung but not in the epithelial tissue of the native tracheas.

Other types of cells active in the immune system are also likely involved in the development of chronic rejection. In an autopsy study, Pittsburgh researchers (29) were able to show an increased incidence of dendritic cells, which in the lung are often conveniently located in the bronchial and bronchiolar epithelium, especially in patients dying of bronchiolitis obliterans. Dendritic cells can be active lymphocyte stimulators and likely function as antigen-presenting cells (29). These cells have been shown to have an important role in the rejection process in other organ systems.

A second and somewhat complementary theory about pathogenesis suggests that it is at least in part a result of ischemia secondary to vascular obstruction, which is a result of chronic vascular rejection, a common finding in other organ system rejection. It is manifested as fibrointimal hyperplasia, sometimes with a component of subendothelial, intimal, or medial mononuclear cell infiltrates (31). The loss of blood supply (secondary to vascular occlusion) could lead to scarring and eventual obliteration of the bronchial lumen. This hypothesis might be supported by the finding (32) in bronchiolitis obliterans that in areas of lung where lesions are not present, often the vascular obliterative changes are not present either, and vice versa. However, it could also be postulated that whatever caused increased antigenicity of the bronchiolar epithelium in that area up-regulated the vascular endothelium class II antigens and that both were targets of recipient lymphocytes.

Other factors related to mechanical aspects of transplantation might also be important in the pathogenesis. The lung is denervated and local defense mechanisms, such as cough, are reduced in the graft. In addition, mucociliary clearance has been shown (33) to be reduced even though beat frequency and pattern remain normal. Studies of the bronchial cartilage (34) have shown changes, likely related to ischemia from loss of the bronchial circulation, which could reduce the structural integrity of the bronchial tree and impair mucosal and submucosal function. Thus, the overall ability of the lung to clear itself of aspiration particles, atmospheric pollutants, and any other inhaled substance is greatly reduced. When all these factors are taken into account, it is clear that local irritation and inflammation could be a contributing factor in the development of bronchiolitis obliterans.

CLINICAL SYMPTOMS AND PHYSICAL FINDINGS

Original reports of bronchiolitis obliterans in heart–lung transplant recipients suggested that the presentation usually consisted of shortness of breath and chronic productive cough. The accompanying radiographs showed interstitial infiltrates (4). Early reports, however, probably reflected the findings of advanced disease with complicating bacterial bronchitis or bronchiectasis.

Bronchiolitis obliterans is now often diagnosed clinically much earlier than in the original reports because of close monitoring with pulmonary function studies and a high index of suspicion in the presence of any respiratory or vague systemic symptoms.

Unfortunately, the symptoms of incipient bronchiolitis obliterans are distressingly nonspecific. Careful review of serial pulmonary function studies will often show the beginning of a decrease in FEF_{25-75} before any symptoms appear (Fig. 1); sometimes histologic evidence is seen on surveillance transbronchial biopsy before either pulmonary function studies or symptoms suggest it. When symptoms do appear, the patients most often feel vaguely unwell, with mild malaise and fatigue sometimes accompanied by a nonproductive cough. Eventually, they experience the insidious onset of mild dyspnea and then often show a decrease in FEV_1 and mild hypoxemia. At this point bacterial bronchitis or bacterial pneumonia may complicate and worsen the underlying process.

Conversely, bacterial and viral pneumonias or bronchitic infections in patients who were previously well may be immediately followed by a decrease in flow rates, which heralds the development of bronchiolitis obliterans. Most commonly, cytomegalovirus infections have been associated with the appearance of bronchiolitis obliterans, although this association remains controversial.

The result of physical examination in early disease is similarly nonspecific. It is most often normal, but patients may have a few crackles or wheezes. Likewise, the chest radiograph initially shows no abnormalities. Early changes include peripheral decreased vascular markings, slight volume loss, and subsegmental atelectasis (35). As the disease advances the radiograph may show a variety of findings, including linear, nodular, reticulonodular, or patchy alveolar densities (36). Many of these changes probably represent organizing pneumonia or

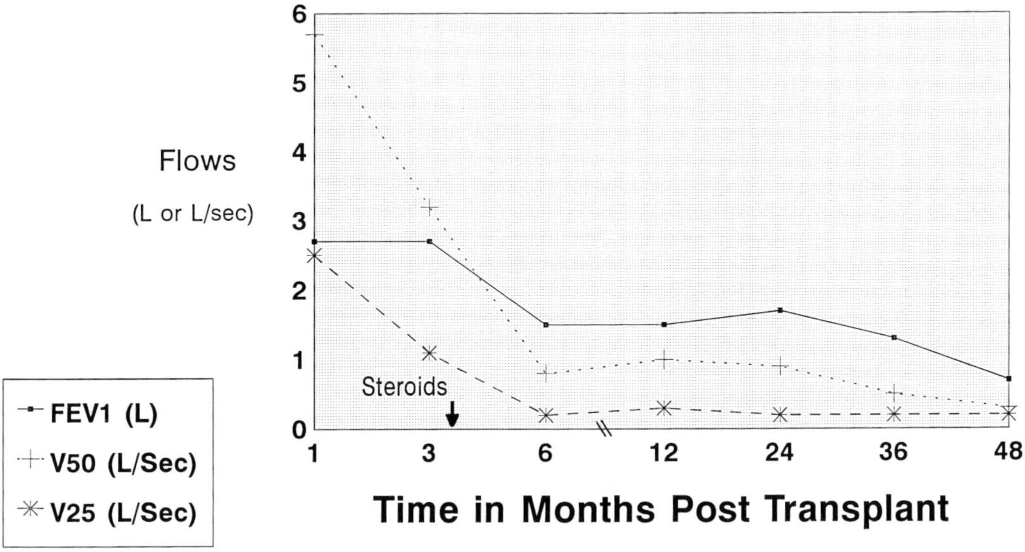

FIG. 1. Development of bronchiolitis obliterans in a double lung transplant patient.

complications secondary to the underlying pathology, such as bronchiectasis, which has been frequently documented both radiographically and histologically. A common radiographic finding in isolated lung transplant recipients with long-standing disease has been the gradual progression of pleural-based densities in the mid to upper lung zones (Fig. 2). On biopsy, these densities appear to be bland fibrosis, possibly scarring secondary to relative ischemia in those areas of the affected lung.

High-resolution chest CT examination shows decreased peripheral vascular markings and peripheral bronchiectasis and can help substantiate the clinical diagnosis (35).

Pulmonary function studies are characteristic in bronchiolitis obliterans. The initial changes are decreases in the flow rates at low lung volumes. These changes characteristically predate symptoms and decreases in FEV_1 (Fig. 1) and may be overlooked by the treating physician. As the disease progresses the decreases in flow rates are accompanied by decreases in volumes and diffusing capacity. Early, there may be an increase in the alveolar-arterial difference. As the disease progresses, hypoxemia develops, and hypercapnia develops in end-stage disease.

Another entity that has been described in lung transplant recipients and that one should be careful to distinguish from bronchiolitis obliterans is bronchiolitis obliterans organizing pneumonia (BOOP). This has been described in isolated lung trans-

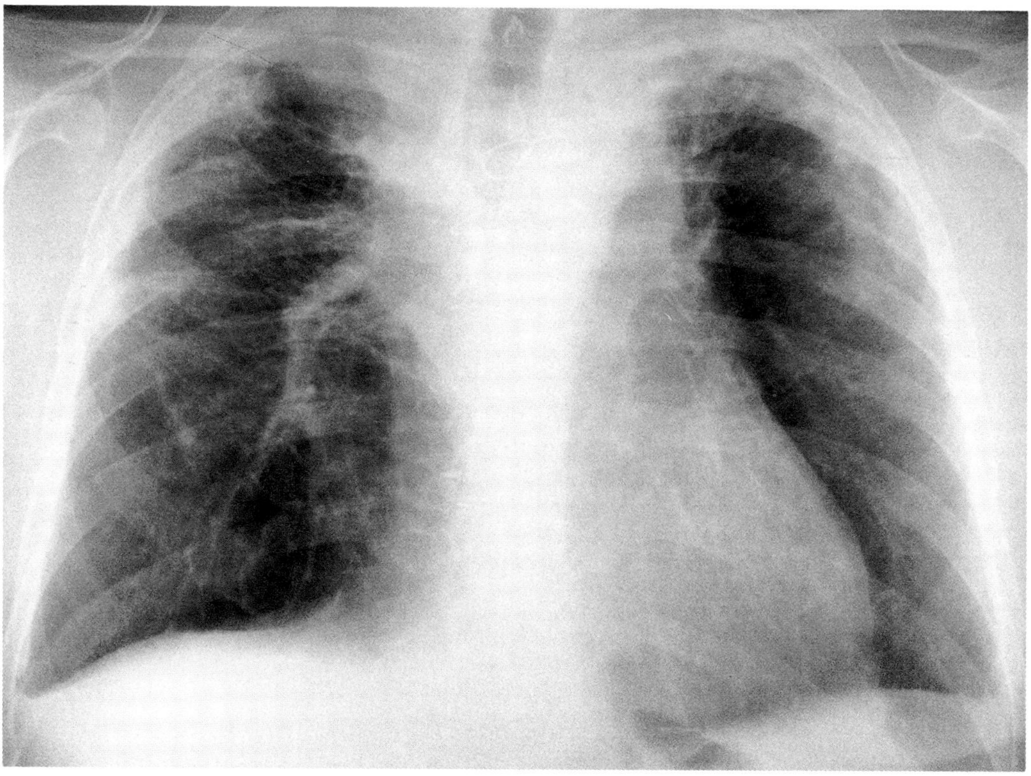

FIG. 2. Chest x-ray examination showing peripheral mid to upper zone densities in advanced bronchiolitis obliterans. Biopsy of these areas revealed subpleural fibrosis of the lung parenchyma with little active inflammation. This may be the result of ischemia secondary to the vascular lesions that often accompany severe bronchiolitis obliterans.

plants (11) and in heart–lung recipients (37). In the report on heart–lung recipients, the histology reported is from autopsy specimens, and the authors comment that bronchiolitis was seen in 7 of 11 sets of lungs. Of the 7, 3 were believed to have classic bronchiolitis obliterans, but the others had lesions consistent with BOOP. Each of these had an accompanying aspiration or infection or some other reason for developing this lesion.

The isolated lung transplants were reported to have a clinical picture of acute or subacute progressive pulmonary infiltrates and hypoxemic respiratory failure occurring 3 to 9 months after transplant. These cases, which sometimes developed after a respiratory tract infection, were documented by open lung biopsy. The patients presented with predominantly restrictive pulmonary function studies and responded well to high-dose corticosteroid therapy (11).

DIAGNOSIS

Unfortunately, the clinical picture of incipient bronchiolitis obliterans is nonspecific and therefore not very useful in making early diagnosis. Because of the impact of this entity on long-term functional outcome, a number of measures have been suggested in an attempt to detect early clinical or preclinical disease, mostly by means of frequent pulmonary function measurement.

The ideal approach would be to identify pre-onset high-risk patients; this would likely need to be done with immunologic markers. The Pittsburgh researchers (27) have found that the presence of positive primed lymphocyte testing against recipient cells in bronchoalveolar lavage fluid in well patients with negative transbronchial biopsy histology identifies many patients who will subsequently develop bronchiolitis obliterans. Unfortunately, this finding is not present in peripheral blood, and the lavage immunologic predictor has not yet been confirmed by other investigators; nor has any other easily measured marker been identified that would allow early intervention in bronchiolitis obliterans.

Thus, the state of the art remains close observation. Currently most programs use careful home monitoring, with patients measuring their own FEV_1s with hand-held spirometers at least daily; any decrease of 5 to 10% lasting at least 2 days is generally considered to warrant more formal evaluation. The researchers in Papworth initially reported the usefulness of home monitoring (38) and reported that decreases in flow rates occurred with both infection and rejection. A decrease in FEV_1 thus requires more evaluation to establish a definite diagnosis. This type of monitoring has since been widely adopted for both isolated lung recipients and heart–lung recipients; however, selected groups of recipients may not be followed easily this way. In unilateral lung recipients with obstructive disease, for example, the usefulness of this technique is somewhat problematic; nevertheless, if a post-transplant baseline is carefully established, decreases in flows may be helpful (39). Likewise, recipients with hyperreactive airways disease may undergo an excessive number of additional investigations because of diurnal changes in flow rates related to that problem. A schema for home monitoring of post-transplant patients is shown in Fig. 3.

Typical histology is considered to be diagnostic of bronchiolitis obliterans. Tissue can be obtained by transbronchial biopsy or open lung biopsy. In the absence of typical histology, and when bronchoscopy specimens have eliminated infectious etiologies, clinical diagnosis can be made on the basis of typical pulmonary function studies and clinical course with sufficient confidence to institute augmented immunosuppression.

Bronchoscopy is routinely performed in patients who develop pulmonary function changes or symptoms. Bronchoalveolar lavage and transbronchial biopsy can essen-

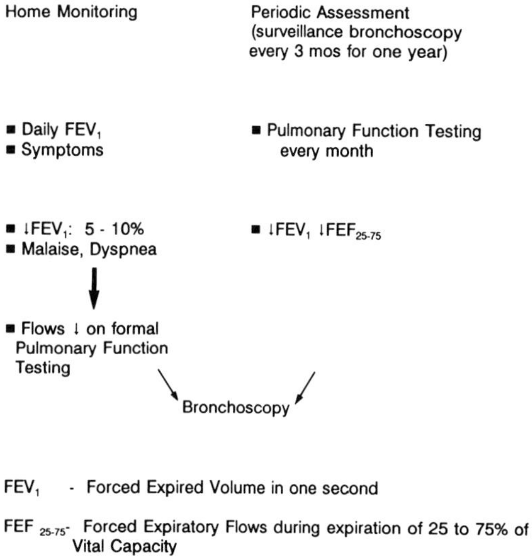

FIG. 3. Chronic rejection strategy for monitoring diagnosis.

tially diagnose or eliminate opportunistic infection. When adequate pieces of tissue are obtained, acute rejection can be diagnosed with a sensitivity of more than 80% and a specificity approximating 100% (40). Bronchioles, however, are more difficult to sample, and the sensitivity of diagnosing bronchiolitis obliterans via transbronchial biopsy is not clear. One report (41) in heart–lung recipients suggests a sensitivity of 66%, but the sensitivity approaches 100% with repeated bronchoscopies and biopsies. In the Toronto group of 20 patients with bronchiolitis obliterans, 13 (65% sensitivity) had lesions on transbronchial biopsy specimens, although all 20 had at least one bronchoscopy after clinical disease was suspected. In this population, sensitivity also increases with more than one bronchoscopy. It should be mentioned that acute rejection may accompany bronchiolitis obliterans histologically; specimens must be carefully assessed for acute rejection as the approach to treatment and likelihood of significant response is often different.

It is also critically important that adequate numbers of biopsies be taken in order to avoid sampling error. The Lung Rejection Study Group (42) recommends at least five pieces of tissue, including lung parenchyma, be taken. Some institutions have recommended at least twice that many.

In addition, several patients among the Toronto transplant recipients have been found, on surveillance bronchoscopy biopsy, to have isolated bronchiolitis obliterans lesions without pulmonary function changes or clinical symptoms. The meaning of such "false-positive" biopsies is not clear, but it is conceivable that localized areas of rejection or other bronchiolar injury that have been arrested could arise and have no consequence in the long-term function or survival of the transplant recipient. Alternatively, this finding in asymptomatic patients might represent the incipient phase of the disease, and this may be a useful predictor. Prospective observation of such patients is necessary.

Open lung biopsy is the gold standard and has a sensitivity of 100% in diagnosing bronchiolitis obliterans, but it is rarely indicated. Physicians at most centers agree that clinical and pulmonary function evidence of obstructive airways disease and absence of infection is adequate information to initiate therapy for bronchiolitis obliterans. Open lung biopsy is probably necessary only when the usual studies are unclear, e.g., atypical pulmonary function studies or chest radiograph findings, atypical clinical course, or consideration for retransplantation.

Bronchoalveolar lavage cell counts and cell differentials have not been useful in the diagnosis of bronchiolitis obliterans. Lymphocytes appear to be significantly increased in most cases of acute rejection, but this is often not true in bronchiolitis obliterans (43). Increased neutrophils usually reflect predominant larger airway sampling, which in turn reflect the occluded smaller airways. Probably the most consistent finding in bronchiolitis obliterans is that lavage fluid return is markedly reduced from normal.

PREDISPOSING FACTORS TO THE DEVELOPMENT OF BRONCHIOLITIS OBLITERANS

Since the initial descriptions of bronchiolitis obliterans, predisposing factors to its development have been sought (Table 3). One of the first associations was the use of two-pronged chronic immunosuppression (44). After noting a decreased incidence of bronchiolitis obliterans following a change to three-pronged therapy, researchers at Stanford University became convinced that two-pronged regimens were inadequate and represented a significant predisposing factor in the heart–lung recipients. Since then, most but not all programs have used a three-pronged approach with cyclosporine, azathioprine, and prednisone. The benefit of three-pronged versus two-pronged chronic therapy has not been evaluated in a randomized prospective study. It remains possible that the improvement seen with three-pronged therapy reflects better awareness of bronchiolitis obliterans and more aggressive, earlier monitoring and therapy.

Several investigators (40,45,46) have attempted to correlate early acute rejection with the development of bronchiolitis obliterans. One of these studies (46) has shown that early acute rejection with bronchiolar injury and persistent or recurrent acute rejection is a significant predictor of bronchiolitis obliterans. These findings have led to the widespread use of surveillance bronchoscopy in an attempt to diagnose occult acute rejection, which appears to be present in about 20% of patients at grade II or greater severity (43,47,48). It is not yet clear, however, that treating this asymptomatic acute rejection makes any difference in the development of bronchiolitis obliterans.

TABLE 3. *Lung transplant obliterative bronchiolitis*

Predisposing Factors
Likely Predisposing Factors
Recurrent episodes of acute rejection
Severe acute rejection
Inadequate or fluctuating maintenance immunosuppression
Infections, especially recurrent, of any etiology
Possible Predisposing Factors
Positive cytomegalovirus serology, with or without disease
Positive Epstein-Barr virus serology or conversion
Two or more HLA loci mismatches
Age less than 50 years
Non-cytolytic induction immunosuppression

A second, widely accepted predisposing factor is infection. Every physician involved in transplantation has anecdotal examples of previously well patients who, in the wake of a bacterial or other pneumonia or bronchitis, has appeared to develop bronchiolitis obliterans. The most studied infection in this regard is cytomegalovirus infection. Researchers from Pittsburgh (49) have evaluated a combined group of 20 heart–lung recipients and 7 double lung recipients and found that histologic bronchiolitis obliterans developed in a surprising 18 of 27 patients. It developed in 12 of 13 patients who either were seropositive at transplant or were transplanted with a seropositive graft. It was also seen in 6 of 14 patients who were seronegative and received seronegative grafts. French investigators (50) have reported that in heart–lung and double lung recipients, the only correlation among several factors tested, including HLA matching with development of bronchiolitis obliterans, was cytomegalovirus serology in which the donor organ was positive and the recipient was negative.

In the first 80 patients who received transplants in Toronto and who survived at least 2 weeks (long enough potentially to suffer from cytomegalovirus infection or other immunologic consequences), 13 patients were noted to have clinically significant bronchiolitis obliterans. Of the 80 patients, 28 had serologic or culture evidence of active cytomegalovirus and 8 of these 28 had developed bronchiolitis obliterans. Only 5 of 53 recipients who had no evidence of active cytomegalovirus infection developed bronchiolitis obliterans.

Although these experiences suggest a relative risk of developing bronchiolitis obliterans in the face of cytomegalovirus infection, this association remains controversial. Studies of at least two other institutions (51,52) have not found a convincing association.

A less studied but interesting viral association has been noted in Pittsburgh's (53) heart–lung recipients, in whom the incidence of Epstein-Barr related post transplant lymphoproliferative disorders (PTLD) has been reported at an astounding 9.4% of recipients. In that population over 80% of those with post transplant lymphoproliferative disorders also had bronchiolitis obliterans. Of interest, 83% of their patients suffering from bronchiolitis obliterans have evidence of Epstein-Barr virus serologic conversion (54). No reports of this association in isolated lung recipient populations have been published.

If bronchiolitis obliterans represents primarily an immunologically mediated complication, one might expect to see higher incidences in recipients who receive poorly HLA matched grafts because lung graft recipient matching is done usually only by blood groups. However, researchers at Stanford University (55) have found a tendency toward better outcomes in more closely matched patients, but the difference is not statistically significant.

Age, sex, or type of induction immunosuppression has not been correlated with the development of bronchiolitis obliterans. Age, however, appears to be associated with more episodes of infection, but fewer episodes of rejection in isolated lung recipients (56). What impact, if any, this has on the development of bronchiolitis obliterans is not known.

PATHOLOGY

Various descriptions of bronchiolitis obliterans were published in the middle 1980s from the early reports in heart–lung recipients (57,58). An elegant description by Billingham (59) of the dynamic process that may be operative in incipient disease states that bronchiolitis obliterans "develops through a sequence of epithelial injury that is initiated by an active cellular phase of lymphocytic bronchiolitis with ulceration and denuding of the mucosa. This may result in luminal ingrowth from the submucosa with organization of intraluminal plaques and the formation of a polypoid massive granulation tissue. . . ."

Certainly, lymphocytic bronchiolitis is observed in acute rejection, but by definition the disease present in acute rejection does not involve granulation tissue or scarring (42). How or whether acute rejection progresses to or predisposes to a more irreversible lesion is not clear. The above description of pathogenesis by Billingham represents a proliferative lesion (or phase of the disease) that ought to respond to treatment. Most commonly, the clinician working with transplants sees a patient whose disease has progressed far beyond this active phase. The lesion in these patients most often is characterized by relatively bland scar tissue "obliterating" the bronchiole lumen, and this is not likely to respond to treatment. Advanced and irreversible disease can appear within a few days to weeks, which suggests that some patients may never have a proliferative phase. Occasionally in the same patient bronchiolitis obliterans lesions of different stages are seen; this may explain why some patients appear to respond much better to therapy than others.

It must also be remembered that Billingham's description of bronchiolitis obliterans is not unlike the sequence of events that occurs in any type of bronchiolitis obliterans from a variety of insults; the underlying foreign tissue as an initiating factor (or target) is what distinguishes transplant obliterative bronchiolitis from any of the other causes of bronchiolitis obliterans.

In mid-1990 a group of pathologists (42) from major heart–lung and lung transplant centers formed the Lung Rejection Study Group and subsequently published a description of the various histologic changes seen in acute and chronic lung rejection. This is now the accepted framework for describing the pathologic changes seen in post lung transplant biopsy specimens, derived from either transbronchial biopsy or larger pieces of tissue.

In this report, bronchiolitis obliterans is described as chronic airway rejection and is "restricted to membranous and respiratory bronchioles having evidence of submucosal scarring that may be eccentric, concentric, or associated with total obliteration of the bronchiolar lumens; it may be associated with foam cells in distal air spaces." (However, this is not to be confused with BOOP.)

Obliterative bronchiolitis is divided into subtotal and total forms and further subdivided in each case into active and inactive (Table 4). Subtotal refers to incomplete obliteration of the lumen of the airway with scar tissue. Destruction of the smooth-muscle wall may occur, and fibrosis may extend outside the bronchiole. In total disease, the lumen is totally occluded. Active disease, either subtotal or total, implies the presence of mononuclear cells that may be causing ongoing epithelial damage.

Vascular changes often are noted in conjunction with bronchiolitis obliterans and usually consist of fibrointimal thickening of arteries and veins with or without an active inflammatory component. A true vasculitis occasionally has been seen.

It is important to distinguish the bronchial or bronchiolar lesion of acute rejection from that of chronic rejection. It is not uncommon to see in airways a submucosal and/or mucosal infiltrate obtained during episodes of acute rejection. These specimens may show epithelial injury, but they show neither scarring of the airway nor obliteration of the lumen and appear potentially completely reversible. In addition, histologically acute perivascular and chronic airway rejection may coexist in the same biopsy specimens.

The issue of BOOP pneumonia was also addressed by the Lung Rejection Study Group. The histology of this entity, which the Lung Rejection Study Group members believed distinguished it from chronic airway injury, included the extension of pathology distally into the alveolar ducts and air spaces, unlike obliterative bronchiolitis, which is localized to the terminal and respiratory bronchioles. The authors suggested that BOOP might represent a response to infection or aspiration as opposed to rejection; but the etiology of this process, which has been reported from both heart–lung and isolated lung centers, is not clear (11,37).

TABLE 4. *Lung transplant obliterative bronchiolitis lung rejection study group nomenclature/description*[a]

Chronic Airway Rejection
Bronchiolitis Obliterans-subtotal
Active
Inactive
Bronchiolitis Obliterans-total
Active
Inactive

[a]Yousem, et al, J Heart Transplant 1990;9:177–86.

TREATMENT AND OUTCOME

Reports of effective treatment to reverse bronchiolitis obliterans have been largely anecdotal; often the most that can be achieved is to arrest the underlying process. An approach is shown in Fig. 4.

Allen and colleagues (60) in 1986 published a case report in which a patient with heart–lung transplant appeared to have a dramatic response to corticosteroid therapy. However, it is not clear from this report that the patient had true bronchiolitis obliterans as opposed to BOOP, which one might expect to have a better response.

Shortly after that report, Stanford University researchers (44) published a report in which azathioprine was added to immunosupression therapy with cyclosporine and prednisone in patients with bronchioli-

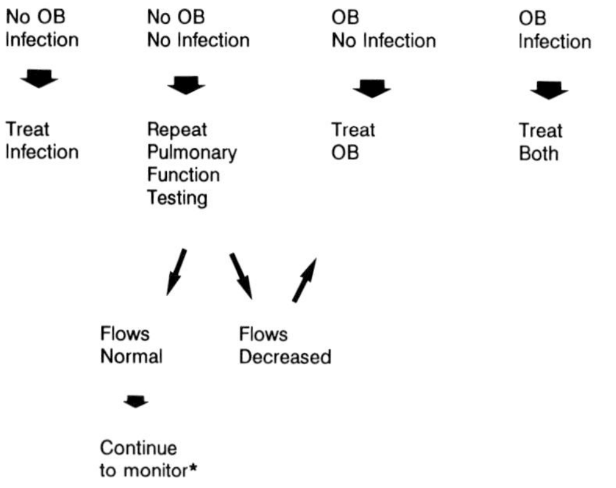

*Repeat Pulmonary Function Testing every one to two week intervals until the patient is stable

OB - Obliterative Bronchiolitis

FIG. 4. A suggested approach to management of treatment to reverse bronchiolitis obliterans, depending upon results of bronchoscopy (see Fig. 3).

tis obliterans. They showed that the progression of the disease could be dramatically slowed. This report has since been used by many centers to justify the routine use of three-pronged chronic immunosuppression.

In the late 1980s, the impact of aggressive monitoring and treatment became evident in terms of reduced morbidity and mortality: at the Stanford University transplant program between 1981 and 1986 the prevalence of bronchiolitis obliterans was 68.4% percent and the cumulative three-year survival 77.3%; between 1986 and 1989 the prevalence was 20% and there were no deaths (6). During the first 5 years of the Stanford University program, patients who died lived a mean of 1 year after diagnosis. Papworth Hospital has reported a rate of less than 20%, while investigators at Pittsburgh continue to report a rate of more than 50% (14).

This wide variation in reported incidences may reflect differences in definition of what constitutes disease and the more aggressive use of surveillance bronchoscopy and transbronchial biopsy in some centers than others. Isolated lesions without a clinical syndrome or small changes in pulmonary function might be classified as bronchiolitis obliterans in one center but not in another. A standard definition of what is reported as "bronchiolitis obliterans" has never been agreed upon by transplant centers.

No studies have been published with regard to outcomes of isolated lung transplant recipients with respect to bronchiolitis obliterans. All patients in the Toronto transplant program diagnosed with histologic and clinical bronchiolitis obliterans or with clinical bronchiolitis obliterans (all eventually confirmed by biopsy) received temporary enhanced immunosuppression in the form of increased oral corticosteroid therapy or intravenous bolus and oral corticosteroids. In most patients this appeared to slow the progression of the disease; in no case was the disease completely reversed except in those patients who had BOOP rather than bronchiolitis obliterans. Occasional patients (two in this group) had a relentless loss of function in the face of multiple attempts at augmented immunosuppression. Another anecdotal report (61) described a patient who had a similar progressive decline to death.

Despite slowing of the rate of decline of flows in most patients, the prognosis is poor. Only 5 of 10 patients with double lung transplants and 3 of 10 patients with single lung transplants remain alive (Table 1). One each of the surviving patients with single and double lung transplants has received a retransplant; whether or not bronchiolitis obliterans will recur with increased incidence in retransplanted lungs is an unanswered question.

About 50% of all patients who die after the first year post transplant die of bronchiolitis obliterans. Thus it is our impression that augmented immunosuppression can slow the progression of this complication, but lung function continues to deteriorate slowly and is an important cause of late deaths in isolated lung recipients. This deterioration is often worsened by the development of bronchiectasis (58,62) and recurrent infections, usually with pseudomonas species.

It seems likely that with the development of bronchiolitis obliterans, loss of functional lung may have more clinical consequences in single lung recipients than in double lung recipients. We have recently compared the impact of bronchiolitis obliterans on the 6-minute walk test in single lung recipients and double lung recipients. Double lung recipients had a decrease in meters walked from mean before bronchiolitis obliterans of 676 ± 120 m to a mean 6 to 12 months after bronchiolitis obliterans of 494 ± 153 m ($p = 0.03$). Single lung recipients had a decrease from 584 ± 66 m to 328 ± 141 m ($p = 0.0006$). These numbers suggest that single lung recipients who develop bronchiolitis obliterans are likely to suffer more loss of exercise capacity than double lung recipients who develop the complication.

The best approach to augmented immunosuppression is not clear. Certainly, if a two-pronged approach is used for chronic maintenance, adding a third drug may be most helpful. But for those patients already on three drugs, the choices are fewer. Increasing the dose of one of the drugs already being used is often the approach taken, although some anecdotal reports suggest success with cytolytic therapy or even total lymphoid irradiation. It is probably not necessary to continue the augmented immunosuppression indefinitely; this in fact may predispose the patient to complicating bacterial infections. One or two limited courses of augmented immunosuppression will likely treat elements of the process that remain reversible.

New immunosuppressive agents are being evaluated that may become first-line maintenance agents or useful in this type of rescue therapy. The best solution to bronchiolitis obliterans will be preventing it, and that will require sorting out the answers, immunologic and otherwise, to its etiology.

SUMMARY

Bronchiolitis obliterans is the most important factor in impaired outcome in lung transplant recipients. Although the reported incidence of this complication has decreased from more than 50% to about 20% in most transplant centers, affected patients can often expect impaired function and a shortened survival. Early detection of the disease by immunologic markers may be the best hope of identifying at-risk recipients, and this will allow interventions that will reverse the incipient inflammatory process.

REFERENCES

1. Toronto Lung Transplant Group. Unilateral lung transplantation for pulmonary fibrosis. *N Engl J Med* 1986;314:1140–1145.
2. Patterson GA, Cooper JD, Goldman B, et al. Technique of successful clinical double lung transplantation. *Ann Thorac Surg* 1988;45:626–633.
3. Report of the St. Louis International Lung Transplant Registry, May 1993.
4. Burke CM, Theodore J, Dawkins KD, et al. Post-transplant obliterative bronchiolitis and other late lung sequelae in human heart–lung transplantation. *Chest* 1984;86:824–829.
5. Chan CK, Hyland RH, Hutcheon MA. Pulmonary complications following bone marrow transplantation. *Clin Chest Med* 1990;11(2):323–332.
6. Theodore J, Starnes VA, Lewiston NJ. Obliterative bronchiolitis. *Clin Chest Med* 1990;11(2):309–322.
7. Paradis I, Dummer S, Dauber J, et al. Risk factors for the development of chronic rejection of the human lung allograft. *Am Rev Respir Dis* 1989;139:A529.
8. Scott JP, Higenbottam TW, Clelland C, et al. The natural history of obliterative bronchiolitis and occlusive vascular disease of patients following heart–lung transplantation. *Transplant Proc* 1989;21(1):2592–2593.
9. McCarthy P, Starnes V, Theodore J, et al. Improved survival following heart–lung transplant. *J Thorac Cardiovasc Surg* 1990;99:54–58.
10. Toronto Lung Transplant Group. Experience with single lung transplantation for pulmonary fibrosis. *JAMA* 1988;259:2258–2263.

11. deHoyos AL, Patterson GA, Maurer JR, et al. Pulmonary transplantation: early and late results. *J Thorac Cardiovasc Surg* 1992;103:295–306.
12. Bolman RM, Shumway SJ, Estrin JA. Lung and heart–lung transplantation: evolution and new applications. *Ann Surg* 1991;214:456–470.
13. Anzueto A, Levine SM, Bryan CL, et al. Obliterative bronchiolitis in single lung transplant recipients. *Am Rev Respir Dis* 1992;145:A700.
14. Keenan RJ, Bruzzone P, Paradis IL, et al. Similarity of pulmonary rejection patterns among heart–lung and double-lung transplant recipients. *Transplantation* 1991;51:176–180.
15. Burke CM, Glanville AR, Theodore J, et al. Lung immunogenicity, rejection, and obliterative bronchiolitis. *Chest* 1987;92:547–549.
16. Romaniuk A, Prop J, Petersen AH, et al. Increased expression of class II major histocompatibility complex antigens in untreated and cyclosporine-treated rat lung allografts. *J Heart Transplant* 1986;5:455–460.
17. Romaniuk A, Prop J, Petersen AH, et al. Expression of class II major histocompatibility complex antigens by bronchial epithelium in rat lung allografts. *Transplantation* 1987;44:209–214.
18. Chang S-C, Hsu H-K, Perng R-P, et al. Increased expression of MHC class II antigens in rejecting canine lung allografts. *Transplantation* 1990;49:1158–1163.
19. Taylor PM, Rose ML, Yacoub MH. Expression of MHC antigens in normal human lungs and transplanted lungs with obliterative bronchiolitis. *Transplantation* 1989;48:506–510.
20. Reinsmoen NL, Bolman RM, Savik K, et al. Differentiation of class I- and class II-directed donor-specific alloreactivity in bronchoalveolar lavage lymphocytes from lung transplant recipients. *Transplantation* 1992;53:181–189.
21. Holland VA, Cagle PT, Windsor NT, et al. Lymphocyte subpopulations in bronchiolitis obliterans after heart–lung transplantation. *Transplantation* 1990;50:955–959.
22. Maurer JR, Gough E, Chamberlain DW, et al. Sequential bronchoalveolar lavage studies from patients undergoing double lung and heart–lung transplant. *Transplant Proc* 1989;21:2585–2587.
23. Jutte NHPM, Vandekerckhove BAE, Vaessen LMB, et al. T-cell receptor-positive T-cell clones derived from human heart transplants do not show donor-specific cytotoxicity. *Hum Immunol* 1990;28:170–174.
24. Zeevi A, Rabinowich H, Yousem SA, et al. Presence of donor-specific alloreactivity in histologically normal lung allografts is predictive of subsequent bronchiolitis obliterans. *Transplant Proc* 1991;23:1128–1129.
25. Zeevi A, Rabinowich H, Paradis I, et al. Lymphocyte activation in bronchoalveolar lavages from heart–lung transplant recipients. *Transplant Proc* 1988;20:189–192.
26. Dauber JH, Zeevi A. Lung transplantation: local immune function and pulmonary defense mechanisms. In: Daniele RP. *Immunology and immunologic diseases of the lung*. Boston: Blackwell Scientific Publications, 1988.
27. Griffith BP, Paradis IL, Zeevi A, et al. Immunologically mediated disease of the airways after pulmonary transplantation. *Ann Surg* 1988;208:371–378.
28. Hruban RH, Beschorner WE, Baumgartner WA, et al. Diagnosis of lung allograft rejection by bronchial intraepithelial Leu-7 positive T lymphocytes. *J Thorac Cardiovasc Surg* 1988;96:939–946.
29. Yousem SA, Ray L, Paradis IL, et al. Potential role of dendritic cells in bronchiolitis obliterans in heart–lung transplantation. *Ann Thorac Surg* 1990;49:424–428.
30. Faustman DC, Steinman RM, Gebel HM, et al. Prevention of rejection in murine islet allografts by pre-treatment with anti-dendritic cell antibody. *Proc Natl Acad Sci USA* 1984;81:3864–3868.
31. Yousem SA, Paradis IL, Dauber JH, et al. Pulmonary arteriosclerosis in long-term human heart–lung transplant recipients. *Transplantation* 1989;47:564–569.
32. Harjula A, Baldwin JC, Tazelaar HD, et al. Minimal lung pathology in long term survivors of heart–lung transplantation. *Transplantation* 1987;44:852–856.
33. Dolovich M, Rossman C, Chambers C, et al. Mucociliary function in patients following single lung or lung/heart transplantation. *Am Rev Respir Dis* 1987;135:A363.
34. Yousem SA, Dauber JH, Griffith BP. Bronchial cartilage alterations in lung transplantation. *Chest* 1990;98:1121–1124.
35. Morrish WF, Herman SJ, Weisbrod GL, et al. Bronchiolitis obliteran's after lung transplantation: findings at chest radiography and high-resolution CT. *Radiology* 1991;179:487–490.
36. Skeens JL, Fuhrman CR, Yousem SA. Bronchiolitis obliterans in heart–lung transplantation patients: radiologic findings in 11 patients. *Am J Radiol* 1989;153:253–256.
37. Abernathy EC, Hruban RH, Baumgartner WA, et al. The two forms of bronchiolitis obliterans in heart–lung recipients. *Hum Pathol* 1991;22:1102–1110.
38. Outlana BA, Higenbottam TW, Ferrari L, et al. The use of home spirometry in detecting acute lung rejection and infection following heart–lung transplantation. *Chest* 1989;97:353–358.
39. Marshall SE, Lewiston NJ, Kramer MR, et al. Prospective analysis of serial pulmonary function studies and transbronchial biopsies in single-lung transplant recipients. *Transplant Proc* 1991;23:1217–1219.
40. Higenbottam T, Stewart S, Penketh A, et al. Transbronchial lung biopsy for the diagnosis of rejection in heart–lung transplant patients. *Transplantation* 1988;46:532–539.
41. Yousem SA, Paradis IL, Dauber JH, et al. Efficacy of transbronchial lung biopsy in the diagnosis of bronchiolitis obliterans in heart–lung transplant recipients. *Transplantation* 1989;47:893–895.
42. The International Society for Heart Transplantation: Yousem SA, Berry GJ, Brunt EM, et al. A working formulation for the standardization of

nomenclature in the diagnosis of heart and lung rejection: lung rejection study group. *J Heart Transplant* 1990;9:593–601.
43. deHoyos A, Chamberlain D, Schvartzman R, et al. Prospective assessment of a standardized pathological grading system for acute rejection in lung transplantation. *Chest* 1993;103:1813–1818.
44. Glanville AR, Baldwin JC, Burke CM, et al. Obliterative bronchiolitis after heart–lung transplantation: apparent arrest by augmented immunosuppression. *Ann Intern Med* 1987;107: 300–304.
45. Clelland C, Higenbottam T, Otulana B, et al. Histologic prognostic indicators for the lung allografts of heart–lung transplants. *J Heart Transplant* 1990;9:177–186.
46. Yousem SA, Dauber JA, Keenan R, et al. Does histologic acute rejection in lung allografts predict the development of bronchiolitis obliterans? *Transplantation* 1991;52:306–309.
47. Starnes VA, Theodore J, Oyer PE, et al. Evaluation of heart–lung transplant recipients with prospective, serial transbronchial biopsies and pulmonary function studies. *J Thorac Cardiovasc Surg* 1989;98:683–690.
48. Hutter J, Stewart S, Higenbottam TW, et al. Histological changes in heart–lung transplant recipients during rejection episodes and at routine biopsy. *J Heart Transplant* 1988;7:440–444.
49. Keenan RJ, Lega ME, Dummer JS, et al. Cytomegalovirus serologic status and postoperative infection correlated with risk of developing chronic rejection after pulmonary transplantation. *Transplantation* 1991;51:433–438.
50. Cerrina L, Le Roy Ladurie F, Parquin F, et al. Risk factors for obliterative bronchiolitis (OB) after heart–lung (HLT) and double lung transplantation (DLT). *Am Rev Respir Dis* 1992; 145:A700.
51. Burke CM, Glanville AR, Macoviak JA, et al. The spectrum of cytomegalovirus infection following human heart–lung transplantation. *J Heart Transplant* 1986;5:267–271.
52. Fradet G, Scott JP, Sharples L, et al. Five years experience with heart–lung transplantation: analysis of risk factors of rejection. *J Heart Transplant* 1990;9:82.
53. Yousem SA, Randhawa P, Locker J, et al. Posttransplant lymphoproliferative disorders in heart–lung transplant recipients: primary presentation in the allograft. *Hum Pathol* 1989;20: 361–369.
54. Randhawa PS, Yousem SA, Paradis IL, et al. The clinical spectrum, pathology, and clonal analysis of Epstein-Barr associated lymphoproliferative disorders in heart–lung transplant recipients. *Am J Clin Pathol* 1989;92:177–185.
55. Harujla A, Baldwin J, Glanville A, et al. Human leukocyte antigen compatibility in heart–lung transplantation. *J Heart Transplant* 1987;6:162–166.
56. Snell GI, deHoyos A, Winton T, et al. Lung transplantation in patients over the age of 50. *Transplantation* 1992;55:562–566.
57. Tazelaar HD, Yousem SA. The pathology of combined heart–lung transplantation: an autopsy study. *Hum Pathol* 1988;19:1403–1416.
58. Yousem S, Burke C, Billingham M. Pathologic pulmonary alterations in long-term human heart–lung transplantation. *Hum Pathol* 1985;16: 911–923.
59. Billingham ME. The pathologic changes in long-term heart and lung transplant survivors. *J Heart Lung Transplant* 1992;11:S252–S257.
60. Allen M, Burke C, McGregor C, et al. Steroid-responsive bronchiolitis after human heart–lung transplantation. *J Thorac Cardiovasc Surg* 1986; 92:449–451.
61. LoCicero J III, Robinson PG, Fisher M. Chronic rejection in single-lung transplantation manifested by obliterative bronchiolitis. *J Thorac Cardiovasc Surg* 1990;99:1059–1062.
62. Granton J, deHoyos A, Chanberlain D, et al. Bronchiectasis is related to the presence of obliterative bronchiolitis in lung transplant recipients. *Am Rev Respir Dis* 1992;145:A700.

Diseases of the Bronchioles, edited by
Gary R. Epler. Raven Press, Ltd.,
New York © 1994.

19

Miscellaneous Causes of Bronchiolitis Obliterans

Gary R. Epler

Associate Clinical Professor, Boston University School of Medicine; Chairman, Department of Medicine, New England Baptist Hospital, 125 Parker Hill Avenue, Boston, MA.

Bronchiolitis obliterans, the airway disorder, is usually categorized into several major causes or associated disorders: idiopathic, toxic fume exposure, postinfectious, connective-tissue diseases (rheumatologic and immunologic disorders), drug-related and post-transplantation (Table 1). Miscellaneous causes are rare and have been reported on a case-by-case basis. This chapter includes a discussion of these miscellaneous causes.

ASPIRATION

Aspiration of foreign bodies or substances may result in bronchiolitis obliterans. Wegelin (1) described the first such occurrence in 1908. A 2 ½-year-old child was accidentally startled and aspirated a prune pit, resulting in an immediate reaction of a coughing attack, fever, and cyanosis. There was some stabilization early in the course of the illness; but respiratory failure developed, and the child died on the 56th day. At autopsy, the prune pit, measuring almost 1 cm by ½ cm, was seen in an ulcerated region of the trachea, 2 cm below the tracheostomy site. The major and moderate sized bronchi were filled with purulent masses. Most airways of about 1 mm in diameter were completely filled with plugs of exudate. These exudative plugs consisted of leukocytes and occasional epithelial cells. The small airways up to the respiratory bronchioles showed a totally different picture. The airway wall was often disrupted. There were strange plugs reaching into the lumen of the airway and filling it almost completely. The plug had a different appearance than the exudates of the bronchi and consisted of newly formed connective tissue. Cells rich in cytoplasm were predominant, while the background consisted of spindle cells and collagen, resulting in the appearance of granulation tissue.

Talcum powder aspiration has been reported as a cause of acute bronchiolitis and may result in bronchiolitis obliterans. In 1962, there was a report (2) of a 22-month-old boy whose mother heard him choking and found him with talcum powder in his mouth, breathing heavily and coughing. An open can of talcum powder was beside him. He was rushed to the hospital, and about 7 hours after admission, respiratory distress increased with a respiratory rate reaching 90 per minute. Intractable cardiopulmonary failure developed, and he died 20 hours after aspiration of the talcum powder. At autopsy, on the cut surface of the lung several branches of small and medium bronchi were filled with greenish-yellow material of creamy consistency. On microscopic examination, most of the bronchial lumina were found to be obliterated by a slightly

TABLE 1. *Causes and associated disorders of bronchiolitis obliterans*

Idiopathic
Toxic fume exposure
Postinfectious
Rheumatologic disorders
Drug-related
Post-transplantation
Miscellaneous
Aspiration
Stevens-Johnson syndrome

basophilic, somewhat granular mass with refractile particles embedded in the homogenous matrix. The epithelium was completely desquamated in many bronchi with various grades of edema, hyperplasia and squamous metaplasia. In some places the intraluminal mass extended through the respiratory bronchioles, filling the adjacent alveoli. The photomicrograph showed destruction of a terminal bronchiole by the aspirated mass, and examination by polarized light demonstrated the birefringent talc particles. It was noted that the short survival period in this case did not permit organization of the airway process. The authors suggested that within 24 to 48 hours, organization of the intraluminal exudates will begin with active fibroblastic proliferation resulting in bronchiolitis obliterans. The composition of baby powder and other body powders has been changed since 1962; the talcum powder used in 1962 was a mixture of 93% talc, 5% magnesium carbonate, and 2% silicate.

Aspiration was noted in the 1973 report (3) of 52 patients with bronchiolitis obliterans. Eight had bronchiolitis obliterans as a result of toxic-fume inhalation, including 3 with aspiration. No clinical information was available in the report regarding these 3 patients. Whether these lesions resulted from aspiration of materials related to the fume inhalation or aspiration of gastric contents is not known.

Activated charcoal, aspirated during treatment of a drug overdose, was reported as a cause of bronchiolitis obliterans in 1989 (4). A 16-year old woman ingested 60 nortriptyline tablets. On arrival at the emergency room, she was combative. A nasogastric tube was inserted and the stomach lavaged until clear of pill fragments. Activated charcoal, 75 g, was given through the nasogastric tube. Ten minutes later, a grand mal seizure and cardiac arrest occurred. Normal cardiac rhythm was restored, and mechanical ventilation was instituted. Bronchoscopy indicated extensive charcoal staining of both mainstem bronchi. She was eventually extubated 15 days after admission. She was readmitted to the hospital 6 days later because of fever, dyspnea, and hypoxemia. After stabilization, she was discharged home, but she was readmitted 48 hours later with progressive dyspnea. Coarse crackles were heard on examination. She had now developed hypercapnia and a vital capacity of only 0.86 L with a forced expired volume in one second (FEV_1) of 0.64 L. Mechanical ventilation was reinstituted. Respiratory failure progressed, and the patient died 14 weeks after the suicide attempt. Autopsy revealed extensive charcoal deposition along the airways in all regions of the lung. Histologically, this was accompanied by bronchiolitis obliterans with fibrous obliteration and stenosis of most small airways. The charcoal deposition was centered on small airways. Massive amounts of black material associated with a foreign body giant cell reaction were embedded within the bronchiolar scar tissue. No food material was seen, and there was no pneumonia. Several causes of the obliterative lesion were possible in this patient. The charcoal particles alone could be the cause, but particles of the pills adsorbed to the charcoal surface or other gastric contents could also be the cause or contributing factors. The facts that a thorough gastric lavage preceded administration of the activated charcoal, that charcoal was present in massive amounts, and that charcoal was the only material associated with the bronchiolar scarring favors charcoal as a cause of bronchiolitis obliterans.

STEVENS-JOHNSON SYNDROME

Bronchiolitis obliterans was reported (5) in a patient after the onset of Stevens-Johnson syndrome. A 41-year-old woman was treated with oral ampicillin and intravenous cephamandole for a fever, generalized fatigue, and conjunctivitis. The next morning she developed diffuse erythematous lesions associated with blisters that were observed on the face, thorax, back, arms, and legs as well as on the conjunctivae, lips, and buccal mucosa. The dermatological lesions cleared. Twelve days later, the patient developed wheezing and progressive dyspnea. The chest roentgenogram revealed hyperinflation but no infiltrative lesions. Her condition deteriorated, hypercapnia developed, and mechanical ventilation was instituted; but despite intensive management, she died 2 months after admission. Autopsy showed an unusual finding of obliteration of the bronchi with fibrous scar tissue. Bronchiolitis obliterans without an organizing pneumonia component was also seen. It was proposed that the additional obliteration of cartilaginous bronchi made the prognosis worse. These authors noted that a similar conclusion was suggested by Japanese investigators (6), who used the term *bronchobronchiolitis obliterans* in a report of eight patients with obstructive changes of both bronchi and bronchioles at autopsy. The cause was of unknown etiology, although underlying disorders of rheumatoid arthritis and juvenile asthma were present in two patients. All of these eight patients deteriorated rapidly and died.

In summary, miscellaneous causes of bronchiolitis obliterans include aspiration of foreign substances and Stevens-Johnson syndrome. An additional classification of immunological-related bronchiolitis obliterans may be appropriate in the future, but additional reports are needed. More unusual situations will most likely be reported as continued investigation of the bronchiolar disorders proceeds.

REFERENCES

1. Wegelin C. Uber Bronchitis obliterans nach Fremdkorperaspiration. *Beitr Pathol Anat Allg Pathol* 1908;43:438–454.
2. Molnar JJ, Nathenson G, Edberg S. Fatal aspiration of talcum powder by a child. *New Engl J Med* 1962;266:36–37.
3. Gosink BB, Friedman PJ, Liebow AA. Bronchiolitis obliterans: roentgenologic-pathologic correlation. *Am J Roentgenol* 1973;117:816–832.
4. Elliott CG, Colby TV, Kelly TM, Hicks HG. Charcoal lung: bronchiolitis obliterans after aspiration of activated charcoal. *Chest* 1989;96: 672–674.
5. Tsunoda N, Iwanaga T, Saito T, et al. Rapidly progressive bronchiolitis obliterans associated with Stevens-Johnson syndrome. *Chest* 1990;98: 243–245.
6. Yamanaka A, Maeda M, Yamamoto R. Bronchobronchiolitis obliterans. *Jpn Chest Dis* 1986;45: 539–554.

SECTION 3

Bronchiolar Diseases: The Interstitial Disorders

Diseases of the Bronchioles, edited by
Gary R. Epler. Raven Press, Ltd.,
New York © 1994.

20

Respiratory Bronchiolitis-Associated Interstitial Lung Disease

Jeffrey L. Myers

Department of Laboratory Medicine and Pathology, Mayo Clinic, Rochester, MN.

Respiratory bronchiolitis was defined in 1974 by Niewoehner and colleagues (1) as a distinct histopathologic entity characterized by the presence of pigmented intraluminal macrophages within first- and second-order respiratory bronchioles. These investigators examined autopsy lungs from victims of sudden nonhospital deaths and identified respiratory bronchiolitis in 19 of 19 young (25.0 ± 1.6 years) cigarette smokers and 5 of 20 age-matched nonsmoking control subjects. Respiratory bronchiolitis varied in intensity and extent and was frequently associated with peribronchiolar edema, fibrosis, and epithelial hyperplasia. Niewoehner and colleagues hypothesized that respiratory bronchiolitis might contribute to small airways dysfunction in cigarette smokers, and also suggested that respiratory bronchiolitis might be a precursor of centriacinar emphysema.

Most studies (1–6) of respiratory bronchiolitis have continued to focus on the contribution of respiratory bronchiolitis to airflow limitation in cigarette smokers. Other air pollutants have also been incriminated as potential causes of respiratory bronchiolitis (7). In surgical and autopsy specimens, respiratory bronchiolitis is usually considered an incidental finding of little clinical significance except as a marker of cigarette smoking. Recently, however, respiratory bronchiolitis has been linked to a syndrome of diffuse interstitial lung disease referred to as respiratory bronchiolitis-associated interstitial lung disease (RB-ILD) that mimics idiopathic pulmonary fibrosis (IPF) (8–12). This chapter reviews the current understanding of RB-ILD as well as the relationship between this disorder and other smoking-related diseases.

CLINICAL FEATURES

The clinical and radiographic features of RB-ILD are nonspecific (8–12). RB-ILD occurs exclusively in cigarette smokers. It mainly affects current smokers in the fourth or fifth decade of life with average exposures of over 30 packyears of cigarette smoking (Table 1). Men are affected more often than women by a ratio of almost 2/1. Symptoms are usually mild and not disabling. Nearly all patients present with nonspecific respiratory complaints including insidious onset of dyspnea and a new or changed cough. Chest pain is described in only a small number of patients, and a similarly small minority are asymptomatic at the time of diagnosis. Systemic complaints such as weight loss and fever have not been reported. Crackles are heard in the majority of patients and have been described as coarse and prolonged, continuing through-

TABLE 1. *Clinical findings in 24 patients with RB-ILD*

Mean age at diagnosis (range)	36.1 years (22–53 years)
Males/females	15/9
Mean packyears cigarette smoking (range)	33.4 (7–75)
Symptoms	
Dyspnea	70.8%
Cough	58.3%
Chest pain	8.3%
Asymptomatic	8.3%
Signs	
Clubbing	0.0%
Rales	33.3%
Chest radiograph	
Interstitial opacities (reticular/reticulonodular)	75.0%
Linear atelectasis	4.2%
Normal	20.2%
PFTs	
Mild to moderate reduction DL_{CO}	92%
Mild restriction	NA
Mild obstruction	NA

Data summarized from refs. 8 and 10.

out inspiration and even into expiration (12).

Chest roentgenograms are abnormal in 80% of patients and show diffuse fine reticular or reticulonodular opacities in a bibasilar distribution. Lynch and colleagues (12) have described bronchial wall thickening, prominent peribronchiolar interstitial markings, small regular and irregular opacities, and small peripheral ring shadows as characteristic features of RB-ILD. Associated volume loss is usually not seen. A small number of patients have only bibasilar atelectasis or even normal chest radiographs. Holt and co-workers (13) reviewed high-resolution CT scans from five patients with RB-ILD and described nonspecific ground glass opacities in three which were extensive in two and focal in one. Intralobular and interlobular interstitial thickening, emphysema, and peripheral blebs were also seen. One patient had a normal chest roentgenogram and a normal high-resolution CT scan.

Mild to moderate reduction in diffusing capacity is the most consistent abnormality of pulmonary function in patients with RB-ILD (8–12). Mild restriction is seen in most patients and is often characterized by a mildly reduced total lung capacity (8). Total lung capacity and functional residual capacity are preserved in others, with an associated increase in residual volume (12). Mild airflow limitation typical of that seen in cigarette smokers who lack detectable emphysema or chronic bronchitis is common. Gas-exchange studies, reported (8,11) for only a few patients, show normal resting arterial oxygenation with mild desaturation after exercise in one-half. Gallium scanning has shown diffusely increased uptake in two of three patients tested (8). Bronchoalveolar lavage yields increased cellularity compared to control subjects who smoke. The increased cellularity is due to an increase in total numbers of macrophages with a minor increase in lymphocytes (8, 11). Neutrophilia and eosinophilia have not been described and may be useful in distinguishing RB-ILD from IPF.

RB-ILD appears to be relatively benign and self-limited. Follow-up for 1 month to 20 years after diagnosis in a total of 22 patients indicated that 18 (82%) were asymptomatic and 4 (18%) had stable disease (8,10). Progressive pulmonary fibrosis has not been documented. The number of patients studied to date is relatively small, however; and additional long term follow-up is required before the potential implications of this entity are firmly established.

Most patients with RB-ILD experience symptomatic improvement after smoking cessation alone (10). Of interest, patients who continue to smoke have shown complete symptomatic, radiographic, and physiologic recovery with corticosteroid therapy (8). Symptomatic improvement has also been seen in untreated patients who continue to smoke (8). On the basis of this limited anecdotal experience, it seems that although smoking cessation is probably an important factor in treating RB-ILD, the precise roles of smoking cessation and corticosteroid therapy remain uncertain.

The incidence of RB-ILD is unknown. Four reported series (8,10,11,13) of this condition describe a total of only 40 patients. These studies were limited to patients who had undergone lung biopsy and represent a highly selected group. Various investigators (14–16) have shown that subtle linear and nodular interstitial opacities appear in the majority of cigarette smokers, suggesting that RB-ILD may be more prevalent than is commonly recognized. It seems likely that respiratory bronchiolitis is associated with a spectrum that ranges from asymptomatic individuals with normal chest roentgenograms to asymptomatic individuals with radiographically detectable interstitial lung disease and a smaller subset of symptomatic patients with clinically significant disease. It is the last group that is most likely to be confused with patients with IPF, and these are the patients most likely to undergo lung biopsy.

PATHOLOGIC FEATURES

Respiratory bronchiolitis is defined by the presence of pigmented macrophages within the lumina of respiratory bronchiolitis. The changes are patchy at low magnification and have a bronchiolocentric distribution (Fig. 1). Respiratory bronchioles, alveolar ducts, and peribronchiolar alveolar spaces contain clusters of dusty-brown macrophages (Fig. 2). The lightly pigmented cells have abundant cytoplasm that contains finely granular golden-brown particles (Fig. 3). The cytoplasmic particles are PAS-positive and also stain with Prussian blue. Positive staining with Prussian blue,

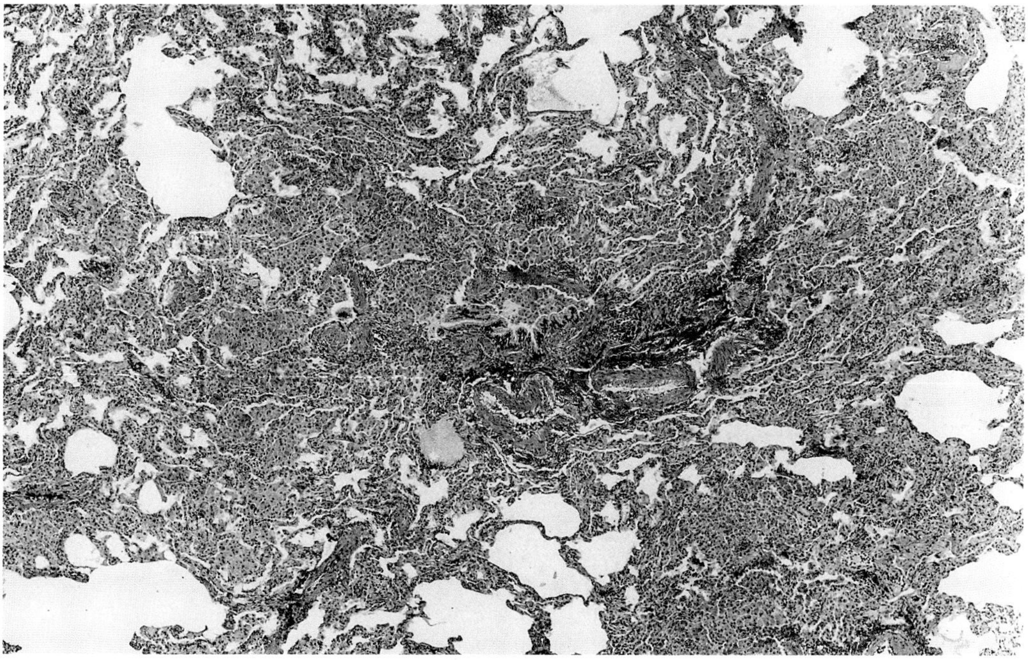

FIG. 1. Low-magnification photomicrograph showing respiratory bronchiolitis in a patient with RB-ILD. The lesion is bronchiolocentric and demonstrates clusters of intraluminal macrophages filling bronchioles, peribronchiolar alveolar ducts, and alveoli.

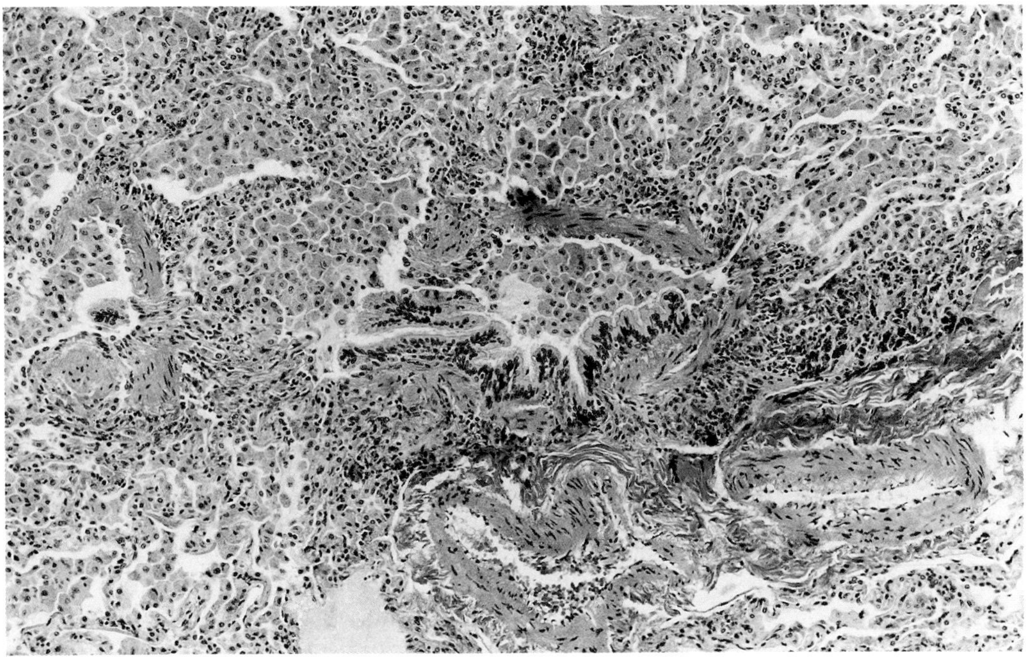

FIG. 2. Higher magnification photomicrograph from patient with RB-ILD illustrated in Fig. 1. Plump, lightly pigmented macrophages fill the centrally located respiratory bronchiole and spill into contiguous alveolar ducts and alveolar spaces.

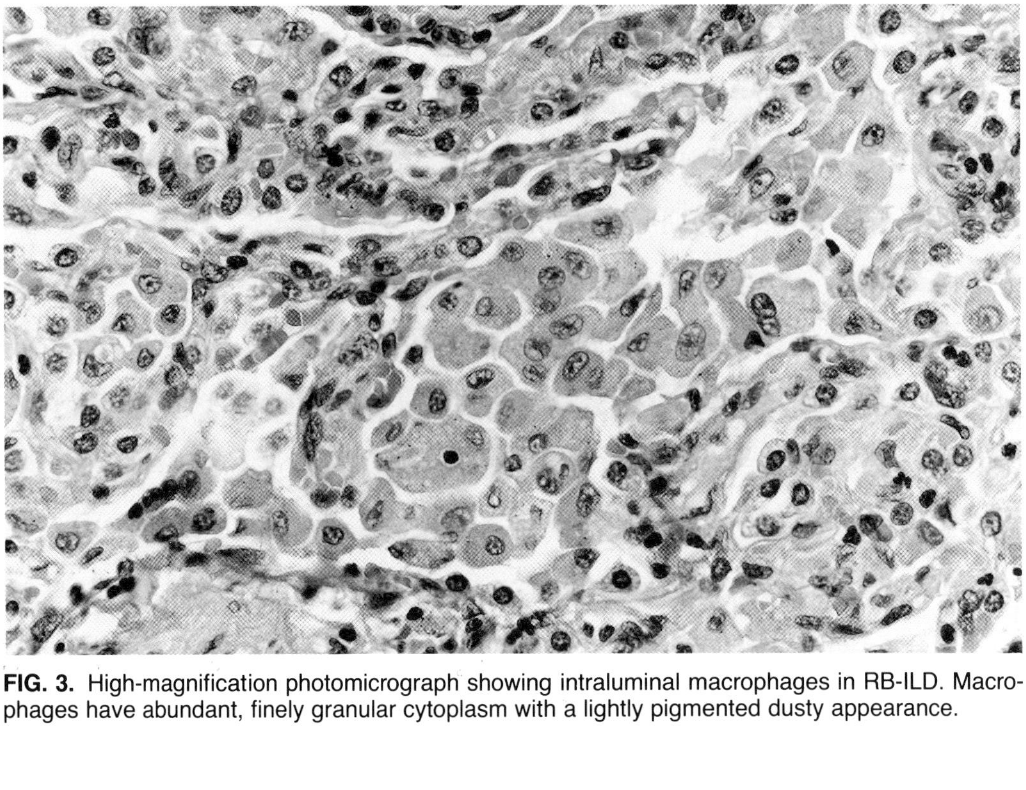

FIG. 3. High-magnification photomicrograph showing intraluminal macrophages in RB-ILD. Macrophages have abundant, finely granular cytoplasm with a lightly pigmented dusty appearance.

an iron stain, correlates with observations of increased iron content in alveolar macrophages from cigarette smokers (17).

Patients with RB-ILD have an associated chronic bronchiolitis characterized by a patchy submucosal and peribronchiolar infiltrate of lymphocytes and histiocytes (Fig. 4). The interstitial histiocytes may contain dusty-brown cytoplasmic pigment identical to that seen within the intraluminal macrophages, or they may contain coarse black anthracotic pigment. Peribronchiolar fibrosis is also seen and expands contiguous alveolar septa, which are lined by hyperplastic type 2 cells and cuboidal bronchiolar-type epithelium (Fig. 5) (8–10). The combination of alveolar septal thickening, epithelial hyperplasia, and pigmented intraluminal macrophages mimics the appearance of desquamative interstitial pneumonia (DIP), but RB-ILD differs in that the changes are patchy and are limited to peribronchiolar zones (Fig. 6).

Ultrastructurally, intraluminal macrophages in RB-ILD contain complex phagolysosomes (8,9). The phagolysosomes contain amorphous electron-dense debris as well as needle-shaped electron-lucent "smokers' inclusions." Several investigators (18,19) have shown that these particles have a platelike configuration when viewed in three dimensions, and that they are composed of kaolinite, an aluminum silicate present in some cigarette smoke.

The histopathologic differential diagnosis of RB-ILD includes a number of interstitial lung diseases. Peribronchiolar fibrosis coupled with hyperplasia of peribronchiolar epithelium may mimic the appearance of usual interstitial pneumonia (UIP), the "usual" histologic finding in patients with IPF. UIP differs from RB-ILD in that the interstitial changes are randomly distributed and include alternating areas of inflammation, fibrosis, and honeycomb change, imparting a variegated appearance to the

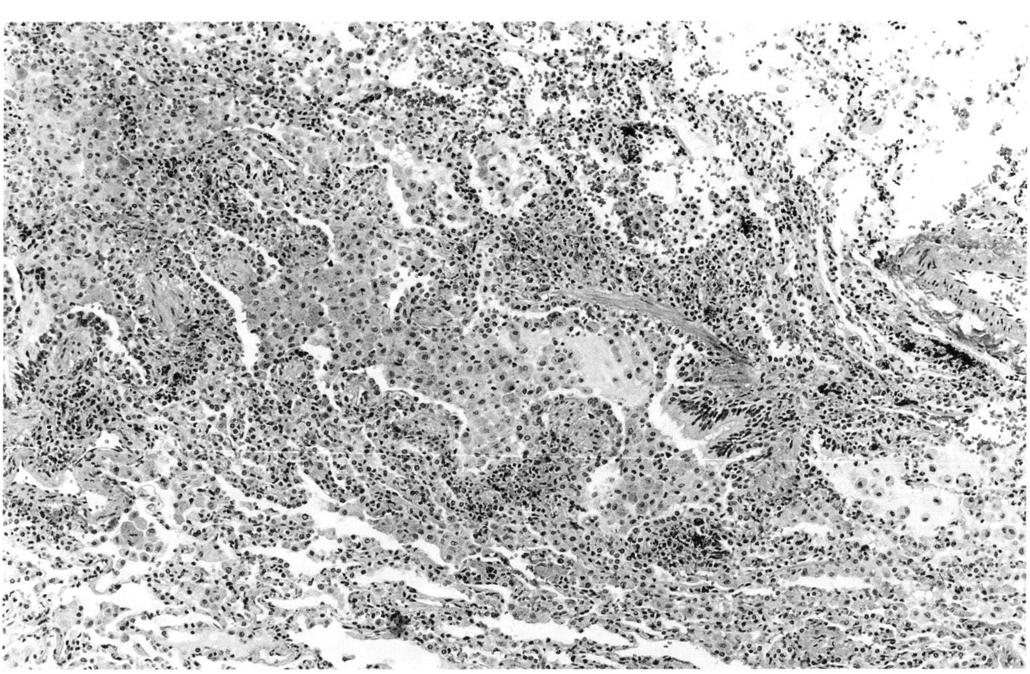

FIG. 4. Photomicrograph illustrating respiratory bronchiolitis in a patient with RB-ILD. The centrally located respiratory bronchiole is filled with pigmented macrophages. There is an associated chronic bronchiolitis characterized by a peribronchiolar infiltrate of chronic inflammatory cells.

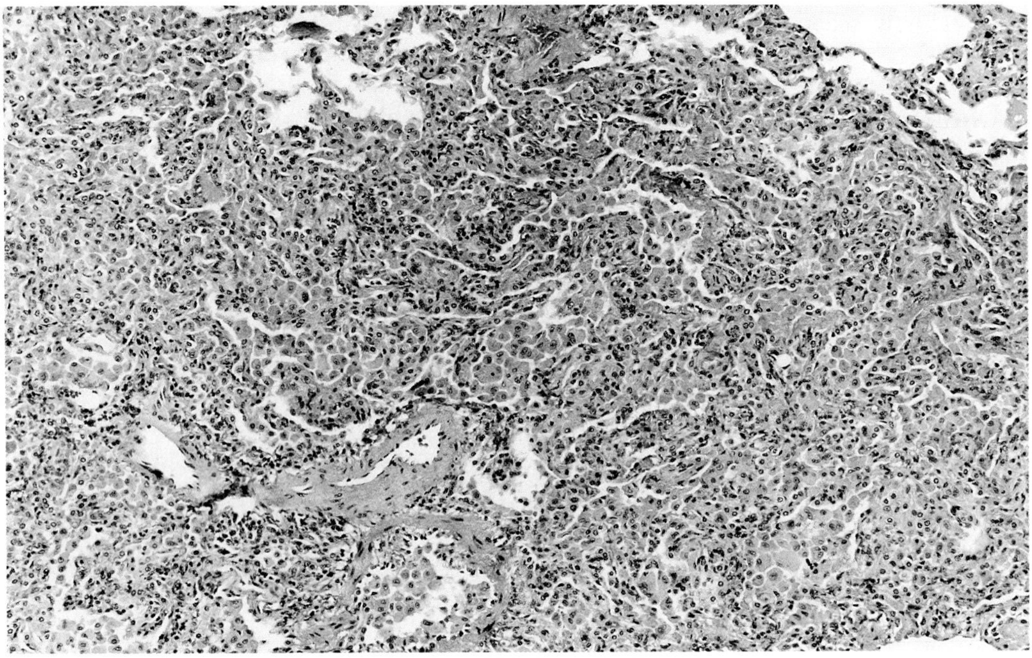

FIG. 5. Photomicrograph showing a DIP-like area in RB-ILD. A respiratory bronchiole and surrounding air spaces are filled with clusters of macrophages with associated thickening of peribronchiolar alveolar septa resulting in a DIP-like appearance.

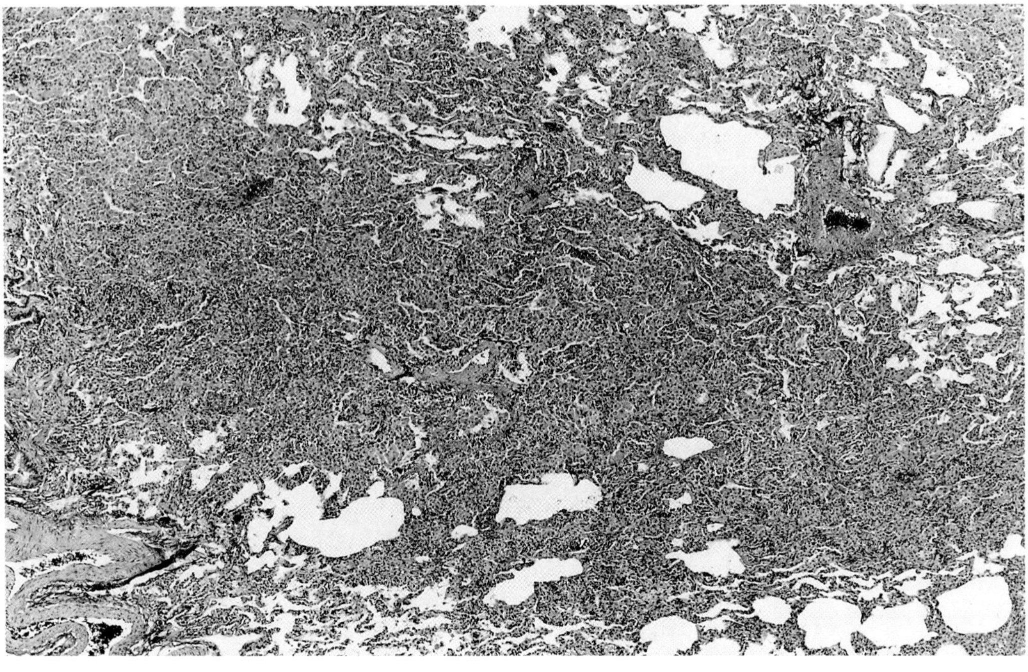

FIG. 6. Lower magnification photomicrograph of biopsy illustrated in Fig. 5, demonstrating patchy bronchiolocentric distribution of the histological changes in RB-ILD.

tissue at low magnification (20). In contrast, fibrosis is mild in RB-ILD and honeycomb change does not occur.

RB-ILD also can closely mimic DIP. DIP is an uncommon finding in patients with IPF and is characterized by diffuse alveolar septal thickening, prominent hyperplasia of alveolar epithelium, and accumulation of intra-alveolar macrophages (10,21). The intraluminal macrophages in DIP frequently contain dusty-brown pigment identical to that seen in RB-ILD and show the same positive staining reactions with PAS and Prussian blue. The main feature that distinguishes DIP from RB-ILD is that DIP affects the lung in a uniform diffuse manner and lacks the bronchiolocentric distribution seen in RB-ILD. Eosinophilic granuloma (histiocytosis X, Langerhans' granulomatosis) is frequently associated with a DIP-like reaction and also can resemble RB-ILD (23). At low magnification, however, eosinophilic granuloma is a predominantly interstitial lesion characterized by the presence of centrally scarred stellate nodules containing a polymorphic inflammatory infiltrate. Diagnosis of eosinophilic granuloma is predicated on recognition of characteristic Langerhans' cells within the inflammatory infiltrate in the appropriate histological context. Of interest, both DIP and pulmonary eosinophilic granuloma are strongly associated with cigarette smoking, and the potential relationship between RB-ILD and these entities is discussed below.

Pulmonary hemorrhage is also characterized by the presence of pigment-laden macrophages and can be confused with RB-ILD. Indeed, two patients reported by Myers and colleagues (8) were initially thought to have pulmonary hemorrhage syndromes on the basis of lung biopsy findings. Low-magnification examination is helpful in distinguishing these conditions because the pigmented macrophages have a bronchiolocentric distribution in RB-ILD, as opposed to a more diffuse random distribution in pulmonary hemorrhage. Other histological clues are often present in alveolar hemorrhage syndromes, including the presence of intra-alveolar erythrocytes with associated fibrin, and areas of organization resembling organizing pneumonia. The pigment in RB-ILD, like the pigment in DIP and DIP-like reactions, is finely dispersed and indistinct, imparting a dusty appearance to the cells. In contrast, hemosiderin pigment in pulmonary hemorrhage forms large refractile granules that often have a gold-green hue. Both pigments stain positively with Prussian blue, but hemosiderin stains darker.

RELATIONSHIP OF RB-ILD, DIP, AND PULMONARY EOSINOPHILIC GRANULOMA

RB-ILD and DIP are similar in that both develop almost exclusively in cigarette smokers, the histological hallmark of both is the presence of pigmented intraluminal macrophages, and both are associated with a relatively good prognosis (8–12,21). Indeed, the initial description (22) of DIP noted a bronchiolocentric distribution of the changes (i.e., respiratory bronchiolitis) in less involved areas of some biopsies. Yousem and co-workers (10) compared RB-ILD with DIP and found that nearly one-half of their patients with RB-ILD had initially been diagnosed as having DIP or possible DIP. These authors found that patients with DIP tended to be older, had more severe respiratory symptoms, and were more likely to have evidence of restriction on pulmonary function testing. Clubbing and "ground glass" alveolar opacities occurred only in patients with DIP and were seen in 44% and 42% of patients, respectively. Only two patients with RB-ILD had persistent symptoms after biopsy, and both of these individuals continued to smoke. In contrast, 32% of patients with DIP for whom follow-up was available died of progressive respiratory disease. Although Yousem and colleagues concluded that RB-ILD and DIP are separate and distinct conditions, the possibility that RB-ILD is a precursor of DIP or a less severe form of the same fundamental lesion cannot be resolved on the basis of the available data. Regardless, it is useful to separate RB-ILD and DIP because of obvious differences in outcome.

Pulmonary eosinophilic granuloma also arises almost exclusively in cigarette smokers and is usually associated with a DIP-like reaction (23). The histological changes in eosinophilic granuloma also tend to be distributed in a bronchiolocentric pattern. Several investigators (24,25) have noted increased numbers of pulmonary Langerhans' cells in cigarette smokers, further suggesting a cause-and-effect relationship between smoking and pulmonary eosinophilic granuloma. Of interest, immunohistochemical studies using antibodies to S-100 protein have identified increased numbers of peribronchiolar Langerhans' cells in patients with RB-ILD (S. Yousem; personal communication). These results indicate that respiratory bronchiolitis and eosinophilic granuloma probably represent independent but overlapping sequelae of cigarette smoking.

SUMMARY

RB-ILD should be suspected in current or former cigarette smokers who present with mild interstitial lung disease. The clinical and radiographic findings are nonspecific, and most patients are thought to have some form of IPF prior to lung biopsy. It is imperative to separate RB-ILD from IPF because of important differences in treatment and natural history. Patients with RB-ILD have a good prognosis, and the disease frequently responds to smoking cessation. Corticosteroids may also be useful, particularly in patients who continue to smoke. DIP and pulmonary eosinophilic granuloma represent additional interstitial lung diseases that develop almost exclusively in cigarette smokers; however, the precise relationship among RB-ILD, DIP, and eosinophilic granuloma is unresolved.

REFERENCES

1. Niewoehner D, Kleinerman J, Rice D. Pathologic changes in the peripheral airways of young cigarette smokers. *N Engl J Med* 1974;291:755–758.
2. Cosio M, Hale K, Niewoehner D. Morphologic and morphometric effects of prolonged cigarette smoking on the small airways. *Am Rev Respir Dis* 1980;122:265–271.
3. Wright J, Lawson L, Pare P, Wiggs B, Kennedy S, Hogg J. Morphology of peripheral airways in current smokers and ex-smokers. *Am Rev Respir Dis* 1983;127:474–477.
4. Wright J, Hobson J, Wiggs B, Pare P, Hogg J. Effect of cigarette smoking on structure of the small airways. *Lung* 1987;165:91–100.
5. Jeffery P. Histologic features of the airways in asthma and COPD. *Respiration* 1992;59[Suppl 1]:13–16.
6. Adesina A, Vallyathan V, McQuillen E, et al. Bronchiolar inflammation and fibrosis associated with smoking: a morphologic cross-sectional population analysis. *Am Rev Respir Dis* 1991;143:144–149.
7. Tyler W, Julian M, Hyde D. Respiratory bronchiolitis following exposures to photochemical air pollutants. *Semin Respir Med* 1992;13:94–113.
8. Myers J, Veal C Jr, Shin M, Katzenstein A-L. Respiratory bronchiolitis causing interstitial lung disease: a clinicopathologic study of six cases. *Am Rev Respir Dis* 1987;135;880–884.
9. Myers J. Respiratory bronchiolitis with interstitial lung disease. *Semin Respir Med* 1992;13: 134–139.
10. Yousem S, Colby T, Gaensler E. Respiratory bronchiolitis-associated interstitial lung disease and its relationship to desquamative interstitial pneumonia. *Mayo Clin Proc* 1989;64:1373–1380.
11. Bogin R, Niccoli S, Waldron J, et al. Respiratory bronchiolitis: clinical presentation and bronchoalveolar lavage findings. *Chest* 1988;94[Suppl]: 21S.
12. King T Jr, Mortenson R. Syndromes that mimic idiopathic pulmonary fibrosis. *Immunol Allerg Clin North Am* 1992;12:461–489.
13. Holt R, Schmidt R, Godwin J, Raghu G. High resolution CT in respiratory bronchiolitis-associated interstitial lung disease. *J Comput Assist Tomogr* 1993;17:46–50.
14. Weiss W. Cigarette smoking and diffuse pulmonary fibrosis. *Am Rev Respir Dis* 1969;99:67–72.
15. Weiss W. Smoking and pulmonary fibrosis. *J Occup Med* 1988;30:33–39.
16. Carilli A, Kotzen L, Fischer M. The chest roentgenogram in smoking females. *Am Rev Respir Dis* 1973;107:133–136.

17. Wesselium L, Flowers C, Skikne B. Alveolar macrophage content of isoferritins and transferrin: comparison of nonsmokers and smokers with and without chronic airflow obstruction. *Am Rev Respir Dis* 1992;143:311–316.
18. Brody A, Craighead J. Cytoplasmic inclusions in pulmonary macrophages of cigarette smokers. *Lab Invest* 1975;32:125–132.
19. Choux R, Pautrat G, Viallat J, Farisse P, Boutin C. Inorganic cytoplasmic inclusions in alveolar macrophages: the role of cigarette smoking. *Arch Pathol Lab Med* 1978;102:79–83.
20. Katzenstein A-L, Askin F. *Surgical pathology of non-neoplastic lung disease: major problems in pathology.* 2nd ed. Philadelphia: W B Saunders;1990:59–75.
21. Carrington C, Gaensler E, Coutu R, FitzGerald M, Gupta R. Natural history and treated course of usual and desquamative interstitial pneumonia. *N Engl J Med* 1978;298:801–809.
22. Liebow A, Steer A, Billingsley J. Desquamative interstitial pneumonia. *Am J Med* 1965;369–404.
23. Colby T, Lombard C. Histiocytosis X in the lung. *Hum Pathol* 1983;14:847–856.
24. Casolaro M, Bernaudin J-F, Saltini C, Ferrans V, Crystal R. Accumulations of Langerhans' cells on the epithelial surface of the lower respiratory tract in normal subjects in association with cigarette smoking. *Am Rev Respir Dis* 1988;137:406–411.
25. Soler P, Moreau A, Basset F, Hance A. Cigarette smoking-induced changes in the number and differentiated state of pulmonary dendritic cells/Langerhans cells. *Am Rev Respir Dis* 1989; 139:1112–1117.

Diseases of the Bronchioles, edited by
Gary R. Epler. Raven Press, Ltd.,
New York © 1994.

21

The Global View of Idiopathic Bronchiolitis Obliterans Organizing Pneumonia

Takateru Izumi

Department of Medicine and Environmental Respiratory Disease, Chest Disease Research Institute, Kyoto University, Shogoin-Kawaramachi 53, Sakyo-ku, Kyoto 606-01, Japan.

The term idiopathic bronchiolitis obliterans organizing pneumonia (BOOP) was proposed by Epler and colleagues (1) in 1985 for a clinicopathological disease entity with a relatively good prognosis and a favorable response to corticosteroid treatment. BOOP is a disease with the following histopathological findings in the lung: patchy bronchiolitis obliterans with organizing pneumonia, interstitial cell infiltrates that are variable in density, foamy cells in the alveolar space, and absence of honeycombing or extensive interstitial fibrosis. This so-called BOOP pattern is nonspecific and relatively common and can be seen in various other disorders, such as organizing infections; organizing diffuse alveolar damages; drug and toxic fume exposures; allergic reactions; organizing chronic eosinophilic pneumonia; connective-tissue diseases; organizing pneumonias associated with chronic obstructive pulmonary diseases; cystic fibrosis; bronchiectasis and other diseases with organizing pneumonias distal to obstruction; organizing pneumonias following aspiration; and vasculitides such as Wegener's granulomatosis (2). In this chapter, the term BOOP is used to designate the idiopathic disease entity with no known pathogen or specific disease. BOOP is not a new disease, and since the first report about this disease by Lange (3) in 1901, several synonyms have been used. BOOP has been included in past reports with terms such as bronchiolitis obliterans with organizing interstitial pneumonia or organizing diffuse alveolar damage (4), bronchiolitis obliterans (5,6,7), organizing pneumonia-like process (8), and cryptogenic organizing pneumonitis (9) (Table 1).

Many physicians have encountered patients with fever, sputum, respiratory difficulties, and patchy infiltrating shadows on the chest radiograph suggesting pneumonia who do not respond to antibiotic treatment. Bronchoalveolar lavage performed for the suspicion of eosinophilic pneumonia reveals no increase in eosinophils. The physician finds corticosteroid therapy effective in such cases. Furthermore, many physicians concerned with interstitial lung diseases have encountered patients with clinical symptoms and chest radiographic findings suggesting idiopathic pulmonary fibrosis, but with symptoms and abnormal shadows that eventually disappear.

There is ongoing discussion (10–12) with regard to which is the better name for the disorder: BOOP or cryptogenic organizing pneumonitis. To avoid confusion regarding the terms bronchiolitis obliterans and BOOP, and to stress the fact that the major pulmonary lesion is in the alveolar areas, cryptogenic organizing pneumonitis was suggested (10,12) to be a better term. However, partly because an article (1) on BOOP

TABLE 1. *Synonyms for BOOP*

1901	Bronchitis et bronchiolitis obliterans (Lange, ref. 3)
1969	Bronchiolitis obliterans with organizing interstitial pneumonia or organizing diffuse alveolar damage (BIP) (Liebow, Carrington, ref. 4)
1973	Bronchiolitis obliterans (Gosink, Friedman, Liebow, ref. 5)
1981	Organizing pneumonia-like process (Grinblat, Mechlis, Lewitus, ref. 8)
1983	Bronchiolitis obliterans (Segger, Mason, Worthen, Stanford, Fernandez, ref. 7)
1983	Cryptogenic organizing pneumonitis (Davison, Heard, McAllister, ref. 9)
1985	Bronchiolitis obliterans organizing pneumonia (Epler, Colby, McLoud, Carrington, Gaensler, ref. 1)
1986	Bronchiolitis obliterans (Katzenstein, Myers, Prophet, Corley, Shin, ref. 6)

appeared in the prestigious *New England Journal of Medicine,* partly because this article covers the largest series of patients, and partly because BOOP is fun to pronounce (10), the term BOOP has been used worldwide. As a result, several reports with comparable numbers of patients have been published out of North America (6,13–17), Europe (18–22), and Japan (23).

In this article, the clinical features of BOOP are described on the basis of results obtained from patients around the world. Important differential diagnoses are discussed.

CLINICAL PROFILE OF BRONCHIOLITIS OBLITERANS ORGANIZING PNEUMONIA IN THE WORLD

Demographics, Symptoms, and Physical Findings

There is no sexual predominance (Table 2) in BOOP. The mean age at onset of the disease is about 57 years, ranging from 21 to 80 years. Less than 50% of the patients were smokers, and no correlation was detected between smoking and BOOP.

The initial symptoms were cough (72 to 76%), fever (49 to 68%), and dyspnea (49 to 90%). Most patients had two or more of these symptoms. Crackles were heard in more than 74% of patients, but clubbing was rare and present in less than 5%.

Laboratory Findings

An increase in the erythrocyte sedimentation rate and a positive C-reactive protein

TABLE 2. *Clinical data from studies of BOOP*

	North America[17] (*n* = 112)	Europe[22] (*n* = 38)	Japan[23] (*n* = 34)
Males/Females	60/52	17/21	17/17
Mean age, years (range)	58 (21–80)	57 (27–74)	57 (41–69)
Smoking history			
Nonsmoker	43%	—	56%
Current smoker	25%	26%	26%
Ex-smoker	32%	—	18%
Symptoms			
Length of symtoms, months	3.6	5.5	7.5
Cough	72%	74%	76%
Fever	49%	68%	53%
Dyspnea	49%	90%	47%
Physical findings			
Crackles	74%	79%	79%
Clubbing	5%	5%	3%
Physiological findings			
Abnormal vital capacity[a]	52%	—	59%
Abnormal diffusing capacity[a]	74%	—	80%

[a]Less than 80% predicted.

were observed in 70 to 80% of patients, whereas an increase in blood leukocyte count was seen in only 30 to 40 %.

Physiological Findings

The physiological tests showed a restrictive impairment with a reduced vital capacity in 52 to 59% of patients, except in a small number of patients who smoked. Impaired gas exchange, as reflected by a decrease in the diffusing capacity, was seen in 80% (Table 2). A decrease in PaO_2 was seen in 70 to 80% of patients.

Chest Radiographic Findings

Bilateral shadows were detected (13,14) in most patients. The patients rarely had unilateral shadowing. The shadows are located in the lower zones of the lung in 60% or more. The pattern of the shadow was patchy in 60 to 80% of patients. The radiographs showed both patchy infiltration and reticulonodular opacities in 30 to 40% of patients. A high frequency of patients showed migration of opacities.

Computed Tomography Findings

On high-resolution chest computed tomography (CT), BOOP consisted of a combination of areas exhibiting either marked air space consolidation or slight ground glass increase in lung density. Air space consolidation and ground glass opacities can be distinguished by the presence of inner vascular images in the ground glass opacities. In some patients, ground glass opacities covered extensive areas of the lung. Both air space consolidation and ground glass opacities seemed to be distributed within the whole secondary lobule.

Bronchoalveolar Lavage Fluid Cell Findings

The main feature of BOOP is an increase in percentage of lavage lymphocytes (17, 23,26). The percentages of neutrophils and eosinophils may also be increased to 5 to 15% and 2 to 10%, respectively. The extent of increase, however, differs from patient to patient. The $CD4^+/CD8^+$ ratio often shows a value of less than 1.

CLINICAL COURSE

Corticosteroids are administered to many patients and have been proven effective. Although the observation period varied, the symptoms, chest radiographic findings, and clinical findings all showed an improvement in more than 60% of our patients. However, in about 30% of the patients whose symptoms had disappeared, some shadows still remained on the radiograph. Some patients showed a spontaneous remission. The overall mortality rate was less than 5%. In our experience, after corticosteroid therapy the symptoms of cough, fever, and dyspnea often disappear within a few days.

Regarding responsiveness to corticosteroid therapy, there are no apparent differences between patients showing patchy shadows and those showing a reticulonodular pattern on the chest radiograph.

DIAGNOSIS AND DIFFERENTIAL DIAGNOSIS

BOOP is suspected when the following findings are seen:

1. subacute onset with cough, fever, and dyspnea
2. crackles on auscultation
3. bilateral patchy infiltrates and sometimes patchy and reticulonodular infiltrates radiographically
4. pulmonary function tests showing a restrictive impairment with decreased diffusing capacity and occasionally hypoxemia
5. an elevated erythrocyte sedimentation rate and positive C-reactive protein
6. a mixed bronchoalveolar lavage cellu-

larity with increased percentages of lymphocytes, neutrophils, and eosinophils

For a definite diagnosis, the findings described above must be confirmed by open lung biopsy. However, from a clinical standpoint, if, in addition to the above features, the transbronchial lung biopsy reveals bronchiolitis obliterans and organizing pneumonia, the clinical diagnosis of BOOP can be made because the possibility of other disease is small.

The entities that must be distinguished from BOOP are shown in Table 3. The first is a disease group showing similar clinical findings, chest radiographic findings, and laboratory findings. BOOP can be distinguished from these entities as follows.

In infectious pneumonia, antibacterial agents are effective for the treatment of most infectious pneumonias except pneumonia from a viral cause. These agents are not effective in BOOP.

In Wegener's granulomatosis, there are extrapulmonary lesions, and a positive antineutrophil cytoplasmic antibody is valuable for the diagnosis. These findings do not occur in BOOP.

In idiopathic pulmonary fibrosis, honeycombing, which is not observed in BOOP, is seen on chest radiograph and chest CT (15); the bronchoalveolar lavage cytology in idiopathic pulmonary fibrosis shows no increase in lymphocytes.

Chronic eosinophilic pneumonia is difficult to distinguish from BOOP via the clinical findings, chest radiographic and CT findings, and laboratory findings (23,27,28). It may be distinguished via the histopathologic findings obtained from the lung. Whether chronic eosinophilic pneumonia and BOOP are the same or different diseases remains to be elucidated. However, clinically it may not be important to differentiate between the two, as both have a good prognosis with a high response rate to corticosteroid therapy.

The second disease group in Table 3 shows an increased percentage of lymphocytes in bronchoalveolar lavage fluid (29). Sarcoidosis and chronic beryllium disease can usually be distinguished by the chest radiographic findings and the high lavage $CD4^+/CD8^+$ ratio.

Hypersensitivity pneumonitis is a disease that shows the same lavage cell findings; however, it can be distinguished by chest radiographic findings, the history of antigen exposure, and the presence of positive serological tests.

The third disease group in Table 3 shows histopathologically the same findings as in BOOP. Idiopathic BOOP must be differentiated from various diseases that may show the so-called BOOP pattern. Rarely, the patients are diagnosed as having unclassified interstitial pneumonia when usual interstitial pneumonia and the BOOP pattern both exist (30).

TABLE 3. *Diseases to be differentiated from BOOP*

Group 1: Diseases showing similar clinical symptoms, chest radiographic and CT findings, and laboratory findings
Infectious pneumonia
Wegener's granulomatosis
Idiopathic pulmonary fibrosis
Chronic eosinophilic pneumonia
Group 2: Diseases showing similar findings in bronchoalveolar lavage cytology
Sarcoidosis
Chronic beryllium disease
Hypersensitivity pneumonitis
Group 3: Diseases showing similar histopathological findings
Various diseases showing the BOOP pattern
Unclassified interstitial pneumonia

TREATMENT

Not all patients with idiopathic BOOP require corticosteroid therapy because some show spontaneous remission. If there are complaints of dyspnea, a distinct decrease in PaO_2, and progressive infiltrates, corticosteroid therapy should be administered. There is no agreement about method of administration, dosage, and duration of corticosteroid treatment. If the treatment period is less than 3 months, however, relapse occurs in one-third of the patients (1).

Our experience suggests that patients can be initially treated with prednisolone, 0.5 mg/kg/day, and the dose is reduced when improvement is detected. Corticosteroid therapy should be continued for at least 6 months. The dose should be increased when recurrence is detected radiographically and, rarely, symptomatically.

SUMMARY

The clinical features, diagnosis, and treatment of BOOP are discussed. Ever since Epler proposed the name bronchiolitis obliterans organizing pneumonia (BOOP) for this disease in 1985, the clinical features, chest radiographic, and CT findings of patients reported around the world show similarities. This is evidence that BOOP should be classified as an independent clinicopathological entity.

REFERENCES

1. Epler GR, Colby TV, McLoud TC, Carrington CB, Gaensler EA. Bronchiolitis obliterans organizing pneumonia. *N Engl J Med* 1985;312: 152–158.
2. Colby TV. Pathologic aspects of bronchiolitis obliterans organizing pneumonia. *Chest* 1992; 102:38S–43S.
3. Lange W. Über eine eigenthümliche Erkrankung der kleinen Bronchien und Bronchiolen (Bronchitis et Bronchiolitis obliterans). *Dtsch Arch Klin Med* 1901;70:342–364.
4. Liebow AA, Carrington CB. The interstitial pneumonias. In: Simon M, Potchen EJ, LeMay M, eds. *Frontiers of pulmonary radiology*. New York: Grune & Stratton; 1969:102–104.
5. Gosink BB, Friedman PJ, Liebow AA. Bronchiolitis obliterans. *AJR* 1973;117:816–831.
6. Katzenstein ALA, Myers JL, Prophet WD, Corley LS III, Shin LS III. Bronchiolitis obliterans and usual interstitial pneumonia: a comparative clinicopathologic study. *Am J Surg Pathol* 1986; 10:373–381.
7. Seggev JS, Mason UG III, Worthen S, Stanford RE, Fernandez E. Bronchiolitis obliterans: report of three cases with detailed physiologic studies. *Chest* 1983;83:169–174.
8. Grinblat J, Mechlis S, Lewitus Z. Organizing pneumonia-like process: an unusual observation in steroid responsive cases with features of chronic interstitial pneumonia. *Chest* 1981;80: 259–263.
9. Davison AG, Heard BE, McAllister WAC, Turner-Warwick MEH. Cryptogenic organizing pneumonitis. *Q J Med* 1983;52:382–393.
10. Geddes DM. BOOP and COP. *Thorax* 1991;46: 545–547.
11. Costabel U, Guzman J. BOOP: what is old, what is new? *Eur Respir J* 1991;4:771–773.
12. du Bois RM, Geddes DM. Obliterative bronchiolitis, cryptogenic organizing pneumonitis and bronchiolitis obliterans organizing pneumonia: three names for two different conditions. *Eur Respir J* 1991;4:774–775.
13. Chandler PW, Shin MS, Friedman SE, Myers JL, Katzenstein ALA. Radiographic manifestations of bronchiolitis obliterans with organizing pneumonia vs. usual interstitial pneumonia. *AJR* 1986;147:899–906.
14. Guerry-Force ML, Mueller NL, Wright JL, et al. A comparison of bronchiolitis obliterans with organizing pneumonia, usual interstitial pneumonia, and small airways disease. *Am Rev Respir Dis* 1987;135:705–712.
15. Müller NL, Guerry ML, Staples CA, et al. Differential diagnosis of bronchiolitis obliterans with organizing pneumonia and usual interstitial pneumonia: clinical, functional, and radiologic findings. *Radiology* 1987;162:151–156.
16. Bartter T, Irwin RS, Nash G, Balikan JP, Hollingsworth HH. Idiopathic bronchiolitis organizing pneumonia with peripheral infiltrates on chest roentgenogram. *Arch Intern Med* 1989;149: 273–279.
17. King TE Jr, Mortenson RL. Cryptogenic organizing pneumonitis: the North American experience. *Chest* 1992;102:8S–13S.
18. Cordier JF, Loire R, Brune J. Idiopathic bronchiolitis obliterans. *Chest* 1989;96:999–1004.
19. Meister P, Pickl-Pfeffer S, Rabben U. Bronchiolitis obliterans mit organisierender Pneumonia (BOOP). *Pathologe* 1989;10:43–45.
20. Patel U, Jenkins PF. Bronchiolitis obliterans organizing pneumonia. *Respir Med* 1989;83:241–244.
21. Alegre-Martin J, Fernandez de Sevilla T, Garcia F, Falcó V, Martinez-Vazquez JM. Idiopathic bronchiolitis obliterans with organizing pneumonia: presentation of three cases with morphologic studies. *Eur Respir J* 1991;4:902–904.
22. Costabel U, Teschler H, Schoenfeld B, et al. BOOP in Europe. *Chest* 1992;102:14S–20S.
23. Izumi T, Kitaichi M, Nishimura K, Nagai S. Bronchiolitis obliterans organizing pneumonia: clinical features and differential diagnosis. *Chest* 1992;102:715–719.
24. Müller NL, Staples CA, Miller RR. Bronchitis obliterans organizing pneumonia: CT features in 14 patients. *AJR* 1990;154:983–987.
25. Nishimura K, Itoh H. High-resolution computed tomographic features of bronchiolitis obliterans organizing pneumonia. *Chest* 1992;102:26S–31S.

26. Costabel U, Teschler H, Guzman J. Bronchiolitis obliterans organizing pneumonia (BOOP): the cytological and immunocytological profile of bronchoalveolar lavage. *Eur Respir J* 1992;5: 791–797.
27. Müller NL, Miller RR. Computed tomography of chronic diffuse infiltrative lung disease. *Am Rev Respir Dis* 1992;142:1440–1448.
28. Mayo JR, Müller NL, Road J, Sisler J, Lillington G. Chronic eosinophilic pneumonia: CT findings in six cases. *AJR* 1989;153:727–730.
29. Reynolds HY. Bronchoalveolar lavage. *Am Rev Respir Dis* 1987;135:250–263.
30. Colby TV, Lombard C, Yousem SA, Kitaichi M. Unclassified interstitial pneumonia. In: *Atlas of pulmonary surgical pathology*. Philadelphia: WB Saunders; 1991:268–270.

Diseases of the Bronchioles, edited by
Gary R. Epler. Raven Press, Ltd.,
New York © 1994.

22

Bronchiolitis Obliterans Organizing Pneumonia as a Model of Inflammatory Lung Disease

Jean-Francois Cordier,* S. Peyrol,† and R. Loire‡

**Department of Pneumology, Louis Pradel Hospital, Claude Bernard University, Lyon, France.*
‡Department of Pathology, Louis Pradel Hospital, Claude Bernard University, Lyon, France.
†Cellular Pathology Laboratory, CNRS URA 602, Institut Pasteur, Lyon, France.

Bronchiolitis obliterans organizing pneumonia (BOOP) is defined pathologically by the presence within the lumen of distal air spaces (bronchioles, alveolar ducts, and alveoli) of granulation tissue mainly composed of fibroblasts and connective matrix.

BOOP is a nonspecific pathological hallmark of various pulmonary disorders that have an inflammatory character as a common denominator. Some of these disorders are secondary to injury by a known etiological agent (for example *Streptococcus pneumoniae* in pneumococcal pneumonia). In others, no definite etiological agent is detected, but BOOP occurs in the context of an inflammatory disease of unknown origin (as in the connective-tissue diseases). BOOP may also develop as an isolated idiopathic process in patients with a characteristic clinicoradiological syndrome associated with stigmata of inflammation, both clinical (as fever) and biological (as assessed by an extremely increased sedimentation rate).

INFLAMMATORY REACTIONS IN THE LUNG

Inflammation has been defined as "the reaction of vascularized living tissue to local injury" (1). It was recognized initially by the clinical association of redness, swelling, heat, and pain of the inflamed tissues. Later, microscopic studies allowed characterization of the cellular process of inflammation, particularly the demonstration that cells are attracted to the site of injury where they show cellular functional activity (such as phagocytosis). During the past 20 years, a burst of investigation has dissected the basic biochemical mechanisms of inflammation. In vitro studies have provided major advances in the knowledge of cell biology in inflammation, but how these may be extrapolated to tissue pathobiology remains somewhat speculative.

Several pathophysiological elementary mechanisms are common to the inflammatory reaction, which is further modulated according to the involved organ and the origin of injury. In acute injury, an early crucial event is the increase of vascular permeability with exudation of plasma proteins and especially coagulation factors. Accumulation of leucocytes, especially neutrophils and monocytes, at the site of injury results from their response to chemotactic agents. Leucocytes and resident cells of the lung are capable of releasing a wide range of mediators of inflammation, in addition to those resulting from necrosis of damaged cells and those exuded from plasma. The mediators that have been implicated in pulmonary inflammation comprise several groups of substances such as vasoactive amines (histamine, serotonin), plasma and lysosomal proteases (including the coagulation–fibrinolytic system), arachidonic acid metabolites, oxygen-derived free radicals, platelet activating factor, and cytokines (1–4).

Cytokines are peptide growth factors or biological response modifiers that signal the replication, phenotypic change, and functional capacities of cells (2,5). The cell-to-cell interactions mediated by cytokines occur in a local microenvironment, and rarely involve distant organs as do the endocrine hormones. In paracrine interactions, a cell secretes a cytokine that acts on a nearby target cell. In juxtacrine interactions, one cell provides the ligand as a membrane-bound precursor of growth factor to a contiguous target cell that provides the receptor. In autocrine mechanisms, the active peptides act on their own producer cell, either after extracellular secretion (external autocrine) or within the cell itself (internal autocrine) (6). Cytokines may be stored in an active form by bonding to the extracellular matrix, thus being available to cells (7). The action of cell modifiers is thus extremely complex, and the cell-to-cell communication is further complicated by the fact that the synergistic effect of several cytokines may markedly differ from the single action of the different cytokines implicated in the "cytokine network" connecting the different cells (6,8). It is thus somewhat artificial to extrapolate the effects of one cytokine on one cell to a complex biopathological process occurring in the lung. The role of adhesion molecules (and especially integrins) in tissue inflammation is presently not precisely established (9–11) but may be important.

The outcomes of acute inflammation in the lung are (a) complete resolution without sequelae (as in most acute infections in the nonimmunocompromised host), (b) necrosis (either by abscess formation as in infection by pyogenic microorganisms, or by aseptic necrosis as in Wegener's granulomatosis), (c) healing with scarring, and (d) progression to chronic inflammation (which may also occur as an insidious process without any recognizable acute onset).

Sometimes, the inflammatory process, instead of limiting the extent of injury and repairing its consequences, contributes of itself to the perpetuation and progression of injury. The loss of homeostatic control of inflammation may result in lung fibrosis by a "fibroproliferative" disease (12,13) in which fibroblasts, which are responsible for collagen and other connective matrix production (14,15), play a key role.

Studies focusing on chronic inflammatory interstitial disorders of the lung (especially sarcoidosis or idiopathic pulmonary fibrosis) have emphasized the concept of alveolitis (16,17), whereby inflammatory cells (mainly macrophages) release inflammation mediators and cytokines acting on mesenchymal interstitial cells to induce them to proliferate and deposit collagen in excess. The concept of alveolitis as the key to fibrosis was reinforced by in vitro studies that used cells recovered by bronchoalveolar lavage. For example, these demonstrated that alveolar macrophages from patients with fibrosing interstitial disease spontaneously synthesize and release increased amounts of growth factors for fibroblasts (18–20).

The characterization of idiopathic BOOP by both clinical and pathological criteria renewed some pathogenic concepts of lung fibrosis. Although the concept of fibrosis as a result of maladapted repair after lung injury had never been abandoned, it had nevertheless been overshadowed by the prevailing concept of alveolitis. BOOP, by focusing attention on intraluminal organization, stimulated several directions of research because it transforms the alveoli into an in vivo pathobiology laboratory: an almost empty space (the lumen of distal airspaces) is filled with exudates, which are then colonized by fibroblasts and progressively replaced by collagen deposits (in a manner similar to the formation of granulation tissue after injury in other sites of the organism). Furthermore, BOOP is a unique model of reversible fibrosis, since most patients with the typical form of the syndrome heal completely after corticosteroid therapy.

LESSONS FROM THE PAST: FROM ACUTE PNEUMOCOCCAL PNEUMONIA TO UNRESOLVED CHRONIC PNEUMONIA

Before the era of antibiotics, pneumococcal pneumonia often led to death, and many pathological studies could be done on autopsy series.

The usual course of lobar pneumococcal pneumonia was defined by Laënnec (21) as following a sequence of congestion, hepatization, and resolution. Congestion is the early stage of pneumonia, lasting generally less than 24 hours. The involved lobe is heavy and hyperemic. Microscopically, the alveolar capillaries are dilated, and some edema rich in pneumococci, red cells, and neutrophils, is present within alveolar airspaces. At the stage of red hepatization (second to third day), the appearance of the involved lobe (red and dense) is similar to that of liver. The alveoli are filled with fibrin that extends from one alveolus to the next through interalveolar pores as described by Kohn (22), who discovered the pores that bear his name in a case of "fibrinous pneumonia." Neutrophils phagocytizing bacteria are numerous. The grey hepatization (fourth to sixth day) characterizes a dry and airless consolidated lobe, the color of which has turned to gray. On histological examination, the fibrin is seen to be invaded by large numbers of neutrophils and macrophages. Pneumococci are rare and degenerated. By the eighth or ninth day of the disease, a favorable outcome is announced by a sudden decrease in fever, profuse sweating, and abundant diuresis. Histologically, resolution of pneumonia corresponds to the liquefaction of the fibrinous exudates by fibrinolytic enzymes from the neutrophils. Alveolar macrophages have also been demonstrated to synthesize and express a plasminogen activator similar to urokinase, but membrane bound (23), which could contribute to the degradation of the fibrin deposits. The fluid is then removed by both expectoration and the macrophages. In pneumococcal pneumonia, the architecture of the lung is preserved and the alveolar walls do not undergo necrosis. Resolution leaves no fibrosis, either interstitial or intra-alveolar.

The failure of resolution results in unresolved chronic pneumonia, which had been extensively studied by the first quarter of the century. The main characters of the histopathology of organizing pneumonia and bronchiolitis obliterans have thus been carefully detailed in this context together with hypotheses related to the pathophysiology of the process. Milne (24) reported 10 cases of "examples of pneumonia where the usual process of resolution has failed and organization of the inflammatory exudate in the air alveoli of the lung by fibrous tissue has resulted." Previous reports had described the main features of chronic pneumonia and addressed the question of the autonomic or secondary (to acute pneumonia) character of organizing pneumonia. In his study, concerning mainly chronic pneumonia secondary to pneumococcal pneumonia, Milne stated that "occasionally some of the smaller bronchi were obstructed, but the process was coincident with the alveolar organization, and certainly did not necessarily precede it," and he questioned: "Is this delayed resolution process then due to a defective emigration of leukocytes which do not remove the foreign material in the air spaces, as is usual by their vital action of phagocytosis, enzyme secretion, and solution, or is it . . . due to defective cellular content in the exudate and consequent failure of the autolytic process of enzyme formation and fibrin solution which are known to follow on the death of cells and so necessitate the development of processes of organization?" Milne also remarked that polymorphonuclear leucocytes were rare in the alveoli and that the new granulation tissue was projected from the alveolar walls into the inflammatory exudate. Auerbach and coworkers (25) also stressed the fact that exudates rich in fibrin and poor in polymorphonuclear leucocytes are more apt to organize.

Further reports (26,27) detailed the morphology of the intraluminal organization and its sequence. Fibrin is deposited first, often extending from one alveolus to the next through the pores of Kohn. Then, "about two weeks after the onset of the pneumonia, cells with elongated nuclei, exhibiting all transitions to fibroblasts, appear within the substance of the fibrin plugs and on their surface. . . . As time passes the fibrin is more or less completely absorbed and replaced by fibrillated connective tissue" (26). However, the origin of the connective tissue was not established, although the fibroblast was recognized as a key cell in the process of organization. Other interesting early observations stressed that the organization process was distinctly predominant within the lumen of the airspaces, with preservation of the delicate alveolar network, which was not destroyed, that the organization was associated with the loss of epithelium of the alveolar walls, and that the bud of connective tissue replaced the fibrin of early exudates (26).

Recently, an experimental model of *Streptococcus pneumoniae* induced BOOP has been obtained by Rhodes and colleagues (28), who induced a nonresolving bronchopneumonia in Wistar rats by strains of *Streptococcus pneumoniae* type 25 of increased virulence delivered into the bronchi. The histological pattern observed at day 8 was quite typical of BOOP. By comparing this model (A) with another model of *Streptococcus sanguis* pneumonia undergoing normal resolution (B) (29), they demonstrated that these differed in several respects. Necrosis of injured type I pneumocytes was observed only in model A, with focal denudation of basal lamina. Furthermore, whereas in model B type II pneumocytes, which are stem cells for the alveolar epithelium (30), transformed into type I pneumocytes and undermined the damaged type I epithelium, this was rarely observed in model A, where type II pneumocytes showed evidence of degeneration. Other changes specific to model A were the presence of endothelial damage (evidenced from days 1 to 8 by widespread focal endothelial cell blebbing and intracellular vacuolation) and persistence of bacterial proliferation. From this comparative study, the authors suggested that the abnormal outcome in their model of *Streptococcus pneumoniae* pneumonia was a consequence of the failure of type II pneumocytes to transform into type I pneumocytes and thus maintain the integrity of the alveolar epithelial surface.

A successful repair after epithelial damage depends largely on an intact epithelial basement membrane (31). Furthermore, the composition of the extracellular matrix (which is altered after lung injury) influences the growth and differentiation of type II cells; for example, fibronectin induces a loss of cell differentiation accompanied by increased keratin expression (as found in type I epithelial cells). Such modulation may play a role in regular reepithelialization by transformation of type II into type I cells (32-34).

Other experimental studies examined the alveolar epithelial cell–fibroblast interactions in lung injury and repair. In mice exposed to 95% oxygen, severe injury with retarded repair of the alveolar epithelium enhanced fibroblast proliferation and collagen production (35). Since no inflammatory cells were present at the time of this proliferation, it was suggested that the proliferation of fibroblasts resulted from a prolonged disruption of their normal close relationship with alveolar cells. Furthermore, when focal type I alveolar epithelial injury was rapidly repaired by type II cell proliferation, no change in fibroblast proliferation was observed (36). On the contrary, after a more severe injury the type II proliferative phase was extended and accompanied by prolonged fibroblast growth. As type II cells persisted where they covered a thick interstitium of fibroblasts and fibrillar collagen, a reciprocal epithelial–fibroblast control was suggested. Hyperoxia blocks the proliferation of type II cells in vitro by altering the expression of at least two late cell cycle growth related genes (histone and thymidine kinase) at the post-transcriptional level (37).

ORGANIZATION OF DIFFUSE ALVEOLAR DAMAGE IN ADULT RESPIRATORY DISTRESS SYNDROME

Intra-alveolar and interstitial fibrosis is a consequence of the diffuse alveolar damage (DAD) associated with the adult respiratory distress syndrome (ARDS). In some cases, the pathological overlap between the proliferation phase of diffuse alveolar damage and BOOP is so evident that the two processes are quite indistinguishable (38). The pathophysiology of DAD is thus of interest in the understanding of the pathogenesis of BOOP.

Diffuse alveolar damage is the pathological pattern of the adult respiratory distress syndrome secondary to acute lung injury by infectious agents, inhalants, ingestants, drugs, radiation, sepsis, shock, and many other etiologic agents (39). DAD has been characterized by a sequential evolution into two stages: the acute early exudative stage (first week) with edema, exudation, and hyaline membranes; and the more chronic proliferative or organizing stage (after 1 to 2 weeks) in which fibrosis predominates (40–43).

Acute Exudative Stage

The acute exudative stage of DAD comprises a high-permeability edema secondary to capillary leakage, with interstitial and intra-alveolar exudation of fluid rich in plasma proteins, and especially coagulation factors leading to fibrin deposits (44). Although the morphologic changes of the endothelial cells are inconspicuous, the endothelial cell layer is considered a major target of the lung injury, allowing exudation of plasma fluid within the interstitium. Because the injured epithelial cells are detached from their basement membrane support, which is disrupted, further exudation within the alveolar spaces ensues. Together with the protein intraluminal exudates, cell debris and inflammatory cells occupy the lumen of the distal air spaces. The microvasculature is impaired by microthrombi with sequestration of leucocytes. The alveolar epithelial damage is the cause of greater alveolar flooding observed in oleic acid–induced low-pressure edema than in high-pressure edema (45). The normal size selectivity, which is preserved in cardiac edema, is severely impaired in patients with ARDS or radiation pneumonitis, who have very high levels of total proteins in bronchoalveolar lavage fluid; furthermore, sodium dodecylsulfate polyacrylamide gel electrophoresis or concomitant polyacrylamide gel electrophoresis and immunoelectrophoresis show that all serum protein species are present in bronchoalveolar lavage fluid, including even such high-molecular-weight proteins as $alpha_2$ macroglobulin and immunoglobulin M (46,47). Within 3 to 7 days following injury, hyaline membranes consisting of cellular debris mixed with fibrin line the alveolar cavities (this being the most characteristic feature of DAD). Inflammation mediators (such as eicosanoids, oxygen products, proteases) responsible for the initial phase of DAD are many. Toxic oxygen free radicals may be released either by resident cells (such as endothelial cells) or by inflammatory cells (monocytes-macrophages, polymorphonuclear cells, lymphocytes, plasma cells) primed and/or attracted by cytokines such as interleukin (IL-8) (3,4,48). Oxygen toxicity (49) contributes to the pulmonary damage in the many patients with ARDS requiring ventilation with a high concentration of oxygen.

The role of neutrophils in this disorder is unclear. These have been suspected to be important, especially by damaging the endothelium of the pulmonary microvasculature (where neutrophils aggregate) and the alveolar structures through the release of toxic oxygen products and/or proteases (4,50–52). However, the fact that ARDS may develop even in the setting of severe neutropenia casts some doubt on a key role for neutrophils in all types of this syndrome (53,54).

Fibrin deposits occurring in the early phase of ARDS are clearly the morphological link between permeability edema and further cell-matrix organization leading to fibrosis. The metabolism of fibrin within intraluminal air spaces results from the balance between procoagulant activity and fibrinolytic processes (Fig. 1) in the alveolar lumen and on alveolar surfaces. Both procoagulant (factor VII and tissue factor) and fibrinolytic (urokinase like plasminogen activator) activities are present in lavage fluid from normal humans (55,56). The procoagulant activity at the alveolar surface is functionally saturated with active complexes of factor VII-tissue factor, and thus the coagulation is regulated by the availability of the factors necessary for thrombin formation (factor X, factor V, prothrombin), which are normally not present on alveolar surface but may exude from plasma (56,57). Human alveolar macrophages synthesize both factor VII activator and a plasminogen activator similar to urokinase but membrane bound (23,58). Rat alveolar epithelial cells express both cell surface and particulate procoagulant activity (59). Rat type II pneumocytes in culture cosecrete plasminogen activator inhibitor type 1 and urokinase-type plasminogen activator (60). Bovine lung capillary endothelial cells produce urokinase-type plasminogen activator (61). Thus, many cell types in the lung are capable of producing both procoagulant and fibrinolysis factors that may contribute to inflammatory processes (57,62,63).

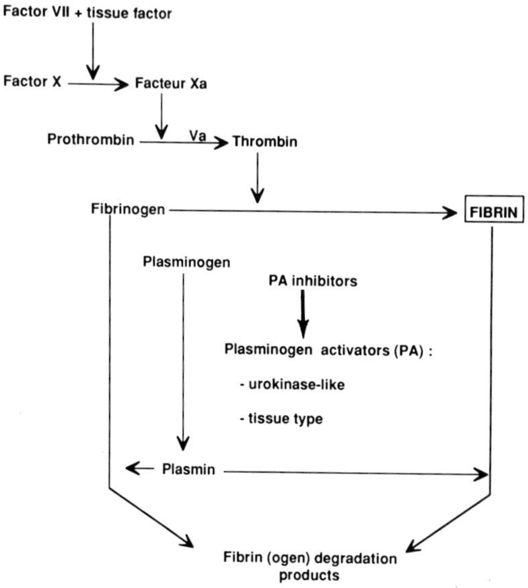

FIG. 1. Schematic summary of the extrinsic pathway of coagulation and fibrinolysis.

Bronchoalveolar lavage fluid of patients with ARDS contains an increased procoagulant activity due to a complex of factor VII-tissue factor. Furthermore, the fibrinolytic activity of lavage fluid is decreased. The reduced fibrinolytic activity is not due to a lack of urokinase, but to the presence of urokinase inhibitors (especially plasminogen-activator inhibitor type 1) (64–66). Similar findings have been reported in experimental models of lung damage. A concomitant increased procoagulant and decreased fibrinolytic activity was found in bronchoalveolar lavage fluid from sheep with oleic-acid-induced lung injury (67) and baboons with evolving diffuse alveolar damage induced by exposure to 100% oxygen (68). On the contrary, a striking increase of the plasminogen activator/procoagulant activity ratio was found in bronchoalveolar lavage fluid of rabbits after phorbol myristate acetate lung injury (69). This change was associated with the clearance of the early intra-alveolar fibrin deposits. Whereas the levels of both procoagulant and plasminogen activator activities associated with alveolar macrophages remained stable, granulocytes expressed similar levels of plasminogen activator to macrophages but almost no procoagulant activity, thus suggesting that granulocytes contributed to fibrinolysis.

Finally, both in human ARDS and in experimental lung injury, an impaired balance between bronchoalveolar lavage fluid procoagulant and fibrinolytic activities favors the formation of fibrin deposits over their dissolution.

Chronic Organizing Stage

The chronic organizing fibroproliferative stage of DAD is characterized by fibroblastic proliferation associated with connective matrix deposits, within both the alveolar lumen and the interstitium (39,70–73). At this stage, there is little persistance of edema or hyaline membranes. Incorporation of the alveolar exudate into the alveolar septa contributes to the process of fibrosis. About 3 to 7 days after injury, hyperplasia of alveolar lining cells develops, consisting of cuboidal cells ultrastructurally identified as type II pneumocytes. Most patients with ARDS who survive the initial stage of respiratory failure die either of sepsis with multiple-organ failure or of pulmonary fibrosis (72,74).

The fibrosis of ARDS may predominate in the interstitium or in the alveolar lumen. It often follows a branching, ramifying pattern similar to alveolar ducts and seems more a consequence of oxygen toxicity than of the process initiating the syndrome (71,75). A pathological study (72) in patients dying of ARDS (treated with extracorporal membrane oxygenation) has shown that the lesions with hyaline membranes predominated in the alveolar duct regions, and that these progressed to fibrosis of the alveolar ducts in patients who survived more than 10 days. The increased damage to the alveolar ducts was interpreted as secondary to high-concentration oxygen ventilation, the inhaled concentration of gas being higher at the level of alveolar ducts than distally, where alveoli received a lesser concentration. For unknown reasons, patients with postsurgical ARDS had significantly more organized pneumonia than patients with the disorder secondary to other conditions.

Fukuda and colleagues (76) studied the role of intra-alveolar fibrosis in the process of pulmonary structural remodeling in patients with diffuse alveolar damage and a clinical diagnosis of ARDS, by immunohistochemical, ultrastructural, and light-microscopic morphometric methods. All patients had been treated by artificial ventilation with a high concentration of oxygen. They distinguished between three stages of DAD: acute, early proliferative, and remodeled. The morphometric analysis showed that intra-alveolar fibrosis predominated over interstitial fibrosis. In the acute stage of DAD, albumin, surfactant apoprotein, fibrinogen, and immunoglobulins (especially immunoglobulins G) were frequently found in the areas of hyaline membrane and were thought to accumulate from plasma. On the contrary, fibronectin, which was initially only scanty, was in later stages abundant in the areas of organizing fibrosis, suggesting a local production by alveolar macrophages. In the early proliferative stage, hyaline membrane formation was associated with further intra-alveolar fibrosis; three types could be distinguished: intra-alveolar "buds" partially filling the air spaces, diffuse intra-alveolar fibrosis completely obstructing the alveolar spaces, and broad-based areas of apposition of the fibrotic mass to the alveolar walls. Activated myofibroblasts (fibroblasts with contractile filaments) were present in the alveolar interstitium and some intra-alveolar spaces, and some of them were seen migrating through gaps in the epithelial basement membrane into the intra-alveolar spaces. In the remodeled stage of DAD, alveoli were fibrotic and obliterated, with covering of the alveolar walls by alveolar epithelial cells and metaplastic stratified squamous epithelium. Finally, this study emphasized intra-alveolar fibrosis as an essential factor in the remodeling of lungs in patients with DAD.

In patients with ARDS, a study (77) demonstrated that a growth- and migration-promoting activity was present in bronchoalveolar lavage fluid; this activity consisted of peptides related to platelet derived growth factor. This growth factor is a most ubiquitous cytokine consisting of peptides A and B encoded by at least two distinct genes. Its active form is usually a disulfide-linked homodimer or heterodimer (AA, AB, or BB) (78). It acts principally as a chemoattractant, especially for fibroblasts (79) and smooth muscle cells (80,81). Platelet derived growth factors AB and BB can also stimulate fibroblasts to contract the collagen matrix with a time course similar to that of wound contraction (82). In pulmonary fibrosis, growth factor gene expression is upregulated in alveolar macrophages, which spontaneously release increased levels of this growth factor (18–20). Furthermore, interferon-gamma increases expression of platelet derived growth factor B mRNA in both normals and patients with interstitial lung disease (83). The peptides related to this growth factor found in bronchoalveolar lavage fluid of patients with ARDS (77) were a 38-kD peptide biophysically and antigenically similar to platelet derived growth factor, a 29-kD peptide identical to this growth factor of platelet origin, and a 14-kD peptide which was the most ubiquitous and abundant peptide, sharing with this growth factor several biophysical, biochemical, receptor-binding, and antigenic properties. The origin of the 14-kD peptide is unknown, and it is not clear if it is produced as such or cleaved from the 29-kD peptide.

Although peptide growth factors probably play a role in attracting and promoting the replication and activity of mesenchymal cells, a more autonomous fibroproliferative phenomenon could occur in the mesenchymal cells themselves. It was demonstrated (84) that mesenchymal cells cultured from patients dying of ARDS (2 to 4 weeks after acute lung injury) proliferated by doubling within 3 days in the absence of any exogenous peptide growth factor, unlike cells from normal individuals. The immediate early cell division cycle genes *c-fos* and *c-jun* (characteristic of proliferating fibroblasts) were constitutively expressed by these cells which had the ultrastructural features of myofibroblasts. The observed proliferative phenotype remained stable for at least five subcultivations and did not appear to depend on autocrine release of trophic factors.

The outcome of ARDS is contrasted, with high mortality but only mild or moderate sequelae in most patients who survive (85). It is thus interesting to note that in some patients fibrosis secondary to DAD undergoes almost complete resolution. The benefit of corticosteroid therapy in ARDS is controversial, and some studies even showed a deleterious effect of the drug. Corticosteroid therapy is thus not currently indicated in patients with ARDS. Nevertheless, Meduri and colleagues (86) have shown that corticosteroid therapy could have a beneficial effect in some patients when given in late chronic ARDS. In their small group of patients, fever and leucocytosis in the absence of any pulmonary or extrapulmonary source of infection were interpreted as resulting from the inflammatory-fibrotic process present in late ARDS. Furthermore, a patient who had diffuse interstitial and alveolar fibrosis on open lung biopsy and who died of sepsis after corticosteroid treatment showed resolution of fibrosis with restoration of normal alveolar architecture on postmortem examination of the lungs.

It is thus clear that fibrosis of ARDS, where the intra-alveolar component is important or predominant, may occasionally regress completely with or without corticosteroid therapy (70) as seen in typical idiopathic BOOP.

CONTRIBUTION OF INTRALUMINAL EXUDATE TO INTERSTITIAL FIBROSIS OF UNKNOWN ORIGIN

Interstitial pneumonias, either acute or chronic, focal or diffuse, are tissue responses in the lung that take place predominantly in the supporting structures, rather than within alveoli (87). However, the role of the intra-alveolar component of inflammation in the pathogenesis of interstitial fibrosis may be prominent, especially in acute interstitial pneumonia, which corresponds to the disease described by Hamman and Rich (88). Hamman-Rich syndrome manifests clinically as ARDS and pathologically as DAD (89). As in ARDS, the outcome of acute interstitial pneumonia is unpredictable, with both a high mortality and the possibility of complete recovery. Finally, acute interstitial pneumonia shows pathologically much resemblance to ARDS, but the two conditions differ by the fact that the initiating cause of the lung injury is not identified in acute interstitial pneumonia (39,89–91).

Acute interstitial pneumonia differs from chronic interstitial pneumonia by its sudden onset with dyspnea, cough, and the development of respiratory failure requiring ventilation within a few days. The course of the disease is more rapid and the mortality rate high. In addition, acute interstitial pneumonias differ from the chronic form in that there is much more interstitial fibroblast proliferation and less collagen deposition. Furthermore, in the chronic form squamous metaplasia of bronchiolar epithelium and adjacent alveolar surface is conspicuous (90,91).

In acute interstitial pneumonia (as in the chronic form) the lung architecture is markedly disorganized, and this could hardly be explained only by the proliferation of fibroblasts and collagen deposition within the alveolar interstitium. Other mechanisms are thus likely to contribute to the pathogenesis of "interstitial" fibrosis: alveolar collapse and the mural incorporation of intra-alveolar exudates (92–96).

Alveolar collapse leads to permanent apposition of alveolar walls and fibrosis (atelectatic induration or collapse induration) (92–94, 96). It may result mainly from a decreased functional surfactant alveolar lining by both inactivation of surfactant by plasma proteins flooding into alveoli (especially fibrin and fibrin peptides) and a decreased production of surfactant by injured pneumocytes II (93,97). Adhesion of intraluminal fibrin and hyaline membranes to the luminal top of denuded and folded basement membrane contributes to the irreversibility of the collapse and allows pneumocyte growth on this support, giving rise to a new epithelial surface. However, this epithelial surface is extremely reduced in comparison with the initial normal surface. Beneath the reepithelialized surface, the apposed infolded basal lamina clefts are incorporated in the connective matrix (96). Alveolar collapse may also play a role in the pathogenesis of usual interstitial pneumonia. Myers and Katzenstein (98) reported focal epithelial necrosis and alveolar collapse in a patient with usual interstitial pneumonia, those changes being associated with fibroblastic foci (aggregates of interstitial fibroblasts embedded within a myxoid stroma).

Together with alveolar collapse, the incorporation of intra-alveolar exudates into alveolar septa leads to an increase of interstitial fibrosis. Spencer (99) characterized this mechanism as one of those leading to chronic interstitial pneumonia, and remarked that it was unaccompanied by capillary proliferation. He also disagreed with Gross (100), who thought that the intra-alveolar plugs of reticulin of organizing pneumonia were not of recent origin. The incorporation of intra-alveolar exudates is mainly due to the growth of type II pneumocytes over the material (cellular debris, fibrin, inflammatory cells, fibroblasts, and collagen) adhering to the denuded epithelial basal lamina. Of interest, two basal laminae are initially present: that produced by the proliferating pneumocytes, and the original alveolar epithelial basal lamina. The two basal laminae are separated by a distance depending on the amount of cell and material trapped beneath the new epithelium. The fragmented original epithelial basal lamina may account for some of the basal lamina pieces incorporated into the initial connective matrix (76,96).

The incorporation of intra-alveolar exudates as a factor of interstitial fibrosis is more evident in the rapidly progressive interstitial pneumonias (Hamman-Rich syndrome) in which hyaline membranes are present, than in the more chronic usual interstitial pneumonia (101). Nevertheless Fukuda and colleagues (102) reported that early fibrotic lesions of idiopathic pulmonary fibrosis were intra-alveolar in location. Furthermore, Basset and colleagues (95) found that intraluminal buds were present in 14% and mural incorporation in 74% of 92 patients with idiopathic pulmonary fibrosis. Kuhn and colleagues (103) considered that fibrosis in chronic idiopathic pulmonary fibrosis results mainly from the organization of exudates within airspaces, for they found that the foci of active collagen synthesis by fibroblasts arose at sites of fibrinous exudate providing the substratum for the invading fibroblasts (the foci were situated outside remnants of basal lamina). They concluded that the fibrosis in idiopathic pulmonary fibrosis was similar to the fibrosis following acute lung injury, although on a smaller and more protracted scale.

Thus, although undoubtedly interstitial inflammation and fibroblast proliferation with collagen deposition are important pathogenic mechanisms in interstitial fibrosis, alveolar collapse and incorporation of alveolar exudates probably contribute more than previously considered (92–94,96,104, 105). In acute interstitial pneumonia (Hamman-Rich syndrome), edematous interstitial widening accompanied by a proliferation of fibroblasts predominates over the deposition of collagen, and organization (often prominent) within airspaces is present in a majority of patients (91). The role of oxygen toxicity in the observed pathological lesions of acute interstitial pneumonia is unclear, but many patients who died of this condition were ventilated with 100% oxygen (91).

Although acute interstitial pneumonia and BOOP are quite distinct entities, in some fields of biopsy specimens of patients with acute interstitial pneumonia the pathological changes are indistinguishable from those of BOOP, suggesting some common pathogenic mechanisms for the two disorders.

IDIOPATHIC BRONCHIOLITIS OBLITERANS ORGANIZING PNEUMONIA AS A MODEL OF LUNG FIBROINFLAMMATORY PROCESS

Clinically, idiopathic BOOP is a stereotype of inflammatory disease (106–111). Most patients have a subacute onset of symptoms, with a flu-like syndrome. Fever, malaise, anorexia, and weight loss give clinical evidence of the inflammatory syndrome. Pulmonary symptoms are generally mild, with persistent nonproductive cough and moderate dyspnea. The most typical imaging pattern of idiopathic BOOP is characterized by multiple alveolar patchy opacities, generally bilateral and sometimes spontaneously migratory. Although idiopathic BOOP may occasionally resolve spontaneously or under antibiotic treatment, most patients remain ill until corticosteroid treatment is undertaken. Within 48 hours, the general condition of the patient improves, and the chest roengenogram and CT scan clear within a few weeks. This dramatic response to corticosteroid therapy and the frequent relapse when corticosteroids are withdrawn too rapidly and sharply is typical of a self-governing inflammatory disease. It is clear in such cases that the inflammatory ongoing process can abate only after prolonged antiinflammatory treatment. Paralleling the clinical inflammatory syndrome of BOOP, the most simple biological test of inflammation, the erythrocyte sedimentation rate, reflects the biological process of inflammation. In typical BOOP, the erythrocyte sedimentation rate is markedly increased, frequently reaching or exceeding 100 mm at the first hour. Furthermore, C reactive protein level is increased (112,113). On bronchoalveolar lavage, alveolitis is constant, the mixed pattern with increased levels of lymphocytes, neutrophils, and eosinophils being rather characteristic (106, 114).

The pathohistophysiology of idiopathic BOOP is probably the best model of a type of inflammatory lung disease. Whatever its origin(s), in idiopathic BOOP the pattern and course of the process is not blurred by such associated factors as the local or general complications of infection, or by oxygen toxicity resulting from the necessity of ventilating patients with high concentrations of oxygen. In idiopathic BOOP, there is no such severe injury that confuses the homogeneous sequence of intraluminal organization. Idiopathic BOOP recapitulates most of the pathophysiological pathways of intra-alveolar organization.

Within the spectrum of infiltrative lung disorders, idiopathic BOOP is histologically quite distinct from the other entities that may comprise intraluminal fibrosis as a component of pulmonary lesions. In the study by Basset and colleagues (95) of intraluminal fibrosis in interstitial lung disorders, idiopathic BOOP ("chronic organizing pneumonia of unknown cause") was characterized by the constant presence of intraluminal buds (which is not surprising since it is a criterion for diagnosis of organizing pneumonia), but these were more frequently moderate or severe than in such other conditions as hypersensitivity pneumonitis or chronic eosinophilic pneumonia, where intraluminal buds were present in about 70% of patients. In idiopathic BOOP,

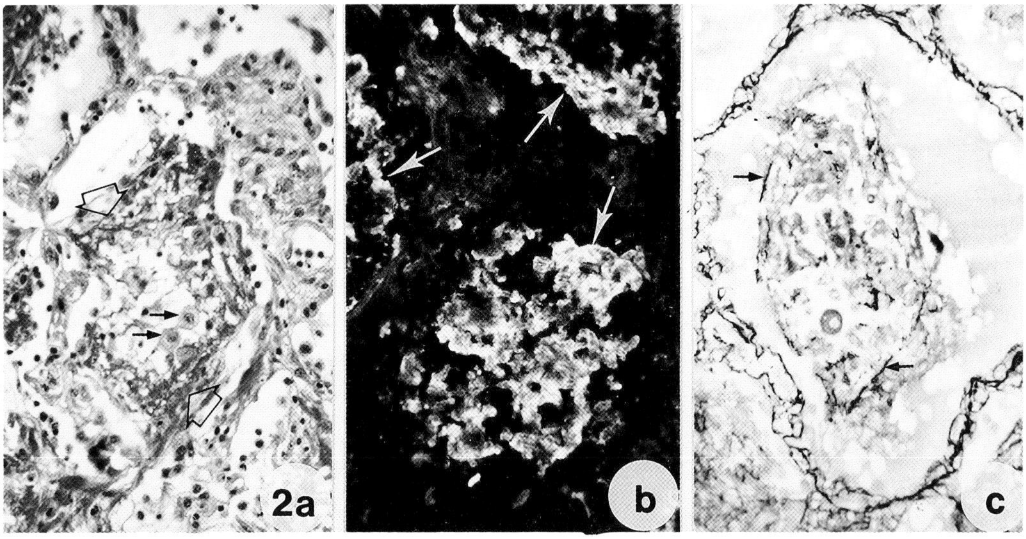

FIG. 2. Fibrinoid inflammatory cell clusters. **a,** Alveolar macrophages (*small arrow*) are closely associated to the fibrin network (*large arrow*) that circumscribes the bud. **b,** Fibrinogen, immunostained with fluorescence, appears as a major component of the buds. From ref. 116 with permission of the American Society for Investigative Pathology. **c,** The reticulin framework of the bud is hardly distinguishable. ×500.

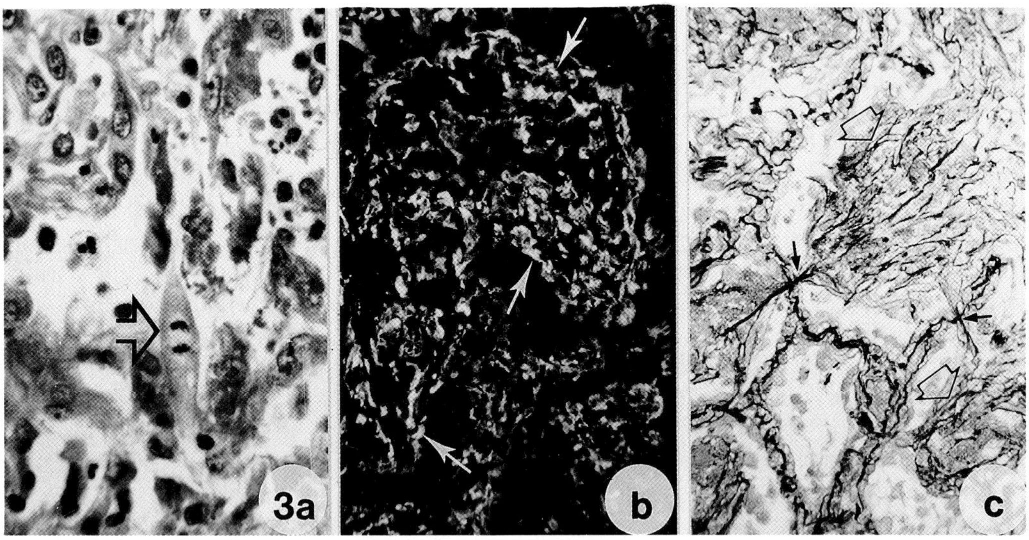

FIG. 3. Fibroinflammatory buds. **a,** A mitotic fibroblast from the alveolar septum is reaching the alveolar lumen. From ref. 116 with permission of the American Society for Investigative Pathology. **b,** Desmin, immunostained with fluorescence, appears as a cytoskeletal component of the intra-alveolar fibroblasts. **c,** The reticulin frameworks of intra-alveolar buds appear distinctly (*large arrow*) and are connected through the Kohn's pores (*small arrow*). ×500.

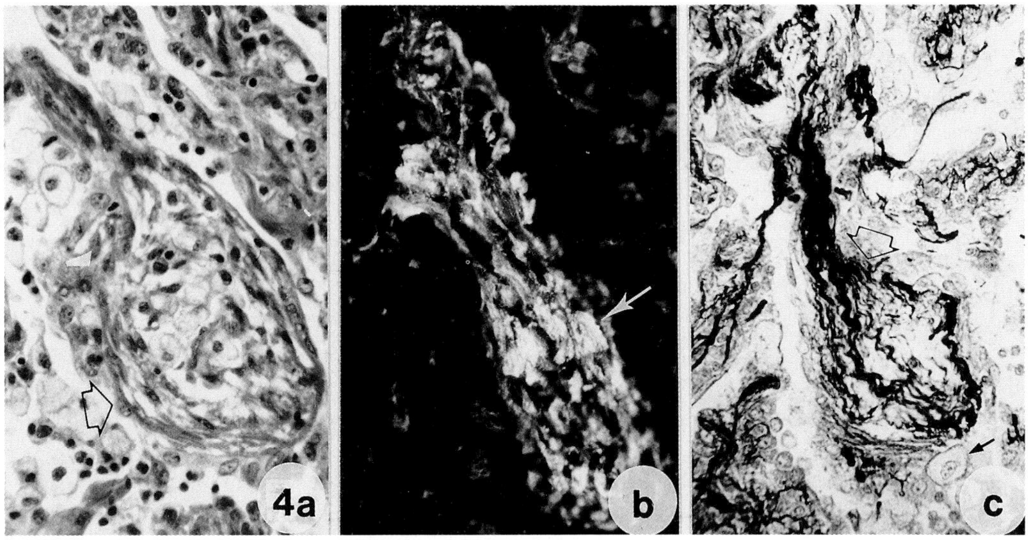

FIG. 4. Mature fibrotic buds. **a,** The bud in encircled by fibroblasts. **b,** Fibronectin, immunostained with fluorescence, is a major matrix component of the bud. **c,** The matrix component consists of a strong reticulin framework (*large arrow*); some alveolar macrophages (*small arrow*) are still present around the bud. ×500. b and c from ref. 116 with permission of the American Society of Investigative Pathology.

the intraluminal buds are most conspicuous and thus distinguish the condition from the other entities, in which intraluminal buds are occasional and accessory findings.

In idiopathic BOOP, the intraluminal organization may involve the distal air spaces (bronchioles, alveolar ducts, alveoli) to a variable extent. Bronchiolitis obliterans is rather uncommon in other infiltrative lung disorders, and is also not constantly found in the clinical syndrome referred to as idiopathic BOOP; most studies emphasize the predominance of intra-alveolar organization (106,115). There is little doubt that the alveolar compartment is a primary site of the inflammatory process, and most studies have focused at this level (95,116). The intraluminal buds only partially fill the lumen of the distal air spaces, and there is generally a space devoid of cells and matrix between the airspace wall and the bud, which is connected to this wall by a narrow stalk or a broader base (Figs. 2,3 and 4). Frequently, the intra-alveolar buds extend from one alveolus to the next through the pores of Kohn, (Fig. 3C). In idiopathic BOOP, complete obliteration of the lumen of distal airspaces and/or extensive mural incorporation of intra-alveolar exudates are not usual. The morphological appearance and sequence of changes leading to the typical histological pattern of BOOP have been recently investigated by ultrastructural and immunostaining studies (95,103,116–118).

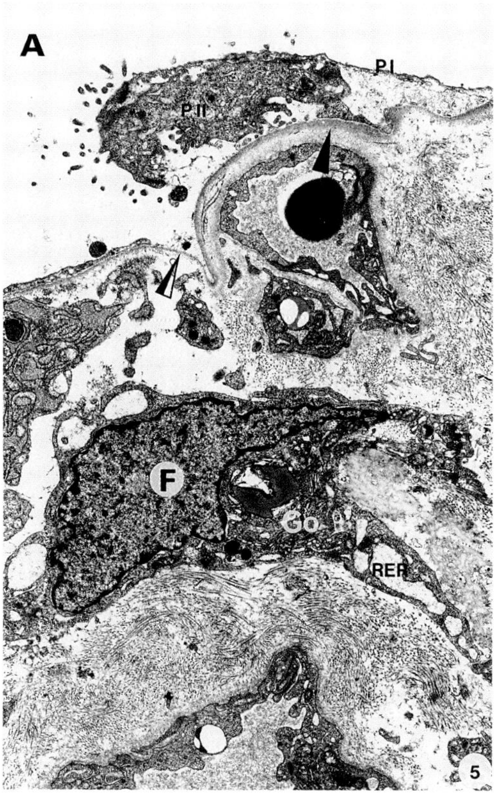

FIG. 5. Alveolar edge of an interstitial septum. Altered type I (*PI*) and type II (*PII*) pneumocytes are being detached from the basal lamina, which appears partially denuded (*open arrow*) and focally thickened (*closed arrow*) at the site of an alveolocapillary junction. An interstitial fibroblast (*F*) shows ultrastructural signs of activation. *Go,* prominent Golgi area; *RER*, rough endoplasmic reticulum. ×8,000.

The initial stage is characterized by a subacute and moderately severe lung injury. Alveolar epithelial injury is constant and prominent at this early stage (116–118). Necrosis and detachment of epithelial cells involving both type I and type II pneumocytes (Fig. 5) result in the denudation of epithelial basal laminae, which are further thickened and locally ruptured (Fig. 6). The severity of epithelial alveolar injury varies among alveoli. Although cell debris and fibrin line the intraluminal side of denuded basal laminae, no hyaline membranes form. The basal laminae may fold and appose and be further incorporated within the alveolar interstitium, but this phenomenon is by far less prominent than in acute interstitial pneumonia. Damage to the endothelial cells of alveolar capillaries may be present especially at the early stage, as evidenced by their cytoplasmic swelling and the multilaminar dissociation of their basal laminae. However, the damage is generally mild, and endothelial necrosis is not a frequent finding (116,118). Altered capillaries frequently bulge into the alveolar lumen (Fig. 7). The respective roles of epithelial and endothe-

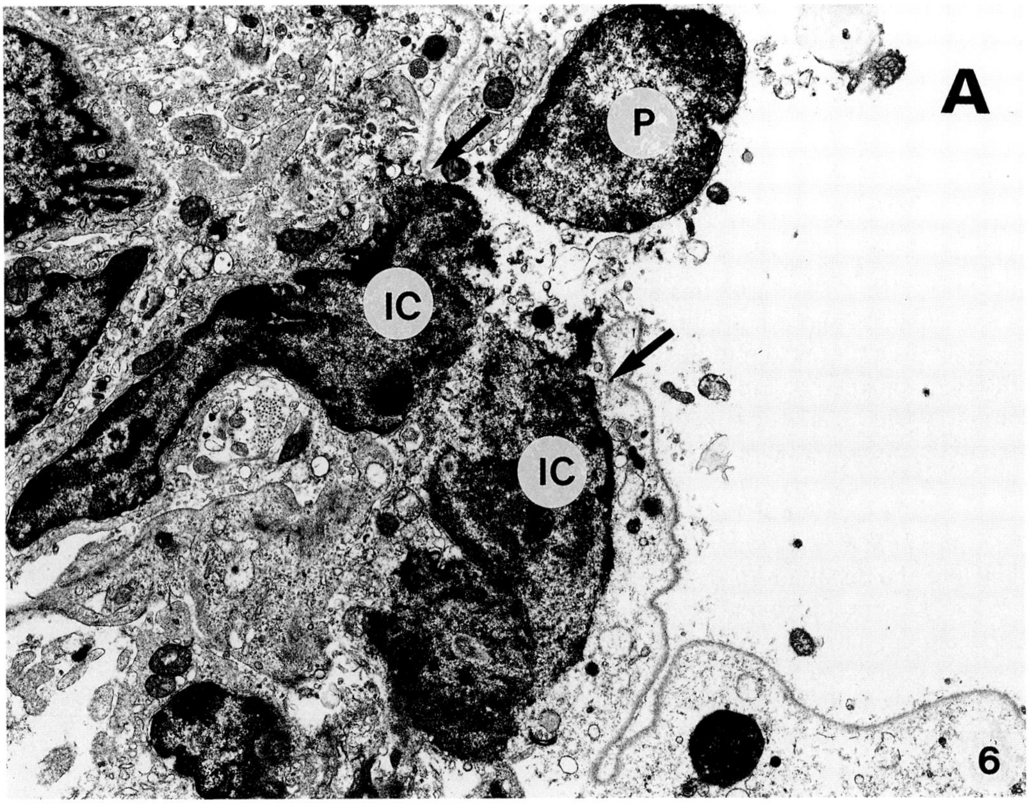

FIG. 6. Denuded basal lamina is interrupted by a gap (*arrows*) coincident with necrosis of a pneumocyte (*P*) and two interstitial cells (*IC*). *A*; alveolar lumen. ×10,000.

lial injury in the pathogenesis of BOOP are unclear. Morphologically, epithelial injury clearly prevails. Within the interstitium, edema containing nonfibrillar material dissociates the preexisting collagen matrix. Inflammatory cells are present, consisting mainly of lymphocytes and polymorphonuclear cells (neutrophils and eosinophils). Mast cells, which are implicated in many pulmonary inflammatory processes (119, 120), are also present. The fibroblastic cell population shows morphological signs of activation: most cells exhibit an electron-dense cytoplasm with conspicuous rough endoplasmic reticulum and Golgi apparatus (Fig. 5). However, within the interstitium, the fibroblastic cell population is not markedly increased and there is no extensive matrix deposition.

Beginning concomitantly with the interstitial inflammation, three distinct sequential intra-alveolar cell-matrix patterns may be described (116): fibrinoid inflammatory cell clusters, fibroinflammatory buds, and fibrotic buds.

Fibrinoid inflammatory cell clusters consist of large, dense fibrillar bundles of fibrin associated with lymphocytes, plasma cells, and occasionally mast cells and polymorphonuclear cells (Fig. 2A). Alveolar macrophages are conspicuous, engulfing and degrading intracellular fibrin bundles (Fig. 8). The intra-alveolar recruitment of inflammatory cells coincides with the presence of

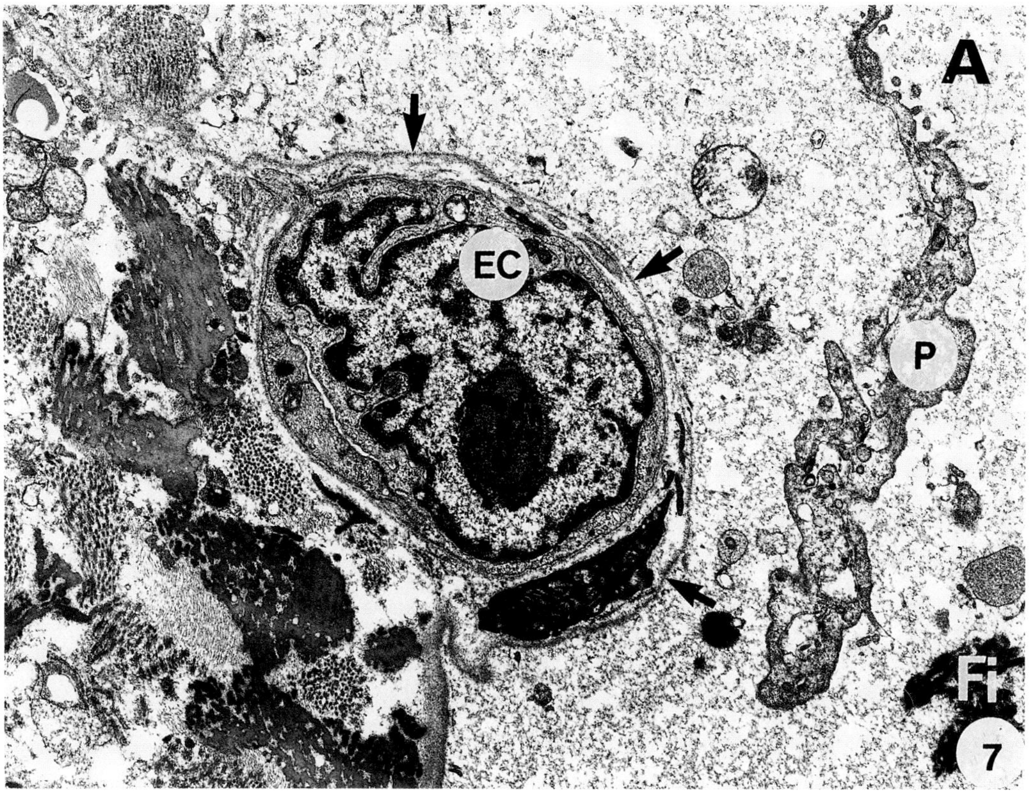

FIG. 7. An alveolar capillary is protruding into the alveolar space (*A*) and pushes forward the denuded basal lamina (*arrow*); a pneumocyte (*P*) is detached in the alveolar lumen (*A*) where fibrin bundles (*Fi*) are deposited. *EC*, endothelial cell of the capillary. ×10,000.

immunoglobulins (mainly G and to a lesser extent A and M) and fibronectin, which may be detected by immunostaining together with procoagulant activity detected as factor VII, factor X, and fibrinogen (Fig. 2B) associated with fibrin deposits. This suggests that, as in ARDS, the activation of the extrinsic coagulation pathways may play a crucial role in the initiation of intra-alveolar organization. The coagulation factors may come from exudation from the capillaries or local cellular release by macrophages, or more probably from both processes. The origin of immunoglobulins may be the plasma cells present in the alveolar lumen, but the contribution of exuded immunoglobulins is likely. At this stage, the reticulin framework of intra-alveolar buds is hardly distinguishable (Fig. 2C).

The *fibroinflammatory buds* follow from the fibrotic involution of the fibrinoid inflammatory cell clusters. Some residual inflammatory cells persist, and fibrinoid deposits appear fragmented. Alveolar macrophages are still present around the buds. Type II pneumocytes begin to proliferate, covering the epithelial laminae and incorporating small amounts of the lining noncellular material into the alveolar wall. The most striking observation at this stage is the migration of the interstitial fibroblasts into the alveolar lumen through gaps in the epithelial basement lamina. Inside the alveolar lumen, the fibroblastic cells infiltrate and

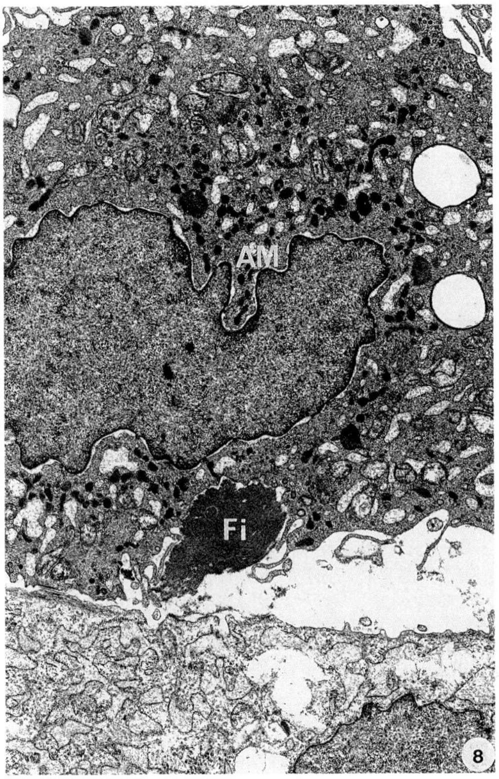

FIG. 8. An alveolar macrophage (*AM*) is engulfing fibrin (*Fi*). ×10,000.

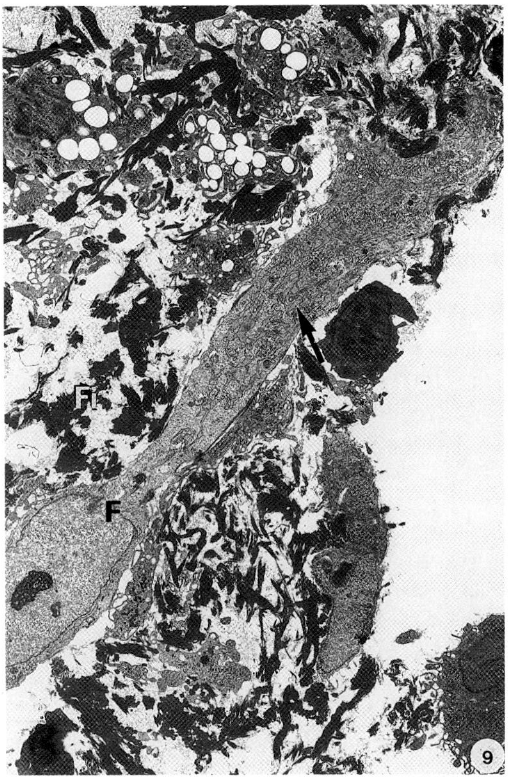

FIG. 9. Bipolar intro-alveolar fibroblast (*F*) migrating among fragmented fibrin deposits (*Fi*); rough endoplasmic reticulum is prominently developed in the major part of cytoplasm (*arrow*). ×3,000.

circumscribe the fibrinoid inflammatory cell clusters. These fibroblasts exhibit conspicuous cytoplasm and nucleolated nucleus (Fig. 9) and occasional mitotic figures, proving their replication may be observed (116) (Figs. 3A and 10). The large bipolar or tripolar shaped cytoplasm of the fibroblasts suggests cell movement. This organization of intracytoplasmic filaments into bundles is conspicuous beneath the cytoplasmic membrane (Fig. 11), and the presence of desmin and alpha smooth muscle actin is demonstrated by immunostaining (Fig. 3B). At this stage, a distinct reticulin framework is visualized in intra-alveolar buds (Fig. 3C).

Mature fibrotic buds progressively replace the fibroinflammatory buds. Inflammatory cells and macrophages are usually absent (some flattened macrophages may line the surface of intra-alveolar fibrotic masses) (95) (Fig 4A). The classical sequence of deposition of matrix components observed in fibrotic disorders (121) occurs in organizing intra-alveolar buds: fibronectin is the earliest deposited component, followed by collagens type III and type I. However, throughout the sequence, fibronectin, procollagen III, and collagen III are codistributed, collagen III usually predominating largely over type I collagen. The fibronectin present in the buds consists of both plasma and cellular fibronectin (103, 122). In the course of fibrotic maturation of the intra-alveolar bud, the matrix fibrillar form of fibronectin prevails (Fig. 4B). Type V collagen participates in the fibrotic organization as early as types III and I collagens

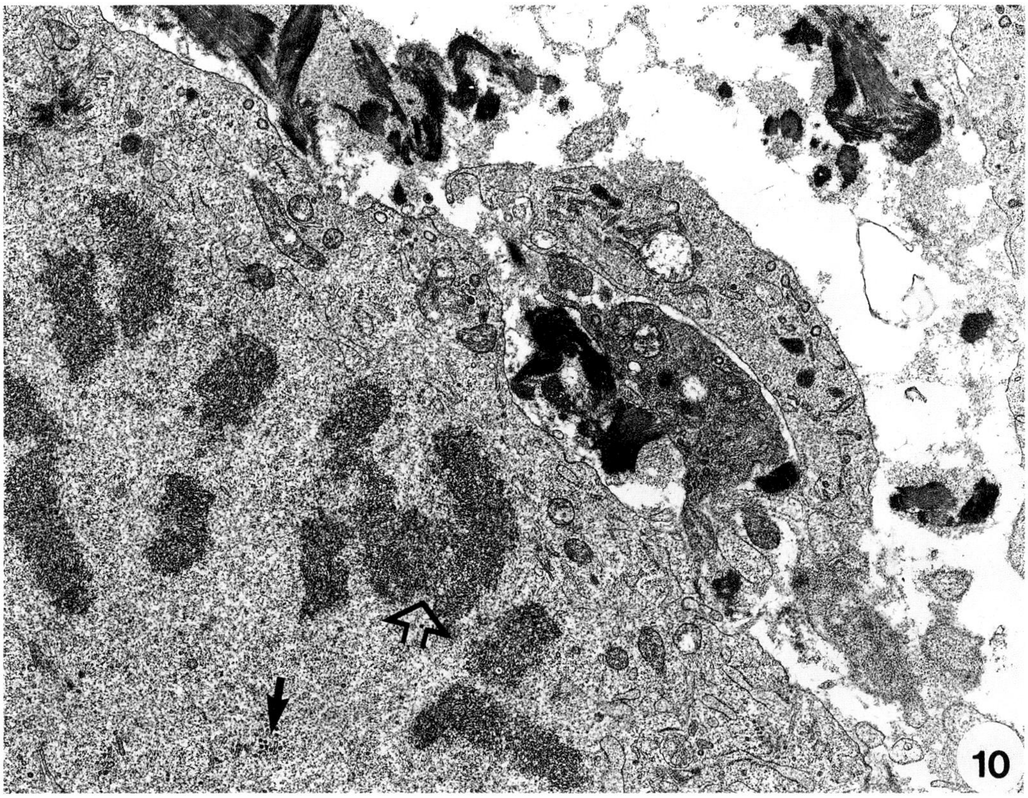

FIG. 10. Mitotic intra-alveolar fibroblast. Nuclear envelope has completely disappeared, condensation of chromosomes is achieved (*open arrow*), and numerous microtubule sections are present (*arrow*). ×10,000.

do. The deposition of all these matrix components leads to the formation of a strong intra-alveolar reticulin framework (Fig. 4C). The fibroproliferative cells are present both at the periphery and at the center of the buds. At the periphery, the fibroblasts are fusiform with two spindle-shaped cytoplasmic processes and they contain an abundant rough endoplasmic reticulum and conspicuous condensations of filaments with focal densifications (Fig. 12). Concentric cellular rings of fibroblasts are separated by a loose polymorphic matrix deposit consisting of thin collagen fibrils (collagen type I and III) and fibrillogranular material (fibronectin, proteoglycans) (Fig. 13). The staining of fibroblasts for procollagen is more intense at the periphery than at the center of the buds (103). At the center of the buds, the fibroblasts are multipolar and form a cellular network across the bud, delineating spaces containing bundles of collagen (Fig. 14).

The fibroblasts, especially at the periphery of the buds, are typical myofibroblasts. They contain bundles of cytoplasmic filaments generally oriented along the axis of the cells, with dense condensations similar to those of smooth muscle cells (103,116) (Figs. 15 and 16). In fact, alpha smooth muscle actin, in association with desmin, appears as a major cytoskeletal component of these cells during the whole fibrotic maturation of intra-alveolar buds (Figs. 17 and

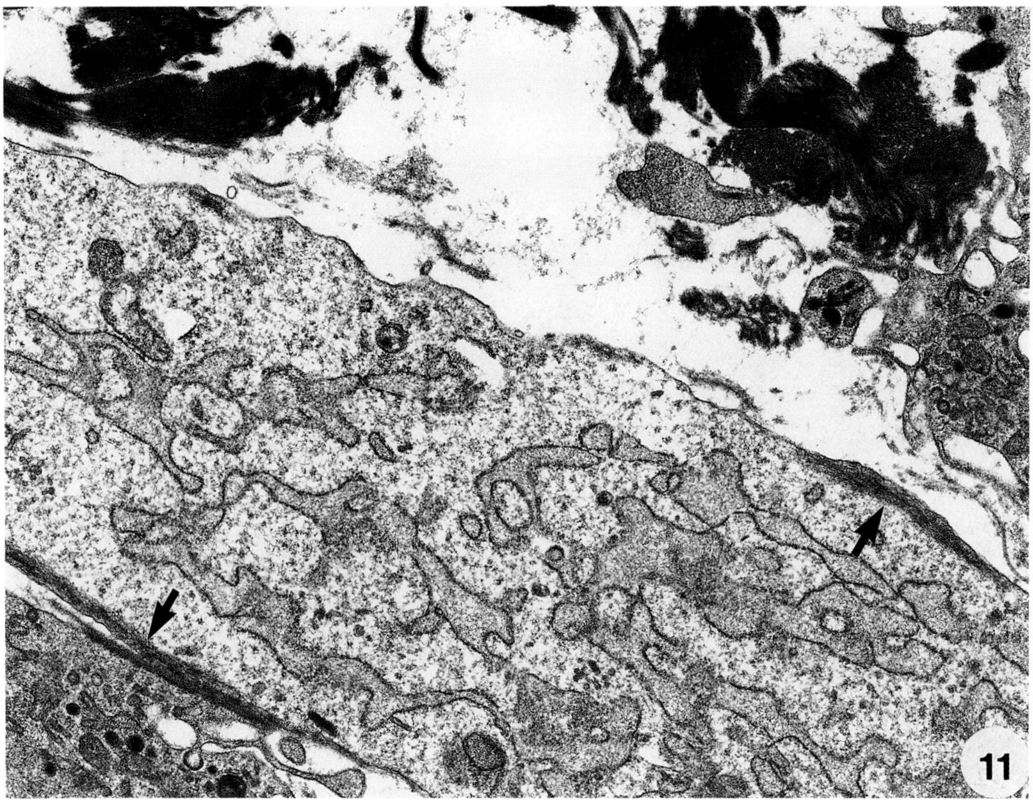

FIG. 11. Detail of the cytoplasm of an intra-alveolar fibroblast (high magnification of Fig. 9) showing its myofibroblastic phenotype. Cytoskeletal filaments are focally organized in bundles beneath the cytoplasmic membrane (*arrow*). ×12,600.

18). In late-stage fibrotic buds, cuboidal epithelialization of the buds may occur, consisting of typical type II pneumocytes or of cells devoid of lamellar bodies (primitive bronchiolar cells?) (95,117). The process of reepithelialization arises from contact between the intraluminal buds and mural structures (95,103).

OTHER MODELS OF BOOP

Paraquat toxicity results in alveolar injury with BOOP. Fukuda and colleagues (123) studied the morphogenesis of intra-alveolar fibrosis after experimental paraquat toxicity administered subcutaneously in monkeys. The sequence of changes leading to intra-alveolar fibrosis was very close to that of idiopathic BOOP, with intra-alveolar migration of interstitial cells differentiating into myofibroblasts, after initial epithelial injury. However, this model differed from idiopathic BOOP by the presence of intra-alveolar smooth muscle cells and the predominance of type I collagen in the newly formed intra-alveolar matrix. The most typical intra-alveolar buds were formed in the group of animals sacrificed 3 to 4 weeks after the first subcutaneous injection of paraquat (which was followed by two weekly injections of the drug). Extensive intra-al-

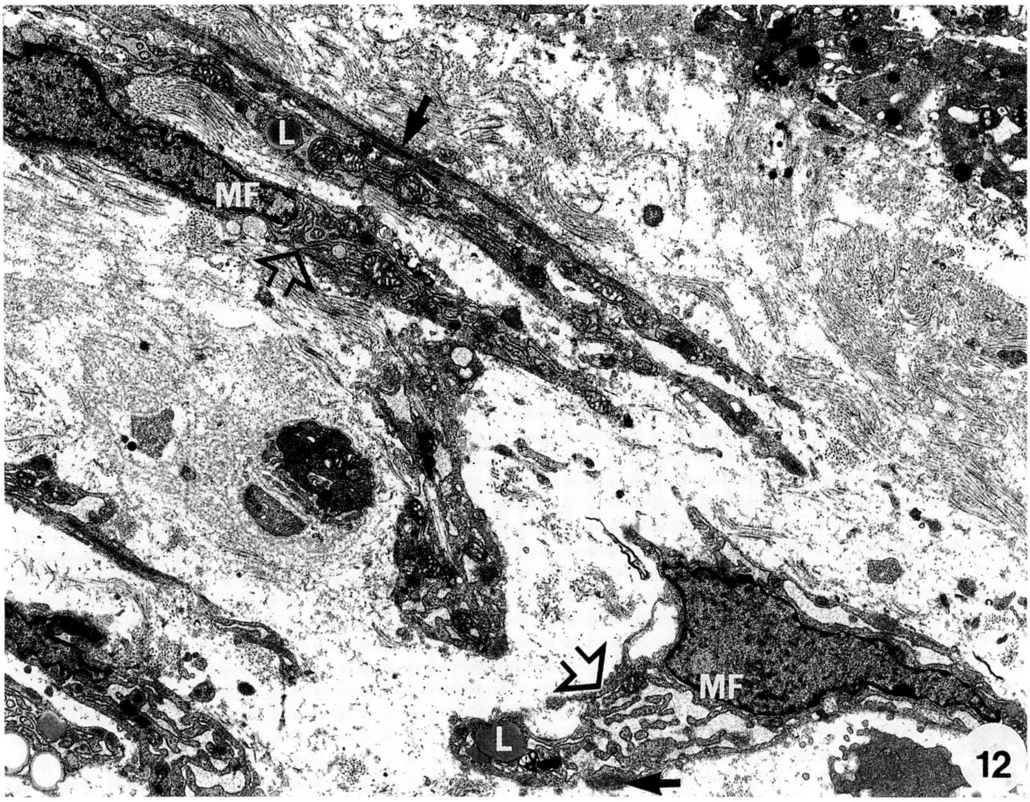

FIG. 12. Myofibroblasts (*MF*) at the periphery of a mature fibrotic bud. They are characterized by prominent ergastoplasmic cisternae (*open arrow*) and lipid droplets (*L*). ×4,400.

veolar fibrosis was also present at autopsy in a patient who died after paraquat ingestion (124).

In experimental models other than paraquat toxicity, intraluminal fibrosis may be prominent, as in intraluminal fibrosis unilaterally induced by lobar instillation of CdCl2 into the rat lung (125). In this model, the lesions developed more rapidly (3 to 7 days) than in the paraquat model, but the sequence of changes was similar.

Lazenby and colleagues (126) studied the pathology of bleomycin-induced pulmonary fibrosis in the rat by staining the basal lamina with antibodies to laminin and collagen IV. Their data suggested that alveolar collapse and intra-alveolar fibrosis play an important role in this model of patchy pulmonary fibrosis. Furthermore, they emphasized the possible role of fibronectin in fibroblast migration into the alveolar lumen, and they suggested that fibronectin found early in the alveolar lumen originated from plasma leakage across the alveolar capillary membrane, whereas fibronectin found in a pericellular distribution at later stages was locally synthesized.

In humans, the causes of BOOP are many. These comprise bacterial and viral infection, drug toxicity, aspiration, and irradiation. BOOP may also be associated with such conditions as connective-tissue diseases, transplantation and inflammatory disorders. All of these are characterized by

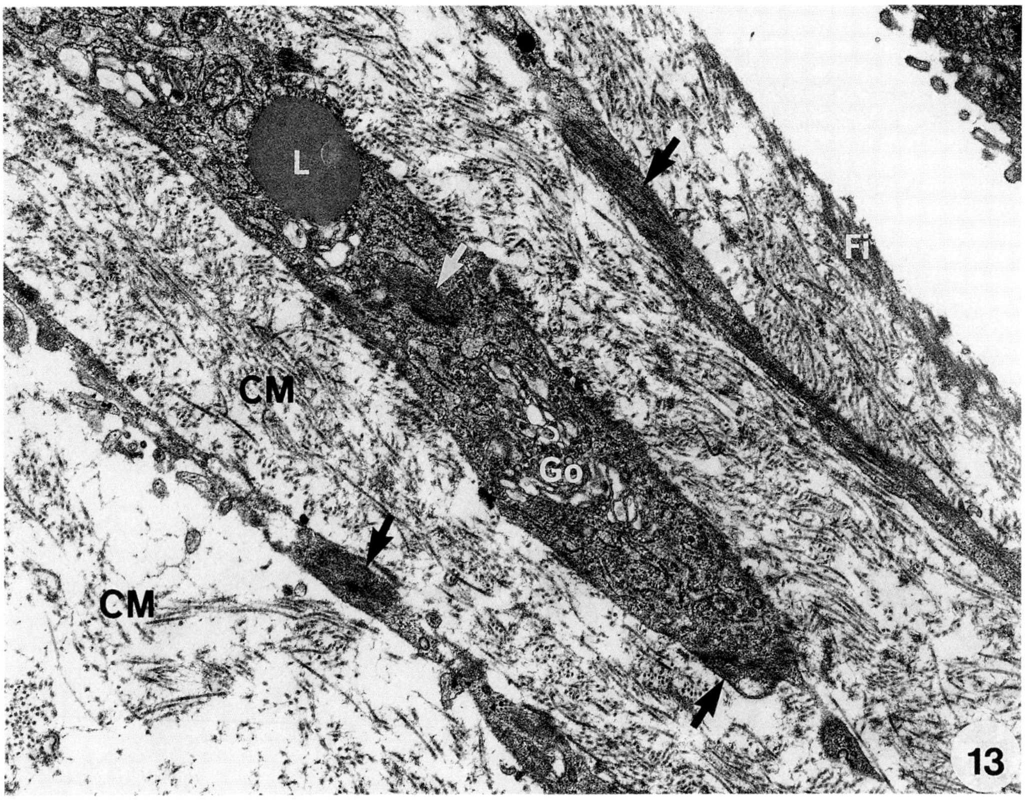

FIG. 13. The myofibroblasts (*MF*) of Fig. 12 are also characterized by a myoid cytoskeleton (*arrow*) and Golgi areas (*Go*). Discrete residual fibrin (*Fi*) is still present. Polymorphic components are associated to collagen fibrils to form a loose connective matrix (*CM*). ×13,600.

acute or subacute inflammation, and they share most of the pathophysiological features previously described (38,127,128).

CHARACTERISTICS OF REVERSIBLE INTRA-ALVEOLAR FIBROSIS

Collagen deposition results from the net effects of collagen synthesis and degradation, which are regulated by complex mechanisms in inflammatory lung disorders (15, 129–132). The striking character of intra-alveolar fibroproliferative organization in a condition such as typical idiopathic BOOP is its reversibility with corticosteroid therapy.

Phenotypic Modulation and Functional Diversity of Fibroblasts

It is clear that the lung fibroblast is not an unvarying cell confined to the function of target cell (14,133,134). On the contrary, it exhibits morphologic plasticity and may also be considered an effector cell. It represents one major cell type of the normal lung interstitium and appears as a spindle-shaped cell with a large nucleus and an available protein synthesis apparatus including mitochondria, rough endoplasmic reticulum, and a Golgi area capable of evolving rapidly to a synthetic fibroblast phenotype.

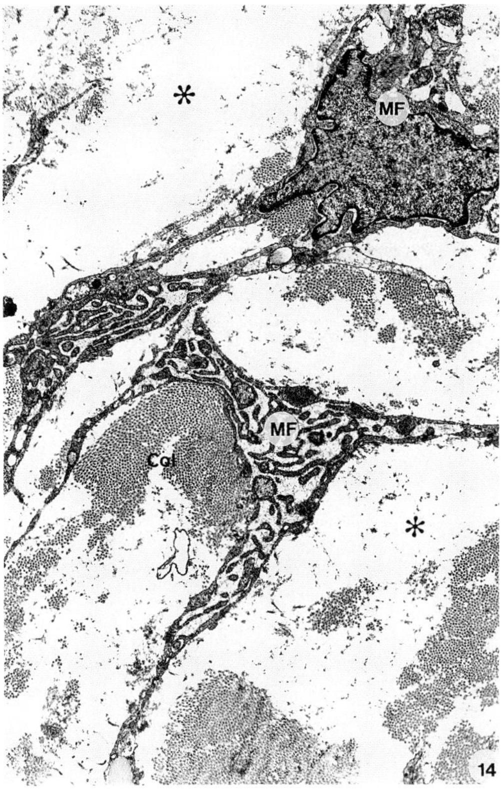

FIG. 14. Multipolar shaped myofibroblasts (*MF*) in the center of a mature fibrotic bud. They are closely associated to collagen fiber bundles (*Col*). An important part of the connective space appears free of any matrix deposit (*asterisk*). ×8,000.

Smooth muscle cells and contractile interstitial cells have a contractile phenotype. Smooth muscle cells are present in the wall of vessels and airways. They are enclosed by basement membrane, contain large amounts of contractile filaments of actin and myosin, but have little morphologic evidence of protein synthesis. Pulmonary capillaries do not have smooth muscle cells in their walls, but they are associated with pericytes enclosed by basement membrane. The contractile interstitial cells present in the thick portion of the air–blood barrier contain both contractile myofilaments and a synthesis apparatus.

The myofibroblast, similar to the contractile interstitial cell, was first described in granulation tissue and is also present in many fibroproliferative conditions. Myofibroblasts are thought to derive locally from resident fibroblasts (134–136), although they may also derive from smooth muscle cells (137). Darby and colleagues (138) studied an experimental wound healing model in the rat. They found that microfilaments in fibroblastic cells accumulated gradually from the sixth up to the fifteenth days, where they were evident in 70% of fibroblastic cells, then regressed progressively and were no longer present in scar fibroblasts on the thirteenth day.

The expression of cytoskeletal proteins has been used as a marker of phenotypic modulation of fibroblastic cells (134). Vimentin (V) is present in fibroblasts. Desmin (D) is expressed in muscular cells. The alpha isoform of actin (A) is expressed in smooth muscle cells (but not in striated muscle cells). The expression of these cytoskeletal proteins has allowed the characterization of four main phenotypes (V, VD, VA, and VAD cells). Darby and colleagues (138) demonstrated that in wound healing, alpha smooth muscle actin was always present in microfilament bundles of myofibroblasts, but not smooth muscle myosin and desmin (VA phenotype), and that the staining paralleled the morphological presence of myofibroblasts. The VA fibroblastic phenotype changes to a V quiescent phenotype when the wound closes. In human hypertrophic scars or scleroderma lesions (including those in the lung), desmin may be expressed in addition to vimentin and actin (139). Expression of alpha smooth muscle actin may be modulated by cytokines (134). In idiopathic BOOP, the myofibroblasts of intra-alveolar buds stain for alpha smooth muscle actin, especially at the periphery of the buds (103, 140, S. Peyrol, unpublished observations). Staining for desmin was negative in one study (103), whereas it was positive in another, espe-

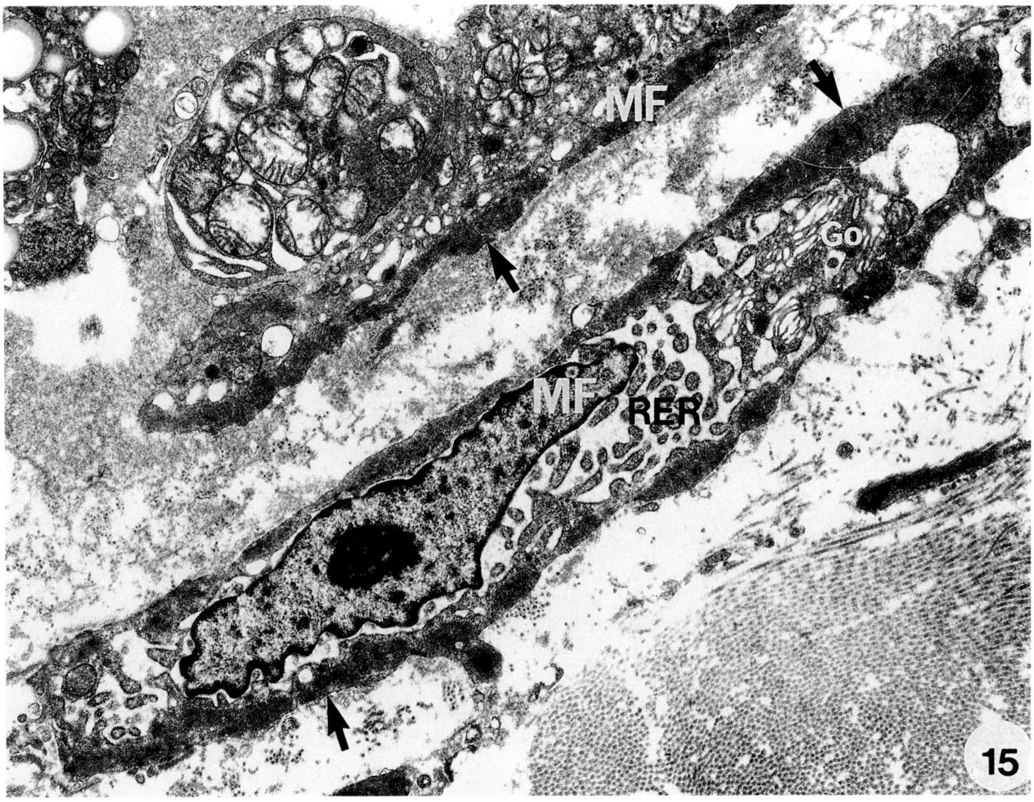

FIG. 15. Myofibroblasts (*MF*) in late fibrotic buds. The myoid cytoskeleton is prominent in the peripheral cytoplasm (*arrows*). Polymorphic components form with collagen fibrils a loose and wavy connective matrix. *Go,* Golgi area. ×9,000.

cially in fibroblasts forming migrating chains from the septa into the alveolar lumen (116).

Taken together, these data show that there is a phenotypic modulation of fibroproliferative cells with expression of a "differentiation repertoire" of cytoskeletal proteins (134). These differences in phenotype, which are present transiently in normally healing wounds and different types of fibrosis, may take a part in the resolution or progression of the fibrotic process. Fibroblasts and extracellular matrix influence each other's morphogenesis, as shown by the remodeling of reconstituted matrix by skin fibroblasts whose ultrastructural morphological features are affected by this matrix (141).

The disappearance of fibroblastic cells in wound healing could occur through the process of apoptosis (programmed cell death) morphologically characterized by the condensation of the nuclear chromatin (138). Our search for apoptotic figures in idiopathic BOOP was negative, whereas we observed such figures in usual interstitial fibrosis (S. Peyrol, unpublished observations).

In intra-alveolar exudate organization, the colonization of the fibrinous exudate by fibroblasts results from their migration from the interstitium into the alveolar lumen. This migration is likely directed by intra-alveolar chemoattractants. Many fibroblast chemoattractants have been identified (142). Some of them are matrix components, such

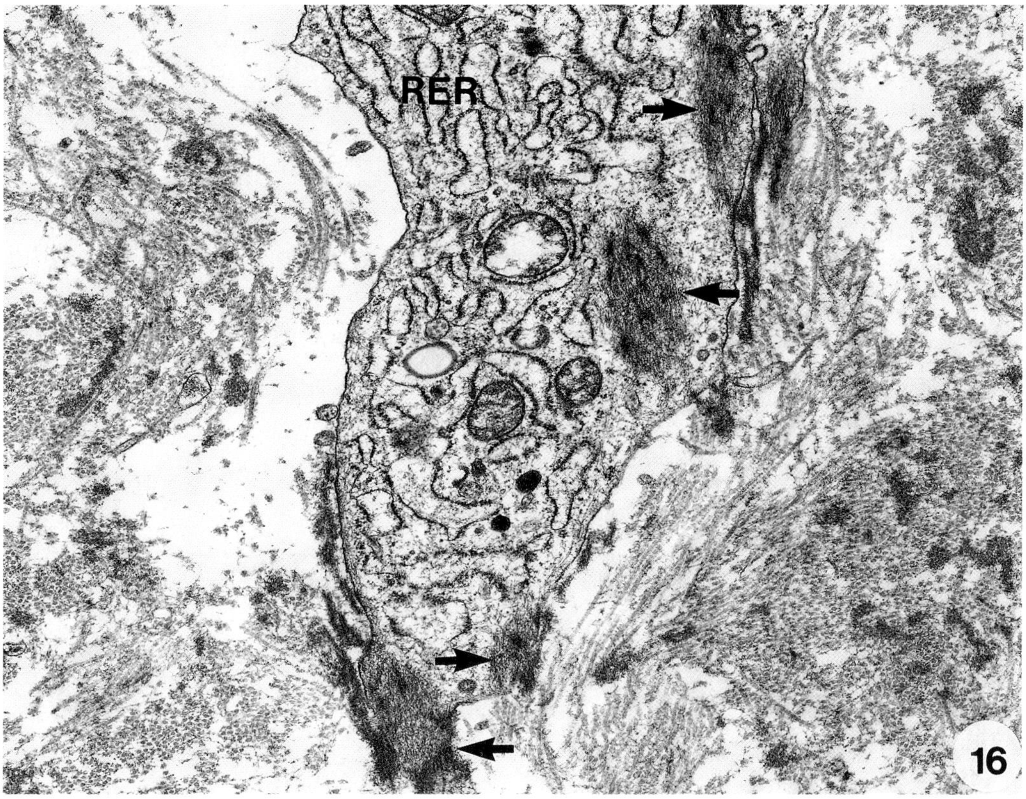

FIG. 16. The myofibroblasts of Fig. 15. The myoid cytoskeleton in the peripheral cytoplasm (*arrows*) is shown. *RER,* rough endoplasmic reticulum. ×13,600.

as collagen or elastin components. Cytokines such as fibronectin are also potent fibroblast and smooth muscle cell chemoattractants. Fibronectin may play a key role in pulmonary fibrosing processes (15).

Both plasma and cellular fibronectin present in intra-alveolar exudates of idiopathic BOOP (103,122) probably play a role in attracting the fibroblasts into the alveolar lumen. Intra-alveolar plasma fibronectin results from exudation from capillaries, while alveolar cells and macrophages are a source of cellular fibronectin. Activated macrophages (143) and alveolar macrophages from patients with idiopathic pulmonary fibrosis (144) release fibronectin. Fibronectin gene expression evaluated by in situ hybridization varies significantly in different populations of macrophages recovered from the lower respiratory tract (145). Fibronectin gene expression is stimulated by such growth factors as platelet derived growth factor, transforming growth factor-beta, gamma-interferon, and interleukin 4 (146,147). Increased fibronectin mRNA was demonstrated in alveolar macrophages of rabbits following in vivo hyperoxia (148). In addition to its chemotactic effect, fibronectin is also a competence factor acting early in the G_1 phase of the cell cycle to promote fibroblast replication (149). Furthermore, fibronectin acts as a substrate for cell adhesion by a membrane receptor (150), and it participates in the organization of collagenous matrices.

Many other cytokines have been implicated in fibroblast attraction, replication, and functional modulation (notably colla-

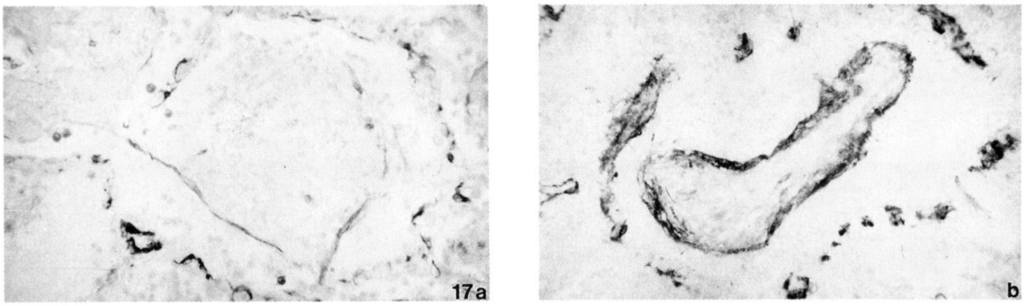

FIG. 17. Immunoperoxydase staining of alpha smooth muscle actin (×700). **a,** in a fibrinoid inflammatory cell cluster; the staining visualizes myofibroblasts coming from the interstitial septum and circumscribing the bud. **b,** in a mature fibrotic bud, heavily stained myofibroblasts form a continuous cellular ring around the bud.

gen production), especially platelet derived growth factor, tumor necrosis factor-alpha (TNF-alpha), insulinlike growth factor I (IGF-I), interleukin (IL)-1, IL-4, IL-6, and transforming growth factor-beta (2,5,147, 151,152).

Transforming growth factor-beta may play a critical role in the processes of repair and fibrosis. This growth factor is an ubiquitous cytokine that has multiple and complex biological effects, resulting especially in fibrosis through both increasing the matrix deposition and blocking its degradation (153, 154). Expression of transforming growth factor-beta is increased at sites of fibrosis in human lungs with pulmonary fibrosis (155). Khalil and colleagues (156) have demonstrated that in the lungs of patients with idiopathic pulmonary fibrosis (IPF), transforming growth factor-beta is increased predominantly in bronchiolar and alveolar epithelial cells and is deposited extracellularly in adjacent subepithelial regions where fibrosis is intense. Of interest, they observed that in an intra-alveolar bud, intracellular transforming growth factor-beta was localized in the hyperplastic type II cells lining the bud whereas extracellular transforming growth factor-beta was distributed in the connective matrix within the intra-alveolar bud. Increased transforming growth factor-beta gene expression is associated with bleomycin-induced pulmonary fibrosis (157). Bleomycin has a direct effect on fibroblasts by increasing transforming growth factor-beta mRNA transcription, followed by transforming growth factor-beta mRNA accumulation, and increased procollagen transcription (158). Transforming growth factor-beta increases collagen mRNA levels and collagen production by normal and fibrotic human lung fibroblasts without increased fibroblast proliferation (159). In addition, this growth factor impairs the fibrinolytic capacity of human lung fibroblasts by increasing plasminogen activator inhibitor-1 and depressing urokinase (160).

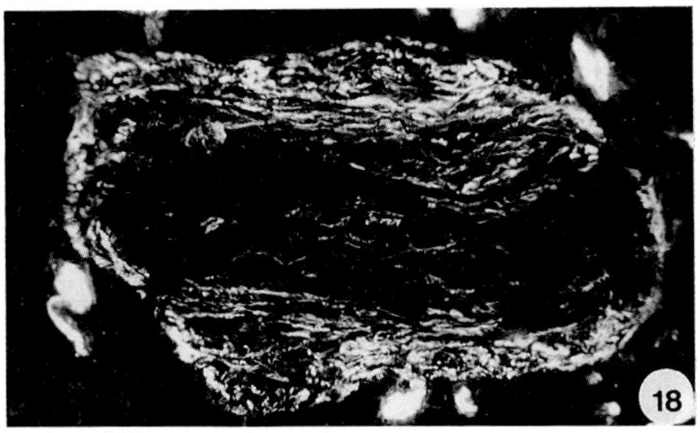

FIG. 18. Immunofluorescent staining of alpha smooth muscle actin in a late mature fibrotic bud. Myofibroblasts, visualized by their cytoskeleton, form a multilayered peripheral ring. There are only few in the center of the bud. ×700.

Connective Matrix of Pulmonary Fibrosis

In typical idiopathic BOOP undergoing complete resolution, the connective matrix organization is characteristically loose, with a codistribution of fibronectin, procollagen type III, type III collagen, and type V collagen. This codistribution is present in all forms of intra-alveolar buds, from the fibroinflammatory buds to the mature fibrotic ones. Type I collagen deposition is also present but is less prominent (116). This pattern of distribution is rather similar to that of the granulation tissue of wound healing. Collagen synthesized in granulation tissue at the early stage when myofibroblasts are present is mainly collagen type III, whereas the phenotypic change of these cells toward a normal fibroblast phenotype coincides with a return to normal proportions of type I collagen (135,161).

On the contrary, in the late stage of interstitial pulmonary fibrosis (and especially in idiopathic pulmonary fibrosis), the fibrotic matrix has a dense connective matrix organization with a high type I/type III collagen ratio (162–165). Furthermore, patients with idiopathic pulmonary fibrosis who have a higher proportion of type III collagen have earlier disease (166,167) and a better response to treatment than those with a lower proportion of type III collagen (166). The presence of type III collagen in biopsy specimens of patients with idiopathic pulmonary fibrosis is associated with disease activity and response to treatment (168). Dense fibrosis, whatever its origin, is generally associated with a marked predominance of type I collagen over type III, whereas the reverse is found in areas of early fibrosis (169).

In the fibrotic lungs of patients dying of ARDS, the proportion of type III collagen was found to be decreased in one study (170) but increased in another (171). Type III collagen accumulation seems indeed associated with an early stage of fibrosis in ARDS (167). The intra-alveolar fibrosis of patients with idiopathic pulmonary fibrosis or ARDS is identical (with regard to collagen I and III distribution) to that of interstitial fibrosis; i.e., it depends on the early or late stage of fibrosis, and it is in direct continuity with the interstitial connective matrix across gaps in the basal lamina (167).

Finally, the intra-alveolar fibrosis of typical idiopathic BOOP is characteristic of a persistent early active stage of fibrosis and thus offers similarities with wound granulation tissue, which is capable of complete healing.

Proteolysis of Intra-Alveolar Fibrosis

The complete resolution of intra-alveolar fibrosis usually occurring in idiopathic BOOP treated with corticosteroid therapy and sometimes in ARDS or acute interstitial pneumonia, suggests that a complete degradation of collagen and other matrix proteins can occur.

The extracellular degradation of deposited collagen requires the action of specific enzymes. The matrix metalloproteinases (MMP) are a family of neutral endopeptidases that have the ability to degrade the components of connective matrices. The collagenases (MMP1, MMP8) are the most specific, cleaving the native triple helicoidal fibrillar collagen molecule of collagens I, II, and III at a single site. The gelatinases degrade other types of collagen and the denatured gelatin forms of collagen, thus acting synergistically with the collagenases. The stromelysins degrade many extracellular matrix proteins. Most of MMP are activated by exogenous proteolytic cleavage of the corresponding propeptide (172,173). Other proteases may participate in the degradation of connective matrix components, but they lack the capacity to break the type I and III collagen molecule. These other neutral proteinases are the elastases (which cleave elastin, but also such other matrix proteins as proteoglycans, fibronectin, type IV collagen) and plasmin. In addition to degrading fibrin, plasmin can activate collagenase from procollagenase by sequential cleavage, and prostromelysin and gelatinase B directly (3).

Neutrophils, monocyte-macrophages, and connective-tissue cells are the main sources of these proteases. Collagenases are secreted mainly by neutrophils (neutrophil collagenase, MMP8) and connective tissue cells (interstitial collagenase, MMP1). The role of neutrophils in fibrosis is unclear. There is some doubt about a major participation of this cell in ARDS. Furthermore, some studies suggest it could limit early fibrogenesis. Collagen deposition in bleomycin-induced pulmonary fibrosis is increased in neutrophil depleted rats (174) and in beige mice whose neutrophils have a defect in degranulation (175). Collagen synthesis is increased in neutrophil-depleted hamsters with bleomycin-induced pulmonary fibrosis (176). Since in idiopathic BOOP neutrophils are rare in the alveolar lumen, it is difficult to maintain that they play a major role in the resolution of fibrosis in this condition, unless corticosteroid treatment was to favor their recruitment within alveolar structures, which is unlikely. Human alveolar macrophages also synthesize and secrete collagenases. Interferon gamma selectively suppresses the lipopolysaccharide-induced production of interstitial collagenase and stromelysin at a pretranslational level (177).

The fibroblasts of intra-alveolar buds may be the main source of collagenase (and stromelysin 1). Of interest, cytokines are capable of modulating the production of collagenase by the fibroblast. For example, IL-1 stimulates the collagenase production (178) and transforming growth factor-beta the expression of collagenase (179). The fibrotic matrix itself may also induce an increased release of proteases. When compared with fibroblasts cultured on plastic, collagen sponge, or collagen-glycosaminoglycan sponge, fibroblasts cultured on an acellular matrix obtained from sarcoid granulomas release increased quantities of collagenase and stromelysin (but not of gelatinase) (180). Whether this occurs through the matrix itself or through mediators trapped on the matrix and available in an active form for the cells is not known. A decrease of protease inhibitors may also favor the matrix degradation.

The major inhibitors of the MMPs are alpha$_2$-macroglobulin and specific tissue inhibitors of metalloproteinases. Due to its size (780 kD), alpha$_2$-macroglobulin is not usually present in alveolar structures, but in severe alveolar damage it may be found in bronchoalveolar lavage fluid (46). The structure of tissue inhibitors of metalloproteinases has been characterized, but their action is still poorly understood in vivo (172). The other proteases capable of degrading the connective matrix are inhibited by the action of specific inhibitors such as alpha$_1$-proteinase inhibitor for elastase, and plasminogen activator inhibitor, which prevents the transformation of plasminogen into plasmin. The availability and functional activity of matrix protease inhibitors results from many mechanisms. For example, in addition to decreasing the synthesis of proteases, transforming growth factor-beta increases the levels of protease inhibitors (179,181). Protease inhibitors may be inactivated by inflammation mediators such as oxidants.

How the balance of the matrix-degrading proteases and their antiproteases is switched from active matrix deposition to matrix dissolution in BOOP is presently not known.

CONCLUSION

BOOP is an original and distinct pattern of inflammatory lung disease. However, it is a nonspecific mode of repair of parenchymal structures after acute or subacute injury, and thus cannot be dissociated from the spectrum of inflammatory reactions that have both alveolar epithelial injury and fibrinous intra-alveolar deposition as a common denominator.

In our opinion, BOOP may be analyzed as a process standing midway between the fibrinous alveolitis of pneumococcal pneumonia undergoing complete resolution and the irreversible parenchymal fibrosis of ARDS or acute interstitial pneumonia, as summarized in Fig. 19. Some striking differences that distinguish between these three types of disorders are as follows:

1. *The degree of severity of initial lung injury* likely determines the capacity of type II pneumocytes to regenerate a normal epithelium if the basal laminae are structurally and spatially intact.
2. *The presence of hyaline membranes* adhering to the devastated epithelium correlates with further mural incorporation of intra-alveolar exudates leading to interstitial fibrosis.
3. *Neutrophil influx* within the alveolar lumen is associated with the resolution of intra-alveolar fibrinous exudates.

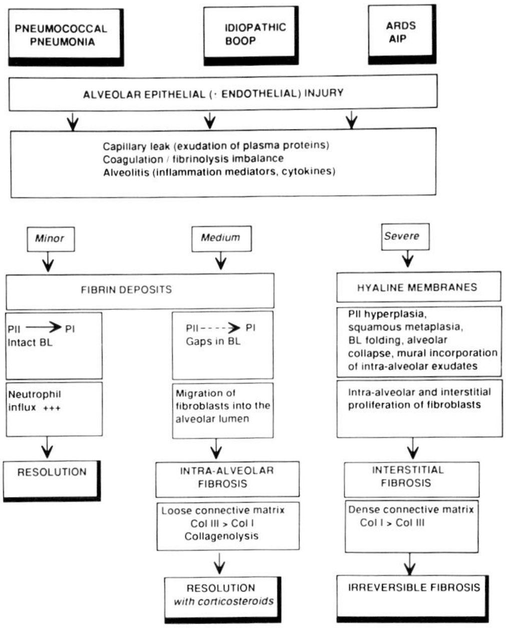

FIG. 19. Comparative pathways of inflammation in pneumococcal pneumonia (resolving), idiopathic BOOP, and ARDS or AIP. *P*, pneumocytes; *BL*, basal lamina; Col, collagen.

4. *Migration of fibroblastic cells* is the crucial mechanism necessary for intra-alveolar organization.
5. *The cell-matrix organization* seems to condition the reversibility of intra-alveolar fibrosis, which likely depends on the phenotypic and functional plasticity of fibroblastic cells, the composition of the matrix, and the occurrence of collagenolytic reactions.

The morphogenic characteristics of intraluminal organization provide a solid basis for further analysis of more basic cellular and extracellular pathobiology. We are aware of an increasing number of basic biological mechanisms involved in inflammation, but these are studied in more and more restrictive models. When analyzed in other or broader contexts, many of them appear to be rather unspecific. Furthermore, these basic biopathological mechanisms are often studied in a single pulmonary disorder (such as idiopathic pulmonary fibrosis) without considering other more common disorders in which they may play a more general role. We are therefore lacking information about the specificity of most basic biopathological mechanisms that need to be integrated into a careful synthetic analysis, and confronted with the clinical and histopathological evidence. Undoubtedly, BOOP may serve as such a model of integrated clinical, pathological, and basic research.

ACKNOWLEDGMENTS

The authors thank M.C. Thevenet for secretarial assistance and T. Greenland for reviewing the translation of the text. Supported by grant HCL–PNRC 005 from the Ministère de la Santé et de l'Action Humanitaire.

REFERENCES

1. Cotran AS, Kumar V, Robbins SL. *Robbins pathologic basis of disease*. 4th ed. Philadelphia: WB Saunders; 1989.

2. Hoogsteden HC, Van Hal PTW. Mediators of the induction of nonallergic pulmonary inflammation. In: Bray MA, Anderson WH, eds. *Mediators of pulmonary inflammation.* New York: Marcel Dekker; 1991:185–277.
3. Ward PA, Morganroth NL, Senior RM, Campbell EJ. Inflammatory mediators of pulmonary tissue injury. In Bray MA, Anderson WH, eds. *Mediators of pulmonary inflammation.* New York: Marcel Dekker; 1991:533–591.
4. Weiss SJ. Tissue destruction by neutrophils. *N Engl J Med* 1989;320:365–376.
5. Kelley J. Cytokines of the lung. *Am Rev Respir Dis* 1990;141:765–788.
6. Sporn MB, Roberts, AB. Autocrine secretion: 10 years later. *Ann Intern Med* 1992;117:408–414.
7. Lortat-Jacob H, Kleinman HK, Grimaud JA. High-affinity binding of interferon-gamma to a basement membrane complex (matrigel). *J Clin Invest* 1991;87:878–883.
8. Elias JA, Zitnik RJ. Cytokine-cytokine interactions in the context of cytokine networking. *Am J Respir Cell Mol Biol* 1992;7:365–367.
9. Albelda SM. Endothelial and epithelial cell adhesion molecules. *Am J Respir Cell Mol Biol* 1991;4:195–203.
10. Montefort S, Holgate ST. Adhesion molecules and their role in inflammation. *Respir Med* 1991;85:91–99.
11. Ruoslahti E. Integrins. *J Clin Invest* 1991;87:1–5.
12. Bitterman PB, Henke CA. Fibroproliferative disorders. *Chest* 1991;99[Suppl]:81S–84S.
13. Sporn MB, Harris ED. Proliferative diseases. *Am J Med* 1981;70:1231–1236.
14. Absher M. Fibroblasts. In: Massaro D, ed. *Lung cell biology.* New York: Marcel Dekker; 1989:401–439.
15. Clark JG, Kuhn C III, McDonald JA, Mecham RP. Lung connective tissue. *Int Rev Connect Tissue Res* 1983;10:249–331.
16. Crystal RG, Gadek JE, Ferrans VJ, Fulmer JD, Line BR, Hunninghake GW. Interstitial lung disease: current concepts of pathogenesis, staging and therapy. *Am J Med* 1981;70:542–568.
17. Keogh BA, Crystal RG. Alveolitis: the key to the interstitial lung disorders. *Thorax* 1982; 37:1–10.
18. Marinelli WA, Polunovsky VA, Harmon KR, Bitterman PB. Role of platelet-derived growth factor in pulmonary fibrosis. *Am J Respir Cell Mol Biol* 1991;5:503–504.
19. Martinet Y, Rom WN, Grotendorst GR, Martin GR, Crystal RG. Exaggerated spontaneous release of platelet-derived growth factor by alveolar macrophages from patients with idiopathic pulmonary fibrosis. *N Engl J Med* 1987;317: 202–209.
20. Nagaoka I, Trapnell BC, Crystal RG. Upregulation of platelet-derived growth factor-A and -B gene expression in individuals with idiopathic pulmonary fibrosis. *J Clin Invest* 1990; 85:2023–2027.
21. Laënnec RTH. Traité de l'auscultation médiate et des maladies des poumons et du coeur. 2nd ed. Paris: Chaudet; 1826.
22. Kohn HN. Zur Histologie der indurirenden fibrinösen Pneumonie. *Münch Med Wochenschr* 1893;8:42–45.
23. Chapman HA, Stone OL, Vavrin Z. Degradation of fibrin and elastin by intact human alveolar macrophages in vitro: characterization of a plasminogen activator and its role in matrix degradation. *J Clin Invest* 1984;73:806–815.
24. Milne LS. Chronic pneumonia (including a discussion of two cases of syphilis of the lung). *Am J Med Sci* 1911;142:408–438.
25. Auerbach SH, Mims OM, Goodpasture EW. Pulmonary fibrosis secondary to pneumonia. *Am J Pathol* 1952;28:69–87.
26. Floyd R. Organization of pneumonic exudates. *Am J Med Sci* 1922;163:527–548.
27. Menetrier P, Pascano A. Transformation fibreuse de l'hépatisation pneumonique ou fibrome végétant intra-alvéolaire post-pneumonique. *Bull Mem Soc Med Hop Paris* 1915; 39:510–524.
28. Rhodes GC, Lykke AWJ, Tapsall JW, Smith LW. Abnormal alveolar epithelial repair associated with failure of resolution in experimental streptococcal pneumonia. *J Pathol* 1989;159: 245–253.
29. Rhodes GC, Tapsall JW, Lykke AWJ. Alveolar epithelial responses in experimental streptococcal pneumonia. *J Pathol* 1989;157:347–357.
30. Voelker DR, Mason RJ. Alveolar type II epithelial cells. In: Massaro D. *Lung cell biology.* New York: Marcel Dekker; 1989:487–538.
31. Rennard SI, Bitterman PB, Crystal RG. Response of the lower respiratory tract to injury: mechanisms of repair of the parenchymal cells of the alveolar wall. *Chest* 1983;84:735–739.
32. Edelson JD, Shannon JM, Mason RJ. Effects of two extracellular matrices on morphologic and biochemical properties of human type II cells in vitro. *Am Rev Respir Dis* 1989;140:1398–1404.
33. Rannels DE, Rannels SR. Influence of the extracellular matrix on type 2 cell differentiation. *Chest* 1989;96:165–173.
34. Woodcock-Mitchell J, Rannels SR, Mitchell J, Rannels DE, Low RB. Modulation of keratin expression in type II pneumocytes by the extracellular matrix. *Am Rev Respir Dis* 1989; 139:343–351.
35. Adamson IYR, Young L, Bowden DH. Relationship of alveolar epithelial injury and repair to the induction of pulmonary fibrosis. *Am J Pathol* 1988;130:377–383.
36. Adamson IYR, Hedgecock C, Bowden DH. Epithelial cell-fibroblast interactions in lung injury and repair. *Am J Pathol* 1990;137:385–392.
37. Clement A, Edeas M, Chadelat K, Brody JS. Inhibition of lung epithelial cell proliferation by hyperoxia. *J Clin Invest* 1992;90:1812–1818.
38. Colby TV, Lombard C. Yousem SA, Kitaichi M. *Atlas of pulmonary surgical pathology.* Philadelphia: WB Saunders; 1991.

39. Katzenstein ALA, Askin FB. *Surgical pathology of non-neoplastic lung disease*. Philadelphia: WB Saunders; 1990.
40. Bachofen M, Bachofen H. Acute lung injury: parenchymal changes. In: Crystal RG, West JB, eds. *The lung: scientific foundations*. New York: Raven Press; 1991:2019–2029.
41. Case Records of the Massachusetts General Hospital (Case 22-1977). *N Engl J Med* 1977; 296:1279–1287.
42. Hasleton PS. Adult respiratory distress syndrome: a review. *Histopathology* 1983;7:307–332.
43. Katzenstein AL, Bloor CM, Liebow AA. Diffuse alveolar damage: the role of oxygen, shock, and related factors. *Am J Pathol* 1976; 85:210–228.
44. Bachofen M, Bachofen H, Weibel ER. Lung edema in the adult respiratory distress syndrome. In: Fishman AP, Renkin EM. *Pulmonary edema*. Bethesda: American Physiological Society; 1979:241–252.
45. Montaner JSG, Tsang J, Evans KG, et al. Alveolar epithelial damage: a critical difference between high pressure and oleic acid–induced low pressure pulmonary edema. *J Clin Invest* 1986;77:1786–1796.
46. Cordier JF, Mornex JF, Lasne Y, et al. Bronchoalveolar lavage in radiation pneumonitis. *Bull Eur Physiopathol Respir* 1984;20:369–374.
47. Holter JF, Weiland JE, Pacht ER, Gadek JE, Davis WB. Protein permeability in the adult respiratory distress syndrome: loss of size selectivity of the alveolar epithelium. *J Clin Invest* 1986;78:1513–1522.
48. Rinaldo JE, Rogers RM. Adult respiratory-distress syndrome: changing concepts of lung injury and repair. *N Engl J Med* 1982;306:900–909.
49. Fanburg BL, Deneke SM. Hyperoxia. In: Massaro D, ed. *Lung cell biology*. New York: Marcel Dekker; 1989:1199–1226.
50. Rinaldo JE. Mediation of ARDS: clinical evidence and implications for therapy. *Chest* 1986; 8:590–593.
51. Rinaldo JE, Rogers RM. Adult respiratory distress syndrome. *N Engl J Med* 1986;315:578–579.
52. Weiland JE, Davis WB, Holter JF, Mohammed JR, Dorinsky PM, Gadek JE. Lung neutrophils in the adult respiratory distress syndrome: clinical and pathophysiologic significance. *Am Rev Respir Dis* 1986;133:218–225.
53. Ognibene FP, Martin SE, Parker MM, et al. Adult respiratory distress syndrome in patients with severe neutropenia. *N Engl J Med* 1986; 315:547–551.
54. Swank DW, Moore SB. Roles of the neutrophil and other mediators in adult respiratory distress syndrome. *Mayo Clin Proc* 1989;64:1118–1132.
55. Chapman HA, Allen CL, Stone OL. Abnormalities in pathways of alveolar fibrin turnover among patients with interstitial lung disease. *Am Rev Respir Dis* 1986;133:437–443.
56. Chapman HA, Stahl M, Allen CL, Yee R, Fair DS. Regulation of the procoagulant activity within the bronchoalveolar compartment of normal human lung. *Am Rev Respir Dis* 1988; 137:1417–1425.
57. Chapman HA, Bertozzi P, Reilly JJ. Role of enzymes mediating thrombosis and thrombolysis in lung disease. *Chest* 1988;93:1256–1263.
58. Chapman HA, Allen CL, Stone OL, Fair DS. Human alveolar macrophages synthesize factor VII in vitro. *J Clin Invest* 1985;75:2030–2037.
59. Gross TJ, Simon RH, Sitrin RG. Tissue factor procoagulant expression by rat alveolar epithelial cell. *Am J Respir Cell Mol Biol* 1992;6:397–403.
60. Parton LA, Warburtow D, Laug WE. Plasminogen activator inhibitor type 1 production by rat type II pneumocytes in culture. *Am J Respir Cell Mol Biol* 1992;6:133–139.
61. Takahashi K, Kiguchi T, Sawasaki Y, et al. Lung capillary endothelial cells produce and secrete urokinase-type plasminogen activator. *Am J Respir Cell Mol Biol* 1992;7:90–94.
62. Sitrin RG. Plasminogen activation in the injured lung: pulmonology does not recapitulate hematology. *Am J Respir Cell Mol Biol* 1992; 6:131–132
63. Vassali JD, Sappino AP, Belin D. The plasminogen activator/plasmin system. *J Clin Invest* 1991;1067–1072.
64. Bertozzi P, Astedt B, Zenzius L, et al. Depressed bronchoalveolar urokinase activity in patients with adult respiratory distress syndrome. *N Engl J Med* 1990;322:890–897.
65. Idell S, Gonzalez K, Bradford H, et al. Procoagulant activity in bronchoalveolar lavage in the adult respiratory distress syndrome: contribution of tissue factor associated with factor VII. *Am Rev Respir Dis* 1987;136:1466–1474.
66. Idell S, James KK, Levin EG, et al. Local abnormalities in coagulation and fibrinolytic pathways predispose to alveolar fibrin deposition in the adult respiratory distress syndrome. *J Clin Invest* 1989;84:695–705.
67. Idell S, Peterson BT, Gonzalez KK, et al. Local abnormalities of coagulation and fibrinolysis and alveolar fibrin deposition in sheep with oleic acid-induced lung injury. *Am Rev Respir Dis* 1988;138:1282–1284.
68. Idell S, Peters J, James KJ, Fair DS, Coalson JJ. Local abnormalities of coagulation and fibrinolytic pathways that promote alveolar fibrin deposition in the lungs of baboons with diffuse alveolar damage. *J Clin Invest* 1989;84: 181–193.
69. Sitrin RG, Brubaker PG, Fantone JC. Tissue fibrin deposition during acute lung injury in rabbits and its relationship to local expression of procoagulant and fibrinolytic activities. *Am Rev Respir Dis* 1987;135:930–936.
70. Lamy M, Fallat RF, Koeniger E, et al. Pathologic features and mechanisms of hypoxemia in adult respiratory distress syndrome. *Am Rev Respir Dis* 1976;114:267–284.
71. Pratt PC. Pathology of adult respiratory dis-

tress syndrome. In: Thurlbeck WM, Abell MR, eds. *The lung: structure, function and disease*. Baltimore: Williams & Wilkins; 1978:43–57.
72. Pratt PC, Vollmer RT, Shelburne JD, Crapo JD. Pulmonary morphology in a multihospital collaboration extracorporeal membrane oxygenation project. *Am J Pathol* 1979;95:191–214.
73. Zapol WM, Trelstad RL, Coffey JW, Tsai I, Salvador RA. Pulmonary fibrosis in severe acute respiratory failure. *Am Rev Respir Dis* 1979;119:547–554.
74. Bell RC, Coalson JJ, Smith JD, Johanson WG. Multiple organ system failure and infection in adult respiratory distress syndrome. *Ann Intern Med* 1983;99:293–298.
75. Effmann EL, Merten DF, Kirks DR, Pratt PC, Spock A. Adult respiratory distress syndrome in children. *Radiology* 1985;157:69–74.
76. Fukuda Y, Ishizaki M, Masuda Y, Kimura G, Kawanami O, Masugi Y. The role of intraalveolar fibrosis in the process of pulmonary structural remodeling in patients with diffuse alveolar damage. *Am J Pathol* 1987;126:171–182.
77. Snyder LS, Hertz MI, Peterson MS, et al. Acute lung injury: pathogenesis of intraalveolar fibrosis. *J Clin Invest* 1991;88:663–673.
78. Ross R. Platelet-derived growth factor. *Lancet* 1989;1:1179–1182.
79. Seppa H, Grotendorst G, Seppa S, Schiffmann E, Martin GR. Platelet-derived growth factor is chemotactic for fibroblasts. *J Cell Biol* 1982; 92:584–588.
80. Grotendorst GR, Chang T, Seppa HEJ, Kleinman HK, Martin GR. Platelet-derived growth factor is a chemoattractant for vascular smooth muscle cells. *J Cell Physiol* 1982;113:261–266.
81. Grotendorst GR, Seppa HE, Kleinman HK, Martin GR. Attachment of smooth muscle cells to collagen and their migration toward platelet-derived growth factor. *Proc Natl Acad Sci USA* 1981;78:3669–3672.
82. Clark RAF, Folkvord JM, Hart CE, Murray MJ, McPherson JM. Platelet isoforms of platelet-derived growth factor stimulate fibroblasts to contract collagen matrices. *J Clin Invest* 1989;84:1036–1040.
83. Shaw RJ, Benedict SH, Clark RAF, King TE. Pathogenesis of pulmonary fibrosis in interstitial lung disease: alveolar macrophage PDGF (B) gene activation and up-regulation by interferon gamma. *Am Rev Respir Dis* 1991;143: 167–173.
84. Chen B, Polunovsky V, White J, et al. Mesenchymal cells isolated after acute lung injury manifest an enhanced proliferative phenotype. *J Clin Invest* 1992;90:1778–1785.
85. Ghio AJ, Elliott G, Crapo RO, Berlin SL, Jensen RL. Impairment after adult respiratory distress syndrome: an evaluation based on American Thoracic Society recommendations. *Am Rev Respir Dis* 1989;139:1158–1162.
86. Meduri GU, Belenchia JM, Estes RJ, Wunderink RG, El Torky M, Leeper KV. Fibroproliferative phase of ARDS: clinical findings and effects of corticosteroids. *Chest* 1991;100:943–952.
87. Liebow AA. New concepts and entities in pulmonary disease. In: Liebow AA, Smith DE, eds. *The lung*. Baltimore: Williams & Wilkins; 1968:332–365.
88. Hamman L, Rich AR. Acute diffuse interstitial fibrosis of the lungs. *Bull J Hopkins Hosp* 1944;74:177–204.
89. Askin FB. Back to the future: the Hamman-Rich syndrome and acute interstitial pneumonia. *Mayo Clin Proc* 1990;65:1624–1626.
90. Katzenstein AL, Myers JL, Mazur MT. Acute interstitial pneumonia: a clinicopathologic, ultrastructural and cell kinetic study. *Am J Surg Pathol* 1986;10:256–267.
91. Olson J, Colby TV, Elliot CG. Hamman-Rich syndrome revisited. *Mayo Clin Proc* 1990; 65:1538–1548.
92. Burkhardt A. Pathogenesis of pulmonary fibrosis. *Hum Pathol* 1986;17:971–973.
93. Burkhardt A. Alveolitis and collapse in the pathogenesis of pulmonary fibrosis. *Am Rev Respir Dis* 1989;140:513–524.
94. Burkhardt A, Cottier H. Cellular events in alveolitis and the evolution of pulmonary fibrosis. *Virchows Arch [B]* 1989;58:1–13.
95. Basset F, Ferrans VJ, Soler P, Takemura T, Fukuda Y, Crystal RG. Intraluminal fibrosis in interstitial lung disorders. *Am J Pathol* 1986; 122:443–461.
96. Katzenstein AL. Pathogenesis of "fibrosis" in interstitial pneumonia: an electron microscopic study. *Hum Pathol* 1985;16:1015–1024.
97. Hamm H, Fabel H, Bartsch W. The surfactant system of the adult lung: physiology and clinical perspectives. *Clin Invest* 1992;70:637–657.
98. Myers JL, Katzenstein ALA. Epithelial necrosis and alveolar collapse in the pathogenesis of usual interstitial pneumonia. *Chest* 1988;94: 1309–1311.
99. Spencer H. Chronic interstitial pneumonia. In: Liebow AA, Smith DE, eds. *The lung*. Baltimore: Williams & Wilkins; 1968:134–150.
100. Gross P, Benz EJ. The concept of organizing pneumonia. *Arch Pathol* 1961;72:607–619.
101. Corrin B, Dewar A, Rodriguez-Roisin R, Turner-Warwick M. Fine structural changes in cryptogenic fibrosing alveolitis and asbestosis. *J Pathol* 1985;147:107–119.
102. Fukuda Y, Basset F, Yamanaka N. Significance of early intraalveolar fibrotic lesions in lung biopsies in idiopathic pulmonary fibrosis. *Am Rev Respir Dis* 1991;143[Suppl]:A770.
103. Kuhn C, Mc Donald JA. The roles of the myofibroblast in idiopathic pulmonary fibrosis: ultrastructural and immunohistochemical features of sites of active extracellular matrix synthesis. *Am J Pathol* 1991;138:1257–1265.
104. Kuhn C. Patterns of lung repair: a morphologist's view. *Chest* 1991;99[Suppl]:11S–14S.
105. Mc Donald JA. Idiopathic pulmonary fibrosis: a paradigm for lung injury and repair. *Chest* 1991;99:87S–93S.

106. Cordier JF, Loire R, Brune J. Idiopathic bronchiolitis obliterans organizing pneumonia: definition of characteristic clinical profiles in a series of 16 patients. *Chest* 1989;96:999–1004.
107. Costabel U, Teschler H, Schoenfeld B, et al. BOOP in Europe. *Chest* 1992;102[Suppl]:14S–20S.
108. Davison AG, Heard BE, Mc Allister WAC, Turner-Warwick MEH. Cryptogenic organizing pneumonitis. *Q J Med* 1983;52:382–394.
109. Epler GR. Bronchiolitis obliterans organizing pneumonia: definition and clinical features. *Chest* 1992;102[Suppl]:2S–6S.
110. Epler GR, Colby TV, Mc Loud T, Carrington CB, Gaensler EA. Bronchiolitis obliterans organizing pneumonia. *N Engl J Med* 1985;312:152–158.
111. King TE, Mortenson RL. Cryptogenic organizing pneumonitis: the North American experience. *Chest* 1992;102[Suppl]:8S–13S.
112. Izumi T, Kitaichi M, Nishimura K, Nagai S. Bronchiolitis obliterans organizing pneumonia: clinical features and differential diagnosis. *Chest* 1992;102:715–719.
113. Nagai S, Aung H, Tanaka S, et al. Bronchoalveolar lavage cell findings in patients with BOOP and related diseases. *Chest* 1992;102[Suppl]:32S–37S.
114. Costabel U, Teschler H, Guzman J. Bronchiolitis obliterans organizing pneumonia (BOOP): the cytological and immunocytological profile of bronchoalveolar lavage. *Eur Respir J* 1992;5:791–797.
115. Colby TV, Myers JL. Clinical and histologic spectrum of bronchiolitis obliterans, including bronchiolitis obliterans organizing pneumonia. *Semin Respir Med* 1992;13:119–133.
116. Peyrol S, Cordier JF, Grimaud JA. Intraalveolar fibrosis of idiopathic bronchiolitis obliterans organizing pneumonia: cell-matrix patterns. *Am J Pathol* 1990;137:155–170.
117. Katzenstein AL, Myers JL, Prophet WD, Corley LS, Shin MS. Bronchiolitis obliterans and usual interstitial pneumonia: a comparative clinicopathologic study. *Am J Surg Pathol* 1986;10:3733–381.
118. Myers JL, Katzenstein AL. Ultrastructural evidence of alveolar epithelial injury in idiopathic bronchiolitis obliterans organizing pneumonia. *Am J Pathol* 1988;132:102–109.
119. Peers SP, Schulman ES, Dvorak AM. Mast cells. In: Massaro D, ed. *Lung cell biology*. New YOrk: Marcel Dekker; 1989:345–399.
120. Vadillo-Ortega F, Gonzalez-Avila G. Mast cells, inflammation, and fibrogenesis. In: Selman M, Barrios R, eds. *Interstitial pulmonary diseases: selected topics*. Boca Raton: CRC Press; 1991:137–153.
121. Gay S, Miller EJ. What is collagen, what is not. *Ultrastruct Pathol* 1983;4:365–377.
122. Kuhn C III, Boldt J, King TE, Crouch E, Vartio T, Mc Donald JA. An immunohistochemical study of architectural remodeling and connective tissue synthesis in pulmonary fibrosis. *Am Rev Respir Dis* 1989;140:1693–703.
123. Fukuda Y, Ferrans VJ, Schoenberger CI, Rennard SI, Crystal RG. Patterns of pulmonary structural remodeling after experimental paraquat toxicity: the morphogenesis of intraalveolar fibrosis. *Am J Pathol* 1985;118:452–475.
124. Copland GM, Kolin A, Shulman HS. Fatal pulmonary intra-alveolar fibrosis after paraquat ingestion. *N Engl J Med* 1974;291:290–292.
125. Damiano VV, Cherian PV, Frankel FR, et al. Intraluminal fibrosis induced unilaterally by lobar instillation of CdCl2 into the rat lung. *Am J Pathol* 1990;137:883–894.
126. Lazenby AJ, Crouch EC, Mc Donald JA, Kuhn C III. Remodeling of the lung in bleomycin-induced pulmonary fibrosis in the rat: an immunohistochemical study of laminin, type IV collagen, and fibronectin. *Am Rev Respir Dis* 1990;142:206–214.
127. Colby TV. Pathologic aspects of bronchiolitis obliterans organizing pneumonia. *Chest* 1992;102[Suppl]:38S–43S.
128. Cordier JF. Cryptogenic organizing pneumonitis (bronchiolitis obliterans organizing pneumonia). *Clin Chest Med (in press)*.
129. Adams SL. Collagen gene expression. *Am J Respir Cell Mol Biol* 1989;1:161–168.
130. Harrison NK, Laurent GJ. Lung collagen metabolism: the link between inflammation and pulmonary fibrosis. In: Selman M, Barrios R, eds. *Interstitial pulmonary diseases: selected topics*. Boca Raton: CRC Press; 1991:47–74.
131. Kelley J. Collagen. In: Massaro D, ed. *Lung cell biology*. New York: Marcel Dekker; 1989:821–866.
132. Laurent GJ. Lung collagen: more than scaffolding. *Thorax* 1986;41:418–428.
133. Raghu G, Kavanagh TJ. The human lung fibroblast: a multifaceted target and effector cell. In: Selman M, Barrios R, eds. *Interstitial pulmonary diseases: selected topics*. Boca Raton: CRC Press; 1991:1–34.
134. Sappino AP, Schurch W, Gabbiani G. Differentiation repertoire of fibroblastic cells: expression of cytoskeletal proteins as marker of phenotypic modulation. *Lab Invest* 1990;63:144–161.
135. Adler KA, Low RB, Leslie KO, Mitchell J, Evans JN. Biology of disease: contractile cells in normal and fibrotic lung. *Lab Invest* 1989;60:473–485.
136. Skalli O, Gabbiani G. The biology of the myofibroblast: relationship to wound contraction and fibrocontractive diseases. In: *The molecular and cellular pathology of wound repair.* New York: Plenum; 1988:373–402.
137. Gown AM. The mysteries of the myofibroblast (partially) unmasked. *Lab Invest* 1990;63:1–3
138. Darby I, Skalli O, Gabbiani G. Alpha-smooth muscle actin is transiently expressed by myofibroblasts during experimental wound healing. *Lab Invest* 1990;63:21–29.
139. Sappino AP, Masouye I, Saurat JH, Gabbiani G. Smooth muscle differentiation in sclero-

derma fibroblastic cells. *Am J Pathol* 1990; 137:585–591.
140. Leslie K, King TE, Low R. Smooth muscle actin is expressed by air space fibroblast-like cells in idiopathic pulmonary fibrosis and hypersensitivity pneumonitis. *Chest* 1991;99:47S–48S.
141. Emonard H, Calle A, Grimaud JA, et al. Interactions between fibroblasts and a reconstituted basement membrane matrix. *J Invest Dermatol* 1987;89;156–163.
142. Albini A, Adelmann-Grill BC, Muller PK. Fibroblast chemotaxis. *Coll Relat Res* 1985;5: 283–296.
143. Tsukamoto Y, Helsel WE, Wahl SM. Macrophage production of fibronectin, a chemoattractant for fibroblasts. *J Immunol* 1981;127: 673–678.
144. Rennard SI, Hunninghake GW, Bitterman PB, Crystal RG. Production of fibronectin by the human alveolar macrophage: mechanism for the recruitment of fibroblasts to sites of tissue injury in interstitial lung diseases. *Proc Natl Acad Sci USA* 1981;78:7147–7151.
145. Adachi K, Yamauchi K, Bernaudin JF, Fouret P, Ferrans VJ, Crystal RG. Evaluation of fibronectin gene expression by in situ hybridization: differential expression of the fibronectin gene among populations of human alveolar macrophages. *Am J Pathol* 1988;133:193–203.
146. Dean DC. Expression of the fibronectin gene. *Am J Respir Cell Biol* 1989;1:5–10.
147. Postlethwaite AE, Holness MA, Katai H, Raghow R. Human fibroblasts synthesize elevated levels of extracellular matrix proteins in response to interleukin 4. *J Clin Invest* 1992; 90:1479–1485.
148. Sinkin RA, Lo-Monaco MB, Finkelstein JN, Watkins RH, Cox C, Horowitz S. Increased fibronectin mRNA in alveolar macrophages following in vivo hyperoxia. *Am J Respir Cell Mol Biol* 1992;7:548–5555.
149. Bitterman PB, Rennard SI, Adelberg S, Crystal RG. Role of fibronectin as a growth factor for fibroblasts. *J Cell Biol* 1983;97:1925–1932.
150. Ruoslahti E, Engvall E, Hayman EG. Fibronectin: current concepts of its structure and functions. *Coll Relat Res* 1981;1:95–128.
151. Elias JA, Freundlich B, Kern JA, Rosenbloom J. Cytokine networks in the regulation of inflammation and fibrosis in the lung. *Chest* 1990;97:1439–1445.
152. Elias JA, Kotloff R. Mononuclear cell-fibroblast interactions in the human lung. *Chest* 1991;99:73S–79S.
153. Border WA, Ruoslahti E. Transforming growth factor-β in disease: the dark side of tissue repair. *J Clin Invest* 1992;90:1–7.
154. Raghow R. Role of transforming growth factor-β in repair and fibrosis. *Chest* 1991;99[Suppl]: 61S–65S.
155. Broekelmann TJ, Limper AH, Colby TV, Mc Donald JA. Transforming growth factor β1 is present at sites of extracellular matrix gene expression in human pulmonary fibrosis. *Proc Natl Acad Sci USA* 1991;88:6642–6646.
156. Khalil N, O'Connor RN, Unruh HW, et al. Increased production and immunohistochemical localization of transforming growth factor-β in idiopathic pulmonary fibrosis. *Am J Respir Cell Mol Biol* 1991;5:155–162.
157. Raghow R, Irish P, Kang AH. Coordinate regulation of transforming growth factor-β gene expression and cell proliferation in hamster lungs undergoing bleomycin-induced pulmonary fibrosis. *J Clin Invest* 1989;84:1836–1842.
158. Breen E, Shull S, Burne S, Absher M, Kelley J, Phan S, Cutroneo KR. Bleomycin regulation of transforming growth factor-β mRNA in rat lung fibroblasts. *Am J Respir Cell Mol Biol* 1992;6:146–152.
159. Raghu G, Masta S, Meyers D, Narayanan AS. Collagen synthesis by normal and fibrotic human lung fibroblasts and the effect of transforming growth factor-β. *Am Rev Respir Dis* 1989;140:95–100.
160. Idell S, Zwieb C, Boggaram J, Holiday D, Johnson AR, Raghu G. Mechanisms of fibrin formation and lysis by human lung fibroblasts: influence of TGF-β and TNF-alpha. *Am J Physiol* 1992;263:L487–494.
161. Gabbiani F, Le Lous M, Bailey AJ, Bazin S, Delaunay A. Collagen and myofibroblasts in granulation tissue. *Virchows Arch [B]* 1976; 21:133–145.
162. Clark JG. The molecular pathology of pulmonary fibrosis. In: Uitto J, Perejda AJ. *Connective tissue disease: molecular pathology of the extracellular matrix*. New York: Marcel Dekker; 1987:321–343.
163. Madri JA, Furthmayr H. Collagen polymorphism in the lung: an immunochemical study of pulmonary fibrosis. *Hum Pathol* 1980;11:353–366.
164. Phan SH. Diffuse interstitial fibrosis. In: Massaro D, ed. *Lung cell biology*. New York: Marcel Dekker; 1989:907–980.
165. Seyer JM, Hutcheson ET, Kang AH. Collagen polymorphism in idiopathic chronic pulmonary fibrosis. *J Clin Invest* 1976;57:1498–1507.
166. Kirk JME, Heard BE, Kerr I, Turner-Warwick M, Laurent GJ. Quantitation of types I and III collagen in biopsy lung samples from patients with cryptogenic fibrosing alveolitis. *Coll Relat Res* 1984;4:169–182.
167. Raghu G, Striker LJ, Hudson LD, Striker GE. Extracellular matrix in normal and fibrotic human lungs. *Am Rev Respir Dis* 1985;131:281–289.
168. Bateman E, Turner-Warwick M, Haslam PL, Adelmann-Grill BC. Cryptogenic fibrosing alveolitis: prediction of fibrogenic activity from immunohistochemical studies of collagen types in lung biopsy specimens. *Thorax* 1983;38:93–101.
169. Bateman E, Turner-Warwick M, Adelmann-Grill BC. Immunohistochemical study of col-

lagen types in human foetal lung and fibrotic lung disease. *Thorax* 1981;36:645–653.
170. Last JA, Siefkin AD, Reiser KM. Type I collagen content is increased in lungs of patients with adult respiratory distress syndrome. *Thorax* 1983;38:364–368.
171. Nerlich AG, Nerlich ML, Muller PK. Pattern of collagen types and molecular structure of collagen in acute post-traumatic pulmonary fibrosis. *Thorax* 1987;42:863–869.
172. Murphy G, Docherty AJP. The matrix metalloproteinases and their inhibitors. *Am J Respir Cell Mol Biol* 1992;7:120–125.
173. Emonard H, Grimaud JA. Matrix metalloproteinases: a review. *Cell Mol Biol* 1990;36:131–153.
174. Thrall RS, Phan SH, McCormick JR, Ward PA. The development of bleomycin-induced pulmonary fibrosis in neutrophil-depleted and complement-depleted rats. *Am J Pathol* 1981;105:76–81.
175. Phan SH, Schrier D, Mc Garry B, Duque RE. Effect of the beige mutation on bleomycin-induced pulmonary fibrosis in mice. *Am Rev Respir Dis* 1983;127:456–459.
176. Clark JG, Kuhn C III. Bleomycin-induced pulmonary fibrosis in hamsters: effect of neutrophil depletion on lung collagen synthesis. *Am Rev Respir Dis* 1982;126:737–739.
177. Shapiro SD, Campbell EJ, Kobayashi DK, Welgus HG. Immune modulation of metalloproteinase production in human macrophages: selective pretranslational suppression of interstitial collagenase and stromelysin biosynthesis by interferon gamma. *J Clin Invest* 1990;86:1204–1210.
178. Postlethwaite AE, Lachman LB, Mainardi CL, Kang AH. Interleukin 1 stimulation of collagenase production by cultured fibroblasts. *J Exp Med* 1983;157:801–806.
179. Edwards DRG, Murphy G, Reynolds JJ, Whitham SE, Docherty AJP, Angel P, Heath JK. Transforming growth factor beta modulates the expression of collagenase and metalloproteinase inhibitor. *EMBO J* 1987;6:1899–1904.
180. Emonard H, Takiya C, Dreze S, Cordier JF, Grimaud JA. Interstitial collagenase (MMP-1), gelatinase (MMP-2) and stromelysin (MMP-3) released by human fibroblasts cultured on acellular sarcoid granulomas (sarcoid matrix complex, SMC). *Matrix* 1989;9:382–388.
181. Laiho M, Saksela O, Keski-Oja J. Transforming growth factor-β induction of type-1 plasminogen activator inhibitor. *J Biol Chem* 1987;262:17467–17474.

Diseases of the Bronchioles, edited by
Gary R. Epler. Raven Press, Ltd.,
New York © 1994.

23

Connective-Tissue Disease Related Bronchiolitis Obliterans Organizing Pneumonia

Fernando J. Martinez and Joseph P. Lynch, III

Division of Pulmonary and Critical Care Medicine, Department of Internal Medicine, University of Michigan Medical Center, Ann Arbor, MI.

Bronchiolitis obliterans (with or without organizing pneumonia) represents a spectrum of inflammatory disorders involving small airways (respiratory and terminal bronchioles), which may occur as a rare manifestation of connective-tissue disorders or in the context of diverse insults to the lower respiratory tract including infectious organisms (e.g., *legionellae,* viruses, *mycoplasma*), smoke or toxic gas inhalation, as a complication of bone marrow or lung allograft transplantation, or as a response to pharmacological or exogenous agents (1–11). In many cases, no specific etiology or underlying disorder can be identified (1–11). The association of bronchiolitis obliterans or bronchiolitis obliterans organizing pneumonia (BOOP) and connective tissue diseases has been recognized for more than two decades (12–22). However, the literature is confusing, as a variety of terms such as organizing pneumonia, cryptogenic organizing pneumonia, bronchiolitis obliterans, obliterative bronchiolitis, constrictive bronchiolitis, and bronchiolitis obliterans with organizing pneumonia have been used often interchangeably to refer to a spectrum of bronchiolar diseases, in both idiopathic and connective-tissue disease variants (1–22). Before the discussion of bronchiolitis obliterans or BOOP in the context of connective-tissue disease, the salient clinical and histopathological features of these disorders are reviewed.

Although bronchiolitis obliterans and BOOP share overlapping features, these disorders differ in several important respects. Histologically, bronchiolitis obliterans is characterized by an exuberant inflammatory and fibrotic process involving terminal and respiratory bronchioles (1–3). Polypoid masses of granulation tissue, admixed with acute and chronic inflammatory cells and immature connective tissue, occlude or even obliterate bronchiolar lumina, resulting in airways obstruction (1–3). When this process extends into the alveolar spaces, with resultant consolidation of lung parenchyma, the term BOOP has been applied (1–3). Histological features of BOOP overlap with those of other chronic interstitial lung disorders, (e.g., usual interstitial pneumonitis and eosinophilic pneumonia), and these diagnoses may erroneously be suspected (3,5). In the pure form of bronchiolitis obliterans (also termed mural or constrictive bronchiolitis), peribronchiolar and submucosal scarring, bronchiolar inflammation, and concentric narrowing of airway lumina are evident; the pulmonary parenchyma is spared or only minimally involved (3). However, the histological spectrum and the extent and mixture of inflammatory and fibrotic components are heterogenous; in some patients, foci of bronchiolitis obliterans and BOOP are present concomitantly (3–5).

Clinically, bronchiolitis obliterans and BOOP behave quite differently. BOOP is usually characterized by focal alveolar infiltrates on chest radiograph, a subacute course, and a high rate of corticosteroid responsiveness (1,2,4,8,10). Cryptogenic organizing pneumonia and organizing pneumonia are synonymous with BOOP (6,7). Recent studies employing thin-section high-resolution CT scans (11) and bronchoalveolar lavage (8,10) have shed additional light on the salient features and pathogenetic mechanisms of BOOP; these diagnostic modalities are discussed in detail elsewhere in this book. Pure bronchiolitis obliterans exhibits a distinctly worse prognosis than does BOOP (1,2,8). The course of bronchiolitis obliterans is usually characterized by progressive, severe airflow obstruction and poor responsiveness to corticosteroid therapy or immunosuppressive agents; chest radiographs typically are normal or demonstrate only hyperinflation (1,2,8). The terms constrictive bronchiolitis, mural bronchiolitis, and obliterative bronchiolitis are synonymous with bronchiolitis obliterans (2–5). Unfortunately, even though the clinical features and prognoses of bronchiolitis obliterans and BOOP are disparate, these terms have often been used interchangeably.

Although both bronchiolitis obliterans and BOOP may complicate connective-tissue diseases, most reports (12–16) citing an association of bronchiolar disorder and connective-tissue diseases have described what appears to represent constrictive bronchiolitis or pure bronchiolitis obliterans. In 1977, Geddes (12) described six women, five of whom had classical rheumatoid arthritis, with severe and progressive air-flow obstruction due to what is now called constrictive bronchiolitis; corticosteroid therapy was ineffective in ameliorating the course of the disease. During the next few years, several investigations (13–22) corroborated the association of bronchiolitis obliterans in patients with connective-tissue diseases either as a primary manifestation or related to complications of pharmacological therapy such as penicillamine or gold salts. Several reports have cited an association of BOOP and connective-tissue diseases. In two comprehensive reviews (1,3) of BOOP confirmed by open lung biopsy, connective-tissue diseases were present in 7 of 57 and 5 of 24 patients, respectively. Guerry-Force and colleagues (5) described 16 patients with typical features of BOOP on open lung biopsy, i.e., intense peribronchiolar inflammation with tufts of loose connective tissue in respiratory bronchioles, alveolar ducts, and alveolar spaces; two of these patients had features consistent with mixed connective-tissue disease. In the original description (6) of cryptogenic organizing pneumonitis, 5 of 10 patients had rheumatoid arthritis. Four of 29 patients with BOOP recently described by Japanese investigators (10) had rheumatoid arthritis; 2 were also receiving gold salts. Sporadic cases of BOOP have been described as a manifestation of polymyositis/dermatomyositis (23,24), systemic lupus erythematosus (25–28), mixed connective-tissue disease (3), progressive systemic sclerosis (29,30), and miscellaneous autoimmune inflammatory disorders (31–39). It should be emphasized, however, that histological confirmation of bronchiolitis obliterans with or without organizing pneumonia has only rarely been obtained in the context of connective-tissue diseases. While open lung biopsies have frequently been performed for the diagnosis of idiopathic BOOP, many clinicians are unwilling to recommend open lung biopsy, the gold standard for the diagnosis of bronchiolitis obliterans or BOOP, in patients with known connective-tissue diseases presenting with pulmonary manifestations. In this context, empirical treatment with corticosteroid therapy or immunosuppressive agents is often initiated, without substantiating a specific histological diagnosis. Thus, limited data are available critically analyzing the prevalence, clinical syndromes, and response to therapy for bronchiolitis obliterans or BOOP occurring in the context of connective-tissue diseases. This chapter focuses on BOOP arising as a manifestation of specific connective-tissue or rheumatologic diseases.

RHEUMATOID ARTHRITIS

Rheumatoid arthritis has been associated with diverse pleuropulmonary manifestations including pleural effusion, rheumatoid (necrobiotic) pulmonary parenchymal nodules, Caplan's syndrome, chronic interstitial pneumonitis, pulmonary vasculitis, and bronchiolitis obliterans (37–40). Toxic or hypersensitivity reactions to pharmacological agents utilized in the treatment of rheumatoid arthritis (e.g., gold salts, methotrexate, cyclophosphamide, penicillamine) may also cause pulmonary parenchymal or bronchiolar injury, primarily in the form of chronic interstitial pneumonitis (39,40). Most studies assessing the pulmonary complications of rheumatoid arthritis have focused on chronic interstitial pneumonitis or "rheumatoid lung" (41–44). Factors associated with an increased prevalence of chronic interstitial lung disease in rheumatoid arthritis include male gender, cigarette smoking, subcutaneous rheumatoid nodules, $alpha_1$-antitrypsin variant phenotype, and prominent extra-articular manifestations (37,41). Of importance, the presence or extent of pulmonary parenchymal disease does not correlate with the activity of the articular or systemic disease process or titer of rheumatoid factor (37,40,41). Chronic interstitial lung disease is typically characterized by symptoms of dyspnea and nonproductive cough, which gradually progress over months or even years, associated with interstitial or reticulonodular infiltrates on chest radiograph and a restrictive ventilatory defect (37,40,41). The course of "rheumatoid lung" is often indolent, and historically most investigators have been reluctant to treat this condition aggressively with corticosteroid therapy or immunosuppressive agents. Recent studies have demonstrated evidence for active alveolar inflammation (e.g., increased intrapulmonary uptake of gallium; increased numbers of inflammatory cells, cytokines, and fibroblast growth factors in bronchoalveolar lavage fluid) in subsets of patients with rheumatoid arthritis (42–44). These data support an aggressive diagnostic and therapeutic approach in at least a subset of patients, particularly in those exhibiting a fulminant or deteriorating course. Open lung biopsy has rarely been performed for the histological diagnosis of chronic interstitial lung disease complicating rheumatoid arthritis, since physicians are often willing to treat patients solely on the basis of a compatible clinical and radiographic course. When open lung biopsy has been performed, histological features are often indistinguishable from those of idiopathic pulmonary fibrosis (38–41). Varying degrees of interstitial cellular infiltrates and fibrosis are noted; honeycombing, smooth-muscle proliferation, and extensive destruction of the alveolar architecture has been noted with advanced cases (38–41).

Although data are limited regarding the prevalence of bronchiolar involvement in rheumatoid arthritis, a recent detailed analysis (21) of 40 open lung biopsies from patients with suspected "rheumatoid lung" detected BOOP in 9. BOOP was the predominant histological pattern in 6 patients and a secondary, incidental pattern in 3 additional patients. In the same study, four additional histological patterns were recognized: pulmonary rheumatoid nodules, lymphoid hyperplasia, usual interstitial pneumonia (UIP), and cellular interstitial infiltrates. Pulmonary vasculitic changes were not observed in any of these patients. Segregating patients into specific clinical or histopathologic patterns was often not possible, however; and more than one histologic pattern was noted in 27 of the 40 patients. This study emphasizes the heterogeneity of histologic patterns seen in "rheumatoid lung disease" but also suggests that BOOP may be more common as a cause of "rheumatoid lung" than had previously been appreciated. Five of 6 patients with BOOP as the predominant pattern were treated with corticosteroids, with generally good response; at the time of followup, 4 of the 6 patients were alive without evidence of lung disease, 1 died of respiratory failure, and 1 died of an unrelated cause.

Other studies have suggested that small airways obstruction may be frequent in rheumatoid arthritis; however, a paucity of histologically confirmed cases of bronchiolitis have been described. Reductions in maximal midexpiratory flow rates consistent with airways obstruction were noted in 26 of 43 patients (61%) with classic rheumatoid arthritis in one prospective study (45); however, any relationship to rheumatoid arthritis is obscured by that fact that 24 of the 26 patients with abnormal pulmonary function were smokers. In addition, lung biopsies were not performed to delineate the site of the obstruction. A subsequent prospective study (46) revealed physiological evidence of airways obstruction in 32 of 100 consecutive patients with rheumatoid arthritis, raising the possibility that bronchiolar involvement may have been present in at least some patients. In 1977, Geddes and colleagues (12) described 6 patients with rapidly progressive airways obstruction, 5 of whom had classical rheumatoid arthritis. Despite treatment with corticosteroids, 5 died of respiratory failure 5 to 18 months after the onset of symptoms. Necropsy performed in 4 patients demonstrated features of obliterative (constrictive) bronchiolitis. Following that sentinel report, several cases of bronchiolitis obliterans complicating rheumatoid arthritis were reported; in some cases, previous therapy with gold salts or penicillamine had been used (1,13–18). In most instances, features were those of a constrictive obliterative bronchiolitis rather than BOOP; in some cases, both lesions were noted. The clinical course was usually characterized by progressive and severe airways obstruction unresponsive to corticosteroid therapy (12–18).

In 1982, Begin and colleagues (47) described open lung biopsy findings from six non-smokers with rheumatoid arthritis, five of whom had associated Sjogren's syndrome, who had physiological evidence for small airways disease. Lung biopsies demonstrated varying degrees of inflammatory bronchiolitis, associated with fibrosis and narrowing of airway lumina. The lesions exhibited a striking predilection for bronchioles, with minimal inflammation or fibrosis in the adjacent lung parenchyma, consistent with constrictive bronchiolitis rather than BOOP.

Thus, while the association of small airways disease and bronchiolitis obliterans complicating rheumatoid arthritis has been well recognized, a true organizing pneumonia-like pattern has only rarely been documented (see Table 1). In four reports (3,6,9,10) of histologically confirmed BOOP encompassing 115 patients, at least 11 patients had classical rheumatoid arthritis. In these patients, the clinical and radiographic features were similar to those of idiopathic BOOP. Flowers and colleagues (4) recently described seven patients with classical radiographic and histological features of BOOP, one of whom had preexisting seropositive rheumatoid arthritis. In the patient with rheumatoid arthritis associated BOOP, corticosteroid therapy resulted in prompt relief. Several additional cases of BOOP complicating rheumatoid arthritis have been described. In 1981, Herzog and colleagues (18) reported a patient with rheumatoid arthritis manifesting progressive airways obstruction and multiple nodular infiltrates on chest radiograph. Open lung biopsy demonstrated acute bronchiolitis and rare foci of organizing pneumonia. Immunofluorescent stains demonstrated linear deposition of IgG along alve-

TABLE 1. *BOOP in rheumatoid arthritis*

Reference	Year	Number of patients
Cooney (17)	1981	1
Yousem et al. (21)	1985	6 with primary pathologic pattern; 3 secondary
Katzenstein et al. (3)	1986	1
Rees et al. (19)	1991	3
van Thiel et al. (20)	1991	1
Flowers et al. (4)	1992	1
Yamamoto et al. (10)	1992	4

olar walls. Ibuprofen was administered, with symptomatic relief; at long-term followup, chest radiographs were clear and the patient was asymptomatic.

Cooney and colleagues (17) described three patients with rheumatoid arthritis who exhibited peripheral pulmonary infiltrates, blood eosinophilia, and restrictive pulmonary defects. Open lung biopsy, performed in two patients, demonstrated polypoid masses of granulation tissue occluding small bronchioles as well as foci of chronic interstitial pneumonitis and eosinophilic pneumonia; the overlapping features of BOOP and eosinophilic pneumonia have been noted by others (1,3,9). Both patients responded well to corticosteroid therapy. The third patient with rheumatoid arthritis had peripheral blood eosinophilia and patchy upper lobe infiltrates, which initially regressed with corticosteroid therapy; no lung biopsy was performed. However, she subsequently deteriorated and died of progressive respiratory failure within 6 months of onset of dyspnea. Necropsy demonstrated bronchiolitis obliterans throughout both lungs. While a detailed description of histology was not provided, this third patient likely had constrictive bronchiolitis.

Rees and colleagues (19) described three patients with BOOP and rheumatoid arthritis, all of whom presented with the subacute onset of dyspnea and cough. Crackles were audible in the lower lungs; pulmonary function tests demonstrated a restrictive defect with impaired diffusion capacity. Bilateral infiltrates were noted on chest radiograph; open lung biopsy confirmed typical changes of BOOP. Corticosteroid therapy produced significant improvement.

In 1991, van Thiel and colleagues (20) described a patient with seropositive rheumatoid arthritis and progressive hypoxemic respiratory failure ultimately requiring mechanical ventilatory support. Chest radiographs revealed bilateral alveolar opacities; open lung biopsy showed typical changes of BOOP. Corticosteroid therapy achieved a prompt remission.

Apart from these sporadic case reports, limited data are available regarding the frequency of BOOP in rheumatoid arthritis. Nonetheless, it is clear that BOOP may complicate rheumatoid arthritis and on occasion may result in fulminant, even fatal, respiratory insufficiency. In light of favorable responses to corticosteroid therapy in some cases, BOOP complicating rheumatoid arthritis should be treated aggressively with corticosteroids. An initial dose of prednisone, 1 mg/kg/day or equivalent, for 3 to 6 weeks is reasonable; once a remission has been achieved, a gradual taper can be initiated. Duration and rate of taper need to be individualized, but a minimum of 9 to 12 months of therapy is recommended to reduce the chance for recrudescent disease.

POLYMYOSITIS/DERMATOMYOSITIS

Polymyositis and dermatomyositis are autoimmune, inflammatory myopathies associated with a wide spectrum of pulmonary abnormalities including aspiration pneumonitis from weakness of the pharyngeal or esophageal musculature, respiratory insufficiency from primary involvement of the respiratory muscles or diaphragmatic dysfunction, opportunistic lung infections in patients on corticosteroids or immunosuppressive medications, chronic interstitial lung disease, and BOOP (23,24,37–40, 48–49). In contradistinction to rheumatoid arthritis or systemic lupus erythematosus, pleural involvement has rarely been described in polymyositis/dermatomyositis. Several studies (23,24,48–51) have examined pulmonary parenchymal involvement, primarily manifesting as chronic interstitial pneumonitis. Clinical evidence for chronic interstitial lung disease has been noted in only 3 to 10% of patients, but the incidence of asymptomatic involvement with chronic interstitial lung disease is much higher (23,24,48,49). The extent and severity of the pulmonary inflammatory/fibrotic process do not correlate with the extent of muscle or systemic involvement; in fact, chronic interstitial lung disease may the presenting or predominant feature of the disease (48,49). Specific serological markers may identify patients at risk for development of chronic interstitial lung disease. For example, circulating autoantibodies to the enzyme histidyl-t-RNA-synthetase (anti-Jo-1, anti-PL7, anti-PL-12), and anti-KJ have been noted in up to 70% of patients with polymyositis and chronic interstitial lung disease, but in fewer than 20% of patients without lung involvement (50,51). No studies have examined these serological markers in patients with bronchiolar involvement.

Limited data are available regarding the prevalence of bronchiolitis or BOOP in polymyositis/dermatomyositis (Table 2). Histologically confirmed cases of BOOP complicating polymyositis or dermatomyositis have only rarely been described. In a classical review of pulmonary manifestations of polymyositis, Schwarz and colleagues (23) described 3 patients with polymyositis and histologic features consistent with BOOP.

TABLE 2. *BOOP in polymyositis/dermatomyositis*

Reference	Year	Number of patients
Schwartz et al. (23)	1976	3
Epler et al. (1)	1985	1
Katzenstein et al. (3)	1986	2
Tazelaar et al. (24)	1990	6

The clinical scenario of dyspnea, patchy chest radiographic findings, and restrictive lung disease also support this diagnosis. Two improved with corticosteroid therapy. One of 7 patients with connective tissue disease-associated BOOP reported by Epler and co-workers (1) had polymyositis. This patient exhibited an "an acute problem superimposed on chronic interstitial pneumonia," which partially responded to corticosteroid therapy. Two of 24 patients with BOOP reported by Katzenstein and associates (3) had polymyositis. The most comprehensive analysis of histological features of pulmonary complications of polymyositis/dermatomyositis was provided by investigators at the Mayo Clinic, based upon open lung biopsies in 14 patients and necropsy in 1 (24). The fact that only 14 patients with polymyositis or dermatomyositis had open lung biopsy performed for evaluation of interstitial lung disease at the Mayo Clinic between 1965 and 1989 underscores the reluctance of most clinicians to biopsy patients with underlying connective-tissue diseases. Three major histological patterns were identified: BOOP, usual interstitial pneumonitis, and diffuse alveolar damage. BOOP was the predominant histological pattern in 6 patients; the hallmark was patchy foci of organizing pneumonia and an associated bronchiolitis obliterans with granulation tissue filling bronchioles and alveolar ducts. Five exhibited predominantly usual interstitial pneumonitis; 3, diffuse alveolar damage. One patient exhibited a nonspecific cellular interstitial pneumonitis, similar to what has been seen in other connective-tissue diseases (21). All patients with BOOP were treated with corticosteroid therapy; 2 died of complications of open lung biopsy, but the remaining 4 were alive and well at prolonged follow-up. Prognosis of the remaining histological groups was poor. Three of 5 patients with usual interstitial pneumonitis and all 3 patients with diffuse alveolar damage died.

In summary, BOOP has rarely been documented as a complication of polymyositis or dermatomyositis, although this in part may reflect the infrequency with which lung biopsies are performed in these disorders. We believe that transbronchial lung biopsies are often adequate to exclude alternative etiologies in the context of connective-tissue disease, and open lung biopsies are warranted only in problematic cases or when findings on transbronchial lung biopsies are inadequate. Although data regarding therapy are limited, corticosteroids are the cornerstone of therapy, with anticipated response rates in excess of 67%.

SYSTEMIC LUPUS ERYTHEMATOSUS

Pleuropulmonary manifestations of systemic lupus erythematosus are protean and include pleuritis, with or without pleural effusion; acute lupus pneumonitis; chronic interstitial pneumonitis; diaphragmatic dysfunction; pulmonary vasculitis; pulmonary hypertension; pulmonary embolism, particularly in association with anticardiolipin antibodies; and alveolar hemorrhage (28,37–39,52–61). Lupus pleuritis, with or without pleural effusion, the most common pleuropulmonary manifestation of systemic lupus erythematosus, is noted in up to 60% of patients at some point in the course of the disease (37–39,52,53). Acute lupus pneumonitis may be observed in up to 5% of patients; chronic interstitial pneumonitis occurs in fewer than 3% (55,56). BOOP has only rarely been reported in association with systemic lupus erythematosus, although its frequency may be underestimated due to the frequent implementation of corticosteroid therapy for "lupus pneumonitis" or other pulmonary manifestations. Since open lung biopsy has rarely been performed in these patients, it is possible that some patients believed to have acute lupus pneumonitis or chronic interstitial pneumonitis may have features consistent with or overlapping with BOOP.

Early comprehensive reviews of pulmonary manifestations of systemic lupus erythematosus described features consistent with bronchiolitis obliterans or BOOP, but a paucity of histologically confirmed cases have been documented (see Table 3). Matthay and colleagues (28) described histological features consistent with obliterative bronchiolitis, or perhaps BOOP, in 1 of 12 patients with acute lupus pneumonitis. In that patient, open lung biopsy documented interstitial pneumonitis with narrowed bronchioles and focal occlusion with "granulation tissue infiltrated by lymphocytes, plasma cells and neutrophils." Although initial radiographic improvement was noted after institution of corticosteroid therapy, the patient subsequently died of extensive pulmonary nocardiosis. One of 24 cases of BOOP described by Katzen-

TABLE 3. *BOOP in systemic lupus erythematosus*

Reference	Year	Number of patients
Matthay et al. (28)	1974	1
Kinney and Angelillo (26)	1987	1
Katzenstein et al. (3)	1986	1
Nadorra et al. (27)	1987	13
Guerry-Force et al. (5)	1987	3(?)
Gammon et al. (25)	1992	2

stein and colleagues (3) had systemic lupus erythematosus. Guerry-Force and colleagues (5) mention 3 patients with BOOP, a positive antinuclear antibody, and features compatible with systemic lupus erythematosus or mixed connective-tissue disease. Nadorra and Landing (27) reviewed 26 open lung biopsies from pediatric patients with systemic lupus erythematosus exhibiting diverse pulmonary manifestations; fibrous tissue plugs within bronchioles and alveoli were noted in 13 patients. However, diffuse alveolar damage and other complicating illnesses were frequently present concomitantly, so the primary role of BOOP was not clear. Kinney and Angelillo (26) described a patient with systemic lupus erythematosus who had progressive cough and dyspnea, rales, wheezing, and midinspiratory squeaks on chest auscultation, and a mixed obstructive-restrictive defect on pulmonary function tests. Chest radiograph demonstrated an infiltrate in the right middle lobe. Open lung biopsy demonstrated interstitial fibrosis, focal alveolar hemorrhage, fibrinous pleuritis, and focal obliterative bronchiolitis; in some sections, bronchiolar lumina were completely occluded by cellular debris. These histological features, although consistent with BOOP, suggest that additional processes were operative concomitantly. Prompt improvement was noted with high-dose corticosteroid therapy.

More recently, Gammon and others (25) described two patients with systemic lupus erythematosus in whom BOOP was confirmed by open lung biopsy. In both patients, progressive cough, dyspnea, and focal alveolar opacities on chest radiographs were noted. In the first patient, the abrupt onset of cough, chest pain, dyspnea, and fatigue precipitated admission. Despite aggressive antibiotics, rapid deterioration and hypoxemic respiratory failure necessitated mechanical ventilatory support over the next 24 hours. Transbronchial lung biopsy performed on the second hospital day demonstrated organizing pneumonia; because of persistent respiratory failure, open lung biopsy, performed on day 9, demonstrated BOOP. High-dose corticosteroid therapy resulted in marked and prompt improvement. The second patient, a 28-year-old woman in previously excellent health, presented with subacute arthritic symptoms and 2 weeks of dyspnea on exertion, pleuritic chest pain, rash, and profound constitutional symptoms. Mild hypoxemia and bilateral alveolar and interstitial infiltrates on chest radiograph were present. Lupus prep, anti-Smith, anti-RNP, SS-A, and SS-B antibodies and serum complement levels were normal; however, anti-ds DNA was positive with 12% uptake. The combination of anti-ds antibodies, arthritis, leukopenia, and pleuritis fulfilled criteria for systemic lupus erythematosus. Open lung biopsy performed on the sixth hospital day confirmed BOOP with associated interstitial inflammatory infiltrates. Prednisone, 60 mg/day, was associated with resolution of fever and articular symptoms, but respiratory failure ensued. Despite the addition of cyclophosphamide, she died of respiratory failure 2 months after the diagnosis.

In summary, BOOP may rarely complicate systemic lupus erythematosus; the clinical, radiographic, and histological features may be indistinguishable from the idiopathic form. Although data regarding therapy are limited, we recommend corticosteroids as initial therapy; immunosuppressive or cytotoxic agents should be reserved for patients refractory to corticosteroids or experiencing corticosteroid adverse effects.

MIXED CONNECTIVE-TISSUE DISEASE

Mixed connective-tissue disease displays clinical features that overlap with two or more connective-tissue diseases and exhibits such distinctive serological features as high titer serum antibodies to extractable nuclear antigen (ENA) and to ribonucleoprotein (anti-RNP), speckled antinuclear antibody, and lack of antibodies to Sm antigen (62–64). Extrapulmonary features such as Raynaud's phenomenon, sclerodactyly, polyarthritis, esophageal dysmotility, alopecia, malar rash, and myositis typically dominate (62–64). Although pulmonary features were not described in the initial report in 1972 (62), subsequent studies have documented that pulmonary involvement occurs in a majority of patients (63–66). Pleuritis has been noted in one-third and chronic interstitial pneumonitis in 30 to 85% of patients (63–66). Pulmonary hypertension has been noted in 10 to 30% of patients, typically in those with features of scleroderma, and is an important cause of mortality (63,64). The presence of microvascular changes in the nail beds has been predictive of the subsequent development of pulmonary hypertension(64).

Clinical and radiographic features of chronic interstitial pneumonitis complicating mixed connective-tissue disease are indistinguishable from those of the idiopathic variety (40). Open lung biopsies have rarely been performed in the context of mixed connective-tissue disease. However, when lung biopsies have been performed, pulmonary hypertensive changes have usually predominated; coexistent interstitial inflammation or fibrosis may also be evident (64). The prevalence and extent of bronchiolar involvement or BOOP have not been delineated. Bronchiolar involvement was not mentioned in five comprehensive clinical studies of mixed connective tissue disease (62–66). One of 24 patients with BOOP described by Katzenstein and coworkers (3) had mixed connective-tissue disease (Table 4). Corticosteroid therapy may be effective for the inflammatory manifestations of mixed connective-tissue disease such as arthritis, serositis, and myositis; less data are available regarding their efficacy in chronic interstitial pneumonitis or other pulmonary manifestations (63,65). Favorable responses were noted in 5 of 9 patients with chronic interstitial pneumonitis complicating mixed connective-tissue disease in one study; (63) there are anecdotal reports of patients responding favorably to cyclophosphamide, including patients refractory to corticosteroids (63).

In view of its rarity, no data are available regarding therapy for BOOP complicating mixed connective-tissue disease. However, we believe management of BOOP in this context should be similar to that of idiopathic BOOP (1). Initial treatment with corticosteroids, 1 mg/kg/day prednisone or equivalent, for 3 to 6 weeks, with gradual taper, is appropriate; immunosuppressive or cytotoxic agents should be reserved for patients who do not respond corticosteroid therapy.

Progressive Systemic Sclerosis

Progressive systemic sclerosis (scleroderma) is a poorly understood autoimmune disorder characterized by extensive fibrosis and vascular abnormalities affecting multiple sites (67–69). Dominant clinical

TABLE 4. *BOOP and miscellanous connective tissue diseases*

Reference	Year	Number of patients	Connective tissue disease
Davison et al. (7)	1983	1	Digital vasculitis
Davison and Epstein (29)	1983	1	Scleroderma
Bridges et al. (75)	1992	2	Scleroderma
Epler and Mark (36)	1986	1	Polymyalgia rheumatica
Matteson and Ike (31)	1990	1	Sjogren's syndrome
Usui et al. (84)	1992	1	Sjogren's syndrome
Yamamoto et al. (10)	1992	1	Behçet's disease
Katzenstein et al. (3)	1986	1	Mixed connective tissue disease
Robinson et al. (94)	1992	1	Polyarteritis nodosa
Chien et al. (33)	1991	1	Sweet's syndrome

manifestations are dysphagia secondary to esophageal dysmotility, cutaneous changes such as sclerodactyly or telangiectasia, hypertension of nephrosclerosis, and pulmonary complications (67–69). Pulmonary manifestations of progressive systemic sclerosis include chronic interstitial lung disease, pulmonary hypertension, aspiration pneumonia reflecting esophageal dysfunction, and bronchioloalveolar cell carcinoma (67–69). Pleuritic chest pain or pleural effusions are not a feature of progressive systemic sclerosis. Clinically evident pulmonary fibrosis or pulmonary hypertension has been noted in 20 to 60% of patients; the difference in sensitivity reflects different methods used to detect these aberrations (67–74). Pulmonary symptoms of cough or dyspnea occur in 30 to 60% and chest radiographs are abnormal in 20 to 50% of patients (67–70). When pulmonary parenchymal abnormalities are present, interstitial or reticulonodular infiltrates, small lung volumes, and honeycombing are characteristic (67–70). Abnormalities of pulmonary function studies reflect a restrictive defect, with reduced vital capacity and lung volumes, and impaired gas transfer, as reflected by abnormal diffusing capacity (67–69). Mild degrees of airways obstruction may be observed, but a pure obstructive defect is rare (67–69). These clinical and radiographic features primarily reflect components of fibrosis and derangement of the pulmonary interstitium and pulmonary vasculature.

Open lung biopsies have rarely been performed in progressive systemic sclerosis. However, at necropsy, more than 80% of patients have evidence of chronic interstitial lung disease and pulmonary hypertensive changes are evident in 70 to 95% of patients (67–69). Characteristic histological changes on lung biopsy or necropsy include extensive collagen deposition, destruction and disruption of the alveolar architecture, honeycombing, smooth-muscle hypertrophy, and pulmonary hypertensive and atherosclerotic changes (67–69). Interstitial or intra-alveolar inflammation is usually mild or conspicuously absent, which contrasts with the marked degree of inflammatory cell infiltrate in chronic interstitial lung disease complicating other disorders (37–40,67–69). However, recent studies have demonstrated increased numbers of activated immune effector cells such as alveolar macrophages, lymphocytes, andpolymorphonuclear leukocytes in bronchoalveolar lavage fluid and increased intrapulmonary uptake of gallium in up to 50 to 75% of patients with progressive systemic sclerosis, suggesting that active alveolar inflammation (alveolitis) is present in at least some subsets of patients (70–73).

Peribronchiolar fibrosis may develop in the context of chronic interstitial lung disease complicating progressive systemic sclerosis, but evidence for an acute bronchiolar inflammatory disorder or BOOP appears to be exceedingly rare (67–69). The natural history of chronic interstitial lung disease complicating progressive systemic sclerosis has been a gradual but inexorable decline in pulmonary function, often over several years (67–69). Five-year mortality rates of 30 to 50% have been cited, once pulmonary symptoms or significant radiographic changes have become apparent (67–69).

Historically, the approach to progressive systemic sclerosis has been one of therapeutic nihilism. However, in light of recent studies suggesting that subsets of patients exhibit active alveolitis, corticosteroids, and immunosuppressive and antifibrotic agents such as penicillamine have been tried, with anecdotal successes (69l,71–73). The role and efficacy of therapy in the context of progressive systemic sclerosis remains highly controversial.

Pulmonary hypertension complicating progressive systemic sclerosis has been associated with an increased mortality (67,69). Severe Raynaud's phenomenon, digital ulceration or pitting, peripheral vascular involvement, a diffusing capacity less than 50% predicted, and a history of cigarette smoking have been associated with a greater likelihood of developing pulmonary hypertension (67–69, 74). Unfortunately, there is no evidence that vasodilator agents or other therapies influence or reverse the pulmonary vascular component. Since the lesion appears to be one of progressive vascular obliteration and fibrosis, therapies directly at reversing the pulmonary hypertensive changes will likely be ineffectual.

Currently, no studies have specifically addressed the prevalence of bronchiolar involvement in progressive systemic sclerosis. Although it is possible that subsets of patients exhibiting alveolar inflammation may display concomitant bronchiolar inflammation or bronchiolitis, BOOP has only rarely been described in patients with progressive systemic sclerosis.

In 1983, Davison and colleagues (29) described a patient with primary biliary cirrhosis, CREST (calcinosis, Raynaud's phenomenon, esophageal dysfunction, sclerodactyly, and telangiectasia) syndrome, and chronic pancreatitis who developed recurrent episodes of pneumonia; lung biopsy displayed typical characteristics of cryptogenic organizing pneumonitis.

More recently, two patients with progressive systemic sclerosis, rapidly evolving pulmonary infiltrates, restrictive lung disease, and markedly diminished diffusing capacity were described (75). Open lung biopsy in both patients demonstrated BOOP. One patient responded well to high-dose corticosteroid therapy with marked initial improvement; chest radiographs and pulmonary symptoms resolved, but impairment in diffusing capacity persisted despite improvement in pulmonary mechanics. The second patient exhibited a gradual deteriorating course and died of respiratory failure 12 weeks after open lung biopsy despite high-dose prednisone therapy.

Yousem (30) recently reviewed autopsy and surgical pathology files from the University of Pittsburgh from 1960 to 1989 for all cases of CREST syndrome and pulmonary symptoms or abnormal pulmonary function tests. Histological material (which included four open lung biopsies and 13 necropsies) from 17 patients was reviewed. Changes consistent with pulmonary hypertension or usual interstitial pneumonitis dominated; however, 1 patient had a predominant pattern of chronic small airways injury, with concentric constriction of terminal and respiratory bronchioles. A chronic submucosal inflammatory cell infiltrate was also noted. Eight additional patients had minor changes indicative of small airways disease; all but 1 were smokers, so the relationship of small airways disease to progressive systemic sclerosis is not clear.

Bjerke and colleagues (76) evaluated pulmonary function tests in 39 patients (22 nonsmokers and 17 smokers) with progressive systemic sclerosis to assess the prevalence of small airways disease. Chest radiographs were available for review in 37 and were normal in 20; mild to moderate interstitial fibrosis was evident on chest radiographs in 16 patients; 1 patient had honeycombing. Reductions in diffusing capacity were observed in most; the ratio of forced expiratory volume in one second to forced vital capacity (FEV_1/FVC) was normal in all subjects. More sensitive measurements of small airways dysfunction, including maximal midexpiratory flow rates, closing volume, volume of isoflow, frequency dependence of lung compliance, and other parameters, were obtained in all patients. Only 3 of 22 nonsmokers had abnormalities in more than one test of small airways function; by contrast, one or more parameters were abnormal in the majority of smokers. The authors suggested that functional obstruction of the peripheral airways was an uncommon feature of progressive systemic sclerosis, even among patients with chronic interstitial lung disease; when obstructive changes were found, these could usually be attributed to the effects of cigarette smoking. No lung biopsies were obtained in this study, but it appears that clinically significant bronchiolar involvement is unusual in progressive systemic sclerosis.

Given the rarity of BOOP as a manifestation of progressive systemic sclerosis, optimal therapy is not clear. We have yet to see a patient with BOOP complicating progressive systemic sclerosis, but we believe management of such cases should be similar to that of idiopathic BOOP.

Sjogren's Syndrome

Sjogren's syndrome is characterized by clinical symptoms of xerostomia and xerophthalmia (sicca syndrome), associated with pathological evidence of lymphocytic infiltrates affecting exocrine (such as salivary or lacrimal) glands (39,77–81). Sjogren's syndrome may occur as a primary disorder without associated connective-tissue disease but may also arise in the context of systemic lupus erythematosus, rheumatoid arthritis, progressive systemic sclerosis, polymyositis/dermatomyositis, or primary biliary cirrhosis (39,77–81). Pulmonary complications have been noted in 5 to 25% of patients with Sjogren's syndrome (39,77–81). Lymphocytic interstitial pneumonitis, pseudolymphoma, and lymphoma are rare but well recognized complications (82,83). Chronic interstitial lung disease may also develop but is severe in fewer than 3% of cases (39). However, recent prospective studies have noted evidence of chronic interstitial lung disease in 25 to 38% of patients with primary Sjogren's syndrome (78,79). In addition, subclinical alveolitis appears to be common, as recent studies have demonstrated increased numbers of inflammatory cells, typically lymphocytes, in bronchoalveolar lavage fluids in up to 50% of patients with primary or secondary Sjogren's syndrome (77,79,80). Xerotrachea, due to involvement of the exocrine glands of the trachea and bronchial tree, may result in paroxysmal, irritating dry cough; the frequency of this complication has been highly variable (0 to 17%) (39, 78,80).

The frequency of bronchiolar involvement in Sjogren's syndrome has not been delineated. Reductions in midexpiratory flow rates suggestive of small airways disease were noted in 8 of 36 (22%) patients in one study (80). Transbronchial lung biopsies were performed in only 5 patients in that study: lymphocytic infiltrates and fibrosis were noted within lung parenchyma, but bronchiolar abnormalities were not mentioned. Newball and Brahim (32) reported histological evidence for mononuclear cell infiltration involving bronchioles in 2 patients with Sjogren's syndrome.

To our knowledge, only two reports of BOOP complicating Sjogren's syndrome have been described in the English language literature (31,84). Matteson and Ike (31) described a 52-year-old man with fever, weight loss, cough, and dry eyes and mouth. Retinal vasculitis, posterior uveitis, and patchy, bilateral airspace disease with areas of alveolar confluence were evident (Fig. 1). Pulmonary function tests disclosed a mild mixed obstructive-restrictive ventilatory defect and mild hypoxemia. Open lung biopsy demonstrated organizing pneumonia with marked fibroblastic proliferation and obliteration of the bronchioles by granulation tissue (Fig. 2). No vasculitis was identified. Biopsy of a minor salivary gland supported the diagnosis of Sjogren's syndrome (Tarpley grade IV). High-dose corticosteroid therapy led to dramatic improvement. Symptoms and chest radiographs normalized within 2 months, and corticosteroids were withdrawn after 3 months. At the time of follow-up 18 months later, the patient remained asymptomatic, with only mild evidence of small airways obstruction on pulmonary function tests. Usui and colleagues (84) described a 69-year-old woman with primary Sjogren's syndrome who developed bilateral, peripheral alveolar infiltrates and progressive respiratory failure. She died 3 days after initiation of pulse methylprednisolone 1,000 mg/day. Necropsy demonstrated intrabron-

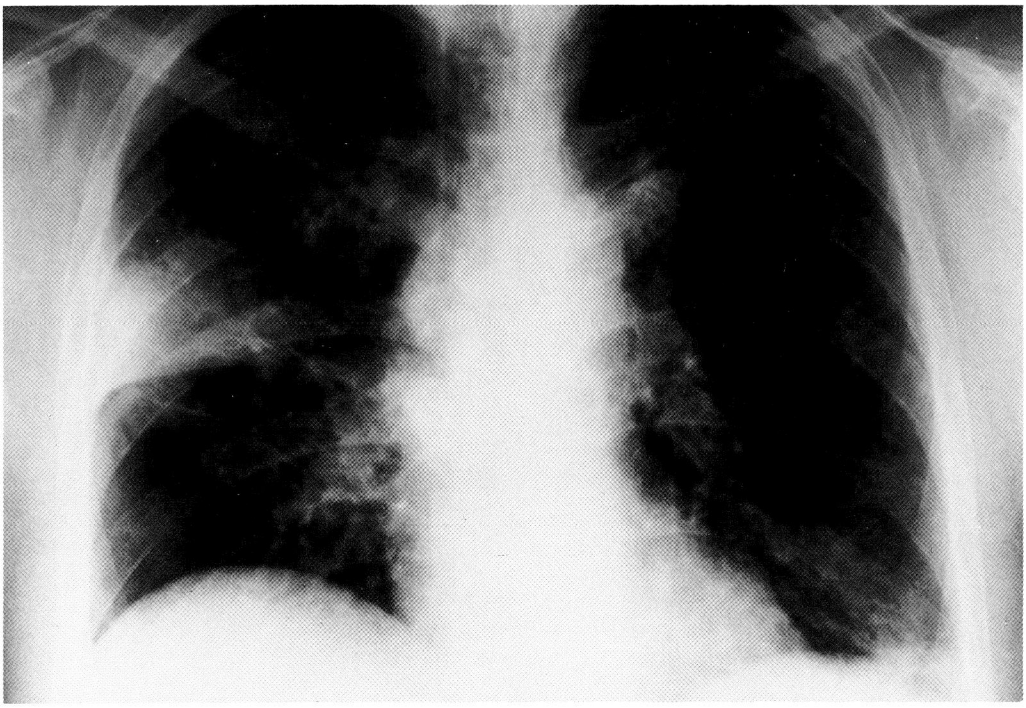

FIG. 1. Posteroanterior chest radiograph demonstrates alveolar infiltrate in the right upper lobe as well as patchy airspace disease in the right and left lower lobes. Open lung biopsy confirmed BOOP. From ref. 31 with permission.

chiolar granulation tissue extending to the alveolar ducts and extensive organizing pneumonia, consistent with BOOP; hyaline membranes and the typical exudative changes of diffuse alveolar damage were present concomitantly. Thus, the clinical and pathological findings of BOOP may be broad and may overlap with concomitant processes.

Sweet's syndrome

Sweet's syndrome (febrile neutrophilic dermatosis), characterized by fever, peripheral blood eosinophilia, multiple cutaneous plaques, and neutrophilic infiltration of the dermis, has rarely been associated with pulmonary complications (85). Malignancy, especially hematological neoplasia, has been observed in up to 20% of patients (85). Extracutaneous features, such as arthralgias, myalgias, conjunctivitis, proteinuria, hematuria, and changes on liver biopsy, may be found in up to 50%, particularly in patients exhibiting concomitant neoplasia (85).

To our knowledge, only five patients have been described with pulmonary manifestations; four had concomitant hematological malignancy (33,85–88). Lung biopsy demonstrated neutrophilic infiltrates and chronic interstitial pneumonitis in three (85,86,88); one patient had no lung biopsy, but pulmonary infiltrates resolved with corticosteroid therapy (87). The remaining patient had BOOP (33). That patient, a 58-year-old man, had a cough, night sweats, fever, and generalized skin eruption for 1 month. Skin biopsy demonstrated typical

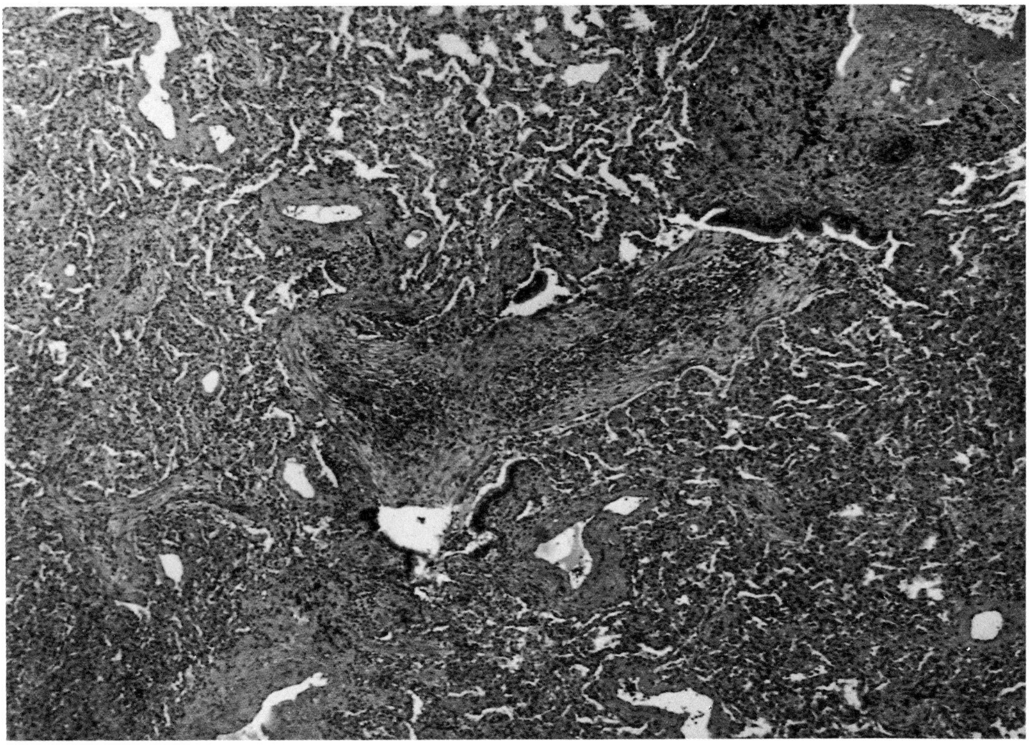

A

FIG. 2. Photomicrographs (open lung biopsy). **A,** Within the center of the field is a bronchiole that has been completely occluded by a chronic inflammatory cellular infiltrate, loose connective tissue, and collagen. Note the extensive inflammatory cellular infiltrates in the surrounding lung parenchyma. These features are indicative of BOOP. **B,** Note the polypoid mass of organizing granulation tissue nearly completly occluding the bronchiolar lumen. From ref. 96 with permission. **C,** Loose connective tissue and mononuclear inflammatory cellular infiltrate completely occlude bronchiolar lumen. The inflammatory process has extended into the adjacent distal lung parenchyma. (Hematoxylin-eosin; high power.)

findings of Sweet's syndrome; open lung biopsy confirmed BOOP. Corticosteroid therapy led to sustained remission. No malignancy or relapse of BOOP was seen during a 6-year follow-up.

Ulcerative colitis

Ulcerative colitis has been associated with diverse pulmonary manifestations, including interstitial pneumonitis, sarcoid-like granulomas, apical infiltrates, lymphocytic bronchitis, chronic bronchitial suppuration and bronchiectasis, and pulmonary vasculitis (39,89–93). While the pathogenetic mechanisms remain to be delineated, circulating immune complexes may elicit a local inflammatory response, with regional lymphatic and pulmonary interstitial inflammatory components. We are aware of only one patient in whom BOOP complicating ulcerative colitis has been documented in the absence of other risk factors. Swinburn and co-workers (34) described a young woman with ulcerative colitis who presented with fever, cough, dyspnea, and pleuritic chest pain 4 years after the initial diagnosis of inflammatory bowel disease. Chest radiographs demonstrated right-sided peripheral infiltrates, and open lung biopsy confirmed BOOP. Prednisone

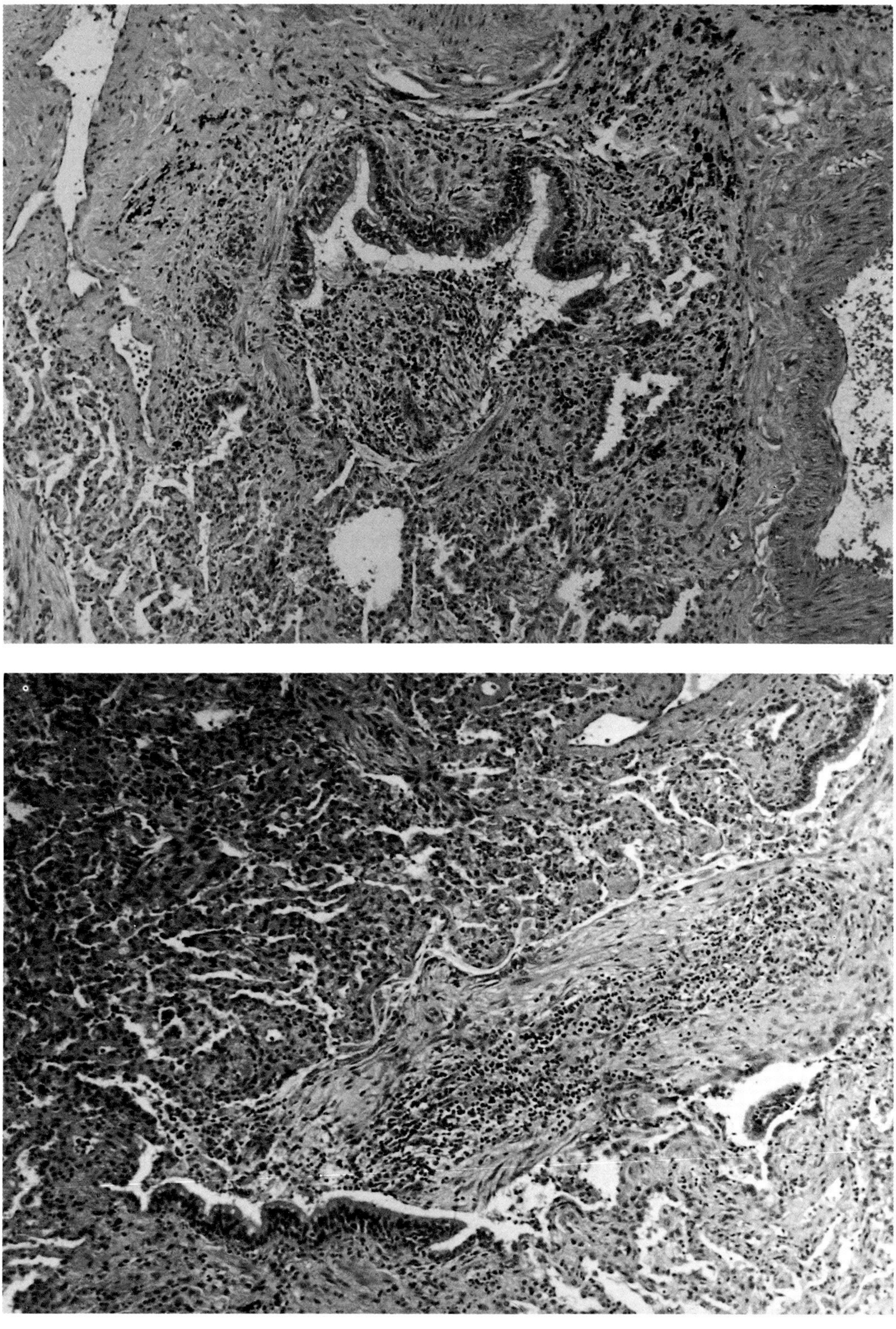

B

C

FIG. 2. *Continued*

therapy resulted in marked, long-lasting, symptomatic relief and radiographic improvement. Williams and associates (35) described a patient with ulcerative colitis who suffered dry cough, fever, night sweats, upper lobe infiltrates on chest radiographs, airflow obstruction, and abnormal diffusing capacity while taking sulfasalazine. Symptoms progressed despite discontinuation of sulfasalazine. Open lung biopsy demonstrated chronic interstitial pneumonitis and marked bronchiolitis obliterans. Rapid improvement was noted after institution of corticosteroid therapy. In this patient, BOOP likely reflected a reaction to sulfasalazine, since this agent has been implicated as a rare cause of interstitial and eosinophilic pneumonias (40,93); however, it is possible that ulcerative colitis may have played a contributory role in the pathogenesis of the lung lesion.

MISCELLANEOUS

BOOP has rarely been reported in association with other connective-tissue or immunologically mediated disorders. Two patients with BOOP complicating polymyalgia rheumatica (3,36) and isolated case reports of BOOP complicating Behçet's disease (10), digital vaculitis (7), and polyarteritis nodosa (94) have been described.

CONCLUSION

BOOP is a well-defined, clinicopathological entity that has occasionally been observed in association with connective-tissue diseases; in that context, rheumatoid arthritis, polymyositis, and dermatomyositis have accounted for most cases. Only anecdotal occurrences of BOOP have been described as a manifestation of systemic lupus erythematosus, progressive systemic sclerosis, and other autoimmune disorders. In various large studies of BOOP, connective-tissue diseases have accounted for 4 to 21% of cases (1,3,5,6,9,10). The clinical and histopathological features of BOOP complicating connective-tissue diseases are similar to those of idiopathic BOOP (1–4). The prognosis of BOOP in connective-tissue diseases has generally been favorable; most patients respond rapidly to corticosteroid therapy. A definitive diagnosis requires lung biopsy; however, in many patients, a presumptive diagnosis can be made by transbronchial lung biopsy and bronchoalveolar lavage. Bronchoscopic procedures are most helpful in excluding alternative disorders such as infection (40,54), but the diagnostic features of BOOP can occasionally be observed even with transbronchial lung biopsies (2,8,40). In view of its potential morbidity and even mortality, the role of open lung biopsy is controversial. However, open lung biopsy is warranted when transbronchial lung biopsies are nondiagnostic and the clinical features are atypical or infection is a significant consideration. Video-assisted thoracoscopy surgery may be performed with less morbidity and may be an acceptable alternative to open thoracotomy biopsy (95). Transbronchial lung biopsies may be adequate in some patients to rule out alternative causes, particularly infectious etiologies, and to allow institution of corticosteroid therapy (54). In this context, favorable responses may be observed as early as 2 to 5 days after onset of treatment. Response to treatment may be used as a diagnostic guide, particularly when transbronchial lung biopsies are equivocal. Corticosteroids are the cornerstone of therapy for BOOP complicating connective-tissue diseases. Although the optimal dose and duration of therapy have not been delineated, we believe an initial dose of prednisone, 1 mg/kg/day or equivalent, for 3 to 6 weeks is usually sufficient to elicit a favorable response. Once a favorable response has been achieved, the dose may be gradually reduced; the rate and extent of taper should be guided by clinical radiographic, and physiological studies. A minimum of 6 to 12 months of therapy is usually required to maintain remission. Patients failing to respond to corticosteroid therapy or experiencing corticosteroid side effects should be treated with alternative immunosuppressive/cytotoxic agents, such as cyclophosphamide or azathioprine, but only if the diagnosis of BOOP is unequivocal. In most situations, this requires an open lung biopsy.

ACKNOWLEDGMENTS

Supported in part by SCOR Research Grant P50-HL 46487 from the National Institutes of Health, Bethesda, MD.

REFERENCES

1. Epler GR, Colby TV, McLoud TC, Carrington CB, Gaensler EA. Bronchiolitis obliterans organizing pneumonia. *N Engl J Med* 1985;312: 152–158.
2. Bartter T, Irwin RS, Nash G, Balikian JP, Hollingsworth HH. Idiopathic bronchiolitis obliterans organizing pneumonia with peripheral infiltrates on chest roentgenogram. *Arch Intern Med* 1989;149:273–279.
3. Katzenstein ALA, Myers JL, Prophet WD, Corley LS, Shin MS. Bronchiolitis obliterans and usual interstitial pneumonia: a comparative clinicopathologic study. *Am J Surg Pathol* 1986;106: 373–381.
4. Flowers JR, Clunie G, Burke M, Constant O. Bronchiolitis obliterans organizing pneumonia: the clinical and radiological features of seven cases and a review of the literature. *Clin Radiol* 1992;45:371–377.
5. Guerry-Force ML, Muller NL, Wright JL, et al. A comparison of bronchiolitis obliterans with organizing pneumonia, usual interstitial pneumonitis and small airways disease. *Am Rev Respir Dis* 1987;135:705–712.
6. Turton CW, Williams G, Green M. Cryptogenic obliterative bronchiolitis in adults. *Thorax* 1981; 36:805–810.
7. Davison AG, Heard BE, McAllister WAC, Turner-Warwick MEH. Cryptogenic organizing pneumonitis. *Q J Med* 1983;52:382–394.
8. Cordier JF, Loire R, Brune J. Idiopathic bronchiolitis obliterans organizing pneumonia: definition of characteristic clinical profiles in a series of 16 patients. *Chest* 1989;96:999–1004.
9. Gosink BB, Friedman PJ, Liebow AA. Bronchiolitis obliterans: roentgenologic-pathologic correlation. *AJR* 1973;117:816–832.
10. Yamamoto M, Ina Y, Kitaichi M, Harasawa M, Tamura M. Clinical features of BOOP in Japan. *Chest* 1992;102[suppl 1]:21S–25S.
11. Muller NL, Staples CA, Miller RA. Bronchiolitis obliterans organizing pneumonia: CT features in 14 patients. *Am J Roentgenol* 1990;154:983–987.
12. Geddes DM, Corrin B, Brewerton DA, Davies RJ, Turner-Warwick M. Progressive airway obliteration in adults and its association with rheumatoid disease. *Q J Med* 1977;46:427–444.
13. Epler GR, Snider GL, Gaensler EA, Cathcart ES, Fitzgerald MX, Carrington CB. Bronchiolitis and bronchitis in connective tissue disease: a possible relationship to the use of penicillamine. *JAMA* 1979;242:528–532.
14. Hakala M, Paako P, Sutinen S, et al. Association of bronchiolitis with connective tissue disorders. *Ann Rheum Dis* 1986;45;656–662.
15. Murphy KC, Atkins CJ, Offer RC, Hogg JC, Stein HB. Obliterative bronchiolitis in two rheumatoid arthritis patients treated with penicillamine. *Arthritis Rheum* 1981;24:557–560.
16. Lahdensuo A, Mattila J, Vilppula A. Bronchiolitis in rheumatoid arthritis. *Chest* 1984;85:705–708.
17. Cooney TP. Interrelationship of chronic eosinophilic pneumonia, bronchiolitis obliterans, and rheumatoid disease: a hypothesis. *J Clin Pathol* 1981;34:129–137.
18. Herzog CA, Miller RR, Hoidal RR. Bronchiolitis and rheumatoid arthritis. *Am Rev Respir Dis* 1981;124:636–639.
19. Rees JH, Woodhead MA, Sheppard MN, duBois RM. Rheumatoid arthritis and cryptogenic organizing pneumonitis. *Respir Med* 1991;85:243–246.
20. van Thiel RJ, van der Burg S, Groote AD, Nossent GD, Wills SH. Bronchiolitis obliterans organizing pneumonia and rheumatoid arthritis. *Eur Respir J* 1991;4:905–911.
21. Yousem SA, Colby TV, Carrington CB. Lung biopsy in rheumatoid arthritis. *Am Rev Respir Dis* 1985;131:770–777.
22. Jacobs P, Bonnyns M, Depierreux M, Duchateau J, Sergysels R. Rapidly fatal bronchiolitis obliterans with circulating antinuclear and rheumatoid factors. *Eur J Respir Dis* 1984;65:384–388.
23. Schwarz MI, Matthay RA, Sahn SA, et al. Interstitial lung disease in polymyositis and dermatomyositis: analysis of six cases and review of the literature. *Medicine* 1976;55:89–104.
24. Tazelaar HD, Viggiano RW, Pickersgill J, Colby TV. Interstitial lung disease in polymyositis and dermatomyositis: clinical features and prognosis as correlated with histologic findings. *Am Rev Respir Dis* 1990;141:727–733.
25. Gammon RB, Bridges TA, Al-Nezir H, Alexander CB, Kennedy JI. Bronchiolitis obliterans organizing pneumonia associated with systemic lupus erythematosus. *Chest* 1992;102:1171–1174.
26. Kinney WW, Angelillo VA. Bronchiolitis in systemic lupus erythematosus. *Chest* 1982;82:646–649.
27. Nadorra RL, Landing BH. Pulmonary lesions in childhood onset systemic lupus erythematosus: analysis of 26 cases, and summary of the literature. *Pediatr Pathol* 1987;7:1–18.
28. Matthay RA, Schwarz MI, Petty TL, et al. Pulmonary manifestations of systemic lupus erythematosus: review of twelve cases of acute lupus pneumonitis. *Medicine* 1974;54:397–409.
29. Davison AG, Epstein O. Relapsing organizing

pneumonitis in a male patient with primary biliary cirrhosis, CREST syndrome and chronic pancreatitis. *Thorax* 1983;38:316–317.
30. Yousem SA. The pulmonary pathologic manifestations of the CREST syndrome. *Hum Pathol* 1990;21:467–474.
31. Matteson EL, Ike RW. Bronchiolitis obliterans organizing pneumonia and Sjogren's syndrome. *J Rheumatol* 1990;17:676–679.
32. Newball HH, Brahim SA. Chronic obstructive airway disease in patients with Sjogren's syndrome. *Am Rev Respir Dis* 1977;115:295–304.
33. Chien SM, Jambrosic J, Mintz S. Pulmonary manifestations in Sweet's syndrome: first report of a case with bronchiolitis obliterans organizing pneumonia. *Am J Med* 1991;91;553–554.
34. Swinburn CR, Jackson CJ, Cobden I, Ashcroft T, Morritt GN. Bronchiolitis obliterans organizing pneumonia in a patient with ulcerative colitis. *Thorax* 1988;43:735–736.
35. Williams T, Eidus L, Thomas P. Fibrosing alveolitis, bronchiolitis obliterans, and sulfasalazine therapy. *Chest* 1982;81:766–768.
36. Case records of the Massachusetts General Hospital (Case 24-1986). *N Engl J Med* 1986;314: 1627–1635.
37. Wise R. Pulmonary complications in collagen vascular disease. In: Lynch JP III, DeRemee RA, eds. *Immunologically mediated pulmonary diseases*. Philadelphia: Lippincott; 1991:40–880.
38. Lynch JP, Hunninghake GW. Pulmonary complications of collagen vascular disease. *Annu Rev Med* 1992;43:17–35.
39. Wiedeman HP, Matthay RA. Pulmonary manifestations of the collagen vascular diseases. *Clin Chest Med* 1989;10:677–721.
40. Lynch JP III, Chavis AD. Chronic interstitial pulmonary disorders. In: Victor L, ed. *Clinical pulmonary medicine*. Boston: Little, Brown; 1992:193–263.
41. Roschmann RA, Rothenberg RJ. Pulmonary fibrosis in rheumatoid arthritis: a review of clinical features and therapy. *Semin Arthritis Rheum* 1987;16:174–185.
42. Gilligan DM, O'Connor CM, Ward K, Moloney D, Brenihan B, Fitzgerald MX. Bronchoalveolar lavage in patients with mild and severe rheumatoid lung disease. *Thorax* 1990;45:591–596.
43. Garcia JG, James HL, Zinkgraf S, Perlman MB, Keogh BA. Lower respiratory tract abnormalities in rheumatoid interstitial lung disease: potential role for neutrophils in lung injury. *Am Rev Respir Dis* 1987;136:811–817.
44. Perez T, Farre JM, Gosset P, et al. Subclinical alveolar inflammation in rheumatoid arthritis: superoxide anion, neutrophil chemotactic activity, and fibronectin generation by alveolar macrophages. *Eur Respir J* 1989;2:7–13.
45. Collins RL. Turner RA, Johnson M, Whitley NO, McLean R. Obstructive pulmonary disease in rheumatoid arthritis. *Arthritis Rheum* 1976; 19:628.
46. Geddes DM, Wegley M, Emerson PA. Airways obstruction in rheumatoid arthritis. *Ann Rheum Dis* 1979;38:222–225.
47. Begin R, Masse S, Cantin A, et al. Airway disease in a subset of nonsmoking rheumatoid patients: characterization of the disease and evidence of an autoimmune pathogenesis. *Am J Med* 1982;72:743–750.
48. Lakhanpal S, Lie JT, Conn DL, Martin WJ II. Pulmonary disease in polymyositis/dermatomyositis: a clinicopathological analysis of 65 cases. *Ann Rheum Dis* 1987;47:23–29.
49. Asura EL, Greenberg AS. Adverse impact of interstitial pulmonary fibrosis on prognosis in polymyositis and dermatomyositis. *Semin Arthritis Rheum* 1988;18:39–47.
50. Marguerie C, Bunn CC, Beynon HL, et al. Polymyositis, pulmonary fibrosis, and autoantibodies to aminoacyl-tRNA synthetase enzymes. *Q J Med* 1990;77:1019–1038.
51. Targoff IN, Arnett FC, Berman L, O'Brien C, Reichlin M. Anti-KJ: a new antibody associated with the syndrome of polymyositis and interstitial lung disease. *J Clin Invest* 1989;84:162–172.
52. Quismorio FP Jr. Clinical and pathologic features of lung involvement in systemic lupus erythematosus. *Semin Respir Med* 1988;9:297–304.
53. Segal AM, Calbrese LH, Ahmad M, et al. The pulmonary manifestations of systemic lupus erythematosus. *Semin Arthritis Rheum* 1985;14: 202–224.
54. Toews GB, Lynch JP III. Pathogenesis and clinical features of pulmonary infections in patients with rheumatoid diseases. In: Cannon GA, Zimmerman GW, eds. *Lung biology in health and disease*. New York: Marcel Dekker; 1990:179–226.
55. Haupt HM, Moore GW, Hutchins GM. The lung in systemic lupus erythematosus: analysis of the pathologic changes in 120 patients. *Am J Med* 1981;71:791–798.
56. Weinrib L, Sharma OP, Quismorio FP Jr. A long-term study of interstitial lung disease in systemic lupus erythematosus. *Semin Arthritis Rheum* 1990;20:48–56.
57. Hedgpeth MT, Boulware DW. Interstitial pneumonitis in antinuclear antibody-negative systemic lupus erythematosus: a new clinical manifestation and possible association with anti-Ro (SS-A) antibodies. *Arthritis Rheum* 1988;31:545–548.
58. Myers JL, Katzenstein AA. Microangiitis in lupus-induced pulmonary hemorrhage. *Am J Clin Pathol* 1985;85:552–556.
59. Churg A, Franklin W, Chan KL, Koop E, Carrington CB. Pulmonary hemorrhage and immune complex deposition in the lung. *Arch Pathol Lab Med* 1980;104:388–391.
60. Carette S, Macher AM, Nussbaum A, Plotz PH. Severe acute pulmonary disease in patients with SLE: ten years of experience at the National Institutes of Health. *Semin Arthritis Rheum* 1984;14:52–59.
61. Asherson RA, Gharavi AE, Harris EN, et al. Pulmonary hypertension in systemic lupus erythematosus: a report of three cases. *J Rheumatol* 1986;13:416–421.

62. Sharp GE, Irving W, Tan E, et al. Mixed connective tissue disease: an apparently distinct rheumatic disease syndrome associated with a specific antibody to an extractable nuclear antigen (ENA). *Am J Med* 1972;52:148–159.
63. Lazaro MA, Maldonado Cocco JA, Catoggio LJ, et al. Clinical and serologic characteristics of patients with overlap syndrome: is mixed connective tissue disease a distinct clinical entity? *Medicine* 1989;68:58–65.
64. Sullivan WD, Hurst DJ, Harmon CE, et al. A prospective evaluation emphasizing pulmonary involvement in patients with mixed connective tissue disease. *Medicine* 1984;63:92–107.
65. Prakash U, Luthra H, Divertie M. Intrathoracic manifestations in mixed connective tissue disease. *Mayo Clin Proc* 1985;60:813–821.
66. Derderian SS, Tellis CJ, Abbrecht PH, Welton RC, Rajagopal KR. Pulmonary involvement in mixed connective tissue disease. *Chest* 1985;88: 45–48.
67. Peters-Golden M, Wise RA, Schneider P, Hochberg MC, Stevens MB, Wigley F. Clinical and demographic predictors of loss of pulmonary function in systemic sclerosis. *Medicine* 1984;63: 221–231.
68. McCarthy DS, Baragar FD, Dhingra S, et al. The lungs in systemic sclerosis (scleroderma): a review and new information. *Semin Arthritis Rheum* 1988;17:271–283.
69. Silver RM, Miller KS. Lung involvement in systemic sclerosis. *Rheum Dis Clin North Am* 1990;16:199–216.
70. Schurawitzki H, Stiglbauer R, Graninger W, et al. Interstitial lung disease in progressive systemic sclerosis: high-resolution CT versus radiography. *Radiology* 1990;176:755–759.
71. Harrison NK, Glanville AR, Strickland B, et al. Pulmonary involvement in systemic sclerosis: the detection of early changes by thin section CT scan, bronchoalveolar lavage and ^{99}Tc-DTPA clearance. *Respir Med* 1989;83:404–414.
72. Rossi GA, Bitterman PB, Rennard SI, Ferrans VJ, Crystal RG. Evidence for chronic inflammation as a component of the interstitial lung disease associated with progressive systemic sclerosis. *Am Rev Respir Dis* 1985;131:612–617.
73. Silver RM, Miller KS, Kinsella MB, Smith EA, Schabel SI. Evaluation and management of scleroderma lung disease using bronchoalveolar lavage. *Am J Med* 1990;88:470–476.
74. Groen H, Wichers G, ter Borg EJ, van der Mark TW, Wouda AA, Kallenberg CM. Pulmonary diffusing capacity disturbances are related to nailford capillary changes in patients with Raynaud's phenomenon with and without an underlying connective tissue disease. *Am J Med* 1990;89:34–41.
75. Bridges AJ, Hsu KC, Dias-Arias AA, Chechani V. Bronchiolitis obliterans organizing pneumonia and scleroderma. *J Rheumatol* 1992;19:1136–1140.
76. Bjerke RD, Tashkin DP, Clements PJ, Chopra SK, Gong H Jr, Bein M. Small airways in progressive systemic sclerosis (PSS). *Am J Med* 1979;66:201–209.
77. Dalavanga YA, Constantopoulos SH, Galanopoulou V, Zerva L, Moutsopoulos HM. Alveolitis correlates with clinical pulmonary involvement in primary Sjogren's syndrome. *Chest* 1991;99:1394–1397.
78. Constantopolous SH, Papdimitriou CS, Moutsopoulos HM. Respiratory manifestations in primary Sjogren's syndrome: a clinical, functional, and histologic study. *Chest* 1985;88:226–229.
79. Hatron PY, Wallaert B, Gosset D, et al. Subclinical lung inflammation in primary Sjogren's syndrome. *Arthritis Rheum* 1987;30:1226–1231.
80. Papathanasious MP, Constantopolous SH, Tsampoulos C, Drosos AA, Moutsopoulos HM. Reappraisal of respiratory abnormalities in primary and secondary Sjogren's syndrome: a controlled study. *Chest* 1986;90:370–374.
81. Wallaert B, Prin L, Hatron PY, Ramon P, Tonnel AB, Voisin C. Lymphocytic populations in bronchoalveolar lavage in Sjogren's syndrome. *Chest* 1987;92:1025–1031.
82. Alkhayer M, McCann BG, Harrison BD. Lymphocytic interstitial pneumonitis in association with Sjogren's syndrome. *Br J Dis Chest* 1988; 82:305–309.
83. Hansen LA, Prakash UB, Colby TV. Pulmonary lymphoma in Sjogren's syndrome. *Mayo Clin Proc* 1989;64:920–931.
84. Usui Y, Kimula Y, Miura H, et al. A case of bronchiolitis obliterans organizing pneumonia associated with primary Sjogren's syndrome who died of superimposed diffuse alveolar damage. *Respiration* 1992;59:122–124.
85. Takimoto CH, Warnock M, Golden JA. Sweet's syndrome with lung involvement. *Am Rev Respir Dis* 1991;143:177–179.
86. Gibson LE, Dicken CH, Flach DB. Neutrophilic dermatoses and myeloproliferative disease: report of two cases. *Mayo Clin Proc* 1985;60:735–740.
87. Soderstrom RM. Sweet's syndrome and acute myelogenous leukemia: a case report and review of the literature. *Cutis* 1981;28:255–260.
88. Lazarus AA, McMillan M, Miramadi A. Pulmonary involvement in Sweet's syndrome (acute febrile neutrophilic dermatosis). *Chest* 1986;90: 922–924.
89. Butland RJA, Cole P, Citron K, Turner-Warwick M. Chronic bronchial suppuration and inflammatory bowel disease. *Q J Med* 1981;197: 63–75.
90. Kraft SC, Earle RH, Roesler M, Esterly JR. Unexplained bronchopulmonary disease with inflammatory bowel disease. *Arch Intern Med* 1976;136;454–459.
91. Theodoropoulos G, Archimandritis A, Davaris P, Plataris J, Melisinos K. Ulcerative colitis and sarcoidosis: a curious association—report of a case. *Dis Colon Rectum* 1981;24:308–310.
92. Isenberg JI, Goldstein H, Korn AS, Ozeran RS, Rosen V. Pulmonary vasculitis: an uncommon

complication of ulcerative colitis. *N Engl J Med* 1968;279:1376–1377.
93. Mosely RH, Barwick KW, Dobuler K, DeLuca VA. Sulfasalazine-induced pulmonary disease. *Dig Dis Sci* 1985;30:901–904.
94. Robinson BW, Sterrett G. Bronchiolitis obliterans associated with polyarteritis nodosa. *Chest* 1992;102:309–311.
95. Ferson PF, Landreneau RJ, Dowling RD, et al. Comparison of open vs. thoracoscopic lung biopsy for pulmonary diffuse infiltrative disease. *J Thorac Cardiovasc Surg* 1993;106(2):194–199.
96. Neages GR and Lynch JP III. Making sense of bronchiolitis obliterans and related disorders. *J Respir Dis* 1991;12(9);789–814.

Diseases of the Bronchioles, edited by
Gary R. Epler. Raven Press, Ltd.,
New York © 1994.

24

Drug-Related Bronchiolitis Obliterans Organizing Pneumonia

Helen M. Hollingsworth

Division of Pulmonary and Critical Care Medicine, University of Massachusetts Medical School, 55 Lake Avenue North, Worcester, MA.

A variety of drugs (Table 1) have been associated with clinical, radiographic, and pathologic features identical to those of idiopathic bronchiolitis obliterans organizing pneumonia (BOOP) (1,2). This is a relatively recent observation: BOOP was not listed among the types of drug-induced pulmonary toxicity in the excellent and comprehensive two-part review of drug-induced pulmonary disease written by Cooper and colleagues (3,4) in 1986. This chapter reviews the clinical presentation, time course of drug therapy, radiographic findings, and biopsy data for each of the drugs that has been implicated as a cause of BOOP.

ANTI-INFLAMMATORY AND IMMUNOMODULATORY DRUGS

Because BOOP has been associated with connective-tissue disorders in the absence of drug therapy (Chapter 23) (2,5), evaluating the potential role of anti-inflammatory and immunomodulatory agents in the development of pulmonary toxicity is at times difficult. Drug effects must be differentiated from the effects of the underlying disease for which the drug was prescribed. In addition, certain underlying diseases may predispose a given patient to develop the histopathologic changes of BOOP as the expression of pulmonary toxicity to a particular drug. This section attempts to piece together the circumstantial evidence for drug-induced BOOP in this setting.

Gold

Interstitial lung disease is a well-recognized, although infrequent (1%), complication of gold therapy (4,6–8). The clinical course is usually suggestive of a hypersensitivity reaction with fever (40%), skin rash (40 to 60%), and eosinophilia (25 to 33%) (4,9,10). BOOP appears to be another manifestation of gold-related pulmonary toxicity. Costabel and colleagues (9,11–13) mention five reports of patients with pathologic changes consistent with BOOP associated with gold therapy.

Fort and colleagues (9) reported one patient who developed dyspnea on exertion, cough nonproductive of sputum, and peripheral edema after receiving weekly gold injections for 2 months as well as naproxen 500 mg twice daily. She did not have a rash or eosinophilia. The chest radiograph revealed bilateral (left greater than right), soft, nodular densities that were peripheral in distribution. Open lung biopsy demonstrated BOOP. Treatment consisted of discontinuing gold and instituting methylprednisolone 100 mg intravenously, twice daily, and cyclophosphamide 200 mg intrave-

TABLE 1. *Drugs for which BOOP may be a sign of toxicity*

Drug	Evidence for drug-related BOOP
Anti-inflammatory and immunomodulatory	
Gold	+ + +
Mesalazine	+ +
Methotrexate	+ + +
Naproxen	+
Sulphasalazine	+ + +
Sulphamethoxypyridazine	+ + +
Sulindac	+
Antimicrobials	
Amphotericin-B	+ +
Cepharadine	+ + +
Cardiovascular drugs	
Acebutolol	+ +
Amiodarone	+ + +
Chemotherapeutic drugs	
Bleomycin	+ + +
Mitomycin-c	+
Illicit	
Cocaine	+ + +

+, weak; + +, fair; + + +, strong.

nously for 3 days, followed by 100 mg orally. The hospital course was complicated by a pneumothorax and empyema, but she eventually improved with the cyclophosphamide and a tapering course of prednisone. Cyclophosphamide was discontinued after 12 months, and prednisone was continued at 5 mg daily. By this time, the pulmonary infiltrates had resolved and the patient remained free of respiratory disease.

A patient with a similar presentation was described by Morley and co-workers (13). After 6 weeks of weekly intramuscular injections of gold, the patient developed malaise, low-grade fever, and a nonproductive cough. After 4½ more months of gold therapy, she was admitted because of progressive dyspnea and bilateral, lower lobe, peripheral alveolar and interstitial infiltrates. Neither skin rash nor eosinophilia was present. Transbronchial lung biopsy revealed a mild infiltrate of lymphocytes and plasma cells, parenchymal fibrosis, and an organizing alveolar exudate. Gold was discontinued and prednisone, 40 mg daily, was given with almost complete clearing of the chest radiograph after 2 months.

McCormick and colleagues (12) reported two patients with gold-associated pneumonitis, one of whom had pathologic changes on open lung biopsy consistent with BOOP. This patient developed a nonproductive cough and dyspnea after 1 month of gold therapy. Diffuse, predominantly bibasilar infiltrates were noted on chest radiograph. She had no skin rash, fever, or eosinophilia. She died of necrotizing bacterial pneumonitis 2 months later after treatment with intravenous corticosteroids and, subsequently, dimercaprol and cyclophosphamide. Peripheral blood lymphocytes were obtained from this patient and from another patient with pulmonary infiltrates associated with gold therapy who did not undergo lung biopsy. The lymphocytes from both patients elaborated the cytokines, migration inhibition factor and macrophage chemotactic factor, when incubated with gold salts, suggesting a cell-mediated pathogenesis of the pulmonary toxicity.

In their review of the Japanese experience with BOOP, Yamamoto and co-workers (5) reported two patients with rheumatoid arthritis who developed BOOP while receiving gold therapy. The specific details of the clinical presentation of these particular patients were not delineated, except that they improved with corticosteroid therapy, as did the other two patients with rheumatoid arthritis who did not receive gold therapy.

Mesalazine

Mesalazine (5-aminosalicylate) is sometimes used in the treatment of inflammatory bowel disease. Swinburn and colleagues (14) described the course of a 20-year-old patient who developed fever, anorexia, nonproductive cough, breathlessness on exertion, and central pleuritic chest pain after 1 year of therapy with mesalazine for ulcerative colitis. She had previously taken sulfasalazine for 3 years. Peripheral blood eosinophilia was noted, but this had antedated drug therapy. Chest radiograph revealed extensive, nonsegmental peripheral consolidation in the right middle and lower lung zones. Open lung biopsy revealed the histopathologic changes of BOOP. Discontinuation of mesalazine and institution of prednisone, at 40 mg daily, resulted in rapid clinical and radiographic improvement in 1 week. Complete clearing of the chest radiograph was noted at 1 month. Rechallenge with mesalazine was not undertaken, so it remains unclear whether BOOP in this patient was related to her underlying disease or to mesalazine.

Methotrexate

Methotrexate is a folic acid analog that induces an intracellular deficiency of folate coenzymes, thus inhibiting cell growth (3). Several different manifestations of pulmonary toxicity have been attributed to methotrexate, including acute noncardiogenic pulmonary edema after intrathecal administration, acute pleuritis, pulmonary hypersensitivity with interstitial pneumonitis, granuloma formation and bronchiolitis, diffuse alveolar damage and nonspecific lung injury, progressive fibrosis and BOOP (3,10, 15,16). The overall incidence appears to be on the order of 4 to 7% (3,10).

In their description of 168 patients with arthritis who received long-term, low-dose methotrexate therapy, Carson and colleagues (15) reported that 7 had probable methotrexate-induced pulmonary toxicity and 12 had possible methotrexate-induced pulmonary toxicity. They described 5 patients in detail, 3 of whom underwent open lung biopsy. The description of the clinical presentation and lung pathology of one of these is suggestive of BOOP: mild interstitial fibrosis, ill-formed interstitial granulomas, and bronchiolitis. In this patient, the onset of fever, chills, breathlessness, and productive cough occurred after 54 weeks of methotrexate therapy and simultaneous reduction in the prednisone dose from 10 to 5 mg daily. Chest radiograph revealed bilateral interstitial infiltrates. In comparison, another patient who had severe dyspnea, but no constitutional complaints, had interstitial infiltrates with chronic inflammatory cells, eosinophils, and microgranulomata. The third patient experienced breathlessness, right-sided pleuritic chest pain, fever, malaise, and a productive cough. Lung biopsy revealed focal emphysematous changes (consistent with known history of cigarette smoking) and organizing diffuse alveolar damage with chronic interstitial inflammation. All 3 patients had diffuse bilateral infiltrates on chest radiograph. Although the clinical presentation did not seem to be predictive of the exact histopathology, all 3 patients improved with discontinuation of methotrexate and administration of or increase in the dose of prednisone.

Another patient with rheumatoid arthritis who was receiving low-dose oral weekly methotrexate developed a somewhat different presentation of BOOP (17). After 8 months of therapy, he developed fatigue, weight loss, and a nonproductive cough. The chest radiograph was reportedly normal. One month later, he noted acute, lancinating right lateral chest pain while coughing. The chest radiograph now revealed right upper lobe triangular consolidation in the axillary area with an air bronchogram, as well as an eighth-rib displaced fracture. Blind transbronchial lung biopsy revealed BOOP. Eight months later the patient was subjectively improved and the lung consolidation was partially resolved. Methotrexate therapy had been interrupted for only 1 month; corticosteroids were not given.

Naproxen

A patient discussed in the Case Records of the Massachusetts General Hospital, Case 24-1986 (18), developed BOOP while being treated with naproxen for knee and shoulder pain. The white blood cell count revealed 8% eosinophils. The chest radiograph showed bilateral, patchy alveolar densities more marked in the upper lung zones, with relative sparing of the bases. Her history was suggestive of polymyalgia rheumatica and, possibly, giant cell arteritis in the more distant past. She improved with corticosteroid treatment and, presumably, discontinuation of naproxen.

Naproxen has also been associated with pulmonary infiltrates in patients presenting with cough, a flu-like syndrome, and either peripheral blood or sputum eosinophilia (19,20). Transbronchial biopsy in one of these patients (19) showed interstitial fibrosis, fibrous thickening of the alveolar septa, proliferation of alveolar macrophages, and an inflammatory interstitial infiltrate composed of eosinophils, lymphocytes, and histiocytes. Because this was not an open lung biopsy, it is possible that BOOP was missed. The other three patients (20) did not have a biopsy. Two patients improved with discontinuation of naproxen alone (19, 20). The other two patients improved with corticosteroid administration. Two of the four patients were challenged with naproxen again: one developed cough and chest heaviness, which resolved after naproxen was stopped (20); the other experienced transient fever, cough, and wheezing (19). The clinical similarity of these four patients with the Massachusetts General Hospital patient raises the possibility that one or more of them may have had undiagnosed BOOP.

Sulphasalazine

Williams and colleagues (21) reported a patient with BOOP occurring during sulfasalazine therapy. Six months into treatment with sulfasalazine for ulcerative colitis, the 66-year-old ex-smoker developed shortness of breath. Four months later, a nonproductive cough, malaise, and a temperature of 38.5°C were noted. Sulfasalazine was stopped. The white blood cell count and differential were normal, but the sedimentation rate was elevated at 60 mm per hour. Extensive upper lung zone triangular infiltrates were seen on chest radiograph. Gallium scan revealed increased uptake over the same areas. Pulmonary function tests showed a mild obstructive ventilatory defect and a mild reduction in diffusing capacity.

Despite discontinuing sulfasalazine, the patient experienced progressively worsening dyspnea, cough, fever, and night sweats over the next 6 weeks. Pulmonary function tests then showed a combined restrictive and obstructive ventilatory defect, as well as a moderately severe reduction in diffusing capacity. Open lung biopsy showed chronic interstitial pneumonia and marked bronchiolitis obliterans. Occasional granulomas were also noted.

Administration of prednisone, 60 mg daily, resulted in subjective improvement in 1 week. Prednisone was tapered down to 10 mg daily with progressive improvement. Although subsequent studies revealed improvement in lung volumes and air flow, the diffusing capacity remained reduced and the chest radiograph showed biapical pleural thickening and upper lung zone fibrotic stranding. Whether a longer course of higher doses of prednisone would have led to further improvement is not known. The observation that the patient's condition continued to deteriorate for 6 weeks after sulphasalazine was discontinued could be evidence against the hypothesis that sulphasalazine was an etiologic agent. In this vein, it would have been interesting to know how active the patient's ulcerative colitis was at the time.

Another patient who developed predominantly interstitial infiltrates while taking sulphasalazine for ulcerative colitis was reported by Jordan and Cowan (22). Symptoms included dyspnea, cough, and night sweats. Lung biopsy was not performed. The patient improved after sulphsalazine was discontinued; corticosteroids were not given. The patient subsequently tolerated mesalazine without respiratory symptoms.

Sulphamethoxypyridazine

Treatment with sulphamethoxypyridazine has also been associated with BOOP (23). A patient who was being treated with sulphamethoxypyridazine for linear IgA dermatitis developed increasing dyspnea over 5 months, despite concomitant prednisolone, 15 mg daily. Chest radiograph revealed diffuse interstitial infiltrates, and an open lung biopsy showed BOOP. Sulphamethoxypyridazine was discontinued and prednisolone increased to 60 mg daily. Within 5 weeks the chest radiograph had cleared and the arterial oxygenation had normalized, but breathlessness on exertion persisted. Rechallenge was not attempted. The previously reported association (21) of sulphasalazine with bronchiolitis obliterans and alveolitis was believed to support a role for sulphamethoxypyridazine in the pathogenesis of BOOP in this patient (23).

Sulindac

A single patient who developed a clinical syndrome and chest radiograph suggestive of BOOP while taking sulindac has been described by Takimoto and colleagues (24). After 5 months of therapy with sulindac for degenerative arthritis, the patient developed low-grade fevers, sweats, chills, a nonproductive cough, and dyspnea. Complete blood count and differential were normal. The chest radiograph showed bilateral, patchy alveolar infiltrates. Twelve days after sulindac was discontinued, the infiltrates had improved significantly. Rechallenge with sulindac 8 days later resulted in the return of her initial symptoms within hours, as well as diffuse alveolar consolidation. Discontinuing sulindac again resulted in prompt symptomatic and radiographic improvement. No bronchoalveolar lavage or biopsy information was reported.

Two other patients with pulmonary infiltrates related to sulindac therapy have been reported (25,26). Fein (25) described an elderly woman receiving sulindac for osteoarthritis who developed fever, myalgias, and a dry cough. The differential blood count revealed 8% eosinophils. The chest radiograph showed diffuse interstitial disease with areas of consolidation in the upper and lower lobes on the right. Transbronchial lung biopsy showed thickened alveolar walls infiltrated with monocytes and polymorphonuclear cells. High-dose corticosteroid therapy resulted in gradual but complete clearing. Rechallenge with sulindac resulted in a return of her symptoms and pulmonary infiltrates. This time she improved without any treatment other than stopping sulindac.

Smith and Lindberg (26) reported a young man with rheumatoid arthritis who developed fever, headache, sore throat, and abdominal pain during therapy with sulindac. Chest radiograph revealed bilateral lower lobe infiltrates. Improvement was associated with discontinuation of sulindac. Transient pruritus, fever, and hypotension followed a single dose of sulindac given 10 days later.

Although none of the patients with pulmonary toxicity related to sulindac had documented BOOP, the clinical picture is quite similar to that of the patient with BOOP related to naproxen therapy (18).

ANTIMICROBIAL DRUGS

Amphotericin B

Amphotericin B is frequently added to the medical regimen of febrile neutropenic patients when they are unresponsive to broad-spectrum antibiotics. Roncoroni and co-workers (27) reported one patient who was treated with amphotericin B because of a localized infiltrate seen on chest radiograph and persistent fevers despite use of broad-spectrum antibiotics. Fever, chills, and dyspnea developed in association with the amphotericin B infusions. Transbronchial biopsy was performed because of progressive hypoxemia and worsening, diffuse, interstitial infiltrates. In addition to histopathologic findings consistent with BOOP, a scant growth of *Candida* species was detected in one of the bronchoscopy specimens.

The diffuse infiltrates improved when ketoconazole was substituted for amphotericin. Four months later, amphotericin was again infused, but had to be discontinued because of dyspnea. Although the recurrence of dyspnea on rechallenge with amphotericin supports the hypothesis that amphotericin B contributed to the development of BOOP in this patient, the presence of a localized infiltrate on the chest radiograph prior to initiation of amphotericin B raises the possibility that BOOP was caused by a viral or, possibly, candidal infection.

Cephalosporins

Cephalosporins have been associated with histopathologic changes consistent with BOOP in two reports. The first instance was reported by Grinblat and colleagues (28). Their patient developed worsening shortness of breath and a nonproductive cough in the midst of subacute thyroiditis. Her respiratory status appeared to deteriorate acutely with the addition of cephalexin. Percutaneous lung biopsy revealed a few plugs of fibrin with organization filling alveoli, mild to moderate collagenous thickening of alveolar walls, and infiltration by lymphocytes and histiocytes. Of note, after initial improvement following administration of prednisone, 30 mg daily, challenge with cephalothin resulted in increasing dyspnea and extension of lung infiltrates. Rapid improvement followed discontinuation of cephalothin. A positive migration inhibition factor test to cephalosporin was mentioned.

Dreis and co-workers (29) described another patient with a history of skin rash associated with cephalexin who developed a pruritic erythematous rash, dyspnea, a nonproductive cough, and malaise 4 days after an oral course of cephradine for a urinary tract infection. Cephradine was discontinued, but her respiratory symptoms progressed over the next 3 days. The chest radiograph showed patchy, somewhat peripheral, midlung and basilar infiltrates. Peripheral eosinophilia was not present. The sedimentation rate was elevated at 62 mm per hour. Pulmonary function tests revealed restriction and a reduced single breath diffusing capacity. Transbronchial biopsy was consistent with BOOP. Approximately 20 days after discontinuing cephradine, she remained unimproved. Prednisone, 30 mg twice daily, resulted in prompt subjective improvement. After 2 weeks of prednisone therapy, her chest radiograph had cleared. Prednisone was tapered over 2 months. Rechallenge with cephradine 4 months later resulted in return of cough, dyspnea, and a lingular infiltrate, in addition to reductions in vital capacity and diffusion capacity. Her symptoms continued to progress after cephradine was stopped, and steroid therapy was again required.

CARDIOVASCULAR DRUGS

Acebutolol

After receiving acebutolol for 2 years, a patient developed nonproductive cough, increasing dyspnea, weight loss, and a low-grade fever (30). The chest radiograph revealed peripheral, basilar and mid-lung zone infiltrates. Transbronchial lung biopsy revealed changes consistent with BOOP. With discontinuation of acebutolol, he became afebrile. Two months later the chest radiograph had improved significantly, and by 8 months the lung function was normal. He did not receive corticosteroid therapy.

Amiodarone

Pulmonary toxicity develops in 1 to 6% of patients taking amiodarone, an iodinated, benzofuran derivative (4,10). The time of onset of symptoms has varied from 1 month to 9 years after initiation of therapy. The typical histopathologic features are intra-alveolar accumulation of foamy alveolar macrophages, alveolar septal thickening, and hyperplasia of type II pneumocytes (4). More recently, several patients have been described in whom the histopathologic findings were characteristic of BOOP (11,30,32).

One of the four patients with amiodarone-induced pulmonary toxicity described by Marchilinski and co-workers (32) may have had BOOP. This particular patient was admitted to the hospital with progressive exertional dyspnea, a nonproductive cough, anorexia, and weight loss after 8 months of amiodarone therapy. He was afebrile and had fine basilar crackles and a pleural rub. Chest radiograph showed diffuse interstitial infiltrates with confluence in the mid-lung zones and in the periphery of the right upper lobe, as well as pleural thickening adjacent to the peripheral alveolar process. Open lung biopsy revealed patchy areas of widening of the alveolar septae, with connective tissue and numerous foamy macrophages in the airspaces. Early organization of the infiltrate was noted within some of the alveolar spaces and terminal bronchioles. The patient experienced rapid deterioration of his respiratory status 4 days after surgery and died.

Camus and colleagues (30) described a patient who had received amiodarone for 3 years with a cumulative dose of 190 g in addition to isosorbide dinitrate, aminophylline, canrenone (an antialdosterone diuretic), and frusemide. The patient developed weight loss, fever, dyspnea, and a cough productive of yellowish sputum. Chest radiograph showed right upper lung confluent infiltrates and volume loss. Amiodarone was discontinued. One month later a chest radiograph was repeated because of similar symptoms. The right upper lung zone infiltrate had resolved, but new alveolar infiltrates were noted in the right lower lung field. An exudative pleural effusion was also present. Lung biopsy obtained at thoracoscopy showed ". . .severe interstitial pneumonitis and extensive obliteration of alveolar ducts by typical 'bourgeons conjunctifs.' Occasional foci of foamy cells were also present." This sounds quite consistent with BOOP. Prednisolone, 40 mg daily, was administered, with progressive improvement in symptoms and chest radiograph but not pulmonary function tests.

Costabel and colleagues (11) mentioned that in their group of 14 patients with BOOP, 1 received amiodarone. BOOP was idiopathic in the other 13 patients. They report that the clinical course, chest radiograph, and biopsy in this patient were not different from those of the patients with idiopathic BOOP. Specific details were not given.

CYTOTOXIC DRUGS

Bleomycin

Bleomycin, an antitumor antibiotic isolated from a strain of *Streptomyces verticillus,* appears to act by inhibiting DNA synthesis (3,33). It is associated with pulmonary toxicity that occurs in 6 to 43% of patients (3,10,33). Several different patterns of pulmonary toxicity have been attributed to bleomycin: chronic progressive fibrosis (3,10), adult respiratory distress syndrome (ARDS) in patients receiving supplemental oxygen 30% (10), hypersensitivity pneumonitis with an eosinophilic infiltrate (3,10), and BOOP (10,33–36).

The most common radiographic pattern of bleomycin-related BOOP appears to be a nodular infiltrate (33,34). Patients were frequently asymptomatic at the time of identification of pulmonary nodules on routine radiographs. The pulmonary nodules were either shaggy or well marginated, but irregular in shape (33,34). Cavitation was reported (34). Histopathologic examination of these nodules showed varying degrees of interstitial and/or intra-alveolar fibrosis. Hyperplasia of type II pneumocytes was common (33). A significant eosinophilic infiltrate was occasionally present, although eosinophilic microabcesses were not reported (33). Because bleomycin-related nodules develop during therapy for malignancy, invasive procedures are frequently indicated to exclude metastatic lesions. However, waiting 4 to 6 weeks for a repeat chest CT scan may be reasonable to determine whether the nodules are stable or regressing (33), suggesting a benign lesion.

Peripheral interstitial infiltrates have also been described in bleomycin-related BOOP by Bartter and colleagues (35). Their patient had received bleomycin, cisplatinum, and vinblastin for seminoma. Four months after bleomycin had been omitted from the chemotherapeutic regimen because of a decrease in single breath diffusing capacity, the patient presented with progressive dyspnea, low-grade fevers, and a nonproductive cough. The chest radiograph revealed bilateral (right greater than left), peripheral, irregular linear infiltrates. The diagnosis of BOOP was made on the basis of a transbronchial lung biopsy, which revealed the appropriate histopathologic changes as well as some eosinophils. Despite a trial of prednisone, 60 mg daily, he suffered progressive respiratory failure over the next several months. There was no evidence of recurrent seminoma at autopsy.

Yousem and colleagues (36) reported three patients with "eosinophilic pneumonia" related to therapy with bleomycin. The first patient had breathlessness; a cough productive of white phlegm; and faint, fluffy alveolar infiltrates in the left lower lobe. The second patient was asymptomatic, and chest tomograms revealed a patchy alveolar density and several poorly defined nodular lesions. The third patient experienced a nonproductive cough and breathlessness without flu-like symptoms or fever. The chest radiograph revealed bilateral, lower lobe patchy alveolar infiltrates. Open lung biopsy specimens of these three patients revealed consolidative alveolar infiltrates with varying proportions of eosinophils and histiocytes, bronchiolitis obliterans "with polyps of connective tissue occluding the lumens of the terminal and respiratory bronchioles," and metaplastic alveolar pneumocytes lining alveolar walls. Eosinophilic microabscesses with granular central necrosis were described in the specimens from the first and second patients. No additional bleomycin was given, and no corticosteroid therapy was used; all three patients remained free of pulmonary disease. The histopathologic description suggests an overlap between eosinophilic pneumonia and BOOP.

Mitomycin-C

Mitomycin-C was listed by Rosenow and colleagues (10) in a table of agents for which BOOP may be a sign of toxicity, but further details were not given.

ILLICIT DRUGS

Free-base cocaine

Patel and co-workers (37) described one patient who had used free-base cocaine for a number of weeks when he presented with a 10-day history of nonproductive cough, fever, and dyspnea. He experienced continued respiratory deterioration despite not having used cocaine for at least 4 days. After he developed respiratory failure, an open lung biopsy was performed and revealed a pattern consistent with BOOP. Treatment with methylprednisolone resulted in improvement in lung function and extubation on the tenth hospital day. Methylprednisolone therapy was continued for 6 months. Eighteen months after this episode, he had normal exercise tolerance. This report indicates clinical features typical of BOOP and the typical histologic pattern. The pathogenesis is not known but may be on the basis of a toxic inflammatory response related to the toxins generated by the combustion of the cocaine or unknown contaminants in the mixture.

SUMMARY

Several features are common to both idiopathic and drug-related BOOP: the most common respiratory symptoms are cough, usually nonproductive, and then dyspnea; the clinical presentation ranges from asymptomatic to respiratory failure; flu-like symptoms of fever and malaise are common; the sedimentation rate may be increased; the radiographic pattern varies from diffuse interstitial and alveolar infiltrates to peripheral triangular-shaped consolidation and peripheral nonsegmental infiltrates; and corticosteroid therapy is usually successful.

The observation that many of the drugs associated with BOOP have been associated with other types of pulmonary toxicity may eventually yield helpful information about the nature of the host–drug interaction and how this results in pulmonary toxicity. The wide range of drugs that have been associated with BOOP makes it likely that with time additional drugs will also be found to be related to this lesion.

REFERENCES

1. Davison AG, Heard BE, McAlister WAC, et al. Cryptogenic organizing alveolitis. *Q J Med* 1983; 52:382–394.
2. Epler GR, Colby TV, McCloud TC, Carrington CB, Gaensler EA. Bronchiolitis obliterans organizing pneumonia. *N Engl J Med* 1985;312: 152–158.
3. Cooper JAD, White DA, Matthay RA. Drug-induced pulmonary disease: cytotoxic drugs. *Am Rev Respir Dis* 1986;133:321–340.
4. Cooper JAD, White DA, Matthay RA. Drug-induced pulmonary disease: noncytotoxic drugs. *Am Rev Respir Dis* 1986;133:488–505.
5. Yamamoto M, Ina Y, Kitaichi M, et al. Clinical features of BOOP in Japan. *Chest* 1992;102:21S–25S.
6. Podell TE, Klinenberg JR, Kramer LS, Brown HV. Pulmonary toxicity with gold therapy. *Arthritis Rheum* 1980;23:347–350.
7. Evans RB, Ettensohn DB, Fawaz-Estrup F, Lally EV, Kaplan SR. Gold lung: recent developments in pathogenesis, diagnosis, and therapy. *Semin Arthritis Rheum* 1987;16:196–205.
8. Levinson ML, Lynch JP, Bowers JS. Reversal of life-threatening gold hypersensitivity pneumonitis by corticosteroids. *Am J Med* 1981;71:908–912.
9. Fort JG, Scovern H, Abruzzo JL. Intravenous cyclophosphamide and methylprednisolone for the treatment of bronchiolitis obliterans and interstitial fibrosis associated with crysotherapy. *J Rheumatol* 1988;15:850–854.

10. Rosenow EC, Myers JL, Swenson SJ, Pisani RJ. Drug-induced pulmonary disease: an update. *Chest* 1992;102:239–250.
11. Costabel U, Teschler H, Schoenfeld B, et al. BOOP in Europe. *Chest* 1992;102:14S–20S.
12. McCormick J, Cole S, Lahirir B, Knauft F, Cohen S, Yoshida T. Pneumonitis caused by gold salt therapy: evidence for the role of cell-mediated immunity in its pathogenesis. *Am Rev Respir Dis* 1980;122:145–152.
13. Morley TF, Komansky HJ, Adelizzi RA, Guidice JC. Pulmonary gold toxicity. *Eur J Respir Dis* 1984;65:627–632.
14. Swinburn CR, Jackson GJ, Cobden I, Ashcroft T, Morritt GN, Corris PA. Bronchiolitis obliterans organizing pneumonia in a patient with ulcerative colitis. *Thorax* 1988;43:735–736.
15. Carson CW, Cannon GW, Egger MG, et al. Pulmonary disease during the treatment of rheumatoid arthritis with low dose pulse methotrexate. *Semin Arthritis Rheum* 1987;16:186–195.
16. Green L, Schattner A, Berkenstadt H. Severe reversible interstitial pneumonitis induced by low dose methotrexate: report of a case and review of the literature. *J Rheumatol* 1988;15:110–112.
17. Garcia-Vicuna R, Diaz-Gonzalez F, Castaneda S, Arranz M, Lopez-Bote JP. Rheumatoid disease resembling lung neoplasia. *J Rheumatol* 1990;17:1686–1688.
18. Case records of the Massachusetts General Hospital (Case 24-1986). *N Engl J Med* 1986;314: 1627–1635.
19. Nader DA, Schillaci RF. Pulmonary infiltrates with eosinophilia due to naproxen. *Chest* 1983; 83:280–282.
20. Buscaglia AJ, Cowden FE, Brill H. Pulmonary infiltrates associated with naproxen. *JAMA* 1984;251:65–66.
21. Williams T, Eidus L, Thomas P. Fibrosing alveolitis, bronchiolitis obliterans, and sulfasalazine therapy. *Chest* 1982;81:766–768.
22. Jordan A, Cowan RE. Reversible pulmonary disease and eosinophilia associated with sulphasalazine. *J R Soc Med* 1988;81:233–235.
23. Godfrey KM, Wojnarowska F, Friedland JS. Obliterative bronchiolitis and alveolitis associated with sulphamethoxpyridazine (Lederkyn) therapy for linear IgA disease of adults. *Br J Dermatol* 1990;123:125–131.
24. Takimoto CH, Lynch D, Stulbarg MS. Pulmonary infiltrates associated with sulindac therapy. *Chest* 1990;97:230–232.
25. Fein M. Sulindac and pneumonitis. *Ann Intern Med* 1981;95:245.
26. Smith FE, Lindberg PJ. Life-threatening hypersensitivity to sulindac. *JAMA* 1980;244:269–270.
27. Roncoroni AJ, Corrado C, Besuschio S, Pavlovsky S, Narvaiz M. Bronchiolitis possibly associated with amphotericin B. *J Infect Dis* 1990; 161:589.
28. Grinblat J, Mechlis S, Lewitus Z. Organizing pneumonia-like process: an unusual observation in steroid responsive cases with features of chronic interstitial pneumonia. *Chest* 1981;80: 259–263.
29. Dreis DF, Winterbauer RH, Van Norman GA, Sullivan SL, Hammar SP. Cephalosporin-induced interstitial pneumonitis. *Chest* 1984;86: 138–140.
30. Camus P, Lombard JN, Perrichon M, Piard F, Guerin J, Thivolet FB, Jeannin L. Bronchiolitis obliterans organising pneumonia in patients taking acebutolol or amiodarone. *Thorax* 1989;44: 711–715.
31. Gefter WB, Epstein DM, Pietra GG, Miller WT. Lung disease caused by amiodarone, a new antiarrythmic agent. *Radiology* May 1983;147: 339–344.
32. Marchilinski FE, Gansler TS, Waxman HL, Josephson ME. Amiodarone pulmonary toxicity. *Ann Intern Med* 1982;97:839–845.
33. Santrach PJ, Askin FB, Wells RJ, Azizkhan RG, Merten DF. Nodular form of bleomycin-related pulmonary injury in patients with osteogenic sarcoma. *Cancer* 1989;64:806–811.
34. Cohen MB, Austin JHM, Smith-Vaniz A, Lutzky J, Grimes MM. Nodular bleomycin toxicity. *Am J Clin Pathol* 1989;92:101–104.
35. Bartter T, Irwin RS, Nash G, Balikian JP, Hollingsworth HM. Idiopathic bronchiolitis obliterans organizing pneumonia with peripheral infiltrates on chest roentgenogram. *Arch Intern Med* 1989;149:273–279.
36. Yousem SA, Lifson JD, Colby TV. Chemotherapy-induced eosinophilic pneumonia: relation to bleomycin. *Chest* 1985;88:103–106.
37. Patel RC, Dutta D, Schonfeld SA. Free-base cocaine use associated with bronchiolitis obliterans organizing pneumonia. *Ann Intern Med* 1987;107:186–187.

Diseases of the Bronchioles, edited by
Gary R. Epler. Raven Press, Ltd.,
New York © 1994.

25

Infectious-Related Bronchiolitis Obliterans Organizing Pneumonia

James C. Hogg

UBC Pulmonary Research Laboratory, Pulmonary Division, St. Paul's Hospital, 1081 Burrard Street, Vancouver, BC, Canada.

The term bronchiolitis obliterans with organizing pneumonia (BOOP) was introduced in North America (1) to describe a clinicopathologic entity that is similar to, if not the same as, that described by British authors (2) who used the term cryptogenic organizing pneumonia. BOOP is now recognized as an important subclass of interstitial lung disease of unknown origin that accounted for 129 of a series of 910 cases that Corrin (3) reported from the Brompton Hospital. Although many organisms are capable of producing bronchiolitis with focal organizing pneumonia, these agents cannot usually be demonstrated in the majority of cases of BOOP. This could mean that either there is no infectious cause of BOOP, that the responsible organisms disappear between the time they initiate the disease and the time of biopsy, or that the classic techniques of microbial culture and staining are not sensitive enough to identify the microbial agents responsible. Although the newer technologies using in situ hybridization and polymerase chain reaction are beginning to be applied to this problem, it is too early to determine if they will be helpful in sorting it out. This chapter reviews some of the possible interactions between host and parasite that might contribute to the obliterative bronchiolitic organizing pneumonic inflammatory process that characterize this condition.

Body surfaces such as the upper airways and oropharynx are permanently infected with a large number of organisms that make up their natural flora. These organisms exist in a symbiotic relationship with the host without producing harmful effects. Disease is the result of tissue damage produced by organisms capable of invading the natural tissue barriers and resisting the cellular and humoral defense mechanisms of the host. The lower respiratory tract is sterile in healthy humans and almost always becomes infected from a source above the larynx. Aspiration is common even in healthy people, especially during sleep, but is rapidly cleared by the defense mechanisms of the lower airways. Therefore, successful pathogens must have the ability to overcome these defense mechanisms, to damage airway tissue, and to induce an inflammatory process.

BACTERIAL DISEASES

Pathogenic bacteria are able to overcome the local defense of the airways primarily through properties of their cell wall and capsule (4). These protect them by either suppressing phagocytosis, producing toxins that kill phagocytic cells, or by allowing them to resist intracellular destruction after they have been phagocytosed. Pathogenic organisms can also produce both extotoxins, which are soluble proteins released from bacteria as they grow, or endotoxins, which are complex lipopolysaccharides shed from the cell wall of dead or dying bacteria. The abilities to invade tissue (invasiveness) and produce toxins (toxigenicity) varies from species to species and within strains of a single species and combine to determine the degree of virulence of the organism.

Disease in the distal conducting noncartilaginous airways (bronchioles) and in the transition zone to the gas-exchanging surface of the lung (respiratory bronchioles) is determined by a balance between the virulence of the organisms that reach this area and the defense mechanisms that they encounter (5). These defense mechanisms include mucociliary clearance, phagocytosis of the organisms by alveolar macrophages, and clearance of the infected debris by the cough mechanism. They are highly efficient in the healthy state and normally keep this region of the respiratory tract sterile. Infection is associated with a reduction in the defense mechanisms that allows the lower airways to become colonized, followed by invasion of the tissue and production of an inflammatory response. This response delineates the battleground between the host and parasite that sometimes results in an organizing bronchopneumonic process with the histologic appearance described as BOOP or cryptogenic organizing pneumonia.

The bacteria capable of producing organizing bronchopneumonia include *Streptococcus pneumoniae, Staphylococcus aureus, Streptococcus pyogenes, Klebsiella,* and *Hemophilic influenza.* However, the clinical setting of these infections is usually in patients who are debilitated by cancer, uremia, or stroke, or who have chronic respiratory diseases such as cystic fibrosis, bronchiectasis, or chronic bronchitis. Alternatively, bronchoalveolar infection may occur in healthy subjects who have had a surgical procedure under general anesthesia or who have had a recent viral bronchiolitis or bronchopneumonia. These situations contrast with BOOP, in which patients present with a subacute illness of 3 to 6 months duration; the great majority show evidence of restrictive lung disease and gas-exchange impairment. Furthermore, the bacterial causes of the organizing bronchopneumonic process are readily identified by standard culture and staining procedures and are unlikely to respond positively to steroid therapy. Therefore, it is better to refer to each bronchopneumonic process by its demonstrated bacterial etiology and look elsewhere for possible ways in which an infectious process might produce BOOP or cryptogenic organizing pneumonia.

VIRAL BRONCHIOLITIS

Late in the last century, Holt (6) described a condition that he referred to as *acute catarrhal bronchitis,* which he divided into a mild form that involved larger airways and a more severe form, which he called *capillary bronchitis.* He recognized that the pathologic process was an acute inflammation of the peripheral airway wall and described the swelling, desquamation of the epithelium, and exudation of purulent mucus into the smaller airways. He also reported that the lungs from these patients were more often inflated than collapsed at autopsy and that there was enlargement of the lymph nodes at the hilum. He clearly separated this condition from bronchopneumonia, in which there was a much greater exudate into the airspace. Wohl and Chernick (7) credit Engle and Newns (8) for being the first to use the term *bronchiolitis* and for suggesting that it could have a viral etiology. The subsequent development of immunofluorescent techniques and the bedside inoculation of secretions into susceptible cell lines have now shown that bronchiolitis can be initiated by respiratory syncytial virus (9), adenovirus (10), parainfluenza virus (11), rhinovirus

(12), and influenza virus (13). Although the majority of these viral respiratory infections produce an inflammatory process that is limited to the upper respiratory tract, more severe cases extend below the larynx, where they produce various combinations of bronchitis, bronchiolitis, and pneumonia. Therefore, the possibility that the patchy organizing bronchopneumonia that characterizes BOOP might be produced by viral agents is worthy of consideration.

VIRAL INFECTION

Viruses are obligate intracellular parasites that must gain entry to the cell and make use of the cellular machinery to replicate (14). This process is outlined in Fig. 1, which shows the steps of absorption of the virus to the cell surface, penetration into the cell wall, uncoating of the viral nucleic acid, and production of the early viral proteins. These proteins include polymerases, which are essential for the replication of the viral nucleic acid, as well as other enzymes required to express the structural proteins of the virus. Assembly of the complete virus from the nucleic acid and the structural protein follows, and the viruses are either shed from the surface of the cell or are released in large numbers by cell lysis. This allows the virus to produce three basic types of infection: lytic infections, in which the infected cell is destroyed by the replicating virus; persistent infections, in which there is low-level replication of the complete virus with shedding of viral particles from the cell surface without causing cell lysis; and latent infection, in which the viral DNA is integrated into the host DNA. With latent infection viral DNA may be expressed, and the proteins have a deleterious effect on the host without either replication of the entire viral DNA genome or assembly of a complete virus. Viral culture that depends on replication of a complete virus will identify persistent and latent infections but cannot identify latent infections, in which the virus does not replicate. Increased understanding of the molecular mechanisms associated with persistent and latent infection holds the promise of providing new insight into the pathogenesis of several chronic lung diseases of unknown origin, including BOOP.

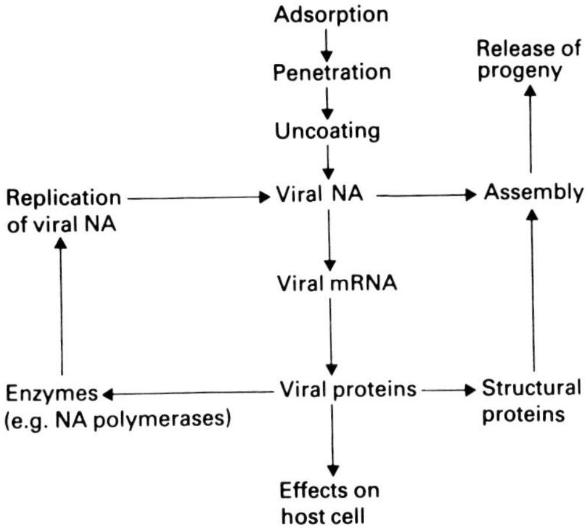

FIG. 1. Steps in the infection of a host cell by a virus. These include absorption onto the cell surface, penetration through the cell wall, uncoating of the viral nucleic acid, and generation of mRNA from the early genes. These early genes include those for the nucleic acid polymerases required to replicate the viral DNA and those required to generate structural proteins. The complete virus is then assembled and released either by lysis of the cell or by shedding from the surface of an intact cell. Viral DNA can also integrate into the host genome and produce important proteins without replication of the complete virus. These latent infections may be particularly important in the production of lung diseases of unknown etiology, such as BOOP. From ref. (14).

CLASSIFICATION OF VIRAL INFECTIONS

Fig. 2 shows a classification of viruses that is based on the nature of their genome (DNA and RNA) and whether or not the nucleic acids are double-stranded or single-stranded (14). Messenger (m) RNA and strands of identical sequence to mRNA are

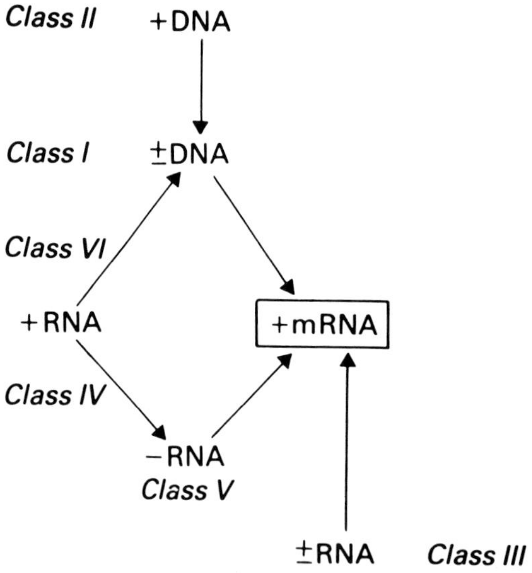

FIG. 2. A classification of viruses based on their nucleic acid. mRNA required for replication of either the viral genome or its structural proteins is designated, + and double-stranded nucleic acids are designated ±. Class I viruses, the double-stranded DNA viruses, include adenovirus and cytomegalovirus, which are important causes of lung disease. Class V, or negative-stranded, RNA viruses, include influenza, parainfluenza, and respiratory syncytial virus, are also important causes of respiratory disease. Class IV viruses, single-stranded RNA viruses such as rhinovirus, produce a great deal of respiratory misery but most is limited to the upper respiratory tract. The AIDS virus, which requires reverse transcriptase to carry it through a DNA step in the host genome, is found in Class VI. From ref. (14).

designated (+), and DNA and RNA complimentary to mMRA are designated (−); double-stranded nucleic acids are designated (±). The major viruses causing respiratory illness are found in class I, which has a double-stranded DNA genome, such as adenovirus and cytomegalovirus; class IV, which has a single-stranded (+) RNA genome and contains the rhinovirus; and class V, which has a single-stranded (−) RNA genome and includes influenza, parainfluenza, and respiratory syncytial virus. In adults, the most likely viruses capable of contributing to the organizing bronchopneumonic process now recognized as BOOP would include the adenovirus and cytomegalovirus found in class I and the influenza, parainfluenza, and respiratory syncytial virus found in class V. Although rhinoviruses are capable of producing much respiratory misery, the bulk of the illness is in the upper respiratory area and therefore is not considered further.

Class I Viral Infections

Adenovirus

The adenovirus is an attractive candidate in the pathogenesis of BOOP because it has the ability to produce bronchiolitis and bronchopneumonia (15,16). However, it is unlikely that its mode of action is straightforward; otherwise the organism would have been isolated in some of the cases. An alternative possibility is that latent adenoviral infection may have the capability of amplifying the inflammatory response to others present in the distal airways.

The adenovirus (14) has an icosohedral shape, which means it has 20 triangular faces, 12 apices, and 30 edges, with an outer coat that consists of 240 hexons (virion protein 2) and 12 penton bases (virion protein 3) located at the apices of the icosohedral structure (Fig. 3). Infection begins when a fiber covalently linked to each penton base (virion protein 4) attaches to a specific receptor on the cell surface to allow the virus to become internalized. Once inside the cell, the capsid is stripped and the double-stranded DNA core is transported to the nucleus, where the viral genes are transcribed. The "early" genes use host cell mechanisms to synthesize viral mRNA and proteins important to subsequent viral DNA replication. The late viral genes are responsible for producing structural proteins, which are synthesized in the cytoplasm and transported to the nucleus for virion assembly. During the late phase, host cell DNA, mRNA, and protein synthesis

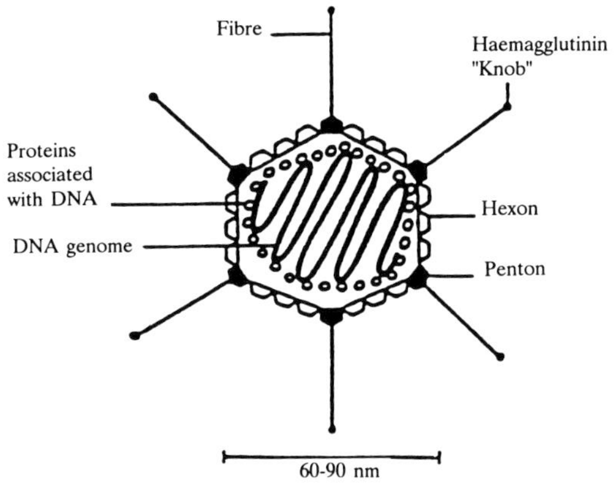

FIG. 3. The structure of an adenovirus. These organisms adhere to host cells by a fiber protein. This then leads to the internalization of the virus, stripping of its coat, and replication of DNA and structural proteins to form a complete virus. The adenovirus is particularly capable of becoming latent by integrating parts of its genome into the human DNA. It is capable of expressing proteins that may have important effects on the host without ever replicating a complete virus. Modified from ref. (17).

are shut off and the cell becomes devoted to the synthesis of the virus. Eventually the cell dies, and the assembled virions are released to infect other cells. In lytic infections the viral yield can rise from zero at the start of the infection up to 10^4 PFU/cell 30 to 35 hours after infection (17).

Fig. 4 shows a histological specimen prepared from a study of postmortem lung in which death was due to acute adenoviral infection (18). It shows both the diffuse alveolar injury with hemorrhagic pulmonary edema (Fig. 4A) and the hyaline membrane formation (Fig. 4B) that occur after tissue injury by the virus. The in situ hybridization studies performed using a probe for the entire length of the adenoviral 5 genome showed that the cells in the peripheral lung are loaded with adenoviral DNA (Fig. 4C). Fig. 5 shows the histology of a peripheral bronchiole from the same lung; there is evidence of epithelial damage and the presence of an inflammatory exudate in the lumen. The in situ hybridization study of this tissue (Fig. 5B) show that many of the airway epithelial cells are loaded with adenovirus.

The histological specimens (Figs. 4 and 5) clearly show diffuse alveolar injury with an inflammatory exudate in the airway lumen that might be expected to develop into a classic picture of BOOP. If this were to happen, one might also expect sufficient diffuse parenchymal disease to produce a restrictive functional defect and local bronchopneumonic processes capable of producing the radiological and histological features of BOOP. The patient would also present with a viral-like prodrome like that described in BOOP or cryptogenic organizing pneumonia, but it is unlikely that the virus would still be readily demonstrable in the tissue. Indeed, when tissue from the same outbreak became available 3 months and 3 years after the infection, no virus could be demonstrated in it. This might be because the technique is too insensitive at detecting low copy numbers of the virus or because no virus was present at that stage.

The possibility that the adenovirus lies dormant in human lung tissue was subsequently investigated by Matsuse and colleagues (19), who found that some of the early regions of the adenoviral DNA were present in excess amounts in human airways; they speculated that proteins produced by these viruses could contribute to an inflammatory process in chronic obstructive pulmonary disease. To understand how this might work requires further consideration of some of the features of the adenoviral genome and the sequence in which it is expressed.

The early genes (20,21) are grouped into six transcription units denoted E1A, E1B, E2A/B, E4, and L1 early. As indicated above, these are referred to as the early genes because they are the first to be expressed during infection and code for proteins that are required to carry out a number of key regulatory functions needed to assemble a new virus. These include the induction of transcription of other regions of

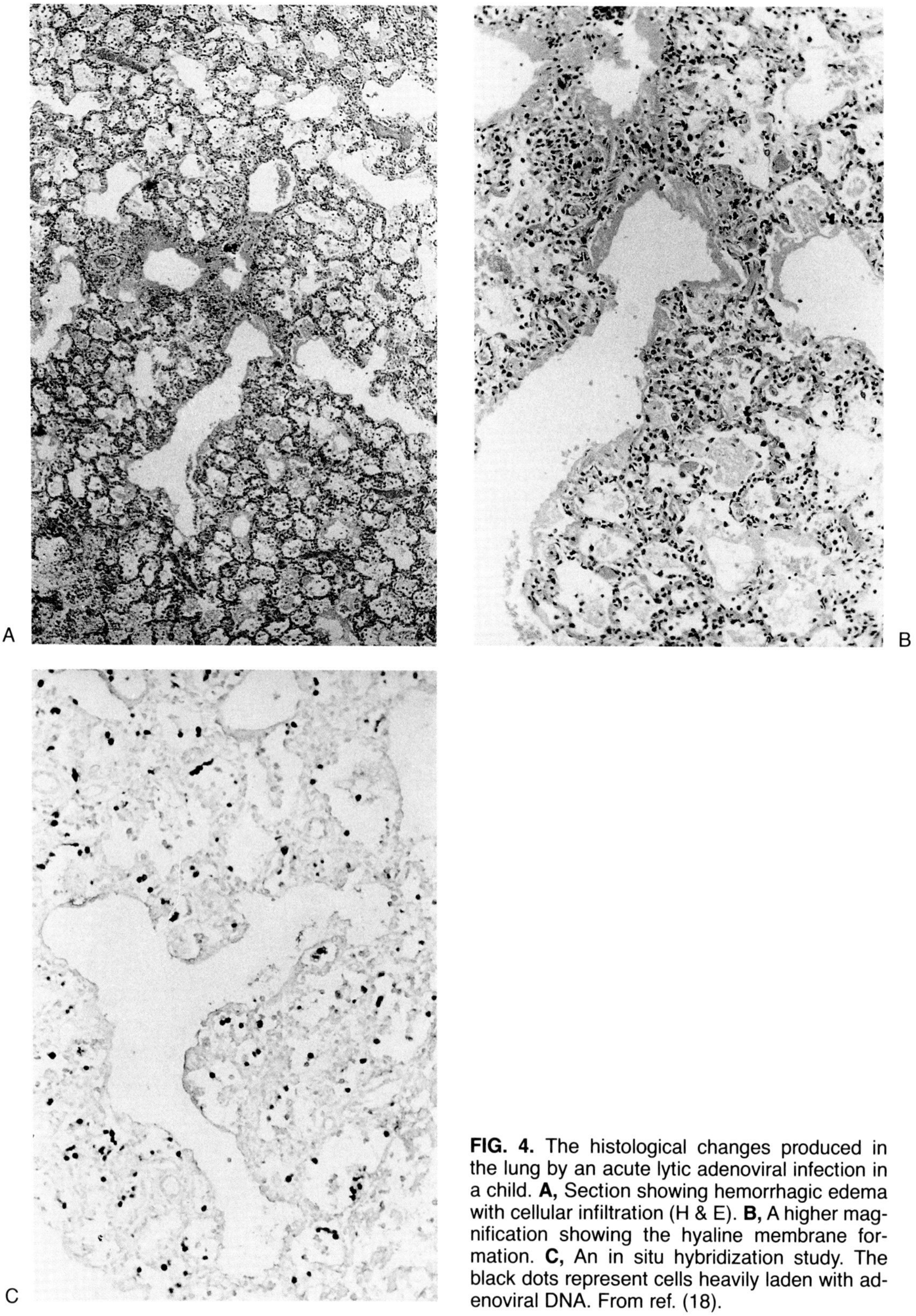

FIG. 4. The histological changes produced in the lung by an acute lytic adenoviral infection in a child. **A,** Section showing hemorrhagic edema with cellular infiltration (H & E). **B,** A higher magnification showing the hyaline membrane formation. **C,** An in situ hybridization study. The black dots represent cells heavily laden with adenoviral DNA. From ref. (18).

A 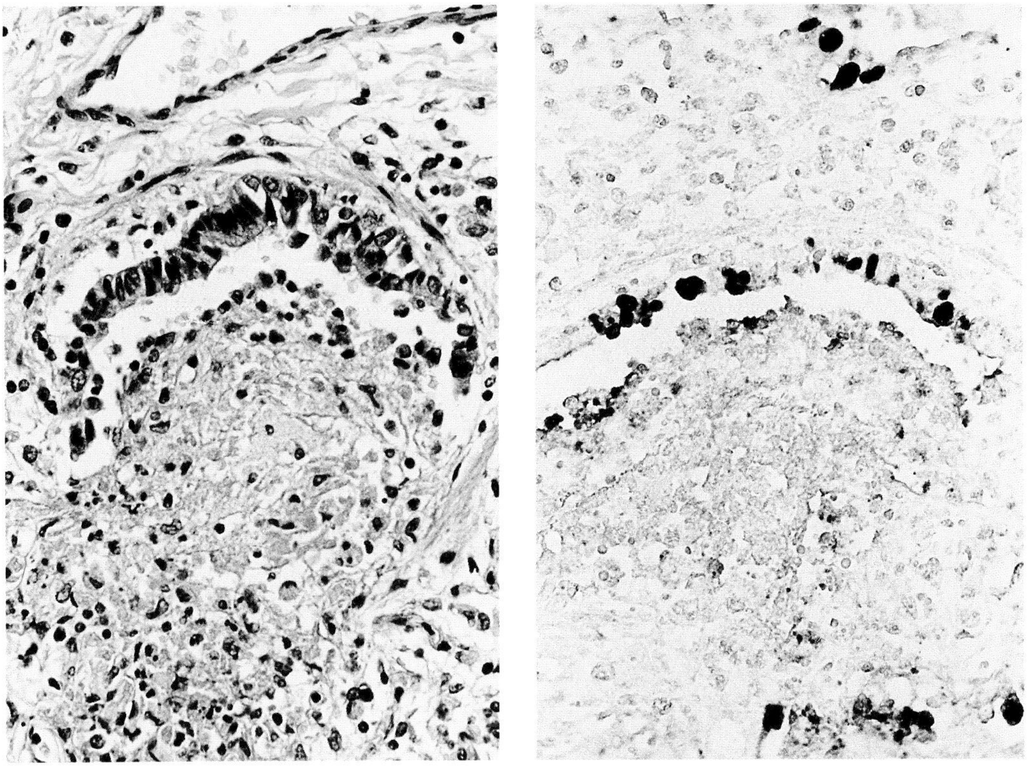 B

FIG. 5. From the same case as Fig. 4. **A,** Destruction of airway epithelium with a polypoid inflammatory exudate present in the airway lumen. **B,** In situ hybridization of the same airway. Many of the epithelial cells are heavily laden with adenoviral DNA. One could easily imagine the polypoid exudative process in A organizing into an obliterative bronchiolitic process that characterizes BOOP. From ref. (18).

the viral DNA code for the structural proteins of the viruses (Fig. 1). The adenovirus has the ability to transform cells using proteins that are coded in the genes of the E1A and E1B regions. These genes can also become integrated at random sites in the DNA of the host cell and be expressed at the protein level. This means that the virus can continue to affect cells without the need to assemble a complete virus. Proteins encoded in the E1A region have been shown to have a variety of interesting functions, including the abilities to interfere with normal inhibitors of cell division and growth and to sensitize cells for destruction by cytokines such as tumor necrosis factor.

The E3 region encodes nine overlapping mRNA with different splicing patterns. One of these proteins, the E3/19K, is capable of blocking the expression of the class I major histocompatibility complex molecule by the infected cell; this allows the cell to evade destruction of cytotoxic T lymphocytes (20–22). Recent studies (21) have shown that the E3/19K protein has different affinities for class I antigen; this means that the pathogenicity of a given adenovirus serotype could be influenced both by the virus and by the host major histocompatibility complex haplotype. In any event, this mechanism serves to protect the adenovirus by preventing destruction of the host cell by the cytotoxic lymphocytes. These protected cells provide an opportunity for the virus to integrate into the host genome.

A normal gene has upstream, proximal

promoter, and activator sequences that assist in regulating transcription. The promoter can be likened to turning on the ignition of a car and the activator to stepping on the gas. In order for transcription to proceed, factors that include RNA polymerase must bind to the upstream gene sequences to turn on the expression of the gene. The function of the product of the retinoblastoma gene is to regulate transcription by binding to these transcription factors and allowing them to be released to the upstream sequences in a controlled fashion (24). The adenoviral E1A protein has the ability to bind to the retinoblastoma protein (25) and compete it away from the transcription factors, allowing them to bind to the upstream regions and initiate gene transcription. Therefore, latent infection of the respiratory tract by adenovirus with expression of the E1A protein could stimulate tissue growth by allowing the expression of genes that amplify the inflammatory process. This might contribute to the connective tissue proliferation in the terminal and respiratory bronchioles and transform the histologic picture of acute bronchiolitis and adult respiratory distress syndrome (ARDS) into one of BOOP. Under these circumstances, one would not be able to culture the virus because it would not be replicating, but the E1A DNA and its protein should be demonstrable.

Cytomegalovirus

The cytomegalovirus also has a double-stranded DNA genome and is perhaps the most widespread member of a widely distributed family of herpes viruses (25). The majority of adults have serum antibodies indicating that they have been exposed to some serotype of the virus. Although the natural reservoir of the virus is in humans, the relationship between host and virus is symbiotic and the vast majority of infections remain subclinical. Both primary and reactivation infections occur in an endemic fashion in certain clinical settings, where they produce disease in salivary glands, renal tract, liver, and lung. The virus can also be transmitted by blood, in which it can be commonly isolated from polymorphonucleocytes, less frequently from monocytes, and occasionally from T lymphocytes. It is frequently responsible for a mononucleosis type of clinical picture in the post-perfusion and post-transfusion setting. Cytomegalovirus infection has become a major problem in immunosuppressed patients, particularly those whose immune system has been compromised either by infection with the AIDS virus or administration of drugs and radiation following organ transplants. Bone marrow transplant patients are particularly susceptible to cytomegalovirus infection, which is associated with prolonged cytomegalovirus viremia in over half of these patients. Cytomegalovirus pneumonia has been implicated in the highly lethal severe respiratory failure that develops in the early phase of bone marrow transplantation. Bronchiolitis obliterans seen in the transplant setting usually occurs as a later complication and may be more closely associated with graft-versus-host disease.

Grundy and associates (26) have suggested that both pneumonitis and obstructive bronchiolitis may be related to an immunopathological mechanism that may not require viral replication. They postulate that the enhanced expression of class I and II major histocompatibility complex antigens in a graft-versus-host reaction could lead to an aggressive T-cell response against cells infected with cytomegalovirus. They suggest that because the cytomegalovirus protein is affectively presented by class I antigens, the combination of viral infection and increased class I expression could cause an exaggerated cell-mediated immune response. This hypothesis is attractive in that it would also explain the ineffectiveness of antiviral agents in this setting because these agents block only viral DNA synthesis after the expression of the early alpha and beta genes. Because these genes can be expressed without replication of the complete virus, the alpha and beta proteins could interact with either host or donor class I molecules to induce an aggressive cytotoxic T-cell mediated inflammatory reaction in the peripheral lung.

Whether or not latent or persistent cytomegalovirus infections are ever responsible for cases of BOOP that occur in the bone marrow transplant setting or in any other clinical situation remains to be determined. Studies of viral DNA expression and interaction between viral proteins and the class I molecules deserve to be explored. It is also possible that an altered presentation of the viral proteins to the immune system could lead to expression of autoantibodies that might cause disease and that certain HLA genotypes would be more susceptible to this than others. Clearly, the interaction of the DNA viruses with the host provides interesting hypotheses, but most of them remain to be tested.

Class V Viruses in the Pathogenesis of Bronchiolitis Obliterans Organizing Pneumonia

The orthomyxoviridae (influenza viruses) (29), paramyxoviridae (parainfluenza viruses) (28), and respiratory syncytial virus (29) have negative single-stranded RNA genomes. However, the genome of the influenza virus is segmented, whereas that of the parainfluenza and respiratory syncytial viruses is not. The segmental nature of the orthomyxoviridae is important because it is responsible for the genetic recombination in the influenza virus, which is rare if it occurs at all in the parainfluenza and respiratory syncytial viruses.

The Influenza Virus

The genome of the influenza virus is divided into eight segments, each of which is surrounded by capsid protein and each of which is a single gene. In the major influenza viruses, types A and B, there are eight segments and ten viral proteins, the extra two proteins being generated by splicing the message for the M protein (segment 7) into three. Classification, based on the internal antigens of the M and nucleo-capsid proteins, allows three independent non-cross-reacting types of influenza virus to be recognized. Strains of influenza type A are found in humans and animals, while B and C are restricted to humans. The segmented nature of the influenza virus genome with its eight pieces of RNA allows the RNA segments of two viruses to become mixed when the co-infect a single cell. This type of genetic recombination and reassortment can form new viral strains or even new species and is the basis or the antigenic shift and drift seen in the influenza virus. Influenza viral infection, probably the most important respiratory disease in humans, is spread by droplet infection and usually establishes infection in the upper respiratory tract before extending into the lower airways. The neuraminidases expressed on the viral surface allow it to penetrate the mucus layer and attach to the cell surface, where it internalizes and replicates.

In uncomplicated influenza infections, bronchoscopic examination of the lower respiratory tract has shown diffuse reddening and swelling of the larynx, trachea, and bronchi. Light microscopic examination of the tissue shows evidence of damage and desquamation of the epithelium frequently exposing a thickened and sometimes hyalinized basement membrane. There is also evidence of submucosal edema with vascular congestion and infiltration of neutrophils and mononuclear cells. Viral antigen can be demonstrated in the epithelial cells and mononuclear cells and occasionally in the basal cell layer. Later in the course of the disease, reparative and destructive processes may be present simultaneously, with complete resolution of the epithelial necrosis occurring over a period of weeks to months. The small peripheral airways are often affected in uncomplicated infection, and abnormalities in peripheral airway function may persist long after the symptomatic illness has subsided. However, in uncomplicated infection there is usually little permanent damage to the lung, even in patients with chronic obstructive lung disease.

The virus can also produce severe pneumonia with diffuse alveolar injury leading to hemorrhagic edema that can be fatal. The edematous phase is followed by formation of hyaline membranes and a slow progressive recovery that can be prolonged. Viral infection predisposes to bronchial infection by several mechanisms (1), including interference with mucociliary clearance, bacterial killing by alveolar macrophages, and the tendency to aspirate mucoid exudate loaded with bacteria from the upper airways. The most commonly involved organisms are the *Streptococcus pneumonia, Staphylococcus aureus,* and *Hemophilus influenza*. This syndrome may be indistinguishable from primary viral pneumonia except that the symptoms of bacterial pneumonia, such as pleuritic chest pain and shaking chills, may signal its onset some time after the influenza symptoms have appeared.

A combined viral and bacterial pneumonia could result in the clinical and pathological syndrome that we recognize as BOOP, which often presents with a prodroma suggesting viral illness. If the virus were diffusely present in the lung and bacterial aspiration occurred into one or more lung regions, a setting might be created suggesting restrictive interstitial lung disease with nodules of a local bronchopneumonic process. However, if this were the case, histological examination and culture should be capable of demonstrating the bacterial pathogens and the virus itself should have been identified by culture. A systematic evaluation of a large series of cases might be useful in determining if there is a role for influenza virus infection in this process.

Parainfluenza and Respiratory Syncytial Virus

The parainfluenza (28) and respiratory syncytial viruses (29) are also major causes of lower respiratory tract disease. They differ from influenza in that their negative single-stranded RNA genome is nonsegmented, although they also have a helical nucleocapsid that is surrounded by a lipid envelope. Both of these viruses have the ability to cause cell fusion giving rise to typical multinucleated giant cells or syncytia when grown in vitro. They also have the ability to establish persistent infection in cultures in which the infected cells survive for long periods while the virus is continuously replicated at low levels that do not produce a typical cytopathic effect. Whether or not this persistence also occurs in vivo is less clear, but if it does, it could be an important reservoir of disease.

Four serologically distinct types of parainfluenza virus produce infections of the respiratory tract, the most dangerous of which is an acute laryngotracheo bronchitis or croup. They are also capable of producing lower respiratory tract infection similar to influenza, which can be complicated by secondary bacterial infection in the same way.

The respiratory syncytial virus differs from influenza and parainfluenza in that it does not express either hemagglutinin or neuraminidases (29). It produces severe life-threatening lower respiratory tract disease in infants and children, in whom it is particularly severe under the age of 6 months. In adults, infection tends to be milder and confined to the upper respiratory tract, although it is a significant cause of viral bronchopneumonia, which can be complicated by secondary bacterial pneumonia. The fact that infants are particularly susceptible when they have circulating maternal IgG antibodies but lack the ability to produce their own local IgA protection has implicated antibody-mediated hypersensitivity in the pathogenesis of the bronchiolitis. The concept that IgG contributed to the bronchiolitis was further supported by an adverse experience in which the administration of a formalin-inactivated vaccine that produced an IgG response in newborns resulted in a more severe bronchiolitis in these children when they were naturally infected in a subsequent epidemic. These findings suggest that the formation of IgG virus complex in the airways could play an important role in the pathogenesis of this form of bronchiolitis and raise the possibility that the host immune system might interact with a virus to produce a chronic organizing bronchopneumonia in some adults.

SUMMARY

This overview of respiratory bacterial and viral respiratory tract infections was designed to outline the possible mechanisms that could produce BOOP. The available data suggest that straightforward bacterial and viral infection is unlikely because attempts to demonstrate the virus with standard microbiological techniques have not been successful to date. Furthermore, some cases of BOOP respond to corticosteroid therapy, which would not be expected if an acute infection were present. However, latent or persistent infection might combine with an altered immune response to produce an organizing bronchopneumonic process. In some cases, latent adenoviral infections are capable of producing viral proteins that could amplify an existing inflammatory process, and cytomegalovirus may induce an aggressive T-cell response that would produce an organizing bronchopneumonic picture. Although the single-stranded RNA viruses are limited to the cell cytoplasm and do not have the ability to integrate into host DNA, they can become persistent by establishing a form of carrier culture in some lung cell population where low levels of replication cause the host to shed virus for prolonged periods. This means that in addition to possibly causing an acute bronchopneumonic process, some of the RNA viruses may persist and induce a more chronic inflammatory reaction. Although there is no clear evidence for any particular mechanism, the nature of the clinical syndrome strongly suggests that persistent and latent viral infection could produce an abnormal host–parasite interaction that might be responsible for BOOP.

ACKNOWLEDGMENTS

Supported by Medical Research Council Grant #7246 and The Respiratory Health Network of Centres of Excellence.

REFERENCES

1. Epler GR, Colby TV, McLoud TC, Carrington CB, Gaensler EA. Bronchiolitis obliterans organizing pneumonia. *N Engl J Med* 1985;312: 152–158.
2. Davison AG, Heard BE, McAllister WA, Turner-Warwick ME. Cryptogenic organizing pneumonitis. *Q J Med* 1983;52:382–394.
3. Corrin B. Pathology of interstitial lung disease. In: Harasawa M, Fukuchi Y, Morinari H, eds. *Interstitial pneumonia of unknown etiology,* Tokyo: University of Tokyo Press; 1989:149–168.
4. Taussig MJ. Processes in pathology and microbiology. In: *Bacterial infection.* 2nd ed. Edinburgh: Blackwell Scientific Publications; 1987: 377–621.
5. Dunnill MS ed. Pulmonary defense mechanisms. In: *Pulmonary pathology.* New York: Churchill Livingston; 1982:1–16.
6. Holt LE. *Diseases of infancy and childhood.* New York: Appleton and Company; 1897:463–466.
7. Wohl MEB, Chernick V. Bronchiolitis: state of the art. *Am Rev Respir Dis* 1978;118:759–781.
8. Engle S, Newns GH. Proliferation mural bronchiolitis. *Arch Dis Child* 1940;15:219.
9. McClelland L, Hilleman MR, Hamparian VV, et al. Studies of acute respiratory illnesses caused by respiratory syncytial virus. 2: Epidemiology and assessment of important. *N Engl J Med* 1961;246:1169–1175.
10. Gold R, Wilt JC, Adhikaria PK, McPherson RI. Adenoviral pneumonia and its complications in infancy and childhood. *J Can Assoc Radiol* 1969;20:218–224.

11. Downham MA, McQuillin J, Gardner PS. Diagnosis and clinical significance of para-influenza virus infections in children. *Arch Dis Child* 1974;49:8–15.
12. Jacobs JW, Peacock DB, Corner BD, Caul EO, Clark SKR. Respiratory syncytial and other viruses associated with respiratory tract disease in infants. *Lancet* 1971;1:871–876.
13. Caul EO, Waller DK, Clark SKR, Corner BD. A comparison of influenza and respiratory syncytial virus infections among infants admitted to hospital with acute respiratory infections. *J Hyg (Camb)* 1976;77:383–392.
14. Taussig MJ. *Processes in pathology and microbiology*. 2nd ed. Oxford, Edinburgh: Blackwell Scientific Publications; 1987:215–375.
15. Brandt CD, Kim HW, Vargoski AJ, et al. Infections in 18,000 infants and children in a controlled study of respiratory tract disease. I: Adenovirus pathogenicity in relation to serologic type and illness syndrome. *Am J Epidemiol* 1969;90:484–500.
16. Becroft DMO. Histopathology of fatal adenovirus infection of the respiratory tract in young children. *J Clin Pathol* 1967;20:561–569.
17. Ginsberg HS, ed. *The adenovirus*. New York, London: Plenum Press; 1984.
18. Hogg JC, Irving WL, Porter H, Evans M, Dunnill MS, Fleming K. In situ hybridization studies of adenoviral infections of the lung and their relationship to follicular bronchiectasis. *Am Rev Respir Dis* 1989;139:1531–1535.
19. Matsuse T, Hayashi S, Kuwano K, Keunecke H, Jefferies WA, Hogg JC. Latent adenoviral infection in the pathogenesis of chronic airways obstruction. *Am Rev Respir Dis* 1992;146:177–184.
20. Ginsberg HS, Lundholm-Beauchamp U, Horswood RL, et al. Role of early regions 3 (E3) in pathogenesis of adenovirus disease. *Proc Natl Acad Sci USA* 1989;86:3823–3827.
21. Gooding LR, Wold WSM. Molecular mechanisms by which adenoviruses counteract antiviral immune defences. *Crit Rev Immunol* 1990; 10:53–71.
22. Burgert HG, Kvist S. An adenovirus type 2 glycoprotein blocks cell surface expression of human histocompatibility class I antigens. *Cell* 1985;41:987–997.
23. Bandara LR, LaThangue NB. Adenovirus E1A prevents the retinoblastoma gene product from complexing with a cellular transcription factor. *Nature* 1991;351:494–497.
24. Whyte P, Buchlovich KJ, Horowitz JM, Friend SH, Raybuck M, Weinberg RA, Harlow E. Association between an oncogene and an antioncogene: the adenovirus E1A proteins bind to the retinoblastoma gene product. *Nature* 1991;351: 494–497.
25. Alford CA, Britt WJ. Cytomegalovirus. In: Field BM, ed. *Virology*. New York: Raven Press; 1985:527–561.
26. Grundy JD, Shanley JD, Griffiths PD. Is cytomegalovirus interstitial pneumonia in transplant recipients an immunopathological condition? *Lancet* 1987:996–999.
27. Murphy BR, Webster RG. Influenza viruses. In: Field BM, ed. *Virology*, New York: Raven Press; 1985:1179–1240.
28. Shanock RM, MacIntosh K. Para-influenza virus. In: Field BM, ed. *Virology*, New York: Raven Press; 1985:1241–1254.
29. MacIntosh K, Shanock RM. Respiratory syncytial virus. In: Field BM, ed. *Virology*, New York: Raven Press; 1985:1285–1304.

Diseases of the Bronchioles, edited by
Gary R. Epler. Raven Press, Ltd.,
New York © 1994.

26

Miscellaneous Causes of Bronchiolitis Obliterans Organizing Pneumonia

Gary R. Epler

Associate Clinical Professor, Boston University School of Medicine; Chairman, Department of Medicine, New England Baptist Hospital, 125 Parker Hill Avenue, Boston, MA.

Bronchiolitis obliterans organizing pneumonia (BOOP) is usually categorized as idiopathic, post-infectious, connective-tissue related (rheumatologic and immunologic disorders), or drug related (Table 1). Several miscellaneous causes or associated disorders have been reported on a case-by-case basis that eventually may lead to a separate classification if sufficiently common. This chapter is a discussion of each of these BOOP-related disorders.

HIV INFECTION

A 40-year-old man who had been HIV positive for 1 year developed dyspnea, nonproductive cough for 4 weeks, and fever, (1). Two weeks before admission, a chest roentgenogram showed subtle infiltrates at the lung bases, and an antibiotic as started. The symptoms progressed. The chest roentogenogram then showed bilateral patchy infiltrates. A bronchoalveolar lavage showed 46% macrophages and 48% lymphocytes. An open lung biopsy was performed because of unexplained progressive respiratory failure. Histologic examination showed BOOP with an interstitial mononuclear cell component. Intravenous corticosteroid therapy was given with defervescence in 48 hours and progressive improvement in oxygenation and the roentgenographic appearance. He was given a total of 6 weeks of corticosteroid therapy. Five months after discharge, he had persistent crackles but no dyspnea. The chest radiograph and arterial blood gases were normal.

It was noted that the lavage findings of increased lymphocytes differed from findings in patients with non-HIV bronchiolitis obliterans, who have increased neutrophils, as reported by Kindt and colleagues (2); however, these patients had bronchiolitis obliterans and not BOOP, as did this patient with HIV infection. Actually, the lavage finding of increased lymphocytes is very consistent with BOOP, as several studies have since shown (3–5).

RADIATION THERAPY

A 61-year-old man with small-cell carcinoma of the lung had a complete remission from six cycles of cyclophosphamide, doxorubicin, and vincristine (6). He then received 5,600 rad for 1 month to the left hilum and mediastinum as well as 1,800 rad of prophylactic brain irradiation. About 2 weeks after the final radiation treatment, he developed dyspnea, cough productive of yellow sputum, and fever. No crackles or wheezes were heard on examination. The chest roentgenogram showed bilateral fluffy infiltrates paralleling the irradiation field.

TABLE 1. *Causes and associated disorders of BOOP*

Idiopathic
Post-infectious
Rheumatological disorders
Drug-related
Miscellaneous
HIV infection
Radiation therapy
Myelodysplastic syndrome
Common variable immunodeficiency syndrome
Chronic thyroiditis
Alcoholic cirrhosis
Seasonal syndrome with cholestasis

The patient was treated with corticosteroid therapy, but symptoms progressed rapidly over 48 hours. Lung biopsy showed obliteration of the bronchiolar lumen by fibroblastic proliferation and organizing pneumonia in alveoli. Despite large doses of corticosteroid therapy, the patient died.

The absence of physical findings was noted but is not unusual, occurring in 25% of patients with idiopathic BOOP (7). The histologic findings were consistent with the typical BOOP patterns except for microthrombi, which is a common finding of radiation pneumonitis.

A second report of BOOP as a result of radiation therapy was noted in a 63-year-old woman who had a radical right mastectomy and postoperative irradiation therapy 18 years before the present hospital admission (8). For 5 years before admission she had recurrent episodes of apparent pneumonia with fever, right-sided pleuritic chest pain, and a nonproductive cough. On her admission to the hospital, the chest radiograph showed poorly defined infiltrates peripherally in the right middle and lower lungs. The chest CT scan showed poorly defined peripheral airspace shadowing confined to the portion of lung that had been irradiated after the mastectomy 18 years before. During several weeks of observation, the infiltrates migrated within this portion of the lung. An open lung biopsy showed BOOP. Corticosteroid therapy resulted in a rapid, sustained, and complete clinical and radiological resolution of the opacities. This report was a response to an article about the radiographic migratory aspects of the patchy infiltrates of BOOP (9), a similar finding observed in the report of idiopathic BOOP by Japanese investigators (10).

MYELODYSPLASTIC SYNDROME

A 58-year-old man developed fever, productive cough, dyspnea and weight loss for 6 weeks (11). A bone marrow biopsy obtained because of pancytopenia showed refractory anemia with excess blasts—a myelodysplastic syndrome. He had bilateral crackles, and the chest roentogenogram showed bilateral infiltrates. After several courses of antibiotics the hypoxemia worsened. The chest roentgenogram showed some clearing of the left lung infiltrate, but progressive alveolar consolidation appeared on the right side. The lung biopsy showed BOOP (photomicrographs were not published). The symptoms and hypoxemia resolved 4 days after prednisone was started. The authors suggested that recognition of BOOP in the immunocompromised patient is critical because of the complete clinical and physiologic recovery seen in the majority of patients.

COMMON VARIABLE IMMUNODEFICIENCY SYNDROME

A 20-year-old woman developed weakness, night sweats, pancytopenia, and massive splenomegaly, and a chest roentgenogram showed linear and patchy densities in both lungs (12). A transbronchial lung biopsy showed interstitial pneumonitis. A splenectomy was performed. The splenic tissue showed non caseating granulomas, suggesting a diagnosis of common variable immunodeficiency syndrome and hypersplenism. Five years later she developed eight episodes of pneumonia over a 1-year period despite monthly injections of gamma globulin. She was treated with various antimicrobial agents but never fully recovered. At age 26, she was admitted to the hospital for diagnosis and management. The chest roentgenograms showed persistent and worsening infiltrates. End-inspiratory crackles were heard on examination. Pulmonary function studies showed a normal vital capacity and flow rates, while the diffusing capacity was decreased to 63% predicted. The lung biopsy showed noncaseating granulomas and plugs of granulation tissue in airways consistent with BOOP. Corticosteroid therapy was begun with gradual improvement in the chest roentgenogram and no recurrence of the episodes of pneumonia.

The authors noted that the features of common variable immunodeficiency syndrome were similar to the X-linked agammaglobulinemias. The usual pulmonary features are bronchiectasis and noncaseating granulomas. Possible etiologies include intrinsic B-cell defect, immunoregulatory T-cell imbalance, and autoantibodies to B or T cells. The relationship of B and T cell dysfunction has not been defined with BOOP; these authors suggested that the improvement with corticosteroid therapy may indicate some alteration or reduction in autoantibodies to B or T cells.

LYMPHOMA

A 58-year-old woman developed a nonproductive cough, fever, and progressive dyspnea for 3 weeks (13). Bilateral inspiratory crackles were heard. The erythrocyte sedimentation rate was 90 mm per hour. The chest roentgenogram showed diffuse, patchy linear and alveolar opacities in both lungs. A transbronchial lung biopsy showed buds of loose connective tissue containing inflammatory cells and fibroblasts filling bronchiolar lumina and alveoli. The findings were consistent with BOOP. Administration of prednisone led to rapid symptomatic and radiological improvement with virtual resolution of shadowing after 1 month of treatment. The prednisone was continued for 13 months. There were two recurrences during the next 2 years.

Four years after the first episode of BOOP, resection of an enlarged lymph node in the neck was resected showed a nodular, diffuse proliferation of small and intermediate lymphoid cells with cleaved and noncleaved nuclei consistent with malignant lymphoma, and diffuse mixed, small, and large cells of intermediate grade of malignancy. There were no respiratory symptoms, abnormal chest radiographic findings, or abnormal physiological tests. Treatment with cyclophosphamide, doxorubicin, vincristine, and prednisone (CHOP) for 5 months achieved complete clinical remission after the sixth week.

Two years later, cough and dyspnea again developed, and the chest roentgenogram showed a lingular infiltrate. Transbronchial lung biopsy was consistent with BOOP. Prednisone treatment was restarted with a striking response. Ten months later, the patient was free of disease, but prednisone, 20 mg every other day, was continued.

The authors discussed the possibility of an autoimmune mechanism as a cause of BOOP but concluded that whether a true pathogenic relationship existed between these two infrequent disease was not known. A previous report of fifty-two patients with bronchiolitis obliterans noted that two patients had lymphoma, one with idiopathic thrombocytopenic purpura and one with diabetes, but the type of bronchiolar lesion and specific details were not available (14). One patient among these fifty-two also had a malignant process of acute lymphocytic leukemia.

CHRONIC THYROIDITIS

Among the report of twenty-nine patients with BOOP by Japanese investigators (10), two patients had chronic thyroiditis. The first was a 61-year-old woman with dyspnea, productive cough, and fever. The chest roentgenogram showed patchy infiltrates. Bronchoalveolar lavage showed 70% neutrophils and no lymphocytes. The illness responded to corticosteroid therapy. The second patient was a 60-year-old woman with cough and dyspnea. The chest radiograph showed micronodular opacities at the lung bases, and the sedimentation rate was 39 mm per hour. The patient recovered without corticosteroid therapy.

ALCOHOLIC CIRRHOSIS

One patient among the twenty-nine patients with BOOP reported by the Japanese investigators had alcoholic-related cirrhosis (10). The patient was a 64-year-old man with fever. The chest roentgenogram showed both patchy infiltrates and micronodular opacities. The sedimentation rate was markedly increased to 146 mm per hour. The patient recovered from BOOP without corticosteroid therapy.

SEASONAL SYNDROME WITH CHOLESTASIS

Most of the miscellaneous causes of BOOP could be classified in the general category of immunologically related. However, there has been a report (15) of eight women and four men aged 34 to 62 years who developed recurring pulmonary symptoms and abnormal liver enzyme studies suggesting intrahepatic cholestasis. These symptoms arose between late February and early May every year and resolved between June and January. Virtually all these patients had a nonproductive cough and dyspnea; one-half had associated fever; and pleuritic-type chest pain was common. In every patient, these features occurred every year in the last weeks of February and resolved by early May or earlier with corticosteroid therapy. Between relapses, all patients were entirely symptom-free and remained in full-time work. Fine end-inspiratory crackles were heard in all patients. No high-pitched squeaks were recorded. Laboratory studies showed elevated erythrocyte sedimentation rate from 43 to 115 mm per hour, elevated bilirubin values from 3 to 16 mg/dl, and alkaline phosphatase from 345 to 1,029 units/L. The chest roentgenograms showed pleural-based shadows with consolidation within the lung parenchyma in all patients, bilateral in all but one, and predominantly in the lower and middle areas. Chest CT scans of eight patients confirmed the peripheral pattern of the pulmonary infiltrates and indicated airspace consolidation with evidence of air bronchograms. During clinical remission there was complete or partial resolution of the radiographic abnormalities, either spontaneous or after treatment. Pulmonary function tests showed reduction in the vital capacity in ten patients from 42 to 79% of predicted and reduction in the diffusing capacity in 9 from 25 to 76% of predicted. Two patients had severe air-flow obstruction with an FEV_1/FVC of 49% and 53%, respectively, and they had never smoked cigarettes. Bronchoalveolar lavage in eight patients showed higher than normal percentages of neutrophils of 10% and lymphocytes of 16%. Three patients had open lung biopsy, four percutaneous biopsy and five transbronchial biopsy, all showing intraalveolar buds of granulation tissue. In the three patients who underwent open lung biopsy, there were areas of infiltration and obstruction of the lumen of the terminal bronchiole by granulation tissue; however, most bronchioles were patent even when there was widespread organizing pneumonia. Liver biopsy in two patients showed nonnecrotizing granuloma within the hepatic parenchyma, unrelated to bile ducts, with no other abnormalities.

The patients reported spontaneous remission of the first episode after a short illness. Eventually, however, the illness became more severe. Corticosteroid therapy, which was often used, provided a rapid and complete resolution of their symptoms. The cause was not determined, although it was thought to be an inhaled agent present in the general environment from late February to early May, at least in England. It most likely is an outcome of an immunologically mediated hypersensitivity response, rather than an infection. Suspected causes were pollen of such trees as hazel, birch, apple, and cherry. Patients were tested but no immediate responses were elicited.

Some of these twelve patients had the typical BOOP pattern histologically. Others, however, had the organizing inflammatory process limited to the alveoli without bronchiolar involvement. This report represents a possible breakthrough in the etiology of idiopathic BOOP in some patients; but continued investigations are required to determine the exact cause.

In summary, there are several miscellaneous causes or disorders associated with BOOP. The clinical findings are similar to those of idiopathic BOOP. Patients with a febrile illness, increased sedimentation rate, and radiographic findings of patchy infiltrates responded to corticosteroid therapy, but others had a fatal outcome. Most of these miscellaneous disorders have an immunologic bases. As additional reports confirm these findings, designating a separate category of immunologically related BOOP will be appropriate.

REFERENCES

1. Allen JN, Wewers MD. HIV-associated bronchiolitis obliterans organizing pneumonia. *Chest* 1989;96:197–198.
2. Kindt GC, Weiland JE, Davis WB, et al. Bronchiolitis in adults: a reversible cause of the airway obstruction associated with airway neutrophils and neutrophil products. *Am Rev Respir Dis* 1989;140:483–492.
3. Cordier JF, Loire R, Brune J. Idiopathic bronchiolitis obliterans organizing pneumonia. *Chest* 1989;96:999–1004.
4. Costabel U, Teschler H, Schoenfeld B, et al. BOOP in Europe. *Chest* 1992;102:14S–20S.
5. Nagai S, Aung H, Tanaka S, et al. Bronchoalveolar lavage cell findings in patients with BOOP and related diseases. *Chest* 1992;102:32S–37S.
6. Kaufman J, Komorowski R. Bronchiolitis obliterans: a new clinical-pathologic complication of irradiation pneumonitis. *Chest* 1990;97:1243–1244.
7. Epler GR, Colby TV, McLoud TC, et al. Bronchiolitis obliterans organizing pneumonia. *N Engl J Med* 1985;312:152–158.
8. Tobias ME, Plit M. Bronchiolitis obliterans organizing pneumonia with migratory infiltrates: a late complication of radiation therapy. *AJR* 1993;160:205–206.
9. Epstein DM, Bennett MR. Bronchiolitis obliterans organizing pneumonia with migratory pulmonary infiltrates. *AJR* 1992;158:515–517.
10. Yamamoto M, Ina Y, Kitaichi M. Clinical features of BOOP in Japan. *Chest* 1992;102:21S–25S.
11. Tenholder MF, Becker GL, Cervoni MI. The myelodysplastic syndrome and bronchiolitis obliterans. *Ann Intern Med* 1990;112:714–715.
12. Kaufman J, Komorowski R. Bronchiolitis obliterans organizing pneumonia in common variable immunodeficiency syndrome. *Chest* 1991;100:552–553.
13. Romero S, Martin C, Massuti B, et al. Malignant lymphoma in a patient with relapsing bronchiolitis obliterans organizing pneumonia. *Chest* 1992;102:1895–1897.
14. Gosink BB, Friedman PJ, Liebow AA. Bronchiolitis obliterans: roentgenologic-pathologic correlation. *Am J Roentgenol* 1973;117:816–832.
15. Spiteri MA, Klenerman P, Sheppard MN, et al. Seasonal cryptogenic organizing pneumonia with biochemical cholestasis: a new clinical entity. *Lancet* 1992;340:281–284.

SECTION 4

Bronchiolar Diseases Among Children

Diseases of the Bronchioles, edited by Gary R. Epler. Raven Press, Ltd., New York © 1994.

27

Bronchiolitis in Children

Mary Ellen Beck Wohl

Professor of Pediatrics, Harvard Medical School; Chief, Division of Respiratory Diseases, Children's Hospital, 300 Longwood Avenue, Boston, MA.

Bronchiolitis is an airway disease primarily located in the small, peripheral airways of the lung. In pediatrics, for the last four decades, the term has referred to a respiratory illness that is acute in onset and is characterized by rhinorrhea, cough, shortness of breath, and often wheezing, occurring in a child under 1 or 2 years of age (1). The commonly implicated infectious agent is respiratory syncytial virus, although other viral agents can cause this clinical syndrome. Uncommonly, a severe necrotizing lesion of small airways can occur in children of any age. This lesion, caused by both infectious and noninfectious agents and often associated with substantial sequelae, is frequently referred to as bronchiolitis obliterans and is discussed elsewhere. This chapter focuses on acute viral bronchiolitis.

ETIOLOGY

In the young child, the most common viral agent causing respiratory distress is respiratory syncytial virus (2,3). In studies of hospitalized infants, respiratory syncytial virus is thought to account for the majority of the admissions (4).

Other viruses, including parainfluenza 1 and 3, influenza A and B, various strains of adenovirus, and rhinovirus and mycoplasma have been associated with a clinical illness indistinguishable from respiratory syncytial virus infections (5–8). In the northern hemisphere epidemics of respiratory syncytial virus occur between October and June (9–11). Infection is widespread in the population. The attack rate is lowest in adults, 17%, in whom it produces nasal congestion and cough. It is higher in infants who have school-age siblings, are hospitalized for other causes, and live in crowded urban settings (10,12,13). The highest attack rate is in infants attending day care centers, where virtually all become infected during an epidemic (14). Nosocomial infections are frequent (15), and strict attention to handwashing can reduce the nosocomial infection rate and the occurrence of bronchiolitis in already ill infants (16).

In infants and young children, respiratory syncytial virus can produce a range of illnesses including mild nasal congestion and rhinorrhea, conjunctivitis, otitis media, tracheitis, bronchitis, bronchiolitis, and pneumonia (17). A number of factors may account for the fact that bronchiolitis, with its attendant respiratory distress and abnormalities of gas exchange, is such a problem in the infant.

FACTORS INFLUENCING SEVERITY

The incidence of bronchiolitis peaks between 2 and 6 months of age. Anatomic features of the infant's lung, loss of immunologic protection from the mother, altered host defenses in the infant compared to the adult, the sites of inflammation, and additional risk factors may all contribute to the nature and severity of viral infections in young children.

The lung of the infant and young child differs from that of the adult (18–20). The total complement of conducting airways is developed early in gestational life, but alveoli are made primarily in the last months of fetal life and the first 2 years after birth. Airways of a given generation are smaller in the infant than in the older child or adult; and peripheral airways, those distal to the tenth generation, may be disproportionately small (21). Physiologic studies (21) conducted on a limited number of excised lungs showed that peripheral airways resistance, expressed as a fraction of lower airway resistance, is higher in the child than in the adult. Airways in children contain more mucus glands than they do in adults (22). At a given generation, the constituents of the airway wall probably occupy a greater share of the maximum external airway wall area in the child than in the adult. Collateral pathways, although present in the infant lung, are less well developed. These anatomic features of the infant's airway suggest that a given amount of edema, airway fluid, or inflammation might produce relatively more airway obstruction in the younger than in the older lung. Elastic recoil is reduced in the young lung (20) and increases with increasing age, at least until young adulthood. Airway closure occurs at higher lung volumes in the child's than in the young adult's lung (23). These factors probably contribute to the development of patchy atelectasis, a prominent feature of pediatric respiratory tract disease including bronchiolitis.

Physiologic measurements of healthy infants in epidemiologic studies before they acquired lower respiratory tract disease support an increased risk for the development of symptomatic lower respiratory infections in young children inferred to have smaller airways (24).

Immunologic mechanisms have been considered both to be protective and to contribute to the pathophysiology of bronchiolitis. The observation (25) in the late 1960s that infants immunized with a killed viral vaccine developed a severe form of bronchiolitis despite high titers of neutralizing antibodies led to the hypothesis that antigen–antibody interaction might contribute to the pulmonary pathology. Recent immunologic and epidemiologic data, however, support the role of neutralizing antibody to F and G glycoproteins on the cell surface in protecting against infection. Other antibodies to cell-surface antigens confer some short-lived protection, although these antibodies are not neutralizing (26). The protection offered by these antibodies is not total, and recurrent infection can take place not only throughout life but also within the same year (27).

Some investigators have focused on the role of bronchial associated lymphoid tissue in the host response to respiratory syncytial virus infection. Intact cellular immunity appears to be required for clearance of the virus (28) but may also be associated with disease-producing effects (29). Indeed, high levels of respiratory syncytial virus specific memory T lymphocytes of the $CD4^+$ lineage in the absence of respiratory syncytial virus specific $CD8^+$ CLT response (26) may account for the severe response to the killed viral vaccine.

Levels of secretory IgA have also been associated with protection from infection and clearing of the virus (28). Infants, who produce secretory IgA in reduced amounts, who have poor serum neutralizing antibody responses, and who may have less well established cell-mediated immune responses, are thus likely to be vulnerable to infection and replication of virus (26) and to experience the greatest morbidity and mortality.

Absence of or minimal breastfeeding, low levels of maternal antibody, sec (male), crowding, and being in day care are all risk factors for acquiring disease during epidemic months (30–32). The group to which the strain of virus belongs may affect the severity of disease (33,34), although group A infections have not been more severe in all studies (35).

Infants born prematurely (36,37), infants with cyanotic congenital heart disease in particular and pulmonary hypertension (38), and infants with underlying lung disease appear to be particularly susceptible to respiratory syncytial virus infection and to have a particularly severe course (37,39,40).

PATHOPHYSIOLOGY

Respiratory syncytial virus is a cytopathic virus that, by the formation of syncytia, involves adjacent cells in the infectious process. The cytopathic changes induced by multiplication of the virus and the accompanying inflammatory response lead to necrosis of the respiratory epithelium, destruction of the ciliated lining layer, and edema of the submucosa and adventitia. The peribronchial and peribronchiolar spaces are infiltrated with inflammatory cells, mainly lymphocytes; and this infiltrate sometimes extends into adjacent lung parenchyma. Respiratory syncytial virus infection, particularly bronchiolitis, does not usually lead to extensive alveolar involvement or destruction of the elastic and collagen of the lung supporting tissues. Airways obstruction is produced by edema of the airway wall, sloughing of the ciliated lining layer, other cellular debris, and secretions (1). Smooth-muscle constriction probably plays a relatively minor role. Depending on whether the obstruction is complete or partial and depending on whether or not collateral ventilation is present, some units will develop atelectasis whereas others will be overdistended.

The resolution of bronchiolitis has been inferred from large classic studies of McLean and others (41–43). Recovery is slow. Basal layers begin to recover in 3 to 4 days; regeneration of the cilia may take more than 2 weeks. Interstitial thickening produced by edema and infiltration of lymphocytes is seen in parenchyma adjacent to the airways. Occasionally there is extensive necrosis of the airway epithelium, which results in sloughing of epithelium and its replacement by layers of stratified, undifferentiated epithelium. Virus continues to be shed in nasal secretions for a week or longer (44).

These pathological processes result in increased pulmonary resistance, decreased compliance, increased lung volumes, and increased work of breathing. The uneven distribution of the lesions producing ventilation/perfusion mismatching, the major cause of hypoxemia, is virtually always present. In previously healthy children, carbon dioxide retention and respiratory acidosis are rare and most likely to be the result of severe mismatching of ventilation and perfusion combined with some degree of respiratory muscle fatigue. Metabolic acidosis caused by inadequate caloric and fluid intake can contribute to the acid–base disturbance. Increased secretions of antidiuretic hormone combined with increased plasma renin activity may result in normal sodium levels in the presence of fluid retention (45).

The clinical features of bronchiolitis reflect the pathophysiology. Tachypnea, often with nasal flaring and chest retraction; tachycardia; and prolonged expirations are virtually always present. Crackles and wheezes are often, but not always, present. The chest is hyperresonant, and the liver may be displaced 2 to 3 cm below the right costal margin. Cyanosis is rarely detected in infants, perhaps because of better cardiac outputs and lower hemoglobin levels than usually observed in adults, but in careful clinical assessment it can be observed in two-thirds of infants with saturations less than 90%. Pulse oximetry provides the best clinical indicator of disease severity and is better than the respiratory rate (46). Chest radiographs often appear deceptively normal because of the hyperinflation. Patchy atelectasis, peribronchial thickening, and subsegmented consolidations may be present. Atelectasis of a segment or of a lobe may develop, particularly during recovery (47–49).

The diagnosis of bronchiolitis is confirmed by the identification of a viral etiology in the appropriate clinical setting. Culture of nasal aspirates promptly inoculated and not frozen, determination of respiratory syncytial virus by direct fluorescent-antibody test, and enzyme immunoassay techniques are all in clinical use to identify the virus (50). Rapid viral diagnostic procedures are also available for the diagnosis of parainfluenza, adenovirus, and influenza antigens (51).

COMPLICATIONS AND SEQUELAE

Apnea is relatively common with respiratory syncytial virus infection in infants (52) and may be the presenting symptom (53). The episodes are usually central in type, and the etiologies probably include hypoxemia, upper airway obstruction, stimulation of laryngeal or airway receptors, and immaturity of respiratory control (54).

Current statistics for the number of infants in the population requiring hospitalization and the number requiring intensive care because of bronchiolitis are not available. A review (40) of 1,584 high-risk hospitalized patients over 3 years from the pediatric centers serving all but 10% of the Canadian population concentrates on children with cardiac disease, chronic lung disease, prematurity, severe hypoxemia, and compromised immune function. Of these high-risk children, 15% required mechanical ventilation and 1% died. Most of the deaths were in the patients with congenital heart disease (40). The morality in these high-risk infants is lower than has previously been observed (38).

Pneumothorax and pneumomediastinum are potential complications of bronchiolitis but are rarely observed (37).

The major indicators for intubation and mechanical ventilation are clinical deterioration manifest by worsening respiratory distress, tachycardia with heart rates greater than 200 beats per minute, listlessness, poor peripheral perfusion, hypercarbia, and apnea (55).

Most infants not requiring intensive care improve within 3 to 4 days, and by 2 weeks after the height of their illness are clinically well with normal respiratory rates and gas exchange. Physiologic and radiographic abnormalities may persist. A subset of hospitalized infants estimated to be about 20% (1) develop a more complicated course with persistent wheezing and hyperinflation.

Since bronchiolitis is one of the leading causes of hospitalization in the first year of life, respiratory infection is a major cause of morbidity and mortality in less well developed countries. Risk factors for chronic lung disease in adults are continuously sought; and considerable attention has been directed toward the relationship between acute viral (usually respiratory syncytial virus) bronchiolitis and subsequent morbidity and abnormalities in lung function. The findings can be summarized under three headings: the development of severe lung damage with fixed airways obstruction (bronchiolitis obliterans), an association of bronchiolitis with the subsequent development of asthma, and the relationship between bronchiolitis and subsequent modest abnormalities in lung function.

Adenoviral infections, particularly types 3, 7, and 21, have been associated with the development of severe bronchiolitis and bronchopneumonia, with a course that waxes and wanes for several months in survivors (1). More than one-half of these youngsters develop chronic lung disease (56–61). The pathology differs from that usually associated with acute viral bronchiolitis. The epithelial lining layers of bronchi are completely destroyed. There is destruction and disorganization of the airway wall accompanied by disruption of collagen and elastin layers. The lumina of bronchioles can be replaced by vascularized connective tissue, and distal bronchioles can be considerably dilated. Areas of fibrosis, atelectasis, and overdistention characterize the alveolar region of the lung. Vessels are narrowed, and there is a reduction in the vasculature to affected areas (1,61). Similar findings are occasionally observed after bronchiolitis and bronchopneumonia caused by influenzae type B (62) and by *Mycoplasma pneumoniae* (63). Substantial airways obstruction has been observed in at least 50% of children studied 12 years after adenovirus type 7 bronchiolitis and pneumonia (64). However, this picture is not observed, or only very rarely observed, as a sequel to respiratory syncytial virus bronchiolitis and appears to require more extensive parenchymal involvement and airway wall involvement than usually occurs in bronchiolitis caused by the virus.

The association between bronchiolitis and the subsequent development of asthma has been investigated since the late 1950s. Most of these studies have demonstrated an increased incidence of asthma or more frequent episodes of wheezing (65–67), increased airway reactivity (68–70), and an increased incidence of lower respiratory tract infections (71–76) in those children who had bronchiolitis as an infant.

Asthma and bronchiolitis may share common pathogenic mechanisms (77). Respiratory syncytial virus specific IgE has been identified in nasopharyngeal secretions after infection (35,78), and elevated plasma levels of histamine and a metabolite of prostaglandin $F_{2\alpha}$ have been observed in patients with acute bronchiolitis (79) and in those with asthma (80).

Abnormalities in lung function have been documented at school age in children with and without clinical evidence of wheezing (68,81–84). In children not ill enough to require hospitalization, the impairment was very modest and of marginal significance (85). The importance of modest alterations in lung function is difficult to determine. If 40 to 95% of infants acquire respiratory syncytial virus infection each year and 5% of these are hospitalized, then the possibility exists that the observed abnormalities in lung function at school age in children who had been hospitalized reflect, at least in part, pre-illness variability in lung function (24). It is possible that infants sick enough to require hospitalization are drawn from a group with small airways and/or increased airway reactivity, and that some of the reported abnormalities do not reflect sequelae of bronchiolitis. Rather, the clinical severity of the infection may be influenced by the underlying anatomy and physiology of the lung.

TREATMENT

Approaches are available to limit viral multiplication, to modify the inflammatory response, to bronchodilate airways to treat the abnormal gas exchange, and to treat the complications of the disease such as apnea, dehydration, and respiratory failure. Among pediatricians there is agreement only about the supportive measures and treatment of disease complications.

Specific antiviral therapy is available to limit viral replication. Ribavirin (1-β-D-ribafuranosyl-1,2,4-triazole-3-carboxamide) is a synthetic nucleoside with a structure similar to that of guanosine. It inhibits viral replication in a number of RNA and DNA viruses. A series of studies (86–91) showed that infants treated with a solution of 20 mg/ml nebulized for 18 or more hours for 3 to 5 days had improved oxygenation, improved clinical scores, and decreased viral shedding when compared to control infants. Initial studies (92) in which a concentrated solution was administered for shorter periods of time appear promising. Since the drug is expensive, cumbersome to use, and possibly associated with as yet undetermined long-term sequelae, treatment is recommended (93–94) only for infants at high risk, those with cyanotic congenital heart disease, bronchopulmonary dysplasia, chronic lung disease, prematurity, those immunosuppressed, those hypoxemic on admission (PaO_2 less than 65 mm Hg), and those with other neurologic and metabolic disease. Several reviews (95–97) question the use of the drug, its costs, and its long-term potential sequelae.

The use of bronchodilators has been considered controversial (98–99). However, three recent, well designed placebo-controlled trials (100–102) demonstrated improvement as judged by clinical scores and improvement of or no decrease in oxygen saturation. In contrast, in two studies (103, 104) oxygen saturation decreased with administration of bronchodilators and in another study forced expiratory flow decreased (105). Two studies report improvement with epinephrine (106) and racemic epinephrine (107). These observations may be accounted for at least in part by relief of airway edema.

The effect of corticosteroid therapy on the course of bronchiolitis has been evaluated in a well designed, controlled study (108) that did not demonstrate any beneficial effect. However, at that time, oxygen saturation could not be conveniently measured. A subsequent study (109) did show improvement in children treated with dexamethasone and inhaled albuterol. In subsequent studies (110–113) the numbers of patients are small and outcomes are highly variable. Ipratroprium bromide has been evaluated in a cohort of wheezy infants using lung function tests to measure outcome. Some infants demonstrate improvement (114). However, ipratroprium bromide, theophylline, and cromolyn have not been well studied either in acute bronchiolitis or in the subset of children with persistent wheezing. At present some data support the use of bronchodilator therapy. Careful observation appears to be the clinician's best approach.

No controversy exists over the importance of supportive measures in the treatment of viral bronchiolitis. For children with mild bronchiolitis, careful observation and feeding may be all that is required. For children with moderate respiratory distress and decreased oxygen saturation, hospitalization is necessary for supportive care. This care includes the administration of humidified oxygen, monitoring to detect apnea and hypoxemia, evaluation for respiratory failure, provision of a thermoneutral environment, and appropriate fluid administration. Inspired concentrations of oxygen of 28 to 35% usually correct the hypoxemia since most is related to ventilation–perfusion mismatch. The growing numbers of patients with chronic lung disease of prematurity and substantial bicarbonate retention require special attention in order not to blunt respiratory drive excessively. Since infants increase oxygen consumption with fever, chilling, and shivering, care must be taken to avoid chilling of the infant in the device used to administer oxygen. A number of infants are dehydrated on admission. Since inappropriate antidiuretic hormone secretion is common (45), care must be taken to avoid excessive fluid retention. The large negative pleural pressure swings, which are probably transmitted to the interstitium, may enhance interstitial fluid accumulation in the lung.

Antibiotics are virtually never indicated in the treatment of viral bronchiolitis. The overall incidence of secondary bacterial infection is 1.2% but it is substantially higher, 9%, in those given parenteral antibiotics for 5 days or more (115). Infants require appropriate cultures of blood, urine, cerebrospinal fluid, and tracheal secretions if clinical deterioration occurs and the clinical features of sepsis develop.

Although the vast majority of children who acquire viral bronchiolitis improve in 3 or 4 days, a subset, perhaps as high as 7%, will require mechanical ventilation (55). Extracorporeal membrane oxygenation has been successfully employed in a small group of infants (116).

PREVENTION

The prevention of respiratory syncytial virus infection and the attendant bronchiolitis has been a goal of a number of investigators. The recent ability to identify subtypes of the virus, the improved information about components of the virus inducing protective antibodies, and the ability to incorporate parts of the virus into a vaccinia vector may assist in vaccine development (26). However, the experience with the killed vaccine, the short-lived protection conferred by antibody, and the spontaneous mutations of temperature-sensitive mutant strains developed as a vaccine have so far impeded the development of effective preventive strategies. Currently, the administration of hyperimmune intravenous gammaglobulin appears safe (117) and effective (118) and may become a strategy for preventing serious disease in high-risk infants.

SUMMARY

Acute viral bronchiolitis occurs in many children, is usually caused by respiratory syncytial virus, and accounts for the major share of serious morbidity in children under 1 year of age. Mortality rates are low, except for children with cyanotic congenital heart disease. Treatment is essentially supportive, except in high-risk infants, in whom the administration of nebulized ribavirin is indicated. Effective protection has been demonstrated in infants given hyperimmune gammaglobulin, and vaccines are under development.

REFERENCES

1. Wohl MEB, Chernick V. Bronchiolitis: state of the art. *Am Rev Respir Dis* 1978;118:759–776.
2. Henderson FW, Clyde WA Jr, Collier AM, et al. The etiologic and epidemiologic spectrum of bronchiolitis in pediatric practice. *J Pediatr* 1979;95:183–190.
3. Avila MM, Carballal G, Rovaletti H, et al. Viral etiology in acute lower respiratory infections in children from a closed community. *Am Rev Respir Dis* 1989;140:634–637.
4. Martin AJ, Gardner PS, McQuillin J. Epidemiology of respiratory viral infection among pediatric inpatients over a six-year period in north-east England. *Lancet* Nov 11 1978;1035–1038.
5. Welliver RC, Wong DT, Sun M, McCarthy N. Parainfluenza virus bronchiolitis. *Am J Dis Child* 1986;140:34–40.
6. Hall CB, Douglas G Jr. Respiratory syncytial virus and influenza. *Am J Dis Child* 1976; 130:615–620.
7. Jennings LC, et al. Acute respiratory tract infections of children in hospital: a viral and *Mycoplasma pneumoniae* profile. *NZ Med J* 1985; 98:582–585.
8. Zollar LM, Krause HE, Mufson MA. Microbiologic studies on young infants with lower respiratory tract disease. *Am J Dis Child* 1973;126:56.
9. Brandt CD, Kim HW, Arrobio JO, et al. Epidemiology of respiratory syncytial virus infection in Washington, D.C. III: Composite analysis of eleven consecutive yearly epidemics. *Am J Epidemiol* 1973;98:355.
10. Glezen WP, Denny FW. Epidemiology of acute lower respiratory disease in children. *N Engl J Med* 1973;288:498.
11. Kim HW, Arrobio JO, Brandt CD, et al. Epidemiology of respiratory syncytial virus infection in Washington, D.C. I: Importance of the virus in different respiratory tract disease syndromes and temporal distribution of infection. *Am J Epidemiol* 1973;98:216.
12. Hall CB, Geiman JM, Biggar R, Kotok DI, Hogan PM, Gouglas G Jr. Respiratory syncytial virus infections within families. *N Engl J Med* 1976;294:414–419.
13. Glezen WP, Paredes A, Allison JE, Taber LH, Frank AL. Risk of respiratory syncytial virus infection for infants from low-income families in relationship to age, sex, ethnic group, and maternal antibody level. *J Pediatr* 1981;98:708–715.
14. Loda FA, Glezen WP, Clyde W Jr. Respiratory disease in group day care. *Pediatrics* 1971;49: 428–437.
15. Hall CB, Douglas RG Jr, Geiman JM, Messner MK. Nosocomial respiratory syncytial virus infections. *N Engl J Med* 1975;293:1343–1346.
16. Leclair JM, Sullivan BF, et al. Prevention of nosocomial respiratory syncytial virus infections through compliance with glove and gown isolation precautions. *N Engl J Med* 1987;317: 330.
17. Reilly CM, Stokes J Jr, McClelland L, Cornfield D, Hamparian VV, Ketler A, Hilleman MR. Studies of acute respiratory syncytial vi-

rus. III: Clinical and laboratory findings. *N Engl J Med* 1961;264:1176.
18. Wohl MEB, Mead J. Age as a factor in respiratory disease. In: Kendig EC Jr, Chernick V, eds. *Disorders of the respiratory tract in children.* 5th ed. Philadelphia: WB Saunders; 1990: 185–181.
19. Brody JS, Thurlbeck WM. Development, growth, and aging of the lung. In: Fishman AP, Macklem PT, Mead J, Geiger SR, eds. *Handbook of physiology: mechanics of breathing.* Baltimore: Williams & Wilkins; 1986:355–386. (*The respiratory system;* vol III).
20. Bryan AL, Wohl MEB. Respiratory mechanics in children. In: Macklem P, Mead J, eds. *Handbook of physiology: mechanics of breathing.* Baltimore: Williams & Wilkins; 1986:179–191. (*The respiratory system;* vol III).
21. Hogg JC, Williams J, Richardson JB, Macklem PT, Thurlbeck WM, Path MC. Age as a factor in the distribution of lower-airway conductance and in the pathologic anatomy of obstructive lung disease. *N Engl J Med* 1970;282:1283–1287.
22. Matsuba K, Thurlbeck WM. A morphometric study of bronchial and bronchiolar walls in children. *Am Rev Respir Dis* 1972;105:908–912.
23. Mansell A, Bryan C, Levison H. Airway closure in children. *J Appl Physiol* 1972;33:711–714.
24. Martinez FD, Morgan WJ, Wright AL, Holberg CJ, Taussig LM, Group Health Medical Associates Personnel. Diminished lung function as a predisposing factor for wheezing respiratory illness in infants. *N Engl J Med* 1988;319:1112–1117.
25. Kapikian AZ, Mitchell RH, Chanock RM, Shvedoff RA, Stewart CE. An epidemiologic study of altered clinical reactivity to respiratory syncytial (RS) virus infection in children previously vaccinated with an inactivated RS virus vaccine. *Am J Epidemiol* 1968;89:405.
26. Chanock RM, Parrott RH, Connors M, Collins PL, Murphy BR. Serious respiratory tract disease caused by respiratory syncytial virus: prospects for improved therapy and effective immunization. *Pediatrics* July 1992;137–143.
27. Glezen WP, Taber LH, Frank AL, Kasel JA. Risk of primary infection and reinfection with respiratory syncytial virus. *Am J Dis Child* 1986;140:543–546.
28. McConnochie KM, Roghmann KJ. Parental smoking, presence of older siblings and family history of asthma increase risk of bronchiolitis. *Am J Dis Child* 1986;140:806–812.
29. Holberg CJ, Wright AL, Martinez FD, Ray CG, Taussig LM, Lebowitz MD, Group Health Medical Associates. Risk factors for respiratory syncytial virus-associated lower respiratory illnesses in the first year of life. *Am J Epidemiol* 1991;133:1135–1151.
30. Pullan CR, Toms GL, Martin AJ, Gardner PS, Webb JKG, Appleton DR. Breast-feeding and respiratory syncytial virus infection. *BMJ* 1980; 281:1034–1036.
31. McConnochie KM, Hall CB, Walsh EE, Roghmann KJ. Variation in severity of respiratory syncytial virus infections with subtype. *J Pediatr* 1990;117:52–62.
32. Hall CB, Walsh EE, Schnabel KC, Long CE, McConnochie KM, Hildreth SW, Anderson LJ. Occurrence of groups A and B of respiratory syncytial virus over 15 years: associated epidemiologic and clinical characteristics in hospitalized and ambulatory children. *J Infect Dis* 1990;162:1283–1290.
33. Stark JM, Fatemi SH, Amini SB, Huang YT. Occurrence of respiratory syncytial virus subtypes in hospitalized children in Cleveland, Ohio, from 1985 to 1988. *Pediatr Pulmonol* 1991;11:98–102.
34. McIntosh K, Rishaut JM. Immunopathologic mechanisms in lower respiratory tract disease of infants due to respiratory syncytial virus. *Prog Med Virol* 1980;26:94–118.
35. Welliver RC, Kaul A, Ogra PL. Cell-mediated immune response to respiratory syncytial virus infection: relationship to the development of reactive airway disease. *J Pediatr* 1979;94:370–375.
36. Shaw KN, Bell LM, Sherman NH. Outpatient assessment of infants with bronchiolitis. *Am J Dis Child* 1991;145:151–155.
37. Lebel MH, Gauthier M, Lacroix J, Rousseau E, Buithieu M. Respiratory failure and mechanical ventilation in severe bronchiolitis. *Arch Dis Child* 1989;64:1431–1437.
38. MacDonald NE, Hall CB, Suffin SC, Alexson C, Harris PJ, Manning JA. Respiratory syncytial viral infection in infants with congenital heart disease. *N Engl J Med* 1982;307:397–400.
39. Groothuis JR, Gutierrez KM, Lauer BA. Respiratory syncytial virus infection in children with bronchopulmonary dysplasia. *Pediatrics* 1988;82:199–203.
40. Navas L, Wang E, de Carvalho V, Robinson J, Pediatric Investigators Collaborative Network on Infections in Canada. Improved outcome of respiratory syncytial virus infection in a high-risk hospitalized population of Canadian children. *J Pediatr* 1992;121:348–354.
41. McLean KH. The pathology of acute bronchiolitis: a study of its evolution. I: The exudative phase. *Aust Ann Med* 1956;5:254.
42. McLean KH. The pathology of acute bronchiolitis: a study of its evolution. II: The repair phase. *Aust Ann Med* 1957;6:29.
43. Monto AS, Bryan ER, Rhodes LM. The Tecumseh Study of respiratory illness. VII: Further observations on the occurrence of respiratory syncytial virus and *Mycoplasma pneumoniae* infections. *Am J Epidemiol* 1974; 100:458.
44. Hall CB, Douglas G Jr, Geiman JM. Quantitative shedding patterns of respiratory syncytial virus in infants. *J Infect Dis* 1975;132:151–209.
45. Gozal D, Colin AA, Jaffe M, Hochberg Z. Water, electrolyte and endocrine homeostasis in infants with bronchiolitis. *Pediatr Res* 1990; 27:204–209.

46. Mulholland EK, Olinsky A, Shann FA. Clinical findings and severity of acute bronchiolitis. *Lancet* 1990;335:1259–1261.
47. Simpson W, Hacking PM, Court SDM, Gardner PS. The radiological findings in respiratory syncytial virus infections in children. I: Definitions and interobservations in the assessment of abnormalities on the chest x-ray. *Pediatr Radiol* 1974;2:97.
48. Simpson W, Hacking PM, Court SDM, Gardner PS. The radiological findings in respiratory syncytial virus infections in children. II: The correlation of radiological categories with clinical and virological findings. *Pediatr Radiol* 1974;2:155.
49. Rice RP, Loda F. A roentgenographic analysis of respiratory syncytial virus pneumonia in infants. *Radiology* 1966;87:1021.
50. Halstead DC, Todd S, Fritch G. Evaluation of five methods for respiratory syncytial virus detection. *J Clin Microbiol* 1990;28:1021–1025.
51. Sarkkinen HK, Halonen PE, Arstila P, Salmi AA. Detection of respiratory syncytial, parainfluenza type 2, and adenovirus antigens by radioimmunoassay and enzyme immunoassay on nasopharyngeal specimens from children with acute respiratory disease. *J Clin Microbiol* 1981;13:258–265.
52. Bruhn FW, Mokrohisky ST, McIntosh K. Apnea associated with respiratory syncytial virus infection in young infants. *Pediatrics* 1977; 90:382.
53. Hall CB, Hall WJ, Speers DM. Clinical and physiological manifestations of bronchiolitis and pneumonia. *Am J Dis Child* 1979;133:798.
54. Anas N, Boettrich C, Hall BC, Brooks JG. The association of apnea and respiratory syncytial virus infection in infants. *J Pediatr* 1982;101: 65–69.
55. Outwater KM, Crone RK. Management of respiratory failure in infants with acute viral bronchiolitis. *Am J Dis Child* 1984;138:1071–1075.
56. Lang WR, Howden CW, Laws J, Burton JF. Bronchopneumonia with serious sequelae in children with evidence of adenovirus type 21 infection. *BMJ* 1969;1:73–79.
57. Gold R, Wilt JC, Adhikari PK, Macpherson RI. Adenoviral pneumonia and its complications in infancy and childhood. *Can Assoc Radiol J* 1969;20:218–224.
58. Cumming GR, Macpherson RI, Chernick V. Unilateral hyperlucent lung syndrome in children. *J Pediatr* 1971;78:250.
59. Strieder DJ, Nash G. Case records of the Massachusetts General Hospital. *N Engl J Med* 1975;292:634.
60. James AG, Lang WR, Liang AY, et al. Adenovirus type 21 bronchopneumonia in infants and young children. *J Pediatr* 1979;95:530.
61. Becroft DMO. Bronchiolitis obliterans, bronchiectasis, and other sequelae of adenovirus type 21 infection in young children. *J Clin Pathol* 1971;24:72.
62. Laraya-Cuasay LR, DeForest A, Huff D, et al. Chronic pulmonary complications of early influenza virus infection in children. *Am Rev Respir Dis* 1977;116:617.
63. Stokes D, Sigler A, Khouri N, Talamo RC. Unilateral hyperlucent lung (Swyer-James syndrome) after severe *Mycoplasma pneumoniae* infection. *Am Rev Respir Dis* 1978;117:145.
64. Sly PD, Soto-Quiros ME, Landau LI, et al. Factors predisposing to abnormal pulmonary function after adenovirus type 7 pneumonia. *Arch Dis Child* 1984;59:935.
65. Wittig HJ, Cranford NJ, Glaser J. The relationship between bronchiolitis and childhood asthma. *J Allergy* 1959;30:20.
66. Eisen AH, Bacal HL. The relationship of acute bronchiolitis to bronchial asthma: a 4- to 14-year follow-up. *Pediatrics* 1963;31:859.
67. Rooney JC, Williams HE. The relationship between proved viral bronchiolitis and subsequent wheezing. *J Pediatr* 1971;79:744.
68. Gurwitz D, Mindorff C, Levison H. Increased incidence of bronchial reactivity in children with a history of bronchiolitis. *J Pediatr* 1981; 98:551–555.
69. Sims DG, Downham MAPS, Gardner PS, Webb JKG, Weightman D. Study of 8-year-old children with a history of respiratory syncytial virus bronchiolitis in infancy. *BMJ* 1978;1:11–14.
70. Tepper RS, Rosenberg D, Eigen H. Airway responsiveness in infants following bronchiolitis. *Pediatr Pulmonol* 1992;13:6–10.
71. Henry RL, Hodges IGC, Milner AD, Stokes GM. Respiratory problems 2 years after acute bronchiolitis in infancy. *Arch Dis Child* 1983; 58:713–716.
72. Stokes GM, Milner AD, Hodges IGC, Groggins RC. Lung function abnormalities after acute bronchiolitis. *J Pediatr* 1981;98:871–874.
73. Hall CB, Hall WJ, Gala CL, MaGill GB, Leddy JP. Long-term prospective study in children after respiratory syncytial virus infection. *J Pediatr* 1984;105:358.
74. Mok JYQ, Simpson H. Outcome for acute bronchitis, bronchiolitis, and pneumonia in infancy. *Arch Dis Child* 1984;59:306–309.
75. McConnochie KM, Roghmann KJ. Predicting clinically significant lower respiratory tract illness in childhood following mild bronchiolitis. *Am J Dis Child* 1985;139:625–631.
76. Carlsen KH, Larsen S, Orstavik I. Acute bronchiolitis in infancy: the relationship to later recurrent obstructive airways disease. *Eur J Respir Dis* 1987;70:86–92.
77. McIntosh K. Bronchiolitis and asthma: possible common pathogenetic pathways. *J Allergy Clin Immunol* 1976;57:595.
78. Welliver RC, Sun M, Rinaldo D, Ogra PL. Predictive value of respiratory syncytial virus-specific IgE responses for recurrent wheezing following bronchiolitis. *J Pediatr* 1986; 109:776–780.
79. Skoner DP, Fireman P, Caliguiri L, Davis H. Plasma elevations of histamine and a prostaglandin metabolite in acute bronchiolitis. *Am Rev Respir Dis* 1990;142:359–364.
80. Skoner DP, Page R, Asman B, et al. Plasma el-

evation of histamine and a prostaglandin metabolite in acute asthma. *Am Rev Respir Dis* 1988;137:1009.
81. Kattan M, Keens TG, Lapierre J-G, Levison H, Bryan AC, Reilly BJ. Pulmonary function abnormalities in symptom-free children after bronchiolitis. *Pediatrics* 1977;59:683–688.
82. Mok JYQ, Simpson H. Outcome of acute lower respiratory tract infection in infants: preliminary report of seven-year follow-up study. *BMJ* 1982;285:333–337.
83. Pullan CR, Hey EN. Wheezing, asthma, and pulmonary dysfunction 10 years after infection with respiratory syncytial virus in infancy. *BMJ* 1982;284:1665–1669.
84. Sims DG, Downham MAPS, Gardner PS, et al. Study of 8-year-old children with a history of respiratory syncytial virus bronchiolitis in infancy. *BMJ* 1978;1:11.
85. McConnochie KM, Roghmann KJ. Predicting clinically significant lower respiratory tract illness in childhood following mild bronchiolitis. *Am J Dis Child* 1985;139:625–631.
86. Taber LH, Knight V, Gilbert BE, et al. Ribavirin aerosol treatment of bronchiolitis associated with respiratory syncytial virus infection in infants. *Pediatrics* 1983;72:613–618.
87. Hall, CB, McBride JT, Walsh EE, et al. Aerosolized ribavirin treatment of infants with respiratory syncytial viral infection. *N Engl J Med* 1983;308:1443–1447.
88. Hall CB, McBride JT, Gala CL, Hildreth SW, Schnabel KC. Ribavirin treatment of respiratory syncytial viral infection in infants with underlying cardiopulmonary disease. *J Am Med Assoc* 1985;254:3047–3051.
89. Barry W, Cockburn F, Cornall R, Price JF, Sutherland G, Vardag A. Ribavirin aerosol for acute bronchiolitis. *Arch Dis Child* 1986;61:593–597.
90. Groothuis JR, Woodin KA, Katz R. Early ribavirin treatment of respiratory syncytial viral infection in high-risk children. *J Pediatr* 1990;117:792–798.
91. Smith DW, Frankel LR, Mathers LH, Tang ATS, Ariagno RL, Prober CG. A controlled trial of aerosolized ribavirin in infants receiving mechanical ventilation for severe respiratory syncytial virus infection. *N Engl J Med* 1991;325:24–29.
92. Knight V, Gilbert BE. Aerosol treatment of respiratory viral disease. *Lung* 1990;[Suppl]:406–413.
93. Committee on Infectious Diseases. Ribavirin therapy of respiratory syncytial virus. *Pediatrics* 1987;79:475–478.
94. Infectious Diseases and Immunization Committee, Canadian Paediatric Society. Ribavirin: indications for use in pediatrics. *Can Med Assoc J* 1986;135:1351–1352.
95. Wald ER, Dashefsky B, Green M. In re ribavirin: a case of premature adjudication? *J Pediatr* 1988;112:154–158.
96. Ray CG. Ribavirin: ambivalence about an antiviral agent. *Am J Dis Child* 1988;142:488–489.
97. Wheeler JG, Wofford J, Turner RB. Historical cohort evaluation of ribavirin efficacy in respiratory syncytial virus infection. *Pediatr Infect Dis J* 1993;12:209–213.
98. Henry RL. Annotation: the use of bronchodilators in the young infant. *Aust Paediatr J* 1988;24:269–270.
99. Milner AD, Murray M. Acute bronchiolitis in infancy: treatment and prognosis. *Thorax* 1989;44:1–5.
100. Schuh S, Canny G, Reisman JJ, Kerem E, Bentur L, Petric M, Levison H. Nebulized albuterol in acute bronchiolitis. *J Pediatr* 1990;117:633–637.
101. Klassen TP, Rowe PC, Sutcliffe T, Ropp LJ, McDowell IW, Li MM. Randomized trial of salbutamol in acute bronchiolitis. *J Pediatr* 1991;118:807–811.
102. Alario AJ, Lewander WJ, Dennehy P, Seifer R, Mansell AL. The efficacy of nebulized metaproterenol in wheezing infants and young children. *Am J Dis Child* 1992;146:412–418.
103. Prendiville A, Rose A, Maxwell DL, Silverman M. Hypoxaemia in wheezy infants after bronchodilator treatment. *Arch Dis Child* 1987;62:997–1000.
104. Ho L, Collis G, Landau LI, Le Soeuf PN. Effect of salbutamol on oxygen saturation in bronchiolitis. *Arch Dis Child* 1991;66:1061–1064.
105. Hughes DM, Lesouef PN, Landau LI. Effect of salbutamol on respiratory mechanics in bronchiolitis. *Pediatr Res* 1987;22:83–86.
106. Lowell DI, Lister G, Von Koss H, McCarthy P. Wheezing in infants: the response to epinephrine. *Pediatrics* 1987;79:939–945.
107. Sanchez I, De Koster J, Powell RE, Wolstein R, Chernick V. Effect of racemic epinephrine and salbutamol on clinical score and pulmonary mechanics in infants with bronchiolitis. *J Pediatr* 1993;122:145–151.
108. Leer JA, Green JL, Heimlick EM, et al. Corticosteroid treatment in bronchiolitis: a controlled, collaborative study in 297 infants and children. *Am J Dis Child* 1969;117:495.
109. Tal A, Bavilski C, Yohai D, Bearman JE, Gorodischer R, Moses SW. Dexamethasone and salbutamol in the treatment of acute wheezing in infants. *Pediatrics* 1983;71:13–18.
110. Webb MSC, Henry RL, Milner AD. Oral corticosteroids for wheezing attacks under 18 months. *Arch Dis Child* 1986;61:15–19.
111. Springer C, Bar-Yishay E, Uwayyed K, Avital A, Vilozni D, Godfrey S. Corticosteroids do not affect the clinical or physiological status of infants with bronchiolitis. *Pediatr Pulmonol* 1990;9:181–185.
112. Carlsen KH, Leegaard J, Larsen S, Orstavik I. Nebulised beclomethasone dipropionate in recurrent obstructive episodes after acute bronchiolitis. *Arch Dis Child* 1988;63:1428–1433.
113. Maayan C, Itzhaki T, Bar-Yishay E, Gross S, Tal A, Godfrey S. The functional response of infants with persistent wheezing to nebulized

beclomethasone dipropionate. *Pediatr Pulmonol* 1986;2:9–14.
114. Hodges IGC, Groggins RC, Milner AD, Stokes GM. Bronchodilator effect of inhaled ipratropium bromide in wheezy toddlers. *Arch Dis Child* 1981;56:729–732.
115. Hall CB, Powell KR, Schnabel KC, Gala CL, Pincus PH. Risk of secondary bacterial infection in infants hospitalized with respiratory syncytial viral infection. *J Pediatr* 1988;113:266–271.
116. Steinhorn RH, Green TP. Use of extracorporeal membrane oxygenation in the treatment of respiratory syncytial virus bronchiolitis: The National Experience, 1983 to 1988. *J Pediatr* 1990;116:338–342.
117. Groothius R, Simoes EAF, Levin M, et al. Respiratory syncytial virus (RSV) immune globulin (IG) prevents severe lower respiratory infection (LRI) in high risk children. *Pediatr Res* 1993;33:169A.
118. Hemming VG, Rodriguez W, Kim HW, et al. Intravenous immunoglobulin treatment of respiratory syncytial virus infections in infants and young children. *Antimicrob Agents Chemother* 1987;31:1882–1886.

Diseases of the Bronchioles, edited by Gary R. Epler. Raven Press, Ltd., New York © 1994.

28

Follicular Bronchiolitis in the Pediatric Population

T. Bernard Kinane and Daniel C. Shannon

Pediatric Pulmonary Unit, Children's Service, Massachusetts General Hospital, Fruit Street, Boston MA.

Lymphoid hyperplasia is a common phenomenon at many sites in the body, and the lung is no exception. There exists a rare group of patients with pulmonary lymphoid hyperplasia, follicular bronchitis, in which no cause is immediately obvious (1–3). In this condition, lymphoid hyperplasia with reactive germinal centers is observed along the bronchioles (4). In adults with this condition, one-third have a connective tissue disease, one-sixth have an autoimmune disease, and the remaining have no known association (1). Most pediatric patients have no recognized association and are said to have idiopathic follicular bronchitis or follicular bronchiolitis.

PATHOPHYSIOLOGY

Follicular bronchitis-bronchiolitis is a condition involving bronchial-associated lymphoid tissue. An understanding of the anatomy and function of this lymphoid tissue provides some insight into this condition. Pulmonary lymphoid cells are compartmentalized into different sites including perihilar lymph nodes, bronchial associated lymphoid tissue, and the lung's interstitial tissue (5,6). Bronchial associated lymphoid tissue is absent at birth but develops at the end of the first week and thereafter increases. It consists of organized follicles in close apposition to the bronchial epithelium. Although gut-associated lymphoid tissue develops months later, the apposition to the epithelium is similar. Bronchial associated lymphoid tissue has been found in many species but is not well developed in humans. These follicles are scattered throughout the airways with a higher frequency at airways' divisions. The localization at sites of particulate deposition suggests that it develops in response to postnatal antigen exposure. However, this localization may also have a genetic component: Milne (7) showed that fetal lungs taken from 18-day-old mouse embryos developed primitive bronchial associated lymphoid tissue follicles when transplanted into the subcutaneous space of syngeneic animals. These follicles are covered by lymphoepithelium similar to that found over Peyer's patches. This specialized epithelial cell layer allows the passage of both soluble and particulate antigenic material from the bronchial lumen to the lymphoid cells. Also, lymphocytes have been shown interdigitating into the lymphoepithelium; and it is accordingly possible that this is the source of lymphocytes that migrate into the airway walls. Both T and B lymphocytes are found within bronchial associated lymphoid tissue, with 20% of cells bearing T-cell markers. Studies of young rats have demonstrated the propensity of these B cells to express IgA. However, as animals age there is a propensity for the number of IgA cells to decrease in comparison to IgM and IgG bearing cells. Nonetheless, bronchial associated lymphoid tissue is thought to be a major source of IgA. A role for bronchial associated lymphoid tissue in systemic immunity has been suggested. Humphrey (8) observed that the contribution by the lung to the antibody pool exceeds the total contribution of the bone marrow, spleen, and lymph nodes after intravenous immunization with pneumococcal antigen—a role made possible by a rich blood supply from the pulmonary artery.

Bronchial associated lymphoid tissue is involved in a number of localized lung diseases as well as systemic disorders. This involvement is compatible with a role in antigen sampling of the airway as well as of the systemic blood. Systemic disorders that cause an enlargement of bronchial associated lymphoid tissue include acquired immunodeficiency syndrome (AIDS), lymphoma, cystic fibrosis, and connective-tissue disorders. Localized causes include infection and carcinoma. Follicular bronchiectasis was used by Whitwell (9) to describe extensive formation of lymphoid follicles in the walls of bronchi with bronchiectasis. He postulated that this type of bronchiectasis was a sequel of such acute infections as measles, whooping cough, or influenza because it was seen most commonly in children. Similar histologic patterns were subsequently demonstrated in association with adenovirus infections. Yousem (1) described similar histologic changes without bronchiectasis and called this entity follicular bronchitis/bronchiolitis. This occurred in patients with autoimmune disease or immunodeficiency states, including AIDS. However in nearly one-half of the patients no microbial or clinical association was found. In the five pediatric patients that we described (3) no association was identified. However, Franchi (10) describes similar histologic findings in the setting of a familial systemic autoimmune disorder in children.

In our group an etiology was not established, but an infectious agent is probable in view of the histologic pattern. Because of the early presentation, an intrauterine origin is suggested. Hydrops fetalis in one of our patients and recurrent pyrexia in others are consistent with this suggestion. A similar histologic picture is seen in animals with infections induced by *Mycoplasma pneumoniae* and a number of viral agents (11,12). Indeed, a survey (13) of bronchial associated lymphoid tissue in the lungs of 200 children who were stillborn or died within 15 days of birth revealed that increased aggregates occur in response to amniotic infection. However the serology and cultures were not helpful in our patients.

This syndrome may also represent a response to nonspecific injury, such as recurrent aspiration. The finding of a similar histologic pattern in autoimmune diseases, tumor, cystic fibrosis, and bronchiectasis would buttress this theory. Two of our patients who were treated surgically for esophageal reflux showed slow improvement. However, this reflux may also reflect the larger than normal transmural esophageal pressure with each breath. The significance of this reflux was further diminished by the lack of lipid-laden macrophages in bronchial alveolar washings. The improvement in lung symptoms after surgery was believed to be coincidental with the normal spontaneous improvement of idiopathic follicular bronchitis. Emery (13) noted a significant increase in bronchial associated lymphoid tissue in children in whom there is neurospinal dysraphism. It was postulated that in such children there was a necrosis of nervous tissue into the amniotic cavity, and it was expected that this material was antigenic to the lung in utero. Another possibility is that the same genetic dysregulation of nervous tissue development may enhance bronchial associated lymphoid tissue development. Also, the finding of this histological pattern in the setting of autoimmunity further broadens the etiology of this disease. It is thus likely that idiopathic follicular bronchitis has multiple etiologies and that the clinical and histologic pattern that describes the syndrome is a reflection of the lung's response to a wide variety of insults.

CLINICAL PICTURE

Idiopathic follicular bronchiolitis is rare in children, but it is probably underrecognized because the diagnosis can be made only with biopsy. The cause is unknown in the first year of life, but later in childhood is associated with autoimmunity. Idiopathic follicular bronchiolitis is similar to viral induced bronchiolitis in clinical presentation, but differs in that crackles persist and recurrence of symptoms is common. In the five patients we identified, all were symptomatic by 6 weeks of age and had peak symptoms between 6 and 18 months. The only other child with this diagnosis had symptoms at 6 months. Cough associated with moderate respiratory distress defined as tachypnea associated with subcostal retractions was seen in all patients. Five of

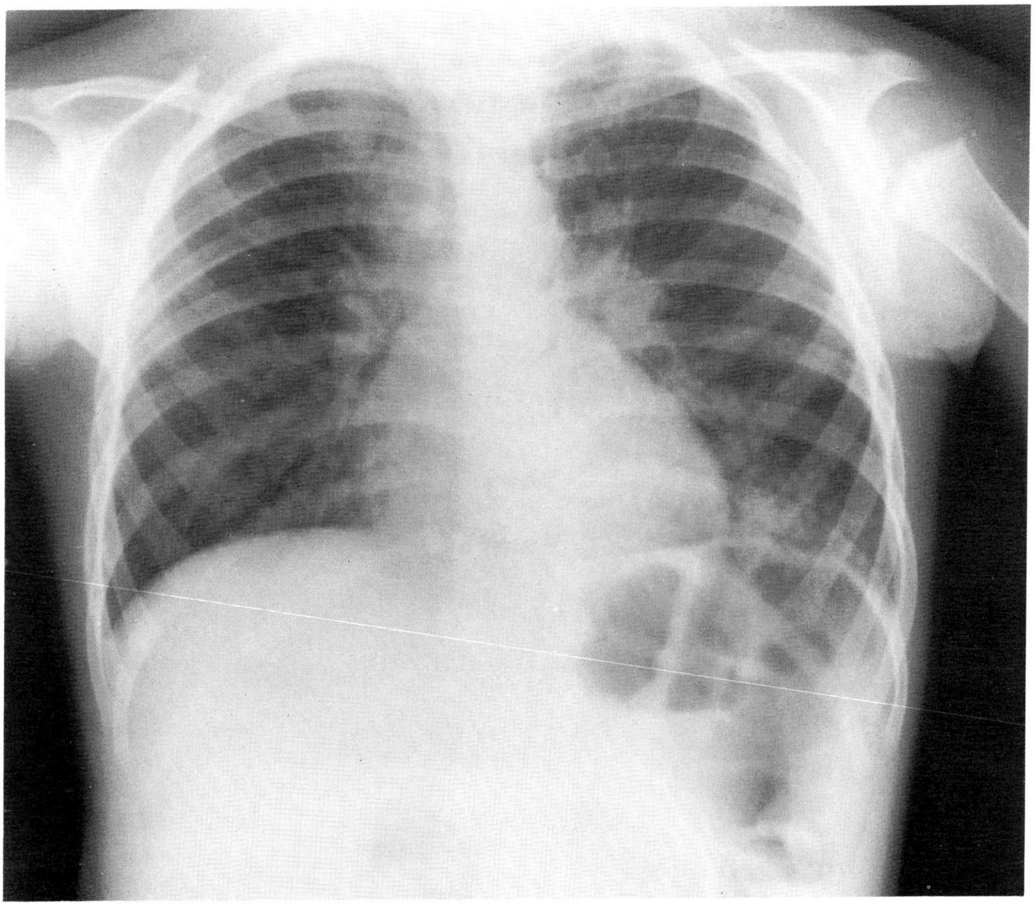

FIG. 1. Chest radiograph with an interstitial pattern of infiltration.

these patients had frequent recurring pyrexia of unknown origin. Two of these patients had unusual perinatal histories: one had hydrops fetalis, and the pregnancy in the other was complicated by maternal surgery for an abdominal abscess during the first trimester and an allergic response to gantrisin. The examination is characterized by diffuse fine crackles, although coarse rhonchi occurred in one patient. The overall pattern of episodic respiratory distress, associated pyrexia of unknown origin, and crackles on examination seems characteristic. The finding of persistent rales, especially in the absence of an infiltrate on chest radiograph, is very unusual in the first year and should suggest this diagnosis. All patients had an interstitial pattern of infiltration on chest radiograph; lung volumes were variable (Fig. 1). Atelectasis of various lobes was intermittently observed.

Laboratory investigations have not been helpful. Viral and bacterial cultures of sputum and lung tissue were negative in our patients. When the diagnosis is suggested, it is prudent to rule out immunodeficiencies, connective-tissue disease, and viral causes because these present with similar clinical and histologic pictures but a different prognosis. The differential diagnosis includes aspiration, but esophageal reflux can be secondary to respiratory distress. Therefore it is recommended that bronchial alveolar washings be performed to establish the existence of significant reflux if abnormal results are obtained on barium swallow or pH probe.

HISTOLOGY

The histology is characteristic, with follicular lymphoid hyperplasia around the

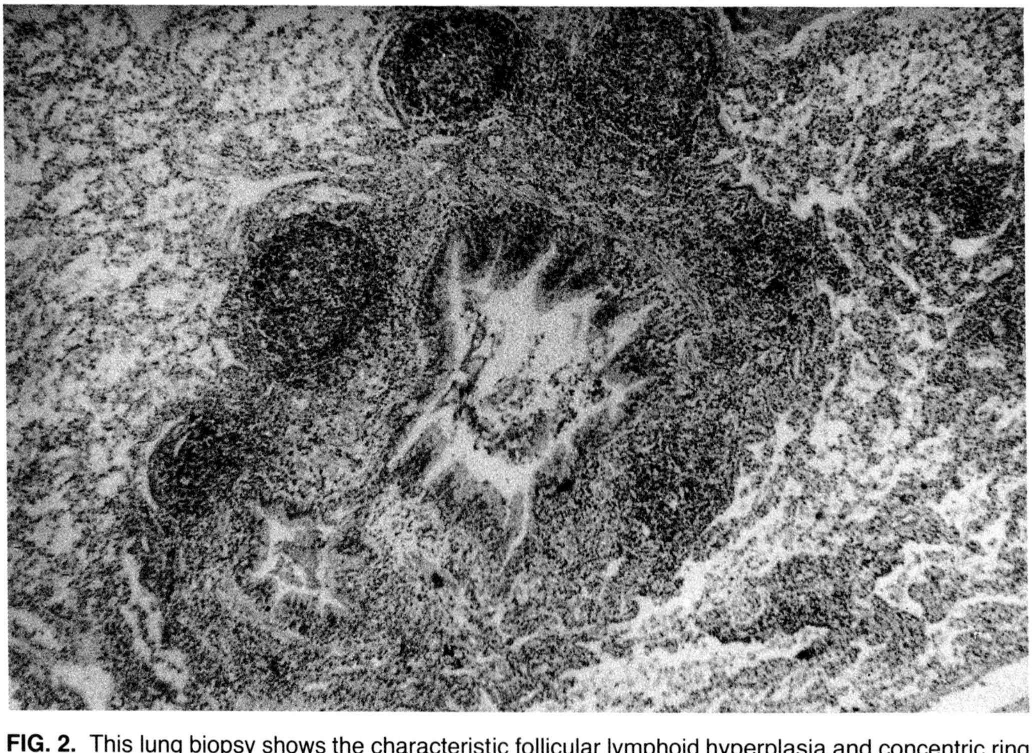

FIG. 2. This lung biopsy shows the characteristic follicular lymphoid hyperplasia and concentric ring of lymphocytes around the bronchiole.

bronchiole (Fig. 2) and between the bronchiole and the pulmonary artery in all patients. These follicles have germinal centers and frequently compress the bronchiolar lumen. A concentric ring of lymphocytes surrounds the bronchioles. The bronchiolar lumen had minimal acute suppurative exudates and rare mucus plugs in two patients. If the diagnosis is suspected, the follicles are best seen by cutting sections in the long axis of the small bronchus or bronchiole, and the overall pattern is best appreciated at low power (as low as 5×).

TREATMENT AND PROGNOSIS

Overall prognosis is very good for eventual recovery, but there is no specific treatment. Our patients were followed up for 2 to 15 years (4 for more than 7 years). Response to bronchodilators and to corticosteroids is minimal. No patient required mechanical ventilation, but one required nasal oxygen between 9 and 12 months of age. All improved between 2 and 3 years of age. Thus the overall treatment is supportive. In the four patients over 7 years of age, serial pulmonary function tests revealed chronic mild airflow obstructive disease (mean FEV_1/FVC of 71%). All patients have a residual of mild airway disease that may arise from airway injury over a protracted period of time. The clinical course also resembles cellular interstitial pneumonitis, which presents at birth and improves gradually over the first 4 years (14). This may reflect either a similar etiology or simply improvement with growth and development. Thus patients with the idiopathic type of process have a more favorable prognosis than those with the follicular bronchiolitis associated with immune deficiency or autoimmune disease. In patients with immune deficiency or autoimmune disease progressive lung disease is frequent.

FUTURE

Because the etiology is likely to be viral in the majority of patients, tissue samples should be explored using the tools of molecular biology. The awareness of this syndrome should increase the frequency of diagnosis.

REFERENCES

1. Yousem SA, Colby TV, Carrington CB. Follicular bronchitis/bronchiolitis. *Hum Pathol* 1985;16:700–706.
2. Grandgeorge S, Wagener JS. On follicular bronchitis without bronchiectasis. *Pediatr Pulmonol* 1987;3:282.
3. Kinane TB, Mansell AL, Zwerdling RG, Lapey A, Shannon DC. Follicular bronchitis in the pediatric population. *Chest* 1993, October.
4. Bienenstock J, Johnson D, Perey D. Bronchial lymphoid tissue: Morphological characteristics. *Lab Invest* 1973;28:6686.
5. Bienenstock J. *Immunology of the lung and upper respiratory tract.* New York: McGraw-Hill; 1984:96–118.
6. Berman SJ, Beer DJ, Theodore AC, Kornfeld H, Bernardo J, Center DM. Lymphocyte recruitment to the lung. *Am Rev Respir Dis* 1990; 142:238–257.
7. Milne RW, Bienenstock J, Perey DYE. The influence of antigenic stimulation on the ontogeny of lymphoid aggregates and immunoglobin containing cells in mouse bronchial and intestinal mucosa. *J Reticuloendolthel Soc* 1981;17:361–369.
8. Humphrey JH, Sulitseanu BD. The use of (^{14}C) amino acids to study sites and rates of antibody synthesis in living hyperimmune rabbits. *Biochem J* 1959;68:146–61.
9. Whitwell F. A study of the pathology and the pathogenesis of bronchiectasis. *Thorax* 1952;7: 213–239.
10. Franchi LM, Chin TW, Nussbaum E, Riker J, Robert M, Talbert WM. Familial pulmonary nodular lymphoid hyperplasia. *J Pediatr* 1992; 121:89–92.
11. Davis J, Cassel G. Murine respiratory mycoplasmosis in Lew and F344 sets. *Vet Pathol* 1982;19:280.
12. Jericho K. Intrapulmonary lymphoid tissue in mink infected with Aleutian disease virus. *Res Vet Sci* 1982;32:206.
13. Emery JL, Dinsdale F. Lymphoreticular aggregates in the newborn lung and their relation to intrauterine infection and neurospinal dysraphism. *Biol Neonate* 1975;26(1–2):44–52.
14. Schroeder SA, Shannon DC, Marks EJ. Cellular interstitial pneumonitis in infants. *Chest* 1992; 101:1065–1069.

Diseases of the Bronchioles, edited by
Gary R. Epler. Raven Press, Ltd.,
New York © 1994.

29

Childhood Bronchiolitis Obliterans

Karen A. Hardy

Pediatric Pulmonary Medicine, California Pacific Medical Center, San Francisco, CA.

Childhood bronchiolitis obliterans is an unusual complication of bronchiolar injury characterized by scarring of the airway lumen. It occurs most commonly after infectious bronchiolitis, but can also follow inhalation of noxious gases or aspiration of gastric acid, charcoal, or foreign bodies. At any age it can be associated with immunosuppression caused by drugs used for transplantation of bone marrow, heart–lung, or lung. Connective-tissue diseases and drugs used to treat them have also been related to bronchiolitis obliterans in some adults. Common features of the clinical course and diagnostic tests facilitate diagnosis. Most children stabilize and improve following injury, depending on their age and the proportion of lung affected. Surprisingly, adequate function can be sustained with very little healthy lung tissue after severe illnesses.

HISTORICAL REVIEW

Bronchiolitis obliterans was defined pathologically at the turn of the century in adults who died rapidly following the inhalation of toxic fumes (1). Shortly thereafter rare discussions appeared in autopsy reports (2) of patients affected after respiratory infections with measles, whooping cough, or scarlet fever. Ladue (3) reviewed 42,038 autopsies in 1941 and found only one case. Bronchiolitis obliterans was then thought to be a disease primarily of young adults. His review emphasized three patterns: irritant or damaging inhalations, postinfection, and idiopathic. The classical course after inhalation of either noxious gases or fumes from fire in an enclosed space was generalized to all patients. Immediate respiratory distress was severe and prompted the patient to seek medical attention. Coarse crackles, coughing, and wheezing were present, and urgent treatment with oxygen was administered. The patient experienced a brief period of improvement before clinical deterioration and chronic symptoms of distress. Most suffered from progressive obliteration with a bronchiolar fibrosis that was so severe they died from inadequate gas-exchanging surface. Patients who suffered a pneumonia could follow a very similar course. Complications included recurrent infection and bronchiectasis, localized air trapping, and areas of atelectasis. Ladue emphasized the well nourished appearance of severely affected patients. The characteristic pathology showed isolated bronchiolar lesions with very little parenchymal abnormality. Grossly, pinpoint nodules could be seen and felt and were difficult ot distinguish from tuberculosis, the common confounding pulmonary illness of that era.

Some patients from the first half of this century were children, although the details of their course was not well described. Diagnostic and treatment options were so different from those today that the most helpful generalizable constants are only those infections that are still likely to be associated with bronchiolitis obliterans today, such as pertussis, influenza, and measles.

Pediatric reports since 1964 emphasize the relationship of pulmonary infection and the uncommon complication of bronchiolitis obliterans. Certain viruses causing necrotizing bronchiolitis were most likely to result in bronchiolitis obliterans and formed the basis of the first case series of pediatric patients. An adenovirus epidemic in Canada resulted in large numbers of native Indian children developing chronic lung disease and bronchiolitis obliterans (4,5,6). Influenza infections and sequelae were reviewed by Laraya-Cuasay (7). Severe pneumonia due to various bacteria were also reported in isolated instances, but the possibility of undiagnosed concurrent viral infection makes it difficult to be certain of the association.

The most comprehensive review of pediatric patients was published in 1988 (8). At St. Christopher's Hospital for children in Philadelphia from 1965 to 1985 2,897 autopsies and 244 lung biopsies or lobectomies were reviewed, and a total of 19 cases were confirmed. Clinical and pathological findings were summarized and associated conditions categorized. These included toxic inhalations, infections, chronic lung diseases, aspiration, and idiopathic. A new category included patients whose immune systems were involved in a primary connective-tissue disease or were altered by drugs for immune suppression after organ transplantation (Table 1). Diagnostic studies were reviewed, and common factors that should help practitioners to suspect the process were specified.

TABLE 1. *Conditions associated with the development of bronchiolitis obliterans*

Inhalation of toxins/fumes
Ammonia chlorine
Chloropierin (trichloronitromethane)
Hydrochloric acid
Mustard gas (dichloroethyl sulfide)
Nitric acid
Nitrogen dioxide (silo fillers' disease)
Phosgene (carbonyl chloride)
Sulfuric acid
Talcum powder
Thermal injury
Zinc chloride
Infection
Viral
Adenovirus (types 1, 3, 7, 21)
Influenza
Measles
Variable-zoster
Bacterial
Bordetella pertussis
Staphylococcus aureus
Streptococcus group B beta hemolytic
Mycoplasma pneumonia
Pneumocystis carinii
Connective-tissue disease/transplantation
Autoimmune hemolytic anemia
Bone marrow transplantation
Eosinophilic fasciitis
Heart–lung transplantation
Lung transplantation
Rheumatoid arthritis
Scleroderma
Sjogren's syndrome
Large lesions
Alveolar proteinosis
Bronchopulmonary dysplasia
Congenital
Congestive heart failure
Cystic fibrosis
Lymphoma
Myasthenia gravis
Penicillamine therapy/rheumatoid arthritis
Sulfasalazine therapy/ulcerative colitis
Aspiration
Foreign bodies (prune pit, amniotic fluid)
Lipids (poppyseed oil)
Stomach contents/gastroesophageal reflux
Idiopathic

Reprinted with author's permission.

Since 1988 a few pediatric case reports (9–12), usually highlighting atypical presentations or possible causes, have been published. Attention paid to the genesis of obliteration has increased because up to 50% of patients who receive heart–lung or lung transplants develop bronchiolitis obliterans (13). These patients undergo frequent biopsy and provide our best source of information to help unravel the process of obliteration.

CLINICAL SYMPTOMS

Bronchiolitis obliterans can develop at any age, although most affected children are toddlers or of primary school age because associated infections are common at these ages. A single case report of bronchiolitis obliterans found at autopsy of a 4-day-old who had not received mechanical ventilation suggests that intrauterine infection can also cause this lesion (14). Symptoms of a flu-like illness with cough, tachypnea, and rhinorrhea are most common. Some children have fever and nonspecific symptoms such as nausea, vomiting, malaise, or anorexia. A viral lower respiratory tract infection is typically diagnosed, and patients are given an antibiotic if physical findings justify administration. Some children remain at home for their initial illness but return to the physician 1 to 2 months later because of prolonged symptoms of coughing, tachypnea, wheezing, or poor exercise tolerance. Most suffer significant respiratory distress and require hospitalization for obvious pneumonia but follow an atypical course. In these patients the airway epithelium does not heal but proceeds to obstruction with organizing cellular masses.

Rarely, other causes of bronchiolitis obliterans are clear, such as an accidental inhalation of toxic fumes resulting in severe coughing and respiratory distress prompting urgent medical care. Children with these exposures follow the course outlined historically by Ladue and others. Persistent cough, wheezing, or exercise intolerance remain the classical symptoms consistent with bronchiolitis obliterans (8).

PHYSICAL FINDINGS

Physical examination signs include crackles, wheezing, or decreased breath sounds. Some patients have diffuse and severe abnormalities, while others suffering a mild initial illness may have only a single segment or lobe involved. Chest deformities secondary to localized or generalized air trapping are common in severely affected patients. Swyer-James syndrome with localized air trapping can also occur (15,16). Affected areas, hyperlucent on radiograph but hypoperfused on perfusion scan or angiography, gradually atrophy. Normal nutritional status and an otherwise healthy appearance without resting respiratory distress typifies patients with this disease and can be confusing. Clubbing is seen only in patients who are severely affected. Sputum production is not typical but can occur as patients develop bronchiectasis of involved segments with poor clearance of secretions.

DIAGNOSTIC TESTING

General Testing

Careful screening to exclude other diseases that may cause chronic obstructive lung disease is important. Cystic fibrosis, tuberculosis, $alpha_1$-antitrypsin deficiency, and immunodeficiencies can confound the diagnosis. The sweat test, Mantoux test, $alpha_1$-antitrypsin levels, and serum immunoglobulins are normal. Gastroesophageal reflux with aspiration and damage to the airways is sometimes associated with bronchiolitis obliterans. This has been more common in patients with congenital tracheoesophageal fistulae who have had surgical repair and then develop achalasia with recurrent aspiration and respiratory symptoms. PH probe testing or bronchoscopy with lavage searching for foreign bodies and lipid-laden macrophages from recurrent aspiration is completed to test for these possibilities. Specific tests to determine the infectious etiology by cultures of nasopharyngeal or lavage fluids, or by fourfold serology titer responses can clarify the viral cause in pediatric patients.

Radiographic Findings

Initial radiograph findings consistently are abnormal, although multiple patterns are seen. Diffuse interstitial and peribronchial infiltrates are common with patchy confluent densities in localized areas (17). Atelectasis of an involved segment can be present and can even involve the entire lung (9,12). Additional studies to characterize the plain film abnormalities have included bronchography, computed tomography (CT) scans, and ventilation–perfusion scans. Bronchography was more often pursued before the technology of CT scanning was available. It classically reveals a characteristic pattern of the "pruned tree" or the "cut-off airway" coinciding with obliteration of the bronchi or bronchioles. Airways can be selectively filled with contrast media using fluoroscopically placed catheters while the patient is anesthetized and ventilated through an endotracheal tube. Positive-pressure insufflation of the lung can demonstrate ballooning of the airways and confirm the lack of passage of contract distally. Alternatively, fiberoptic bronchoscopes now allow more selective positioning of the instrument with instillation of contrast to smaller segments of the lung while the patient breathes spontaneously while sedated. Bronchiectasis, a common complication of obliterative bronchiolitis, is confirmed by bronchography (Fig. 1).

This technique has largely been abandoned in favor of CT. Many authors (18,19) have documented the correlation of bronchiectasis pathologically and radiographically by use of thin-section reconstructions. Patients who are able to voluntarily inspire deeply and hold their breath are well suited for this technique. Young children who are

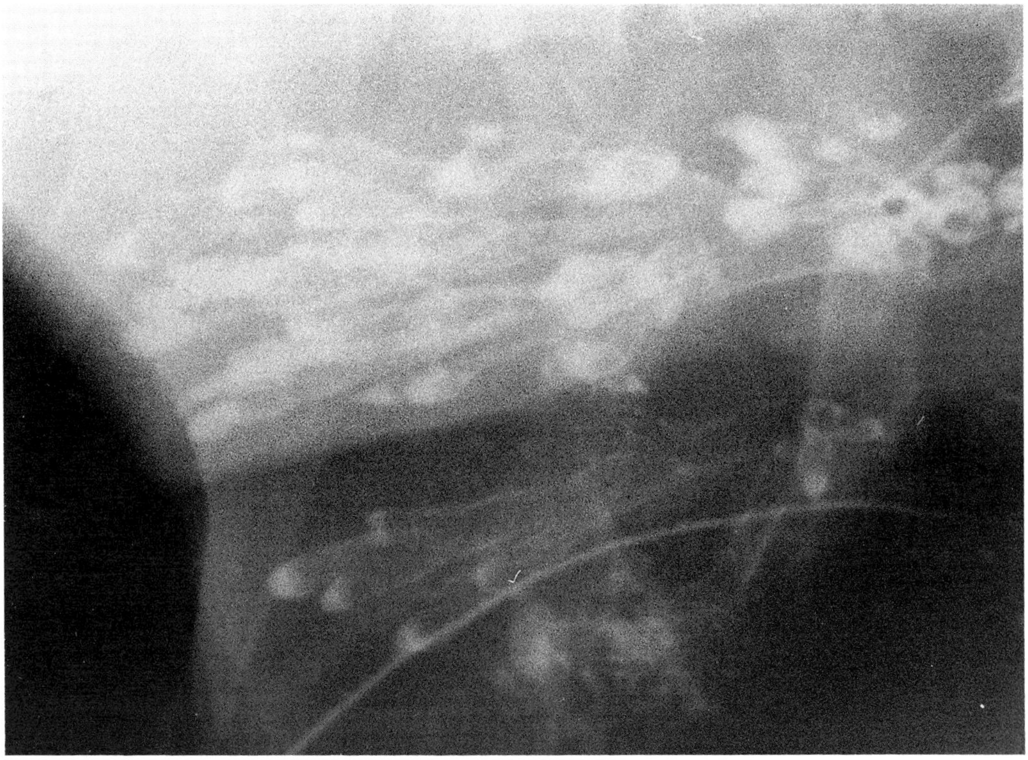

FIG. 1. Bronchogram (lateral view) shows bronchiectasis complicating bronchiolitis obliterans.

unable to hold their breath consciously can still be studied with good correlation if the bronchiectasis is severe (20). High-resolution CT scans that use an ultrafast technique allow the best images to be obtained while the image is freeze-framed during the 50-msec exposure, which avoids motion artifact (21) (limited numbers of these scanners are available in the USA). Ultrafast scanners also allow cinematography from which density calculations can be made to distinguish ventilating areas versus air-trapped areas. Ventilation-perfusion scans show a characteristic pattern of patchy decrease in both ventilation and perfusion (22). These areas are matched and give the two views a moth-eaten appearance (Fig. 2).

Magnetic resonance imaging is not re-

A

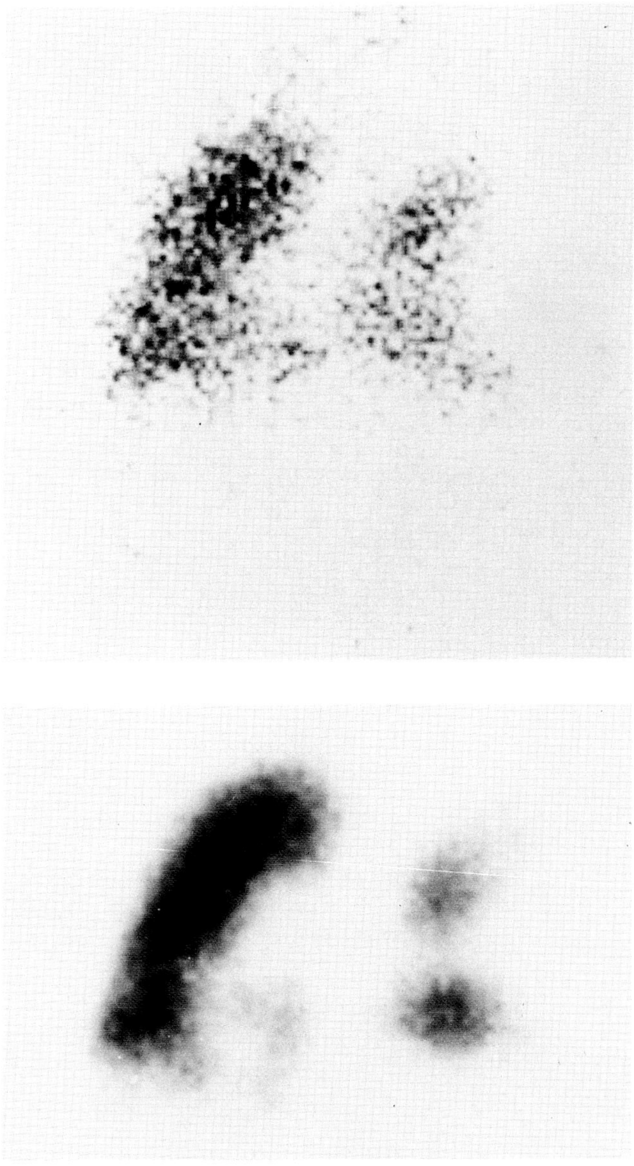

B

FIG. 2. A, Ventilation scan. **B,** Perfusion scan. Note matched defects.

TABLE 2. *Pulmonary function tests in patients with bronchiolitis obliterans*

Patient	Age at onset (years)	Years since onset	FVC	FEV_1/FVC (%)[a]	MMEFR (%)[a]	TLC (H) (%)[a]	RV/TLC (H) (%)[a]
1	13.8	2	89	40	19	106	29.5
2	3.6	12	57	42	13	84	43.5
3	2	7	69	75	42	109	50
4	2.3	8	70	85	112	63	22
5	5.6	9	75	36	15	136	50
8[b]	4.7	9	59	64	34	26	41
9	4	0.8	67	80	70	113	55
10	4	4.5	35	60	11	59	50
Patient	**Age at onset (years)**	**Years since onset**	**FVC**	**FEV_1/FVC (%)[a]**	**MMEFR (%)[a]**	**TLC (P) (%)[a]**	**RV/TLC (P) (%)[a]**
11		3	112	91	136	117	23
12	9	3	50	75	31	84	54
Infant	**Age at onset (months)**	**Years since onset**	**FRC N_2**	**FVL**			
1	7	2	56 ml/kg	obstructed			
2	9	2.7	28 ml/kg	obstructed			

FVC, forced vital capacity; FEV_1, forced expiratory volume in one second; MMEFR, mid maximal expiratory flow rate; TLC (H), total lung capacity helium method; TLC (P), total lung capacity plethysmographic method; RV, residual volume; FRC (N_2), functional residual capacity nitrogen method; FVL, flow volume loop.

[a]Values given as percent of predicted.

[b]Tests done following left lower lobectomy

ported or expected to be useful for diagnosis. Current scanners have slow imaging times, and respiratory motion during each scan effectively blurs each image. If a rapid scanning is performed resolution is unacceptable. If the acquisition is gated to limit motion artifact the length of scanning time increases unacceptably.

Pulmonary Function

Obstructive changes with air trapping are commonly documented by pulmonary function testing. Infant pulmonary function testing has shown the same pattern in younger patients. Resistance and compliance can also be measurably abnormal, depending on the amount of involved tissue. Patients with only segmental involvement occasionally have normal pulmonary function. Restrictive changes as gas trapping becomes severe can also occur (Table 2).

Pathologic Findings

Open lung biopsy provides the gold standard for diagnosis when the characteristic findings of fibroblasts, leukocytes, and fibrin partially or fully obstruct the airway lumen (Fig. 3). Constrictive concentric scarring causing obstruction is also diagnostic (23). "Pure" bronchiolitis obliterans is characterized by airway pathology without parenchymal abnormalities. Organizing pneumonia associated with the classical airway obstruction is diagnosed as bronchiolitis obliterans organizing pneumonia (BOOP) per the observations of Epler (24).

A number of difficulties with lung biopsy are unique to children. The process can be

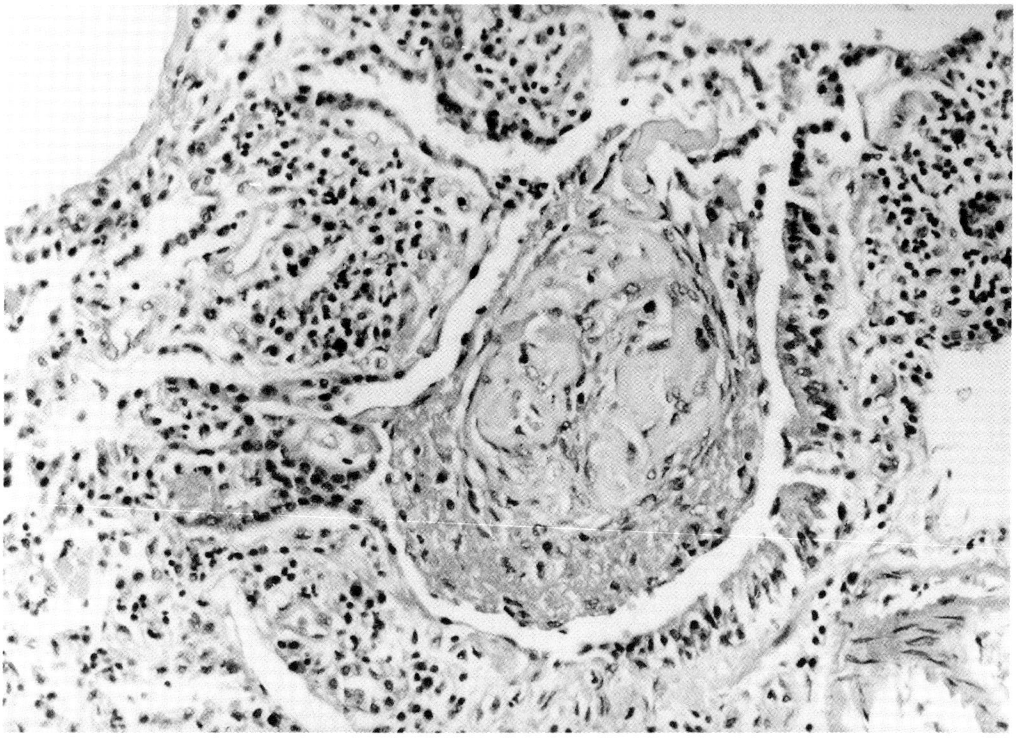

FIG. 3. Obliterated bronchiole.

patchy, and sampling error can occur. Open lung biopsy is needed to gain a large enough sample that has small airways. Many families are unwilling to consent to an invasive procedure that may still miss the diagnosis. Timing of open biopsy is also problematic. Early biopsy may show airways filled with cellular polypoid masses that have not yet organized. Obliteration with fibrosis can develop quickly; the fastest documented case in a child developed 8 days from onset of adenovirus infection to open biopsy (13). Late biopsy may not be useful if severe changes with destruction of the airway walls occur so that few if any remnants of recognizable tissue remain. Transbronchial biopsy forceps are not available for pediatric flexible fiberscopes and would yield too small a sample. Due to these problems, many now base the diagnosis on the charac-

A

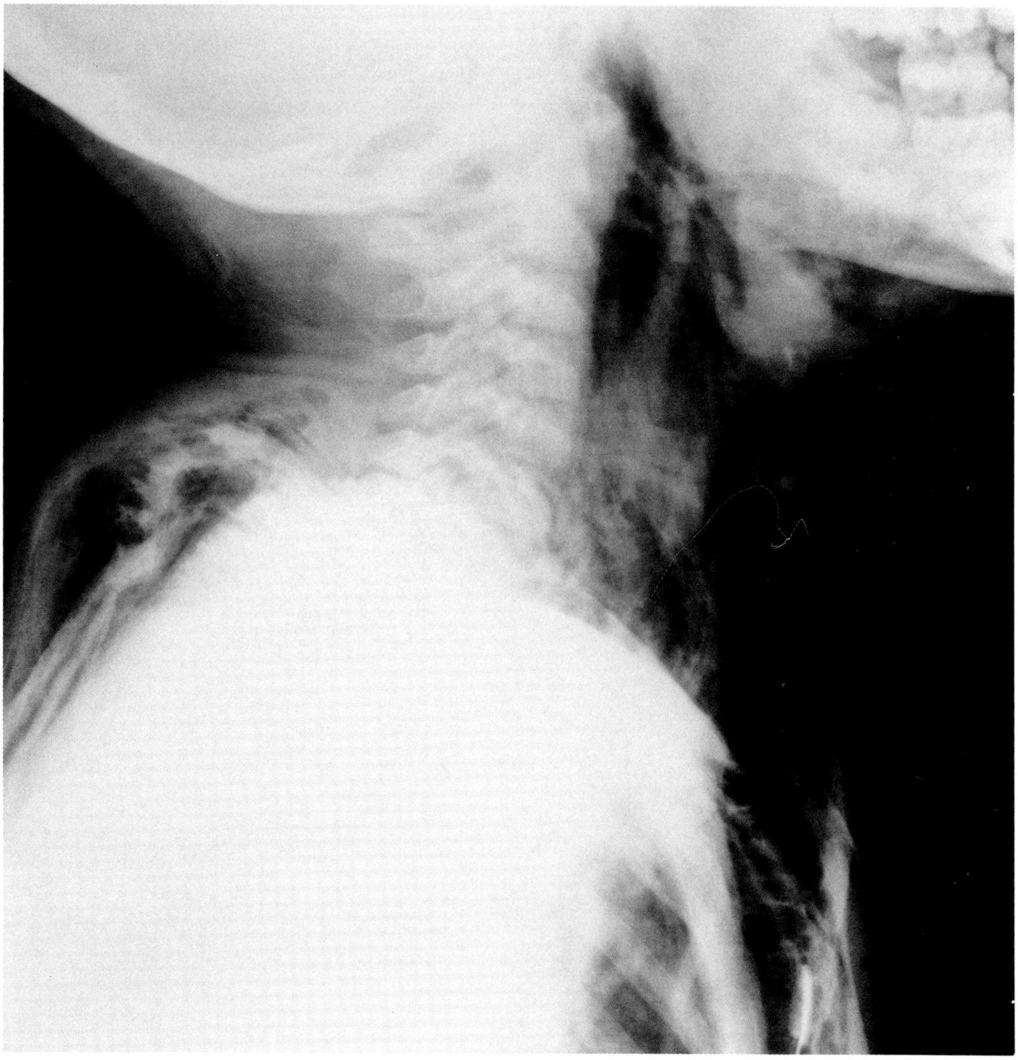

FIG. 4. A, Lateral radiograph and **B,** frontal radiograph documenting severe pneumomediastinum and subcutaneous emphysema.

teristic clinical situation, pulmonary function abnormalities, ventilation–perfusion scan, and bronchographic changes documented by bronchography or CT scan without open lung biopsy.

CLINICAL COURSE

The course following obliteration is variable and relates to the volume of affected tissue. Patients who have a flu-like illness and are initially treated as outpatients usually recover. They often have a period of years of coughing or wheezing and persistent crackles on examination. If areas of atelectasis are present initially they remain. If small, these segments may not cause any further problems, although occasionally they may become secondarily infected and a lobectomy may be required.

Patients who are critically ill at presen-

B

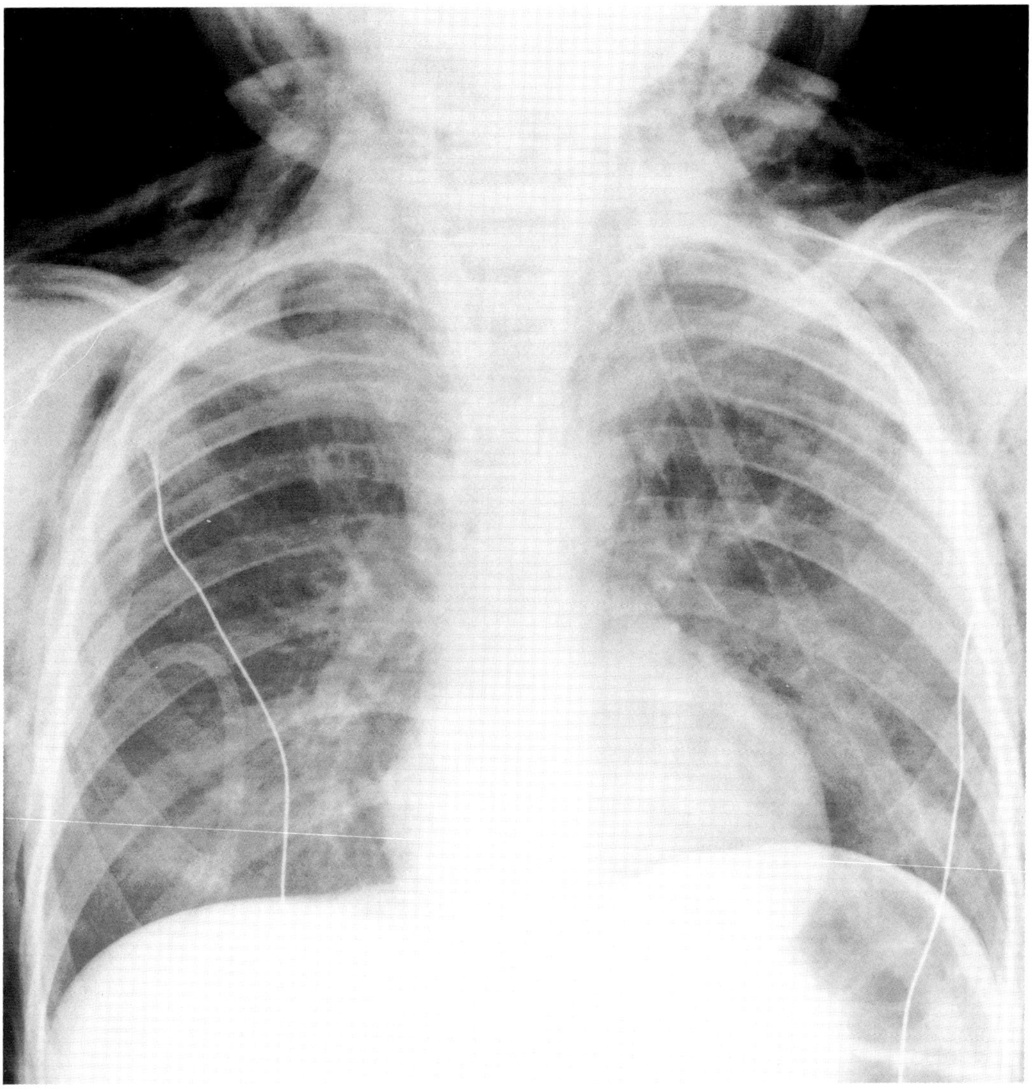

FIG. 4. *Continued*

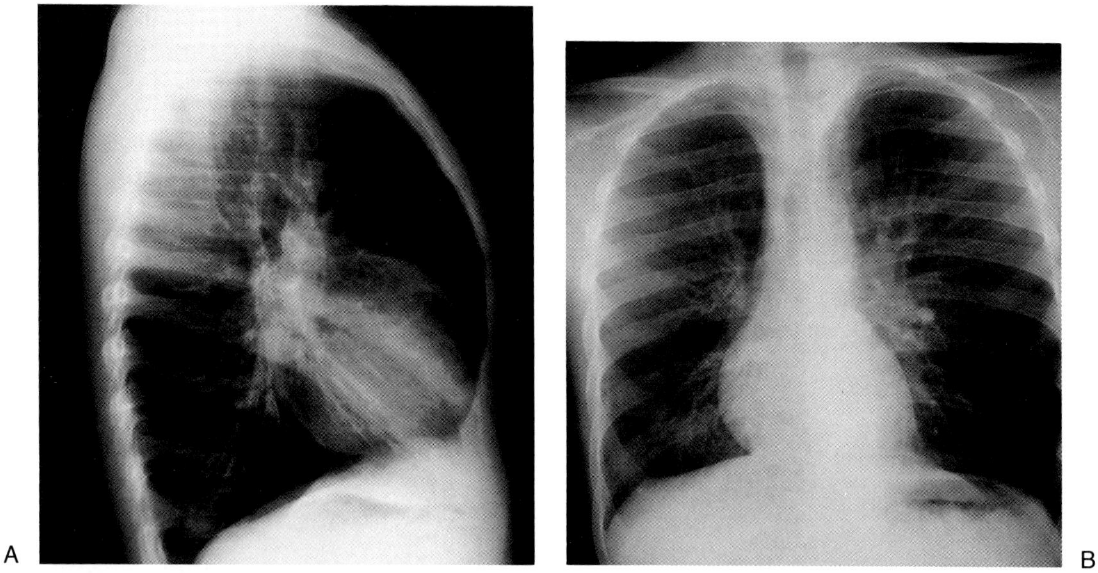

FIG. 5. A, Lateral radiograph and **B,** frontal radiograph of patient shown in Fig. 4, 4½ years after initial insult (influenza). Note severe air trapping.

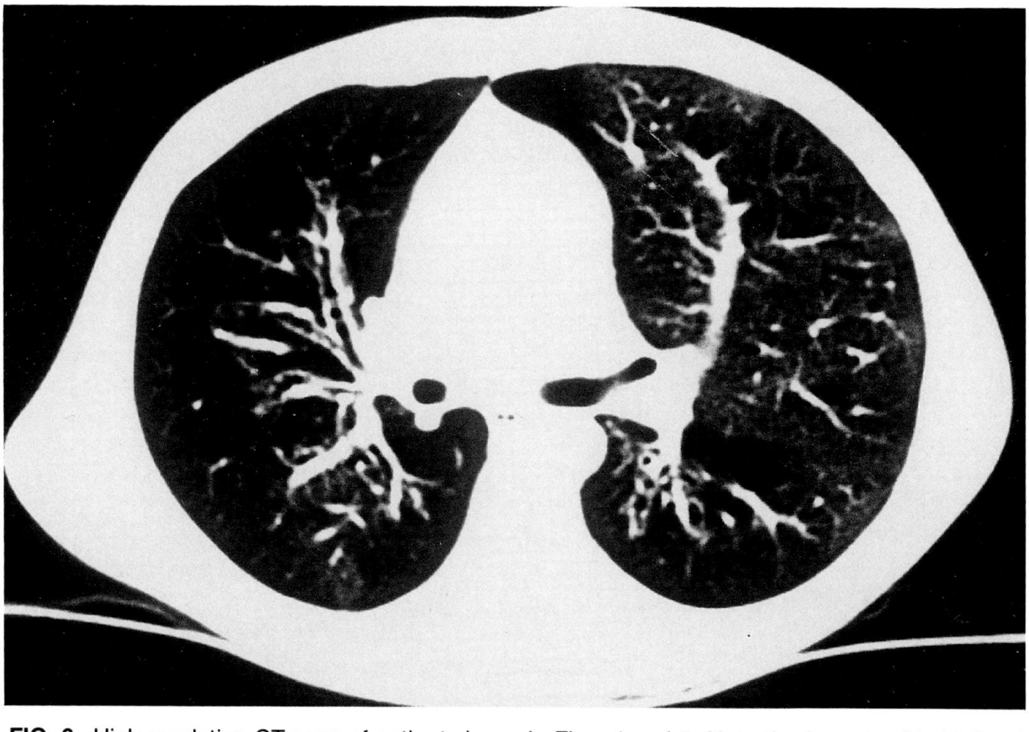

FIG. 6. High-resolution CT scan of patient shown in Figs. 4 and 5. Note the hypertrophied left pulmonary artery, which supplies functional lingula. Note lack of perfusion elsewhere and bronchiectasis of left posterior and right lung fields.

tation fare less well. This group may require mechanical ventilation and may suffer from severe air leaks during the initial pneumonia (Fig. 4). This is due to variable compliance of the unaffected areas, less affected areas, and obstructed areas. Weaning may be a slow and tedious process. These patients ultimately may be liberated from the ventilator but suffer permanent severe obstruction with little remaining functional tissue. They are oxygen dependent and have exercise limitation. Others may have inexorable progression of the airway obliteration, followed by death. Some patients have prominent wheezing and do respond to bronchodilators. If the initial insult occurs while the child is very young, less than 1 or 2 years old, the child may be able to stabilize with very little remaining functional tissue. Some improvement in this population is possible (Figs. 5 and 6).

MANAGEMENT

Treatment is supportive. Once a diagnosis is made, testing of lung function to determine whether bronchodilators will be useful is warranted. The use of corticosteroid therapy is championed for patients who are severely ill. Modifying the fibrotic response with corticosteroids is based on the work of Moran (25), who used a model of bronchiolitis obliterans in rabbits. Due to the small numbers of pediatric patients in any center, a controlled trial of corticosteroid therapy has not been undertaken. Severely ill patients frequently are treated with corticosteroids. Some cases have developed while the patient was undergoing corticosteroid therapy (8). Additional support for its use is present in adults who have bronchiolitis obliterans or BOOP (24). If bronchiectasis occurs, airway clearance techniques including postural drainage, percussion and vibration, positive expiratory pressure, and autogenic drainage can be helpful.

A large and growing population of lung transplant patients are at risk for the development of bronchiolitis obliterans and are carefully studied via frequent tissue sampling. This population has provided the best source of longitudinal information regarding the genesis of bronchiolitis obliterans and its response to treatment. In this group, the disease is thought to represent rejection of the donor lung, and speculation regarding the pathogenesis includes recognition of high rates of acute rejection relating to increased incidence of this lesion (26). Lymphocytic bronchitis in bone marrow transplant recipients and in animal models may be related to the mechanism of injury (27,28). Lymphocytic injury to the epithelial surface may disrupt normal fibroblasts and activate them to proliferate and produce fibrin through various mediators. Prostaglandins, normally secreted by type 2 epithelial cells, may be inhibited in patients who develop this disease (29). The genesis of bronchiolitis obliterans may not be identical with different epithelial injuries.

Patients with a large volume of affected tissue are chronically oxygen dependent and severely limited. At least one 9-year-old patient with severe debilitating disease who underwent lung transplant for primary bronchiolitis obliterans has done well for 1 year (30).

PREVENTIVE MEASURES

Immunizations to prevent common and potentially serious viral and bacterial infections are important. Treatment with prednisone at 2 mg/kg/day is reasonable until the basic cause of abnormal repair of the epithelium is clarified. Bronchodilators may help relieve some patients' dyspnea. Recognition and treatment of bronchiectasis with airway clearance techniques may decrease recurrent infections and further damdage. Suspecting this diagnosis is facilitated by remembering the clues outlined in Table

TABLE 3. *Signs and symptoms suggesting bronchiolitis obliterans*

Persistent cough or wheezing for 6 or more weeks after a pneumonia
Prolonged crackles or wheezing after pneumonia or respiratory failure
Prolonged exercise intolerance after pulmonary injury
Severe respiratory symptoms disproportionate to the abnormalities seen on the chest radiograph
Recurrent aspiration of gastric contents accompanied by clinical signs as above
Hyperlucent lung syndrome
Severe lung disease with localized overaeration

3. Only through recognition of this disease can we learn why bronchiolitis obliterans occurs and develop a more effective treatment strategy.

REFERENCES

1. Fraenkel A. Ueber bronchiolitis fibrosa obliterans, nebst bemerkungen uber lungenhypereamie und inderierende pneumonia. *Dtsch Arch Klin Med* 1902;73:484–488.
2. Blumgart HL, MacMahon HE. Bronchiolitis fibrosa obliterans: a clinical and pathologic study. *Med Clin North Am* 1929;13:197–214.
3. Ladue JS. Bronchiolitis fibrosa obliterans. *Arch Intern Med* 1941;68:663–673.
4. Benyesh-Melnick M, Rosenberg HS. The isolation of adenovirus type 7 from a fatal case of pneumonia and disseminated disease. *J Pediatr* 1964;64:83–86.
5. Becroft DMO. Bronchiolitis obliterans, bronchiectasis, and other sequelae of adenovirus type 21 infection in young children. *J Clin Pathol* 1971;24:72–82.
6. Wenman WM, Pagtakhan RD, Reed MH, Chernick V, Albritton W. Adenovirus bronchiolitis in Manitoba. *Chest* 1982;5:605–609.
7. Laraya-Cuasay LR, DeForest A, Huff D, Lischner H, Huang NH. Chronic pulmonary complications of early influenza virus infection in children. *Am Rev Respir Dis* 1977;16:617–625.
8. Hardy KA, Schidlow DV, Zaeri N. Obliterative bronchiolitis in children. *Chest* 1988;93:460–466.
9. Kargi HA, Kuhn C. Bronchiolitis obliterans unilateral fibrous obliteration of the lumen of bronchi with atelectasis. *Chest* 1988;93(5):1107–1108.
10. Omar AH, Manan A. Bronchiolitis obliterans in children: a report of six cases. *Med J Malaysia* 1989;44(3):204–209.
11. Elliot CG, Colby TV, Kelly TM, Hicks HG. Charcoal lung bronchiolitis obliterans after aspiration of activated charcoal. *Chest* 1989;96: 672–674.
12. Dosanjh A. Unilateral bronchiolitis obliterans: a case report. *Clin Pediatr* 1992:319–320.
13. Abernathy EC, Hruban RH, Baumgartner WA, Reitz BA, Hutchins GM. The two forms of bronchiolitis obliterans in heart–lung transplant recipients. *Hum Path* 1991;22:1102–1110.
14. Sueishi A, Watanabe T, Tanaka K, Shin H. Intrauterine bronchiolitis obliterans. *Virchows Arch [A]* 1974;362:223–229.
15. Swyer PR, James GCW. A case of unilateral pulmonary emphysema. *Thorax* 1953;8:133–136.
16. Macpherson RI, Cumming GR, Chernick V. Unilateral hyperlucent lung: a complication of viral pneumonia. *J Can Assoc Radiol* 1969; 20:225–231.
17. Gosink BB, Friedman PJ, Liebow AA. Bronchiolitis obliterans: roentgenologic-pathologic correlation. *AJR* 1973;117:816–832.
18. Nadich DP, McCauley DI, Khouri NF. Computed tomography of bronchiectasis. *J Comput Assist Tomogr* 1982;6:437–444.
19. Webb WR, Stein MG, Finkbeiner WE, Im JG, Lynch D, Gamsu G. Normal and diseased isolated lungs: high resolution CT. *Radiology* 1988; 166:81–87.
20. Marks J, Hardy K, Garcia-Kennedy, Devries P. Pre and postoperative high resolution computed tomography of severe bronchiectasis in an infant with cystic fibrosis. XI International Cystic Fibrosis Congress WP78.
21. Lynch DA, Brasch RC, Hardy KA, Webb WR. Pediatric pulmonary disease: assessment with high-resolution ultrafast CT. *Radiology* 1990; 176:243–248.
22. Palmer J, Harcke T, Deforest A, Schidlow D, Cuasay L, Huang N. Matched ventilation/perfusion defects in the lung scans of children with obliterative bronchiolitis and long term clinical followup. *Am Rev Respir Dis* 1979;119:280.
23. Katzenstein AL, Askin FB. Miscellaneous I: specific diseases of uncertain etiology. In: Bennington JL, ed. *Surgical pathology of nonneoplastic lung disease*. Philadelphia: WB Saunders; 1982:349–356.
24. Epler GR, Colby TV, McLoud TC, Carrington CB, Gaensler EA. Bronchiolitis obliterans organizing pneumonia. *N Engl J Med* 1985;312: 152–158.
25. Moran TJ, Hellstrom NR. Bronchiolitis obliterans. *Arch Pathol* 1958;66:691–707.
26. Clelland C, Higenbottam T, Otulana B, et al. Histologic prognostic indicators for the lung allografts of heart–lung transplants. *J Heart Transplant* 1990;9:177–186.
27. Bescorner WE, Saral R, Hutchins GM, et al. Lymphocytic bronchitis is associated with graft vs. host disease in recipients of bone-marrow transplants. *N Engl J Med* 1978;299:1030–1036.
28. Lane BP, Habricht GS, Japser GS. Lymphocyte–epithelium interaction during rejection of nonisogeneic rat tracheal grafts. *Am J Pathol* 1977;86:71–80.
29. Adamson IYR, Hedgecock C, Bowden DH. Epithelial cell fibroblast interactions in lung injury and repair. *Am J Pathol* 1990;137:385–392.
30. John Marks M.D.; personal communication.

Subject Index

C

D

G

J

K

L

R

S

T